Neuroscience: Exploring the Brain

Neuroscience: Exploring the Brain

Editor: Oliver Davis

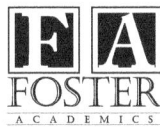

FA
FOSTER
ACADEMICS

www.fosteracademics.com

www.fosteracademics.com

FA FOSTER
ACADEMICS

Cataloging-in-Publication Data

Neuroscience : exploring the brain / edited by Oliver Davis.
    p. cm.
Includes bibliographical references and index.
ISBN 978-1-63242-712-0
1. Neurosciences. 2. Brain. 3. Nervous system. 4. Neurology. I. Davis, Oliver.
RC341 .N48 2019
612.8--dc23

Foster Academics,
118-35 Queens Blvd., Suite 400,
Forest Hills, NY 11375, USA

ISBN 978-1-63242-712-0 (Hardback)

Contents

Permissions

List of Contributors

Index

Preface

Over the recent decade, advancements and applications have progressed exponentially. This has led to the increased interest in this field and projects are being conducted to enhance knowledge. The main objective of this book is to present some of the critical challenges and provide insights into possible solutions. This book will answer the varied questions that arise in the field and also provide an increased scope for furthering studies.

Neuroscience is the study of the nervous system which integrates anatomy, physiology, developmental biology, molecular biology, psychology, mathematical modeling and cytology to understand the functioning of neurons and neural circuits. Such investigations are furthered by cellular and molecular studies of individual neurons, and imaging of sensory motor tasks occurring in the brain. Progress in the fields of electrophysiology, molecular biology and computational neuroscience have advanced the frontiers of neuroscience. Such studies are particularly significant in the medical sciences such as psychosurgery, neurology, neurosurgery, neuropathology, etc. as they allow the diseases of the nervous system to be directly addressed. Psychiatry focuses on the management of behavioral, cognitive, affective and perceptual disorders, while neurology focuses on the conditions of the central and peripheral nervous systems. This book contains some path-breaking studies in the field of neuroscience. It unravels the recent studies in brain exploration. The extensive content of this book provides the readers with a thorough understanding of the subject.

I hope that this book, with its visionary approach, will be a valuable addition and will promote interest among readers. Each of the authors has provided their extraordinary competence in their specific fields by providing different perspectives as they come from diverse nations and regions. I thank them for their contributions.

Editor

Haplotype analysis of *APOE* intragenic SNPs

Vladimir N. Babenko[1,2]*, Dmitry A. Afonnikov[1,2], Elena V. Ignatieva[1,2], Anton V. Klimov[1,2], Fedor E. Gusev[3] and Evgeny I. Rogaev[1,3,4,5]

Abstract

Background: *APOE* ε4 allele is most common genetic risk factor for Alzheimer's disease (AD) and cognitive decline. However, it remains poorly understood why only some carriers of *APOE* ε4 develop AD and how ethnic variabilities in *APOE* locus contribute to AD risk. Here, to address the role of *APOE* haplotypes, we reassessed the diversity of APOE locus in major ethnic groups and in Alzheimer's Disease Neuroimaging Initiative (ADNI) dataset on patients with AD, and subjects with mild cognitive impairment (MCI), and control non-demented individuals.

Results: We performed *APOE* gene haplotype analysis for a short block of five SNPs across the gene using the ADNI whole genome sequencing dataset. The compilation of ADNI data with 1000 Genomes identified the *APOE* ε4 linked haplotypes, which appeared to be distant for the Asian, African and European populations. The common European ε4-bearing haplotype is associated with AD but not with MCI, and the Africans lack this haplotype. Haplotypic inference revealed alleles that may confer protection against AD. By assessing the DNA methylation profile of the *APOE* haplotypes, we found that the AD-associated haplotype features elevated *APOE* CpG content, implying that this locus can also be regulated by genetic-epigenetic interactions.

Conclusions: We showed that SNP frequency profiles within *APOE* locus are highly skewed to population-specific haplotypes, suggesting that the ancestral background within different sites at *APOE* gene may shape the disease phenotype. We propose that our results can be utilized for more specific risk assessment based on population descent of the individuals and on higher specificity of five site haplotypes associated with AD.

Keywords: Alzheimer's disease, *APOE*, ADNI dataset, Haplotype analysis, SNPs, GWAS, PCA, DNA methylation

Background

Alzheimer's disease (AD) is the most frequent case of dementia worldwide, which is manifested by a progressive decline in cognitive function due to loss of neurons, white matter, and synapses. Although it is thought to be caused by progressive accumulation of diffuse and neuritic extracellular amyloid plaques and intracellular neurofibrillary tangles in the brains of AD patients, the etiological mechanisms underlying the neurodegeneration process remain unclear. Since its conception in 2004, Alzheimer's Disease Neuroimaging Initiative (ADNI, http://www.adni-info.org/) has been searching for associations between MRI brain profiles, biomarkers and clinical symptoms. To date, the significant progress has been made for neuroimaging of the ADNI subjects and in identifying potentially predictive biomarkers for AD [1–6]. Importantly, the whole genome sequencing (WGS) has also been performed for > 800 subjects in ADNI cohort, including AD-patients, individuals with Mild

*Correspondence: bob@bionet.nsc.ru
[1] The Federal Research Center Institute of Cytology and Genetics of Siberian Branch of the Russian Academy of Sciences, Center of Neurobiology and Neurogenetics, Lavrentieva str. 10, Novosibirsk, Russia 630090
Full list of author information is available at the end of the article

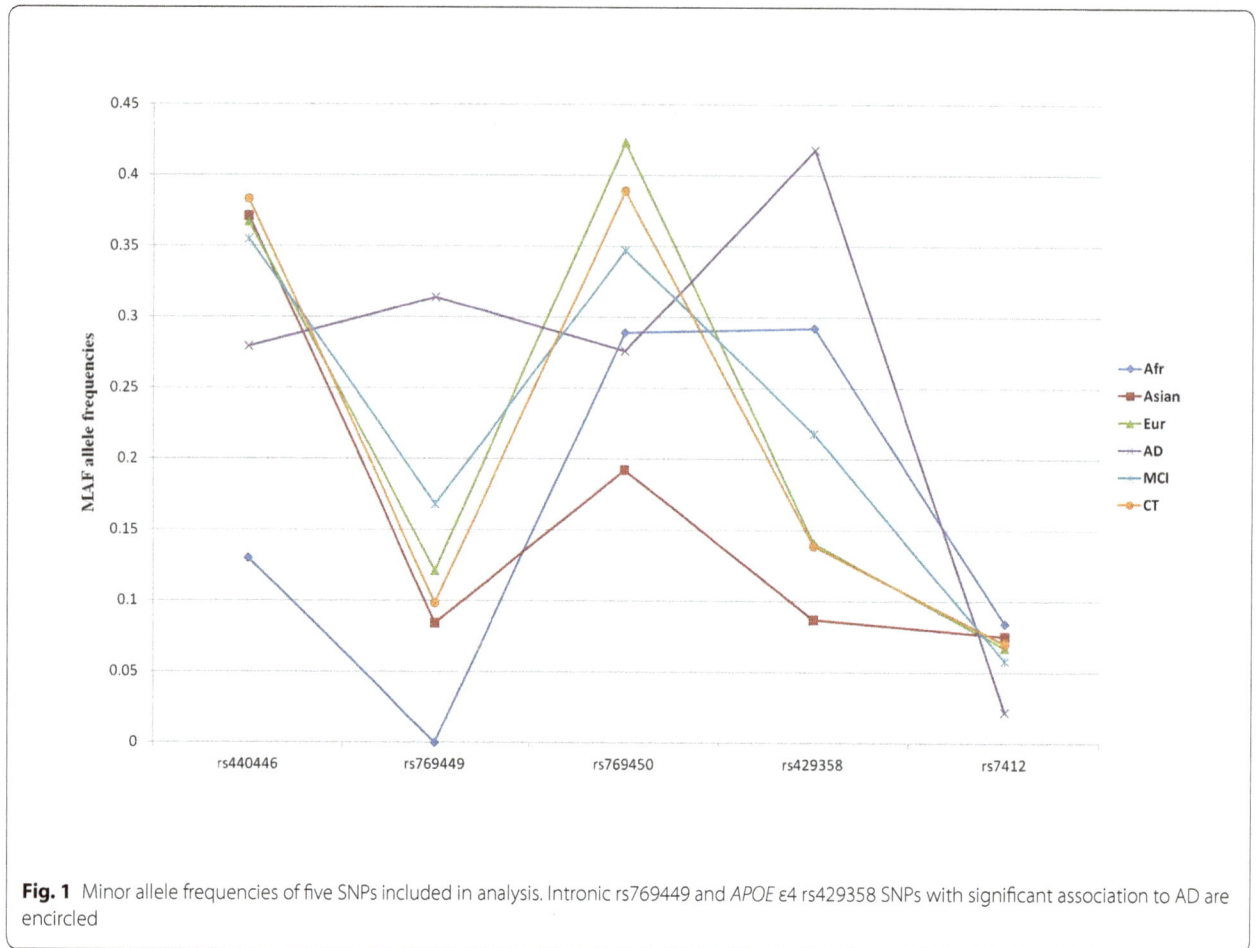

Fig. 1 Minor allele frequencies of five SNPs included in analysis. Intronic rs769449 and *APOE* ε4 rs429358 SNPs with significant association to AD are encircled

Table 2 Minor allele frequencies of 5 SNPs included in analysis. SNPs are sorted by chromosomal position. SNPs with significant association to AD in bold

SNP ID	Alleles (MAF 1st)	Type	Global MAF	1000G (MAF) samples			ADNI (MAF) samples		
				Afr	Asian	Eur	AD	MCI	CT
rs440446	C/G	Noncoding	0.37	0.130	0.371	0.367	0.279	0.355	0.383
rs769449	A/G	Noncoding	0.06	0.000	0.084	0.121	*0.314*	0.168	0.098
rs769450	A/G	Noncoding	0.33	0.289	0.192	0.423	0.276	0.347	0.389
rs429358	C/T	Missense	0.15	0.292	0.087	0.141	*0.418*	0.218	0.139
rs7412	T/C	Missense	0.07	0.084	0.075	0.067	0.022	0.058	0.070
Sample size				185	286	365	183	370	256

frequencies across populations: GGGTC is almost absent in Europeans (<1%) and Asians (<2%), but common in Africans (20%), CGGTC is present in 62% of Asians, but at lower frequencies in Europeans (36%) and Africans (13%). We also observed that two most common ε4—bearing haplotypes have a clear population-specific

patterns. GAGCC is present exclusively in Asian and European populations and absent in African population. In contrast GGGCC is the only ε4—bearing haplotype presented in 29% of African individuals, but occurs at low frequencies in Asian and European groups (<2%). Surprisingly, a protective *APOE* ε2 allele is presented almost

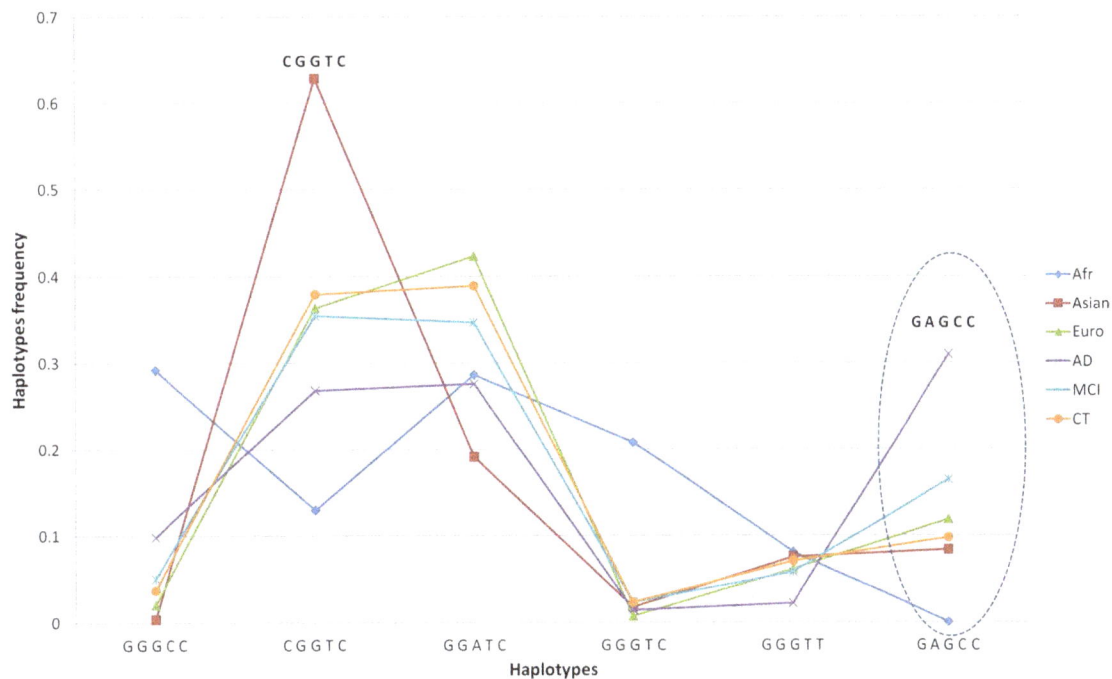

Fig. 2 Haplotype frequencies in human populations and ADNI cohort. X-axis labels represent allelic status of 5 SNPs (rs440446, rs769449, rs769450, rs429358, rs7412; Table 2) in *APOE locus*. Haplotype associated with *APOE* ε4 are in bold italic

exclusively by a single haplotype GGGTT in all human populations with 6–8% frequency. Thus, this allele has a lower population diversity.

Phylogenetic analysis of *APOE* haplotypes revealed that *APOE* ε4 haplotype GGGCC, which is African-specific, is most likely the ancestral variant (Fig. 4). This suggests that a common *APOE* ε3 allele was distributed in human populations after the split with other archaic hominins.

Comparing nucleotide content in the two ε4-bearing haplotypes (GGGCC and GAGCC) we observed that allele G of second SNP (rs769449) separates Africans from individuals of European and Asian ancestry. When we compared these two haplotypes to the most common European haplotype (GGATC), we found that both are significantly associated with AD (Fisher's exact test *P* value < 1e−12 and *P* value < 1e−4), but only GAGCC is associated with MCI. Altogether the data suggests, the state of this SNP might have a modifying effect on

ε4-associated AD/MCI risk development with African-specific allele G being potentially protective, in particular, in African populations.

This SNP is non-coding and therefore might have a regulatory effect on *APOE*. Potentially, A vs G allele in rs769449 can modify the epigenetic state in the *APOE* gene region. Supporting this hypothesis, we observed a robust H3K4Me3 signal using ChIP-seq data in this rs769449-containing region (Fig. 5; encircled) that is common mark of open chromatin. We assessed methylation profile of *APOE* locus based on ENCODE HAIB methylation data performed using Illumina Human Methylation 450 K Bead Arrays (Fig. 5) [18, 27]. While the methylation profile is U-shaped, the region from TSS down to exon 4 is highly sensitive to methylation [18], and comprises a range of transcription factor binding sites (Additional file 1: Table S2). The methylation rate of this region, which includes the SNP rs769449, is

Table 3 Haplotype frequencies in six human cohorts (haplotypes with *f* > 0.001). AD/MCI vs CT:GGATC (last column) represents the association of the haplotype with AD when compared to most common European haplotype (Fisher's exact test); haplotypes with zero frequencies are excluded from analysis

Haplotype	# added CG (positions)	APOE Allele	1000G			ADNI			AD vs CT:GGATC *P* value	MCI vs CT:GGATC *P* value
			Afr	Asian	Eur	AD	MCI	CT		
GGGCC	3 (1,4,5)	ε4	0.292	0.0035	0.0205	0.0984	0.05	0.0371	1.6e-5	0.1975
CGGTC	1 (5)	ε3	0.13	0.628	0.363	0.268	0.354	0.379	1	0.7382
GGATC	2 (1,5)	ε3	0.286	0.191	0.423	0.276	0.346	0.389	NA	
GGGTC	2 (1,5)	ε3	0.208	0.0175	0.00685	0.0137	0.023	0.0234	0.7979	0.8491
GGGTT	1 (1)	ε2	0.0811	0.0752	0.0616	0.0219	0.0581	0.0703	0.039	0.8065
GAGCC	3 (1,4,5)	ε4	0	0.0839	0.119	0.309	0.165	0.0977	2e-13	0.001
GGATT	1 (1)	ε2	0.0027	0	0	0	0	0		
CGATC	1 (5)	ε3	0	0.00175	0	0	0	0		
CGGTT	0	ε2	0	0	0.00411	0	0	0		
GAGCT	2 (1,4)	ε3	0	0	0.00137	0	0	0		
GAGTC	2 (1,5)	ε3	0	0	0	0.00273	0.00135	0		
CGGCC	2 (4,5)	ε4	0	0	0	0.0082	0	0.00391	0.3419	
CAGCC	2 (4,5)	ε4	0	0	0	0.00273	0.00135	0		
GGACC	3 (1,4,5)	ε4	0	0	0	0	0.00135	0		
Total haplotypes			370	572	730	366	740	512		
Sample size			185	286	365	183	370	256		

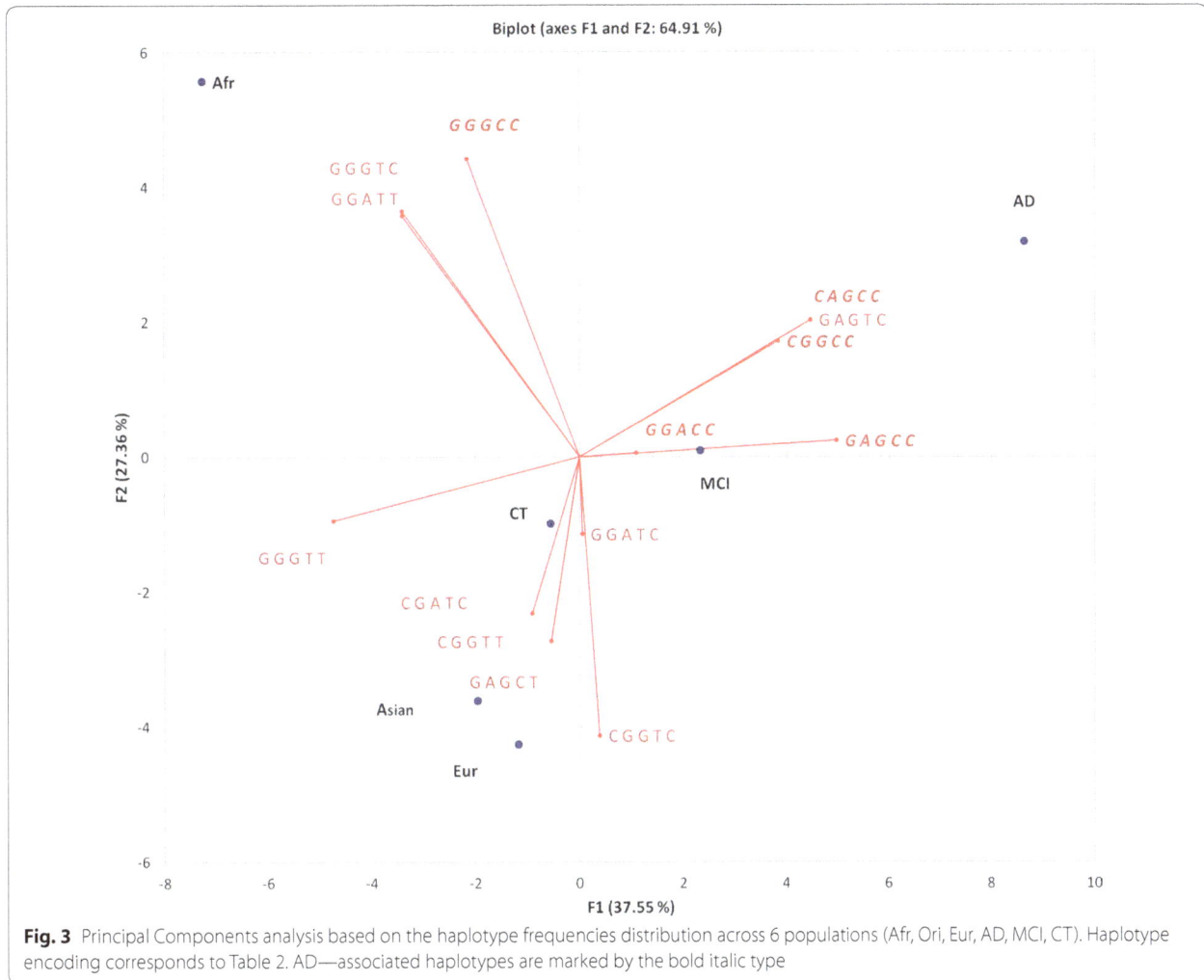

Fig. 3 Principal Components analysis based on the haplotype frequencies distribution across 6 populations (Afr, Ori, Eur, AD, MCI, CT). Haplotype encoding corresponds to Table 2. AD—associated haplotypes are marked by the bold italic type

Table 4 *P* **value for pairwise comparison of populations based on their haplotype frequencies [24]. ADNI Control group and European population don't significantly differ**

	Afr	Ori	Eur	AD	MCI
Ori	< 10E − 4				
Eur	< 10E − 4	< 10E − 4			
AD	< 10E − 4	< 10E − 4	< 10E − 4		
MCI	< 10E − 4	< 10E − 4	< 10E − 4	< 10E − 4	
CT	< 10E − 4	< 10E − 4	*0.5*	< 10E − 4	0.00909

anticorrelated with *APOE* expression rate and is significantly associated with aging [18]. It is also located 78 bp downsteam to second *APOE* exon. The methylation state in this region is changed in aging and associated with *APOE* dysfunction [18]. The rs769449 context is (gGc) and, when turning to A, one of the methylation sites

drops out, thus possibly altering intragenic methylation profile. A set of transcription factor binding sites in the areas of SNPs rs769449 also implies its possible regulatory effect (Additional file 1: Table S2).

It is worth noting that at least three out of five SNPs affect the CG dinucleotide content in *APOE* gene. *APOE* ε4 bears two CG dinucleotides mediated by rs429358 (minor allele) and rs7412 (major allele) that reside in the CpG island of exon 4 (Fig. 5) [18, 28]. rs769450 does not affect CG content (Table 2), while rs440446, the first target haplotype SNP meditates the CG dinucleotide arisen by minor allele, similar to the last ones,. Thus, the *APOE* ε4-bearing haplotypes maintain the largest number of CG dinucleotides within *APOE* (Table 3). Notably, rs769449 mediates CG dinucleotide in the inverse strand. It is resided within hotspot of H3K3me3 region (Fig. 6; encircled), and its C→A transition might affect the binding site of the transcription factor (Additional file 1: Table

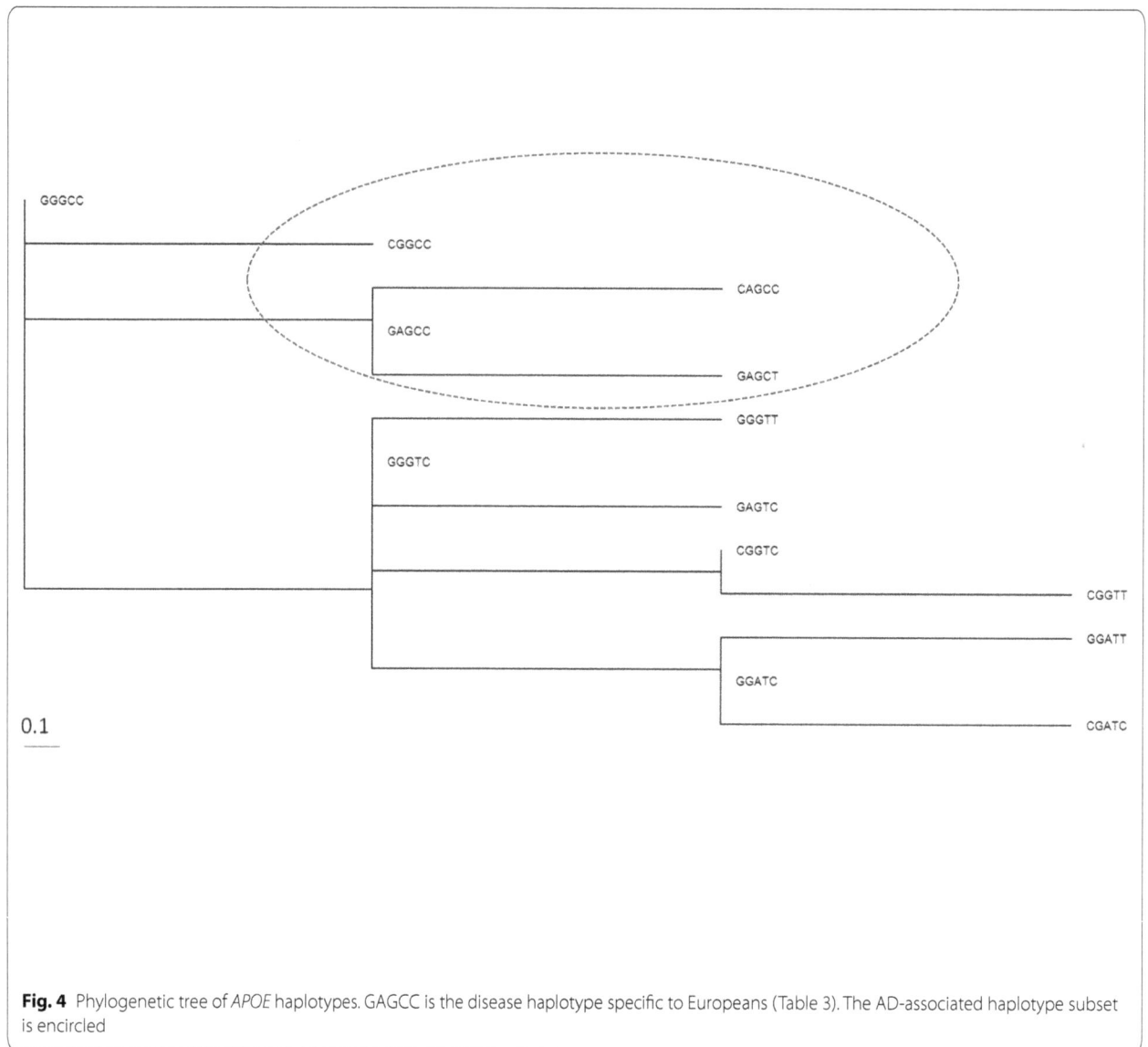

Fig. 4 Phylogenetic tree of *APOE* haplotypes. GAGCC is the disease haplotype specific to Europeans (Table 3). The AD-associated haplotype subset is encircled

S1). Notably, the target Illumina Methylation 450 array CpG site cg06750524 located close to rs769449 (Fig. 6; encircled) methylation status is highly associated with *APOE* ε4 allele: it was reported that its methylation rate is higher for the minor "disease" allele [18].

Discussion

APOE gene maintains the highest genetic association with AD reported to date. However, the association is ethnic- dependent, e.g., the evidence for AD-association with *APOE* is lower for African-Americans, Hispanic or Yoruban-African populatuion [19–21]. We have demonstrated that frequencies of *APOE* haplotypes a significantly different in human populations (Fig. 2, Table 4).

Specifically, the context of *APOE* ε4, which is the AD risk allele, drastically differs in populations (Fig. 3, Table 3). In particular, the two haplotypes for AD-associated *APOE* ε4 variant are GGGCC for African, and CAGCC for European and Asian individuals.

Sequence analysis of the chimpanzee *APOE* gene showed that it is most closely related to human ε4-type haplotypes, differing from the human consensus sequence at 67 synonymous (54 substitutions and 13 indels) and 9 nonsynonymous fixed positions [29]. Our analysis showed further that haplotypes defining the ε3 and ε2 alleles are derived from the ancestral ε4 s and that the ε3 group of haplotypes have increased in European and Asian populations.

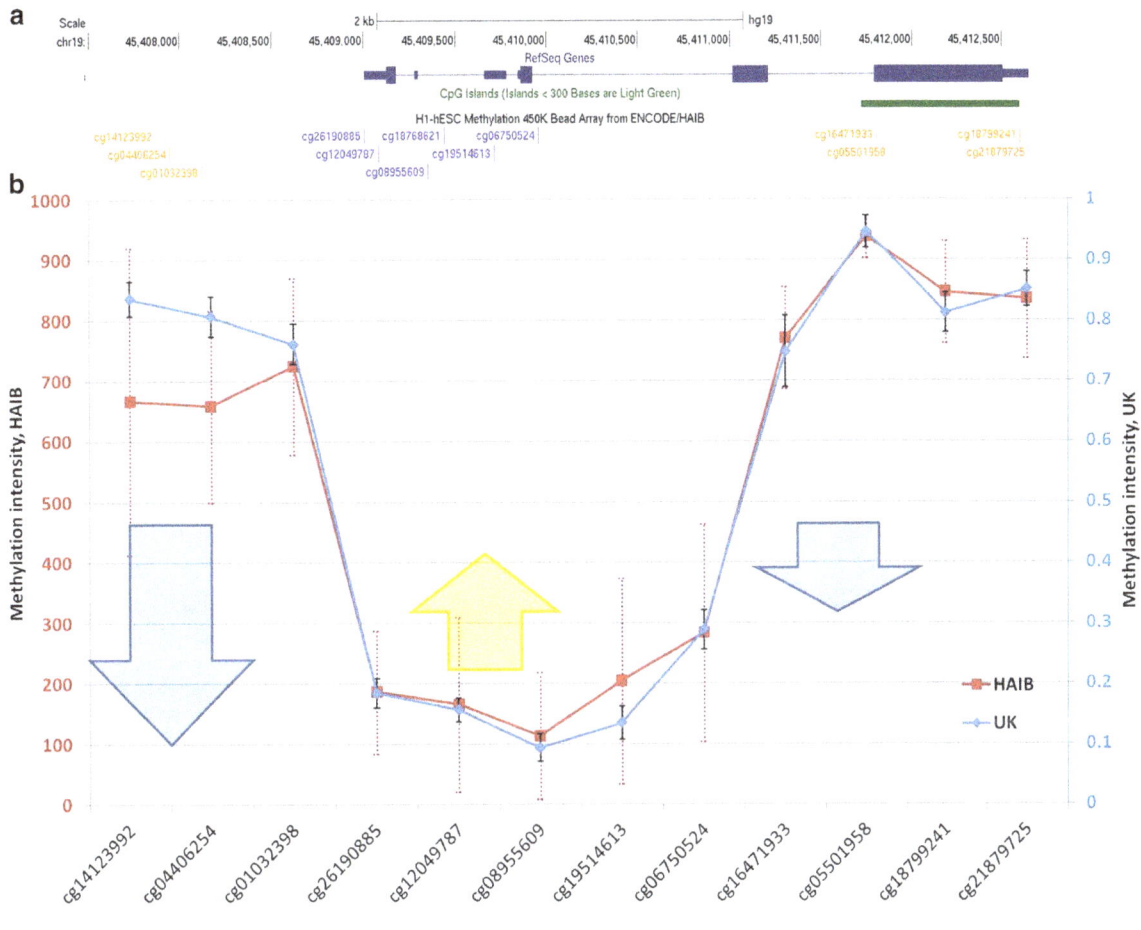

Fig. 5 Methylation profile of the *APOE* locus. **a** Genomic location of Illumina Methyl 450 bead array probes; **b** methylation profile of *APOE* gene based on two methylome projects. 63 HAIB cell lines (HAIB ENCODE methylation data), and 179 fetal brain samples [27] were used. Vertical dotted bars correspond to standard deviation of methylation score. Arrows indicate age related methylation drive [18]

The issue of ancestry of *APOE* ε4 allelotype has been widely discussed [30], and it has been established that the C→ T variant for ε3 allele arose after primate radiation [30]. Its relatively rapid expansion could be attributed to converging to meat diet in ancient human populations [30]. The data suggest also that specific *APOE* haplotypes might have protective effect against AD development potentially via epigenetic reprogramming of *APOE* due to CpG emergence/dropout [18, 28]. Altogether, our data demonstrated that ethnic genetic background defines

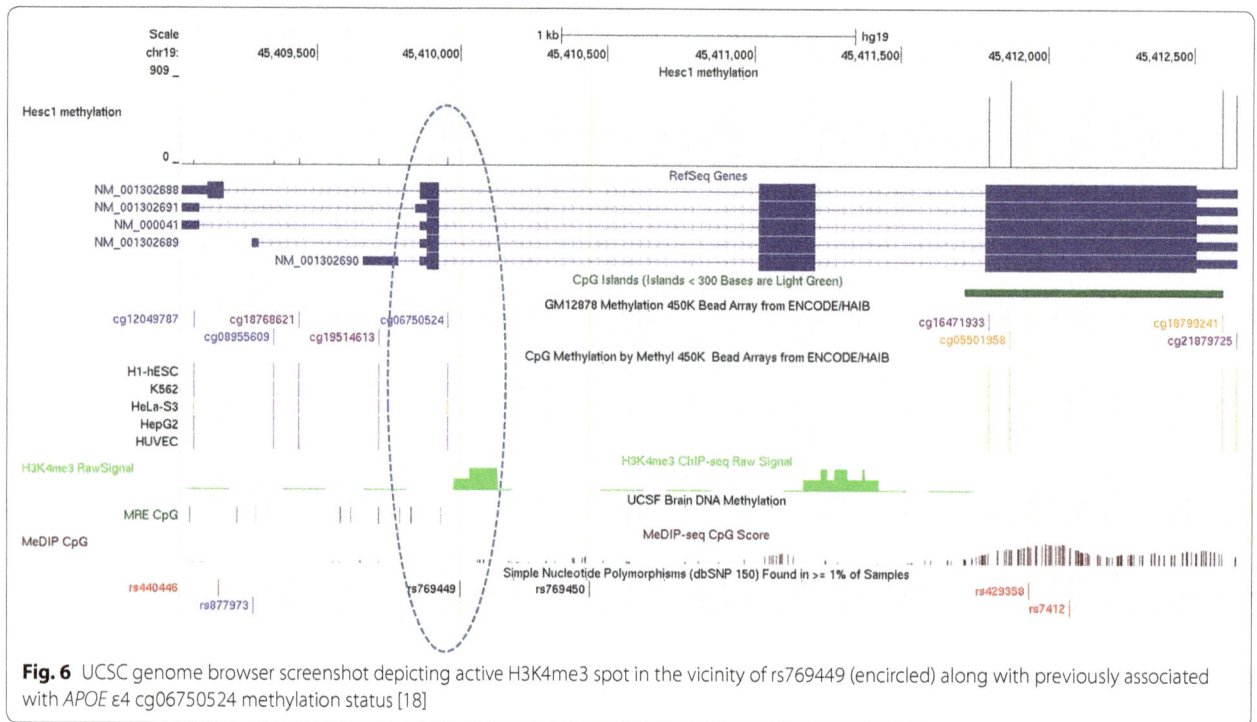

Fig. 6 UCSC genome browser screenshot depicting active H3K4me3 spot in the vicinity of rs769449 (encircled) along with previously associated with *APOE* ε4 cg06750524 methylation status [18]

significant differences in haplotypes for AD- risk alleles in human populations that may potentially be additional factor modifying risk for AD.

Abbreviations
AD: Alzheimer's disease; LOD: Logarithm of odds; SNPs: Single nucleotide polymorphisms.

About this supplement
This article has been published as part of BMC Neuroscience Volume 19 Supplement 1, 2018: Selected articles from Belyaev Conference 2017: neuroscience. The full contents of the supplement are available online at https://bmc-neurosci.biomedcentral.com/articles/supplements/volume-19-supplement-1.

Authors' contributions
E IR, DAA and VNB participated in project conception and in the study design. EIR and FEG coordinated downloading of genotype data from the ADNI web site. VNB and FEG assessed linkage disequilibrium and haplotype inferences in *APOE* locus region; VNB performed PCA analysis and analyzed methylation profiles. DAA and AVK performed statistical analysis with GenABEL program. EVI contributed to data interpretation. All authors read and approved the final manuscript.

Author details
[1] The Federal Research Center Institute of Cytology and Genetics of Siberian Branch of the Russian Academy of Sciences, Center of Neurobiology and Neurogenetics, Lavrentieva str. 10, Novosibirsk, Russia 630090. [2] Novosibirsk State University, Pirogova Str, 2, Novosibirsk, Russia 630090. [3] Vavilov Institute of General Genetics RAS, Gubkina str. 3, Moscow, Russia 119991. [4] Department of Psychiatry, University of Massachusetts Medical School, BNRI, Worcester, MA 15604, USA. [5] Faculty of Biology, Faculty of Bioengineering and Bioinformatics, Lomonosov Moscow State University, Moscow, Russia 119234.

Acknowledgements
The authors are grateful to anonymous reviewers for their valuable comments on our manuscript. Data collection and sharing for this project was funded by the Alzheimer's Disease Neuroimaging Initiative (ADNI) (National Institutes of Health Grant U01 AG024904) and DOD ADNI (Department of Defense Award Number W81XWH-12-2-0012). ADNI is funded by the National Institute on Aging, the National Institute of Biomedical Imaging and Bioengineering, and through generous contributions from the following: AbbVie, Alzheimer's Association; Alzheimer's Drug Discovery Foundation; Araclon Biotech; BioClinica, Inc.; Biogen; Bristol-Myers Squibb Company; CereSpir, Inc.; Cogstate; Eisai Inc.; Elan Pharmaceuticals, Inc.; Eli Lilly and Company; EuroImmun; F. Hoffmann-La Roche Ltd and its affiliated company Genentech, Inc.; Fujirebio; GE Healthcare; IXICO Ltd.; Janssen Alzheimer Immunotherapy Research & Development, LLC.; Johnson & Johnson Pharmaceutical Research & Development LLC.; Lumosity; Lundbeck; Merck & Co., Inc.; Meso Scale Diagnostics, LLC.; NeuroRx Research; Neurotrack Technologies; Novartis Pharmaceuticals Corporation; Pfizer Inc.; Piramal Imaging; Servier; Takeda Pharmaceutical Company; and Transition Therapeutics. The Canadian Institutes of Health Research is providing funds to support ADNI clinical sites in Canada. Private sector contributions are facilitated by the Foundation for the National Institutes of Health (www.fnih.org). The grantee organization is the Northern California Institute for Research and Education, and the study is coordinated by the Alzheimer's Therapeutic Research Institute at the University of Southern California. ADNI data are disseminated by the Laboratory for Neuro Imaging at the University of Southern California.

Evgeny I. Rogaev: For the Alzheimer's Disease Neuroimaging Initiative (ADNI): ADNI data used in preparation of this article were obtained from the Alzheimer's Disease Neuroimaging Initiative (ADNI) database (adni.loni.usc.edu). As such, the investigators within the ADNI contributed to the design and implementation of ADNI and/or provided data but did not participate in analysis or writing of this report. A complete listing of ADNI investigators can be found at: http://adni.loni.usc.edu/wp-content/uploads/how_to_apply/ADNI_Acknowledgement_List.pdf.

Competing interests
The authors declare that they have no competing interests.

Funding
The present study was supported in part by the Government of the Russian Federation, Grant No. 14.B25.31.0033, Resolution No. 220 (assessing linkage disequilibrium and haplotype inferences in *APOE* locus region, haplotype and PCA analysis), in part, E.I.R. supported by R01AG54712-02 and ADDF. Dmitry A. Afonnikov and Anton V. Klimov acknowledge the support of the statistical analysis with GenABEL program by the Federal Agency of Scientific Organizations, Project 0324-2018-0017. This work was also supported in part by Russian Science Foundation #14-44-00077 (ADNI data analysis) and #14-50-00029 (population analysis). The publication costs for this article were funded by the project 0324-2018-0017.

References
1. Takei N, Miyashita A, Tsukie T, Arai H, Asada T, Imagawa M, Shoji M, Higuchi S, Urakami K, Kimura H, Kakita A, Takahashi H, Tsuji S, Kanazawa I, Ihara Y, Odani S, Kuwano R. Japanese genetic study consortium for Alzheimer Disease. Genetic association study on in and around the *APOE* in late-onset Alzheimer disease in Japanese. Genomics. 2009;93(5):441–8. https://doi.org/10.1016/j.ygeno.2009.01.003.
2. Liu M, Bian C, Zhang J, Wen F. Apolipoprotein E gene polymorphism and Alzheimer's disease in Chinese population: a meta-analysis. Sci Rep. 2014;4:4383. https://doi.org/10.1038/srep04383.
3. Lutz MW, Sundseth SS, Burns DK, Saunders AM, Hayden KM, Burke JR, Welsh-Bohmer KA, Roses AD. A Genetics-based biomarker risk algorithm for predicting risk of Alzheimer's Disease. Alzheimers Dement (N Y). 2016;2(1):30–44.
4. Anderson ED, Wahoske M, Huber M, Norton D, Li Z, Koscik RL, Umucu E, Johnson SC, Jones J, Asthana S, Gleason CE. Alzheimer's disease neuroimaging initiative. Cognitive variability-a marker for incident MCI and AD: an analysis for the Alzheimer's Disease neuroimaging initiative. Alzheimers Dement (Amst). 2016;4:47–55. https://doi.org/10.1016/j.dadm.2016.05.003.
5. Luo X, Qiu T, Jia Y, Huang P, Xu X, Yu X, Shen Z, Jiaerken Y, Guan X, Zhou J, Zhang M. ADNI. Intrinsic functional connectivity alterations in cognitively intact elderly *APOE* ε4 carriers measured by eigenvector centrality mapping are related to cognition and CSF biomarkers: a preliminary study. Brain Imaging Behav. 2017;11(5):1290–301. https://doi.org/10.1007/s11682-016-9600-z.
6. Shen L, Kim S, Risacher SL, Nho K, Swaminathan S, West JD, Foroud T, Pankratz N, Moore JH, Sloan CD, Huentelman MJ, Craig DW, Dechairo BM, Potkin SG, Jack CR Jr, Weiner MW, Saykin AJ. Alzheimer's Disease neuroimaging initiative. Whole genome association study of brain-wide imaging phenotypes for identifying quantitative trait loci in MCI and AD: a study of the ADNI cohort. Neuroimage. 2010;53(3):1051–63.
7. Corder EH, Saunders AM, Strittmatter WJ, Schmechel DE, Gaskell PC, Small GW, Roses AD, Haines JL, Pericak-Vance MA. Gene dose of apolipoprotein E type 4 allele and the risk of Alzheimer's disease in late onset families. Science. 1993;261(5123):921–3.
8. Davignon J, Gregg RE, Sing CF. Apolipoprotein E polymorphism and atherosclerosis. Arteriosclerosis. 1988;8(1):1–21.
9. Mahley RW, Weisgraber KH, Huang Y. Apolipoprotein E: structure determines function, from atherosclerosis to Alzheimer's disease to AIDS. J Lipid Res. 2009;50(Suppl):S183–8. https://doi.org/10.1194/jlr.R800069-JLR200.
10. Blum CB, Type III. Hyperlipoproteinemia: still Worth Considering? Prog Cardiovasc Dis. 2016;59(2):119–24. https://doi.org/10.1016/j.pcad.2016.07.007.
11. Hui DY, Innerarity TL, Mahley RW. Defective hepatic lipoprotein receptor binding of beta-very low density lipoproteins from type III hyperlipoproteinemic patients. Importance of apolipoprotein E. J Biol Chem. 1984;259(2):860–9.
12. Mooijaart SP, Berbée JF, van Heemst D, Havekes LM, de Craen AJ, Slagboom PE, Rensen PC, Westendorp RG. *APOE* plasma levels and risk of cardiovascular mortality in old age. PLoS Med. 2006;3(6):e176.
13. Castellano JM, Kim J, Stewart FR, Jiang H, DeMattos RB, Patterson BW, Fagan AM, Morris JC, Mawuenyega KG, Cruchaga C, Goate AM, Bales KR, Paul SM, Bateman RJ, Holtzman DM. Human *APOE* isoforms differentially regulate brain amyloid-β peptide clearance. Sci Transl Med. 2011;3(89):89ra57. https://doi.org/10.1126/scitranslmed.3002156

14. Yajima R, Tokutake T, Koyama A, Kasuga K, Tezuka T, Nishizawa M, Ikeuchi T. *APOE*-isoform-dependent cellular uptake of amyloid-β is mediated by lipoprotein receptor LR11/SorLA. Biochem Biophys Res Commun. 2015;456(1):482–8. https://doi.org/10.1016/j.bbrc.2014.11.111.
15. Caglayan S, Takagi-Niidome S, Liao F, Carlo AS, Schmidt V, Burgert T, Kitago Y, Füchtbauer EM, Füchtbauer A, Holtzman DM, Takagi J, Willnow TE. Lysosomal sorting of amyloid-β by the SORLA receptor is impaired by a familial Alzheimer's disease mutation. Sci Transl Med. 2014;6(223):223ra20. https://doi.org/10.1126/scitranslmed.3007747.
16. Jun G, Vardarajan BN, Buros J, Yu CE, Hawk MV, Dombroski BA, Crane PK, Larson EB; Alzheimer's Disease Genetics Consortium., Mayeux R, Haines JL, Lunetta KL, Pericak-Vance MA, Schellenberg GD, Farrer LA. Comprehensive search for Alzheimer disease susceptibility loci in the *APOE* region. Arch Neurol. 2012;69(10):1270-1279. https://doi.org/10.1001/archneurol.2012.2052.
17. Wang SC, Oelze B, Schumacher A. Age-specific epigenetic drift in late-onset Alzheimer's disease. PLoS ONE. 2008;3(7):e2698. https://doi.org/10.1371/journal.pone.0002698.
18. Ma Y, Smith CE, Lai CQ, Irvin MR, Parnell LD, Lee YC, Pham L, Aslibekyan S, Claas SA, Tsai MY, Borecki IB, Kabagambe EK, Berciano S, Ordovás JM, Absher DM, Arnett DK. Genetic variants modify the effect of age on *APOE* methylation in the genetics of lipid lowering drugs and diet network study. Aging Cell. 2015;14(1):49–59. https://doi.org/10.1111/acel.12293.
19. Barnes LL, Bennett DA. Alzheimer's disease In African Americans: risk factors and challenges for the future. Health Aff (Project Hope). 2014;33(4):580–6. https://doi.org/10.1377/hlthaff.2013.1353.
20. Hendrie HC, Murrell J, Baiyewu O, Lane KA, Purnell C, Ogunniyi A, Gao S. APOE ε4 and the risk for Alzheimer disease and cognitive decline in African Americans and Yoruba. Int Psychogeriatr. 2014;26(6):977–85. https://doi.org/10.1017/S1041610214000167.
21. Tang MX, Stern Y, Marder K, Bell K, Gurland B, Lantigua R, Mayeux R. The APOE-epsilon4 allele and the risk of Alzheimer disease among African Americans, whites, and Hispanics. JAMA. 1998;279(10):751–5.
22. Reiman EM, Webster JA, Myers AJ, Hardy J, Dunckley T, Zismann VL, Joshipura KD, Pearson JV, Hu-Lince D, Huentelman MJ, Craig DW, Coon KD, Liang WS, Herbert RH, Beach T, Rohrer KC, Zhao AS, Leung D, Bryden L, Marlowe L, Kaleem M, Mastroeni D, Grover A, Heward CB, Ravid R, Rogers J, Hutton ML, Melquist S, Petersen RC, Alexander GE, Caselli RJ, Kukull W, Papassotiropoulos A, Stephan DA. GAB2 alleles modify Alzheimer's risk in APOE epsilon4 carriers. Neuron. 2007;54(5):713–20.
23. Aulchenko YS, Ripke S, Isaacs A, van Duijn CM. GenABEL: an R library for genome-wide association analysis. Bioinformatics. 2007;23(10):1294–6.
24. Excoffier L, Lischer HE. Arlequin suite ver 3.5: a new series of programs to perform population genetics analyses under Linux and Windows. Mol Ecol Resour. 2010;10(3):564–7. https://doi.org/10.1111/j.1755-0998.2010.02847.x.
25. Purcell S, Neale B, Todd-Brown K, Thomas L, Ferreira MA, Bender D, Maller J, Sklar P, de Bakker PI, Daly MJ, Sham PC. PLINK: a tool set for whole-genome association and population-based linkage analyses. Am J Hum Genet. 2007;81(3):559–75.
26. Gabriel SB, Schaffner SF, Nguyen H, Moore JM, Roy J, Blumenstiel B, Higgins J, DeFelice M, Lochner A, Faggart M, Liu-Cordero SN, Rotimi C, Adeyemo A, Cooper R, Ward R, Lander ES, Daly MJ, Altshuler D. The structure of haplotype blocks in the human genome. Science. 2002;296:2225–9.
27. Spiers H, Hannon E, Schalkwyk LC, Smith R, Wong CC, O'Donovan MC, Bray NJ, Mill J. Methylomic trajectories across human fetal brain development. Genome Res. 2015;25(3):338–52. https://doi.org/10.1101/gr.180273.114.
28. Yu CE, Foraker J. Epigenetic considerations of the APOE gene. Biomol Concepts. 2015;6(1):77–84. https://doi.org/10.1515/bmc-2014-0039.
29. Fullerton SM, Clark AG, Weiss KM, Nickerson DA, Taylor SL, Stengård JH, Salomaa V, Vartiainen E, Perola M, Boerwinkle E, Sing CF. Apolipoprotein E variation at the sequence haplotype level: implications for the origin and maintenance of a major human polymorphism. Am J Hum Genet. 2000;67(4):881–900.
30. Finch CE. Evolution in health and medicine Sackler colloquium: evolution of the human lifespan and diseases of aging: roles of infection, inflammation, and nutrition. Proc Natl Acad Sci U S A. 2010;107(Suppl 1):1718–24. https://doi.org/10.1073/pnas.0909606106.

2

Arc protein expression after unilateral intracranial self-stimulation of the medial forebrain bundle is upregulated in specific nuclei of memory-related areas

Elisabet Kádár[2,4]*[iD], Eva Vico Varela[1,3][iD], Laura Aldavert-Vera[1][iD], Gemma Huguet[2][iD], Ignacio Morgado-Bernal[1][iD] and Pilar Segura-Torres[1][iD]

Abstract

Background: Intracranial Self-Stimulation (ICSS) of the medial forebrain bundle (MFB) is a deep brain stimulation procedure, which has a powerful enhancement effect on explicit and implicit memory. However, the downstream synaptic plasticity events of MFB-ICSS in memory related areas have not been described thoroughly. This study complements previous work studying the effect of MFB-ICSS on the expression of the activity-regulated cytoskeleton-associated (Arc) protein, which has been widely established as a synaptic plasticity marker. We provide new integrated measurements from memory related regions and take possible regional hemispheric differences into consideration.

Results: Arc protein expression levels were analyzed 4.5 h after MFB-ICSS by immunohistochemistry in the hippocampus, habenula, and memory related amygdalar and thalamic nuclei, in both the ipsilateral and contralateral hemispheres to the stimulating electrode location. MFB-ICSS was performed using the same paradigm which has previously been shown to facilitate memory. Our findings illustrate that MFB-ICSS upregulates the expression of Arc protein in the oriens and radiatum layers of ipsilateral CA1 and contralateral CA3 hippocampal regions; the hilus bilaterally, the lateral amygdala and dorsolateral thalamic areas as well as the central medial thalamic nucleus. In contrast, the central amygdala, mediodorsal and paraventricular thalamic nuclei, and the habenular complex did not show changes in Arc expression after MFB-ICSS.

Conclusions: Our results expand our knowledge of which specific memory related areas MFB-ICSS activates and, motivates the definition of three functionally separate groups according to their Arc-related synaptic plasticity response: (1) the hippocampus and dorsolateral thalamic area, (2) the central medial thalamic area and (3) the lateral amygdala.

Keywords: Arc, Medial forebrain bundle, Intracranial self-stimulation, Memory, Hippocampus, Amygdala, Thalamus, Habenula

*Correspondence: elisabet.kadar@udg.edu
[4] Department of Biology, Sciences Faculty, University of Girona, C/Mª
Aurèlia Capmany 40, Camous Montilivi, 17003 Girona, Spain
Full list of author information is available at the end of the article

Background

Deep brain stimulation (DBS), an electrical current delivered through stereotactically implanted electrodes into specific areas of the brain, is a promising therapeutic option for patients with neurological and psychiatric diseases. To date, DBS has been successfully applied to alleviate movement disorders, such as Parkinson's disease [1]. DBS is now being considered for use as a treatment for neurodegenerative disorders associated with memory impairments such as Alzheimer's disease [2]. However, the mechanisms of action of how DBS affects memory are not yet fully known.

Studies with laboratory animals are required to explore potential targets and to analyze the underlying cellular and molecular brain changes of DBS. Recent studies indicate that bilateral DBS of the fornix/hypothalamic area drives neural activity in the cortico-hippocampal memory circuit with a significant reversal of the impaired cortical glucose utilization observed in patients with Alzheimer's disease [3, 4]. Further experiments in rats have established that forniceal DBS (F-DBS) induces increased hippocampal expression of c-Fos protein, some neurotrophic factors such as BDNF, and other synaptic plasticity markers [5], which are prominent molecular correlates of memory consolidation. These results are consistent with findings from our group which reveal a memory improvement after stimulating the medial forebrain bundle (MFB), the most important pathway of the brain reward system, which passes through the lateral hypothalamus (LH). Activation of brain areas belonging to the reward system generates positive reinforcement, and actions that are positively reinforced are more likely to be repeated than those that do not. Intracranial self-stimulation (ICSS) is a DBS procedure in which subjects self-administer electrical stimulation to brain reward areas by performing an instrumental response, such as pressing a lever in a Skinner box. The use of ICSS in animals allows us to unequivocally ensure that stimulation activates the reward system in a functional manner. In a similar way to F-DBS, ICSS of the LH has a reliable enhancing effect on hippocampus-dependent explicit memory [6–8]. However, while F-DBS affects fornix fibers, ICSS of the LH activates the MFB. Due to the extensive network of the MFB connects, this causes a widespread state of arousal and simultaneous activation of many areas, some of which are associated with different memory systems [9]. This could explain the wide therapeutic effects that MFB-ICSS appears to have in relation to different memory types. In addition to explicit memory, MFB-ICSS also improves performance in implicit memory tasks [10–12]. Most notable are the effects on emotional memory as measured by amygdala-dependent active avoidance tasks, in which ICSS reverses the memory deficit caused by aging [13, 14] and/or brain damage [15, 16].

Consistent with the broad effect of MFB-ICSS on different types of learning tasks, c-Fos expression results suggest ICSS activates multiple regions related to different memory systems, such as the amygdala, the dorsal striatum, the hippocampus and the prefrontal cortex [10, 17–19]. Additionally, MFB-ICSS induces differential time course mRNA expression of some synaptic plasticity-related genes including Arc in the amygdala and the hippocampus [18, 19]. ICSS-treated rats showing a facilitated spatial memory have also long-lasting structural changes including extended dendritic arborization of pyramidal CA1 neurons [6]. Thus, based on the fact that Arc protein is a well-known marker of synaptic plasticity events associated with the memory consolidation process [20] and is also involved in long-term spine enlargement [21], we initially set out to determine the effect of MFB-ICSS has on Arc protein levels in the different sub-regions of the hippocampus and in the retrosplenial cortex. We observed that after 4.5 h of unilateral MFB-ICSS, Arc protein levels increased significantly in the CA1 and DG hippocampal subfields ipsilateral to the stimulated hemisphere [22] but at this time contralateral regions were not analyzed. We also observed that MFB-ICSS increased Arc expression in the granular retrosplenial cortex (RSC), a hippocampus-related region involved in long-lasting memory storage [23]. This study showed a possible lateralization of the ICSS effects on Arc protein levels since changes were only observed in the ipsilateral, but not the contralateral hemisphere.

The current study provides new integrated data of the synaptic plasticity effects of the memory enhancing MFB-ICSS treatment on additional regions related to different memory systems and analyzes hemisphere differences. Arc protein expression was examined by immunohistochemistry in both ipsilateral and contralateral hemispheres 4.5 h after MFB-ICSS in each subject. The studied areas include (1) the hippocampal subfields, involved in spatial memory encoding and consolidation; (2) amygdalar nuclei involved in implicit emotional memory, including the associative lateral amygdala (LA) and the central nucleus (Ce), responsible for the autonomic components of emotions [24]; (3) higher order thalamic nuclei, such as the central medial (CM) and paraventricular (PV) nuclei related to memory through its role in regulation of arousal or attentional levels [25], and the mediodorsal (MD) and dorsolateral (DL) nuclei, considered to be relays to the hippocampus, amygdala and/or associative cortices, as well as being involved in learning and executive functions [26, 27]; and finally (4) the medial and the lateral habenula (MHb and LHb), involved in reward, emotional behavior and cognitive functions [28], which could also be implicated in the circuit in which MFB-ICSS affects memory via the inactivation of structures that project to it [29, 30].

Our findings show that the memory systems engaged by MFB-ICSS include the hilus, the oriens and radiatum layers of CA1 and CA3 hippocampal areas, the LA, DL and CM thalamic nuclei, in accordance with the idea that separate neural systems could operate in parallel to support the effects of ICSS on memory. In addition, a differential hemispheric Arc dependent-synaptic plasticity response to the MFB-ICSS treatment was observed in some of the analyzed regions.

Methods

Subjects

Twenty-five male Wistar rats were used in total, with a mean age of 96.20 days (SD = 2.10) at the beginning of the experiment and an average weight of 361 g (SD = 22.7) at the time of surgery. All were bred at our laboratory and fed ad libitum. Animals were individually housed, kept under controlled temperature (20–22 °C), humidity (40–70%) and subjected to a light/dark cycle of 12/12 h.

Intracranial self-stimulation

Stereotactic surgery

A combination of Ketamine (Imalgene, 150 mg/Kg, Merial, Lyon, France) and Xylazine (Rompun 8 mg/kh, Bayer, Barcelona, Spain) was used to induce deep anesthesia in the subjects. Using a digital stereotactic apparatus (Stoelting Co., 51900, IL, USA), all animals were implanted chronically and unilaterally (right hemisphere) with a 150 µm diameter monopolar stainless steel electrode (PlasticsOne, Roanoke, Va, USA). The tip of the electrode was placed at the LH, within the fibers of the medial forebrain bundle, with the incisor bar set at − 2.7 mm below the interaural line and according to coordinates [31]: AP = − 2.56 mm; ML = 1.8 mm and DV = − 8.5 mm, using the cranium surface as a dorsal reference. ICSS electrodes were anchored to the skull with jeweler's screws and dental cement.

ICSS behavior establishment

After a recovery period of 7 days, subjects were randomly distributed in 2 experimental groups, one that received the ICSS treatment (ICSS group) and their respective control without MFB-ICSS (Sham group). In order to establish self-stimulation behavior behavioral shaping was performed on animals from the MFB-ICSS group using a skinner conditioning box (25 × 20 × 20 cm) (Campden Instruments, Ltd.) with a lever situated on one of the lateral walls and a light switching on in a contingent manner to the stimulation train. The stimulation

consisted of sinusoidal wave currents, of 0.3 s in duration and 50 Hz in frequency, with an intensity ranging from 50 and 250µA. The procedure included the reinforcement of successive approximations to both the lever and to the required action (lever press) by the animal, while attempting to find the minimum current intensity that gave a stable response of 250 lever presses in 5 min, and self-stimulation until 500 reinforcements were reached. Establishment of the optimal intensity (OI) for each animal was performed in the corresponding ICSS treatment session as described in Segura-Torres et al. 1988 [32].

ICSS treatment

Four days after the OI was found, MFB-ICSS treatment was administered. This was done in a single session of 2500 self-administered trains of stimulant current at each particular OI using the same Skinner box where ICSS behavior had been established. The parameters of the stimulation in terms of frequency, intensity and number of trains administered were the same as previous studies since it has been shown to effectively enhance memory, both implicit [33–35] and explicit [6, 8].

Control subjects were placed in the same operant box for 45 min to match the average time it took the ICSS subjects to self-administer the treatment, but without receiving any stimulation (sham session). One of the experimental subjects had to be removed from further analysis at this point in time, due to incomplete treatment.

Arc Immunolocalization

Tissue collection

The animals (ICSS: n = 7, Sham: n = 10) were anesthetized with a lethal dose of pentobarbital (150 mg/kg body weight, i.p.) and perfused transcardially with a solution of 0.1 M phosphate buffer saline (PBS), pH 7.4, followed by a solution of 4% paraformaldehyde in PBS 4,5 h after MFB-ICSS or sham session. This interval has been used previously [22, 23] and chosen as an intermediate point where Arc induction persists after LTP, contextual fear conditioning and reversal learning in a T-maze [20, 21, 36, 37]. Brains were post-fixed in 4% paraformaldehyde in PBS solution for 4 h and then placed in 15% sucrose in PBS for 3 days and 30% sucrose in PBS at 4 °C until they sank. Serial coronal sections of cryopreserved brain (20-µm-thick) were obtained in a cryostat (Cryocut 1800, with 2020 JUNG microtome) at − 20 °C, at coordinates between − 2.50 and − 3.36 AP to Bregma. They were then mounted onto SuperFrost/Plus slides (Menzek-Gläser, Braunschweig, Germany) and stored at − 80 °C until immunohistochemistry staining.

Immunohistochemistry

Frozen coronal sections were washed in 0.05% Tween 20 in PBS 0.1 M (Wash Buffer solution), treated in 1% distilled H_2O_2 for 15 min and incubated in TNB (0,1 M Tris–HCl pH 7.5, 0,15 M NaCl and 0.5% Blocking Reagent; Perkin Elmer Life Sciences, Inc.) as a blocking solution. Sections were incubated in mouse Anti-Arc antibody (sc-166461, Santa Cruz Biotechnology, Inc.; Santa Cruz, CA, USA; diluted 1:50) for 48 h at 4 °C in a humidified chamber. Later the sections were washed and incubated in Biotinylated anti-mouse IgG antibody (Vector Laboratories Inc.; Burlingame, CA, USA; diluted 1:100) ON at 4 °C. Finally, samples were incubated in Streptavidin-peroxidase (Perkin-Elmer Life Sciences, Inc., diluted 1:100) for 2.5 h at room temperature and washed and incubated in DAB (Fisher) for 10 min. Lastly, sections were dehydrated, mounted and cover slipped. No staining was observed in control slides without the primary or secondary antibodies.

Data analysis

Microphotographs were taken with a BX41 Olympus microscope attached to an Olympus DP70 digital camera (Japan) from four regions 1) the hippocampus, including CA1, CA3 and DG; 2) the CeA and LA amygdaloid areas; 3) the PV, CM, DL and MD thalamic nuclei, and 4) the MHb and LHb. The analysis of the hippocampus was further divided by layers and measurements were taken in the oriens, pyramidal and radiatum layers of CA1; the oriens, pyramidal, lucidum and radiatum layers of CA3 and the granular and molecular layers of the medial blade (mbDG) and lateral blade (lbDG) of the DG and the hilus. The image analysis software Image-J 1.43 (http://rsb.info.nih.gov/ij/) was used to assess greyscale intensity levels using circular regions of interest (ROIs). An average of Arc intensity levels from three histological sections between bregma − 2.50 and − 3.36 for all regions. For the CM and PV, ipsilateral and contralateral sides were not taken into account.

Statistics

The statistical computer package program PASW Statistics 17.0 (SPSS) was used to process the data. Analyses of Arc intensity levels/mm^2 were conducted with a mixed ANOVA independent for each brain region. This corresponds to one between-group factor, the *TREATMENT* (sham or ICSS) and one within-group factor, the *HEMISPHERE* (ipsilateral or contralateral to electrode placement). A second within-group factor was considered for the hippocampal regions, the *LAYER* (3 for CA1, 4 for CA3, 5 for DG; see 2.3.3). Student's *t* test was applied to analyze the ICSS effects on Arc expression in the PV and CM nuclei. Additionally, in order to study the underlying

structure of the regions where significant ICSS effects on Arc expression were observed principal components analysis (PCA) with *oblimin* method of rotation was conducted. The α level for all tests was set at.05.

Results

ICSS treatment

The mean values ($\pm$ SD) of the ICSS variables of the ICSS group were: OI (77.14$\pm$42.31 μA), highest response rate (73.92$\pm$13.30 responses/min), treatment duration (50.42$\pm$8.97 min) and number of responses in the treatment session (3052.42$\pm$233.60 lever pressings). Correlation analyses showed no relationship between the ICSS variables and Arc levels in any of the brain areas evaluated.

Arc protein expression in different memory system areas following ICSS

We analyzed the influence of unilateral MFB-ICSS on different memory-related brain areas using Arc protein as a marker of early synaptic plasticity and examined both the ipsilateral and contralateral hemispheres. We compared the expression of Arc protein in both the MFB-ICSS and Sham groups in discrete regions of the hippocampus, amygdala, thalamus and the habenula 4.5 h after treatment.

Hippocampus

ANOVA analysis revealed a statistical significant increase of Arc protein expression in the ICSS group compared to the Sham group in the CA1 region dependent on both hemisphere and layer [*TREATMENT* $\times$ *LAYER* $\times$ *HEMISPHERE*: $F_{(2,30)} = 3.68$; $p = .037$] (see Fig. 1a, b). Further simple effects analysis showed significant effects in the ipsilateral hemisphere ($p = .05$), however, this was dependent on layer [*TREATMENT* $\times$ *LAYER*: $F_{(3,48)} = 2.68$; $p = .007$]. Thus ICSS increased Arc expression in the ipsilateral stratum oriens [$F_{(1,15)} = 4.93$; $p = .042$] and radiatum [$F_{(1,15)} = 5.75$; $p = .03$] layers but not in the pyramidal layer ($p = .07$). In contrast, no effects of the ICSS were observed in the contralateral side ($p = .755$) in any layer (oriens, $p = .360$; radiatum, $p = .319$; pyramidal, $p = .998$).

The increase in Arc protein expression in the CA3 region of the MFB-ICSS group compared to Sham [$F_{(1,15)} = 5,65$; $p = .031$] was independent of both hemisphere and layer [$\times$ *HEMISPHERE*: $p = .442$; $\times$ *LAYER*: $p = .669$] (Fig. 1a). However, since certain hemisphere differences were observed depending on the layer [*HEMISPHERE* $\times$ *LAYER*: $F_{(3,48)} = 3.9$; $p = .034$], simple effects for each hemisphere were studied. Analysis showed significant ICSS effects in the contralateral side ($p = .038$), but not in the ipsilateral ($p = .095$). Specifically, an Arc

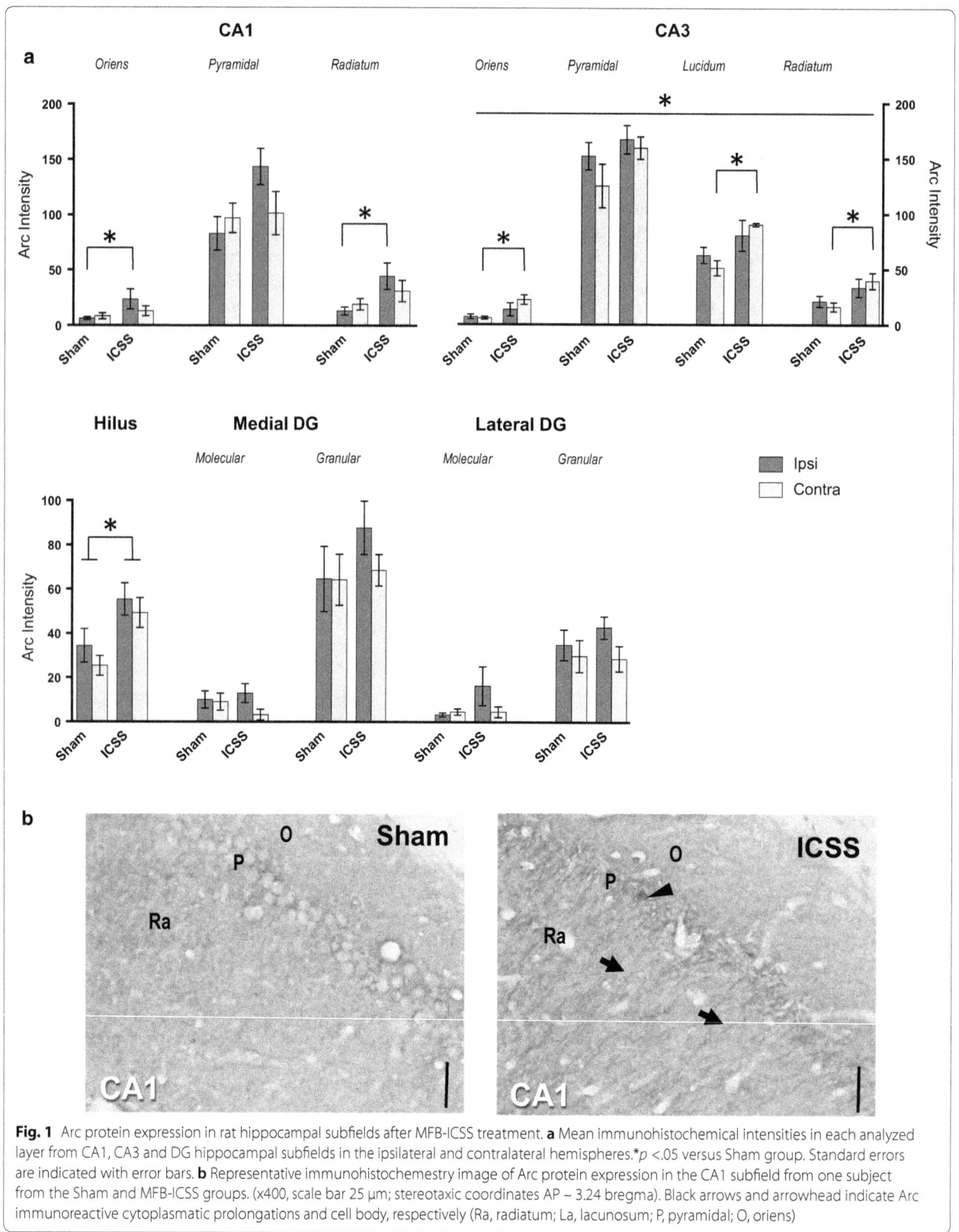

Fig. 1 Arc protein expression in rat hippocampal subfields after MFB-ICSS treatment. **a** Mean immunohistochemical intensities in each analyzed layer from CA1, CA3 and DG hippocampal subfields in the ipsilateral and contralateral hemispheres.*p <.05 versus Sham group. Standard errors are indicated with error bars. **b** Representative immunohistochemestry image of Arc protein expression in the CA1 subfield from one subject from the Sham and MFB-ICSS groups. (x400, scale bar 25 μm; stereotaxic coordinates AP – 3.24 bregma). Black arrows and arrowhead indicate Arc immunoreactive cytoplasmatic prolongations and cell body, respectively (Ra, radiatum; La, lacunosum; P, pyramidal; O, oriens)

increase was observed in the contralateral stratum oriens ($p = 0.004$), lacunosum ($p = .05$) and radiatum ($p = .016$), but not in the pyramidal layer ($p = 0.289$).

Finally, MFB-ICSS treatment had no significant overall effect on the dentate gyrus [$F_{(1,15)} = .663$; $p = .428$] and no significant interactions ($\times HEMISPHERE$: $p = .275$; $\times LAYER$: $p = .250$]. However, a significant difference in Arc protein increase between ICSS and Sham groups was observed in the Hilus [$F_{(1,15)} = 4.73$; $p = .046$] independent of the hemisphere ($p = .683$) and a tendency to significance in the ipsilateral molecular layer of lbDG ($p = .094$), but not in the contralateral ($p = .885$) was found (Fig. 1a).

Amygdala

Since the Box test for equality of covariance matrices was significant ($p = .010$) in the LA, a conservative F correction was therefore applied. ANOVA revealed that the *TREATMENT* had a significant effect [$F_{(1,7)} = 6,51$; $p = .038$], independent of hemisphere ($p = .623$). No significance was found in the CeA (*TREATMENT*: $p = .471$; *TREATMENT* $\times$ *HEMISPHERE*: $p = .407$) (see Fig. 2m).

Thalamus

Student's t-test showed a significant increase in Arc protein levels after MFB-ICSS treatment in the CM [$t_{(9)} = 4.59$; $p = .001$] but not in the PV [$t_{(13)} = 0.910$; $p = .379$] thalamic nuclei (see Fig. 2O). In the DL nucleus, the *TREATMENT* was found to have a significant effect [Box test $p = .027$; F$_{(1,5)} = 7.34$; $p = .042$] independent of hemisphere ($p = .076$). In the MD, no significant effect of the *TREATMENT* factor [Box test $p = .04$; F$_{(1,5)} = 4.013$; $p = .101$], nor the *HEMISPHERE* ($p = .467$) or their interaction ($p = .279$) were detected (see Fig. 2n).

Habenula

ANOVA analysis revealed that the *TREATMENT* had no significant effects on either the medial [$F_{(1,17)} = .331$; $p = .573$] or lateral [$F_{(1,17)} = 1.815$; $p = .196$] habenula, or its interaction with the *HEMISPHERE* (MHb, $p = .847$; LHb, $p = .189$) (Fig. 3).

Relations among Arc expression in different brain regions

Principal component analysis (PCA) was carried out on regions where significant effects of MFB-ICSS were observed, in order to identify whether or not there were any subsets of functionally-related regions to the expression of Arc. First of all, in order to reduce the variables of the analysis, we identified regions with significant correlation values between the ipsilateral and contralateral side (in relation to the electrode implantation) and in which the variable hemisphere did not influence the effects of the treatment. These areas were included in the PCA as the Arc intensity average of both hemispheres (LA, Hilus and DL variables) or in the region (CM). The CA1 and CA3 neurite layers also showed significant MFB-ICSS effects but with very different behavior in each of the hemispheres, however, this was not the case for the pyramidal layers. In this case, the CA1 and CA3 neurite layers were included in the PCA as Arc intensity average in oriens and radiatum layers from ipsilateral CA1 (CA1-neurite-ipsi) and in oriens, radiatum and lacunosum layers from contralateral CA3 (CA3-neurite-contra) variables. Therefore, the PCA included the following variables: LA, H, DL, CM, CA1-neurite-ipsi and CA3-neurite-contra.

Bartlett's sphericity test was statistically significant ($p = .005$). A 3-component model explained 91.83 percent of the variance. Figure 4 shows rotated factor loading. Factor 1 included four items (H, neurite layers of contralateral CA3 and ipsilateral CA1 and the DL thalamus), and could be labeled "hippocampus + associative thalamus". Factor 2 consisted of the lateral amygdala and the unspecific CM thalamus mainly loaded onto the third factor. Factor correlations were low for factor 2 (r $\leq$ .29) and moderated between factor 1 and 3 (r = .59).

Discussion

This study analyzes Arc protein expression in specific memory-related brain regions including the hippocampus, amygdala, thalamus and habenula through which ICSS of the MFB could exert its enhancing effect on memory. Results showed that unilateral MFB-ICSS, delivered with the same parameters with which it facilitates memory, upregulated Arc protein expression in the CA1,

---

(See figure on next page.)

Fig. 2 Arc protein expression in amygdala nuclei (**m**) and thalamic nuclei (**n** and **o**) after MFB-ICSS treatment. Representative immunohistochemistry images of Arc protein expression in the lateral amydala (LA), dorsolateral (DL) and central medial (CM) thalamic nuclei from the Sham (**a** and **b**, **e** and **f**, **i** and **j**) and MFB-ICSS (**c** and **d**, **g** and **h**, **k** and **l**) groups. (scale bar 100 µm in **a**, **c**, **e**, **g**, **i** and **k**, and 25 µm in **b**, **d**, **f**, **h**, **j**, and **l**; stereotaxic coordinates between − 2,50 and − 3.36 AP to Bregma). Arrows indicate Arc immunoreactive cell bodies. (CeA, central amygdala; ec, external capsule; DG, dentate girus; PV, paraventricular thalamic nuclei; IMD, intermediodorsal thalamic nucleus). Bar charts show the mean Arc expression levels in the LA and CeA (**m**) and in the DL and mediodorsal (MD) thalamic nuclei (**n**) from ipsi and contra lateral hemispheres of sham and MFB-ICSS treated groups. **o** mean Arc expression levels in CM and PV thalamic nuclei of sham and MFB-ICSS groups. Standard errors are indicated with error bars

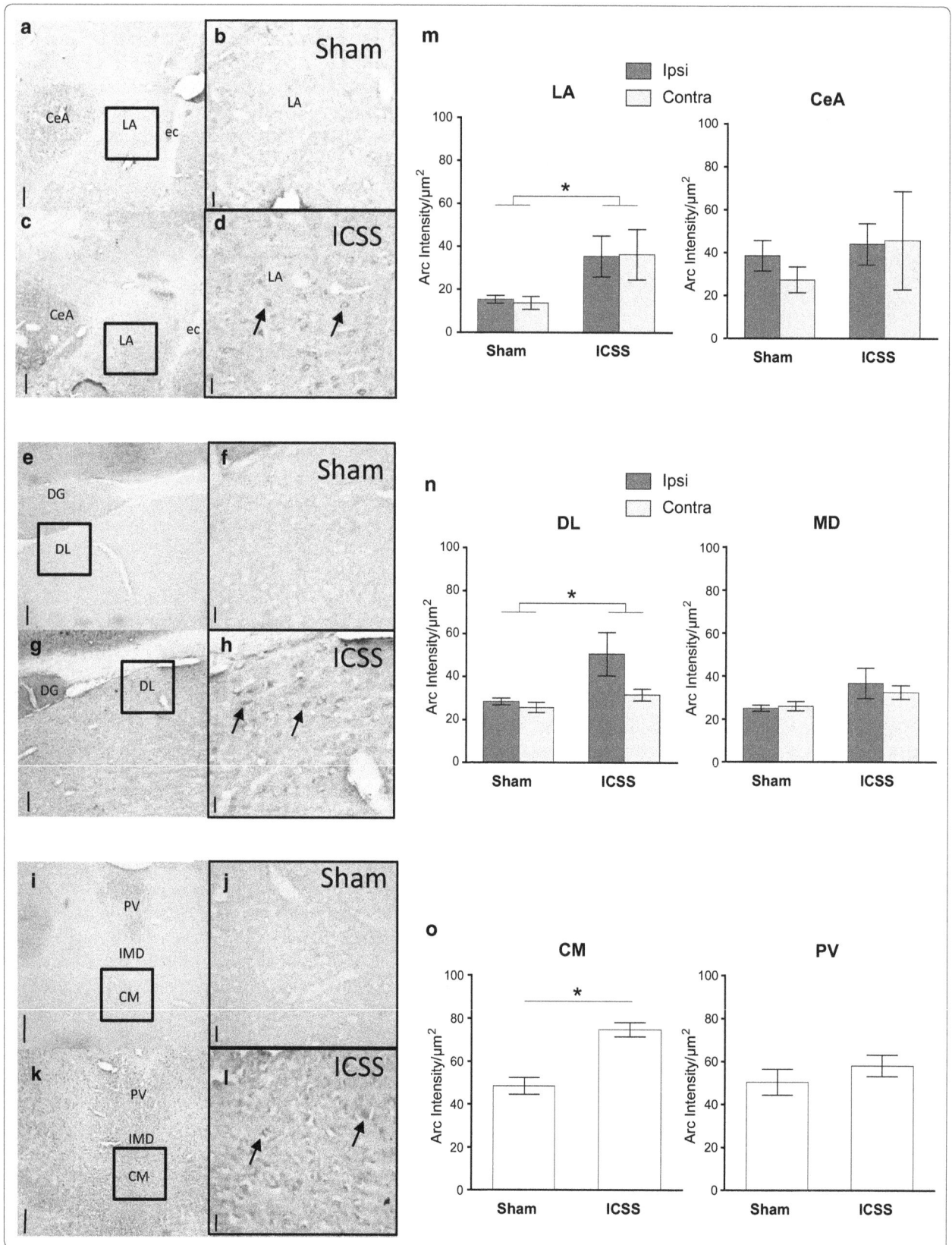

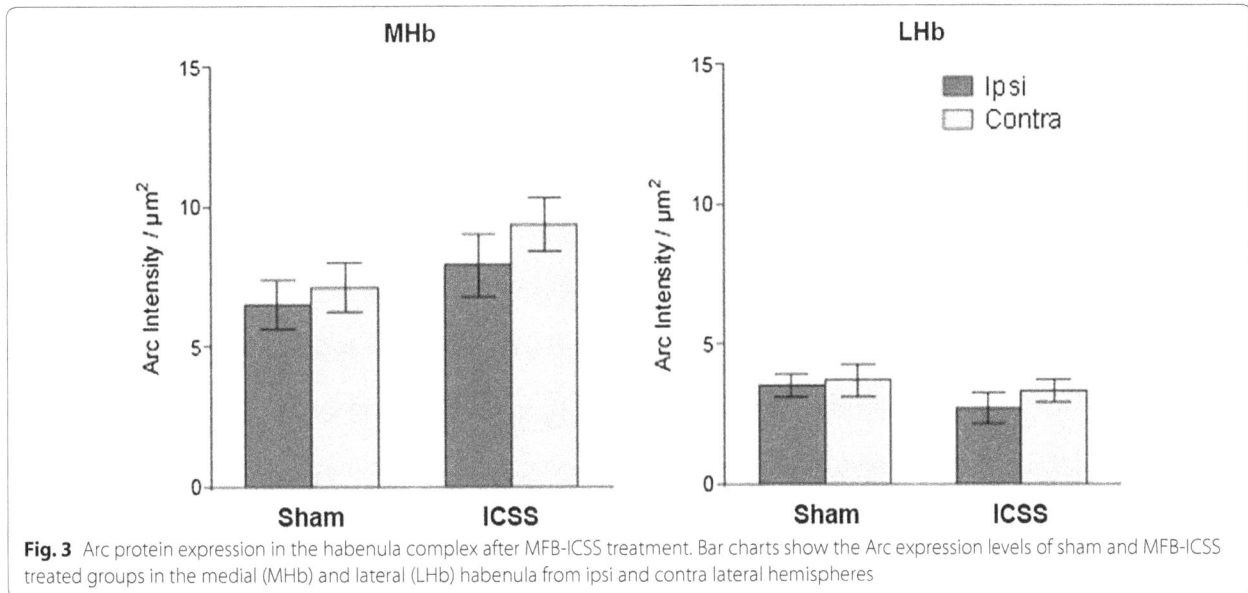

Fig. 3 Arc protein expression in the habenula complex after MFB-ICSS treatment. Bar charts show the Arc expression levels of sham and MFB-ICSS treated groups in the medial (MHb) and lateral (LHb) habenula from ipsi and contra lateral hemispheres

CA3 and hilus hippocampal regions, lateral amygdala, CM and DL thalamic nuclei. A differential hemispheric synaptic plasticity response was observed depending on the analyzed region.

Present results support our previous findings in that they show an overexpression of Arc protein in the neurite layers of the ipsilateral CA1 hippocampal region 4.5 h after MFB-ICSS [22], which is an intermediate time point for Arc protein expression changes [38]. This expression did not increase after the same treatment in contralateral CA1. To support our results further, structural plasticity changes, such as increased spine density and increased size and branching complexity in CA1 dendritic arborizations were also detected, specifically in the ipsilateral CA1 region of the hippocampus, 3 days and 20 days post-MFB-ICSS [6]. In contrast, Arc expression in the CA3 subfield showed predominance in the contralateral hemisphere which indicates that the lack of MFB-ICSS effects previously reported on ipsilateral CA3 is a hemisphere-dependent effect. Previous results of c-Fos expression showing the bilateral activation of CA1 and CA3 after unilateral MFB-ICSS [10] suggest that the hemispheric differences are not a result of higher contralateral hemispheric activation but rather a higher plasticity response. Therefore, differential expression patterns between these two proteins may be a sign of the greater specificity of Arc protein expression in terms of plasticity. Interestingly, hemispheric asymmetry was found in CA3-CA1 pyramidal neuron synapses [39]. This asymmetry has also been observed in long-term memory, where only left CA3 silencing impaired performance in an associative spatial long-term memory task, whereas right CA3

silencing had no effect, suggesting that memory could be routed via distinct left–right pathways within the mouse hippocampus [40]. In the DG, although a global effect was not observed, a significant bilateral increase in Arc expression in the hilus was found, as well as a tendency towards significance in the ipsilateral molecular layer of the lbDG. This reflects sub-regional treatment-induced differences related to synaptic plasticity, similar to previous studies [22].

It has been shown that an analogous MFB-ICSS treatment induces expression changes of different synaptic plasticity-related genes such as Arc and BDNF in the rat amygdaloid complex [19]. However, Arc expression was not analyzed at the protein level in specific amygdala nuclei after MFB-ICSS. Boundaries of expression corresponding to cytoarchitectonically defined amygdala subnuclei have been described in basal conditions [41] and here we observed a significant increase in Arc protein expression 4.5 h after MFB-ICSS treatment in the LA nucleus, whereas no effects were observed in the CeA nucleus. Interestingly, Partin et al. [42] described notable differences in gene expression patterns in the CeA and the LA nuclei. This differential response after MFB-ICSS in LA supports additional experiments in our laboratory in which a differential acetylcholinesterase activity linked to synaptic plasticity events in the LA but not in CeA regions was observed in MFB-ICSS treated lesioned rats. At the behavioral level, MFB-ICSS completely reversed the impairment in the acquisition of an active avoidance task caused by amygdala lesions [15]. There are also functional differences between these two amygdalar regions. The LA is an essential region for fear memory storage

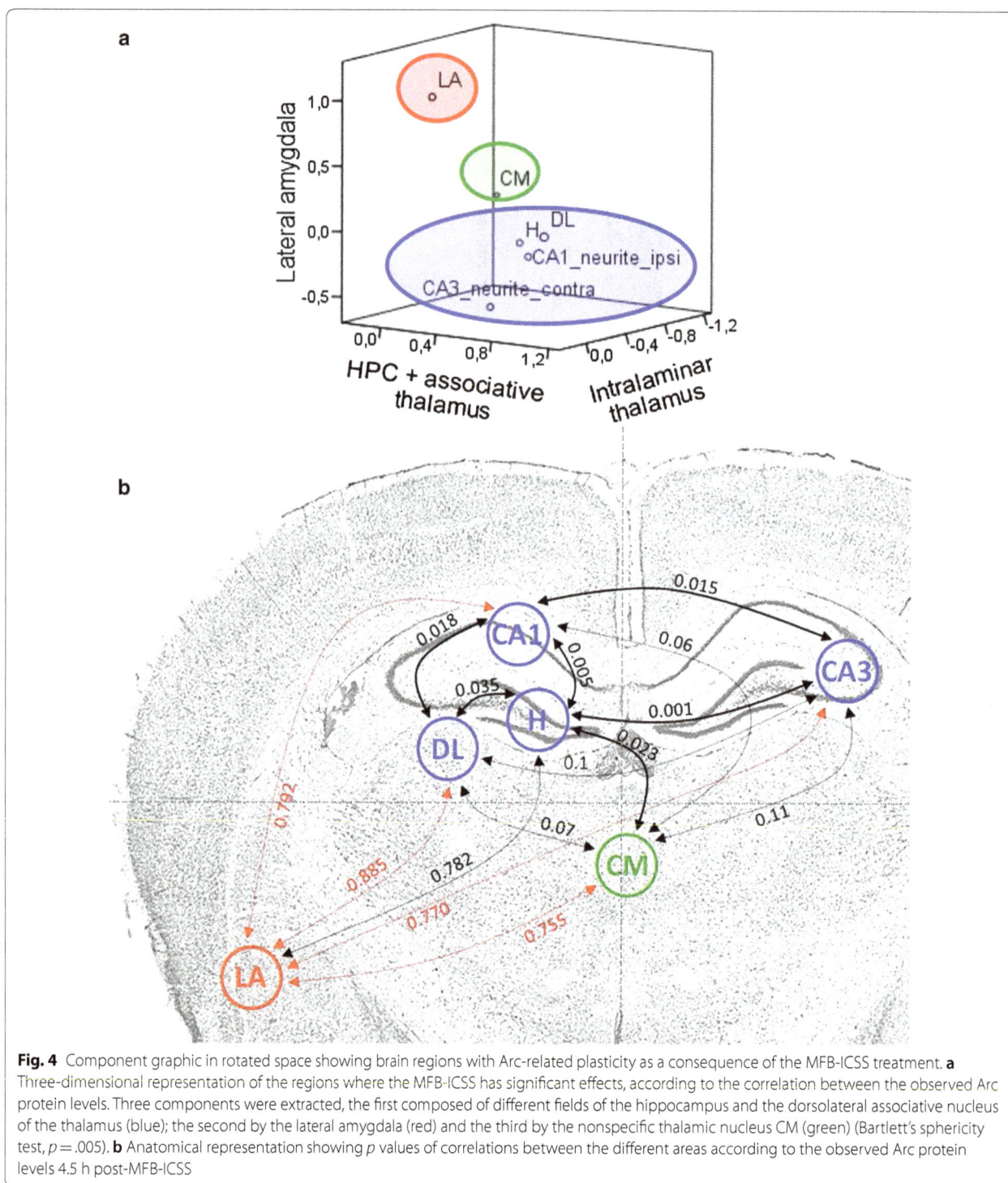

Fig. 4 Component graphic in rotated space showing brain regions with Arc-related plasticity as a consequence of the MFB-ICSS treatment. **a** Three-dimensional representation of the regions where the MFB-ICSS has significant effects, according to the correlation between the observed Arc protein levels. Three components were extracted, the first composed of different fields of the hippocampus and the dorsolateral associative nucleus of the thalamus (blue); the second by the lateral amygdala (red) and the third by the nonspecific thalamic nucleus CM (green) (Bartlett's sphericity test, $p = .005$). **b** Anatomical representation showing p values of correlations between the different areas according to the observed Arc protein levels 4.5 h post-MFB-ICSS

whereas the CeA does not seem to be required for the manifestation of instrumental active avoidance conditioned responses [43]. In agreement with our results, the immediate-early gene Arc has been recognized as a molecular marker for the LA neuronal ensemble recruited during fear learning in mice [44]. Regarding the observed MFB-ICSS hemisphere effects, it is important to point out that while an ipsilateral and contralateral pattern of Arc expression was observed in CA1 and CA3 respectively, a bilateral increased Arc expression was obtained in the LA, in a way that is consistent with the previous cited works, since no hemispheric effects were reported.

Regarding the thalamus, the effects of MFB-ICSS on thalamic synaptic plasticity events related to learning and memory have not been described and few studies have explored this area after electrical stimulation. For instance, LTP and/or LTD have been observed in the anterior thalamus after stimulation of direct and indirect hippocampal projections [45] and Arc protein synthesis has only been explored in relation to the thalamus role as a sensory relay [46, 47]. Present results show that MFB-ICSS induces bilateral Arc expression changes in specific thalamic nuclei including the DL and CM nuclei, whose role in memory may account for improvements in learning tasks. The DL nucleus acts in concert with the anterior nuclei and may serve an important integrative purpose for spatial learning systems [48–50]. The CM nucleus, strongly connected to the mPFC, is likely to be involved in working memory and/or memory consolidation through its modulation of vigilance states [25, 51]. Contrary to expectations, under present conditions MFB-ICSS did not increase Arc protein expression in the DM and PV nuclei, even though they also seem to participate in memory and executive function. The MD nucleus may contribute more to adaptive decision-making, as it is connected to the orbital prefrontal cortex and basolateral amygdala [52]. The PV nucleus, being part of the dorsal midline group, seems to contribute to viscero-limbic functions, reward and defensive behavior, and is a relay station between specific parts of the prefrontal and cingulate cortex, the striatum, and the CeA [25, 53, 54]. Overall, these results indicate that the thalamic nuclei most directly related to memory may mediate the facilitation effects of the MFB- ICSS on memory to some extent. Furthermore, in the same way that MFB-ICSS has proven to potentiate both explicit and implicit memory, the thalamus has also been linked to both memory systems involved. Thus, recent enhancement of c-Fos activity and the alpha4-nicotinic acetylcholine receptor in the hippocampus was observed after central thalamic DBS treatment [55], and expression of genes related to protein synthesis, maturation and degradation are increased in thalamic neurons that project to the LA after fear conditioning [56].

Our results also suggest the existence of certain functional subsystems in regions showing Arc-related plasticity as a consequence of the MFB-ICSS treatment. On the one hand, it is worth noting the autocorrelation between the different parts of the hippocampus and also their functional connection with the DL [57, 58], but not with the CM nucleus of the thalamus. The notion that the latter involves a second subsystem or

component is supported by the described lack of direct anatomical connections between the intralaminar thalamus and the hippocampus [25]. The associative LA is a substrate of action of the MFB-ICSS functionally independent of the hippocampus-DL and CM subsystems. However, since Arc and other plasticity and neuroprotection genes are upregulated in the amygdala before the 4,5 h time point (90 min post MFB-ICSS) [19], we cannot rule out that the activation of the amygdala and hippocampus, or thalamus, could be sequential, yet still related (Additional file 1).

The contribution of the habenular complex to ICSS has been examined in different studies but contradictory results have been observed. While Morissette et al. [59]showed that electrolytic lesions of the habenula attenuate brain stimulation reward, Gifuni et al. [60] showed that neurotoxic lesions of the LHb neurons do not alter the reward-enhancing effect of D-amphetamine in ICSS. Duchesne et al. [61] concluded that mesohabenular dopamine is not an important contributor to brain stimulation reward. Moreover, though recent evidence indicates that the habenular complex plays a role in learning and memory [62], no studies have looked at the effects of ICSS on plasticity-related protein expression in the habenula. Our findings show that MFB-ICSS did not enhance habenular Arc protein expression levels (or c-Fos protein expression- data not shown), at least at the time point analyzed. This supports the idea that the habenular complex may not be involved in the anatomical circuit activated by ICSS.

Finally, all these results taken together support the hypothesis that the stimulation of the reward system activates neural plasticity mechanisms in memory related areas and point MFB as a promising target for memory enhancing treatments. However, an aspect to consider is whether the results obtained with MFB-ICSS could be expected when MFB-stimulation was not self-administered, as it would be in a clinical setting. Although there are no antecedents comparing Arc protein levels caused by passive versus active administration, studies have reported that this variable slightly affects the induction c-Fos expression in the ipsilateral LH, but does not affect other brain memory-related regions [63]. Moreover, Chergui et al. [64] considered that, more than being self-administered or not, a critical parameter of the stimulation could be the temporal organization of the action potentials they generate. Similarly, although at the behavioral level both procedures—self-administered and experimenter-administered- have been shown to facilitate memory [65], the reinforcement component would correlate with the efficiency to potentiate memory [66]. Further studies should be performed to elucidate the differences between these two stimulation paradigms more thoroughly.

Conclusions

Overall, MFB-ICSS upregulates the expression of Arc protein in specific memory related areas including the CA1, CA3 and hilus hippocampal regions, the lateral amygdala and the dorsolateral and central medial thalamic nuclei which showed differential hemispheric response to the treatment. Our findings back up the idea that multiple, separate brain systems, could operate in parallel to support MFB-ICSS behavioral effects with distinct purposes during memory consolidation. Further studies may be performed not only to rule out the contribution from any other long-term storage related areas, such as the medial prefrontal cortex, but also to analyze whether ICSS may reverse the impact that certain brain lesions may have on cognition and memory, by potentiating other functionally related areas.

Abbreviations

Arc: activity-regulated cytoskeleton-associated; CM: central medial; Ce: central nucleus; DBS: deep brain stimulation; DL: dorsolateral; ICSS: Intracranial Self-Stimulation; F-DBS: forniceal DBS; LA: lateral amygdala; lbDG: lateral blade of DG; LHb: lateral habenula; LH: lateral hypothalamus; mbDG: medial blade of the DG; MFB: medial forebrain bundle; MHb: medial habenula; MD: mediodorsal; OI: optimal intensity; PV: paraventricular; PBS: phosphate buffer saline; PCA: principal components analysis; ROIs: regions of interest; RSC: retrosplenial cortex.

Authors' contributions

EV performed Arc immunohistochemistry of all brain sections and contributed in MFB-ICSS procedures with LA and PS. EK, PS, GH and IM analyzed and interpreted data regarding Arc immunolocalization. EK and PS were the major contributors in writing the manuscript and GH, LA, EV and IM revising it critically. All authors agreed to be accountable in ensuring appropriate answer to questions related to the accuracy and integrity of any part of the work. All authors read and approved the final manuscript.

Author details

[1] Departament de Psicobiologia i Metodologia de les Ciències de la Salut, Institut de Neurociències, Universitat Autónoma de Barcelona, 08193 Bellaterra, Barcelona, Spain. [2] Departament de Biologia, Universitat de Girona, 17071 Girona, Spain. [3] Douglas Mental Health University Institute, McGill University, Montreal, QC H4H 1R3, Canada. [4] Department of Biology, Sciences Faculty, University of Girona, C/Mª Aurèlia Capmany 40, Camous Montilivi, 17003 Girona, Spain.

Acknowledgements

We wish to thank Soleil Garcia-Brito, Daniel Rico and Neus Biosca for their excellent technical help, and Dr. Eva Penelo for her selfless aid with the analysis of the principal components.

Competing interests

The authors declare that they have no competing interests.

Funding

This research was supported by a grant support from the Spanish Ministerio de Ciencia e Innovación (I+D projects PSI2013-41018-P; PSI2017-83202-C2-1-P and C2-2-P).

References

1. Ponce FA, Lozano AM. Deep brain stimulation state of the art and novel stimulation targets. Prog Brain Res. 2010;184:311–24.
2. Suthana N, Fried I. Deep brain stimulation for enhancement of learning and memory. Neuroimage. 2014;85(Pt 3):996–1002. https://doi.org/10.1016/j.neuroimage.2013.07.066.
3. Sankar T, Chakravarty MM, Bescos A, Lara M, Obuchi T, Laxton AW, et al. Deep brain stimulation influences brain structure in Alzheimer's disease. Brain Stimul. 2014. https://doi.org/10.1016/j.brs.2014.11.020.
4. Smith GS, Laxton AW, Tang-Wai DF, McAndrews MP, Diaconescu AO, Workman CI, et al. Increased cerebral metabolism after 1 year of deep brain stimulation in Alzheimer disease. Arch Neurol. 2012;69:1141–8. https://doi.org/10.1001/archneurol.2012.590.
5. Gondard E, Chau HN, Mann A, Tierney TS, Hamani C, Kalia SK, et al. Rapid modulation of protein expression in the rat hippocampus following deep brain stimulation of the fornix. Brain Stimul. 2015. https://doi.org/10.1016/j.brs.2015.07.044.
6. Chamorro-López J, Miguéns M, Morgado-Bernal I, Kastanauskaite A, Selvas A, Cabané-Cucurella A, et al. Structural plasticity in hippocampal cells related to the facilitative effect of intracranial self-stimulation on a spatial memory task. Behav Neurosci. 2015. https://doi.org/10.1037/bne0000098.
7. Ruiz-Medina J, Morgado-Bernal I, Redolar-Ripoll D, Aldavert-Vera L, Segura-Torres P. Intracranial self-stimulation facilitates a spatial learning and memory task in the Morris water maze. Neuroscience. 2008;154:424–30.
8. Soriano-Mas C, Redolar-Ripoll D, Aldavert-Vera L, Morgado-Bernal I, Segura-Torres P. Post-training intracranial self-stimulation facilitates a hippocampus-dependent task. Behav Brain Res. 2005;160:141–7.
9. Berthoud H-R, Münzberg H. The lateral hypothalamus as integrator of metabolic and environmental needs: from electrical self-stimulation to opto-genetics. Physiol Behav. 2011;104:29–39. https://doi.org/10.1016/j.physbeh.2011.04.051.
10. Aldavert-Vera L, Huguet G, Costa-Miserachs D, de Ortiz SP, Kádár E, Morgado-Bernal I, et al. Intracranial self-stimulation facilitates active-avoidance retention and induces expression of c-Fos and Nurr1 in rat brain memory systems. Behav Brain Res. 2013;250:46–57. https://doi.org/10.1016/j.bbr.2013.04.025.
11. Coulombe D, White N. The effect of post-training hypothalamic self-stimulation on sensory preconditioning in rats. Can J Psychol. 1982;36:57–66.
12. García-Brito S, Morgado-Bernal I, Biosca-Simon N, Segura-Torres P. Intracranial self-stimulation also facilitates learning in a visual discrimination task in the Morris water maze in rats. Behav Brain Res. 2017;317:360–6. https://doi.org/10.1016/j.bbr.2016.09.069.
13. Aldavert-Vera L, Costa-Miserachs D, Massanes-Rotger E, Soriano-Mas C, Segura-Torres P, Morgado-Bernal I. Facilitation of a distributed shuttle-box conditioning with posttraining intracranial self-stimulation in old rats. Neurobiol Learn Mem. 1997;67:254–8.
14. Redolar-Ripoll D, Soriano-Mas C, Guillazo-Blanch G, Aldavert-Vera L, Segura-Torres P, Morgado-Bernal I. Posttraining intracranial self-stimulation ameliorates the detrimental effects of parafascicular thalamic lesions on active avoidance in young and aged rats. Behav Neurosci. 2003;117:246–56.
15. Kadar E, Ramoneda M, Aldavert-Vera L, Huguet G, Morgado-Bernal I, Segura-Torres P. Rewarding brain stimulation reverses the disruptive effect of amygdala damage on emotional learning. Behav Brain Res. 2014;274:43–52. https://doi.org/10.1016/j.bbr.2014.07.050.
16. Segura-Torres P, Aldavert-Vera L, Gatell-Segura A, Redolar-Ripoll D, Morgado-Bernal I. Intracranial self-stimulation recovers learning and memory capacity in basolateral amygdala-damaged rats. Neurobiol Learn Mem. 2010;93:117–26.

17. Arvanitogiannis A, Tzschentke TM, Riscaldino L, Wise RA, Shizgal P. Fos expression following self-stimulation of the medial prefrontal cortex. Behav Brain Res. 2000;107:123.

18. Huguet G, Aldavert-Vera L, Kádár E, Pena de Ortiz S, Morgado-Bernal I, Segura-Torres P. Intracranial self-stimulation to the lateral hypothalamus, a memory improving treatment, results in hippocampal changes in gene expression. Neuroscience. 2009;162:359–74.

19. Kadar E, Aldavert-Vera L, Huguet G, Costa-Miserachs D, Morgado-Bernal I, Segura-Torres P. Intracranial self-stimulation induces expression of learning and memory-related genes in rat amygdala. Genes Brain Behav. 2011;10:69–77.

20. Korb E, Finkbeiner S. Arc in synaptic plasticity: from gene to behavior. Trends Neurosci. 2011;34:591–8. http://www.pubmedcentral.nih.gov/articlerender.fcgi?artid=3207967&tool=pmcentrez&rendertype=abstract. Accessed 15 Mar 2016.

21. Messaoudi E, Kanhema T, Soule J, Tiron A, Dagyte G, da Silva B, et al. Sustained Arc/Arg3.1 synthesis controls long-term potentiation consolidation through regulation of local actin polymerization in the dentate gyrus in vivo. J Neurosci. 2007;27:10445–55.

22. Kadar E, Huguet G, Aldavert-Vera L, Morgado-Bernal I, Segura-Torres P. Intracranial self stimulation upregulates the expression of synaptic plasticity related genes and Arc protein expression in rat hippocampus. Genes Brain Behav. 2013;12:771–9.

23. Kádár E, Vico-Varela E, Aldavert-Vera L, Huguet G, Morgado-Bernal I, Segura-Torres P. Increase in c-Fos and Arc protein in retrosplenial cortex after memory-improving lateral hypothalamic electrical stimulation treatment. Neurobiol Learn Mem. 2016;128:117–24.

24. Izquierdo I, Furini CRG, Myskiw JC. Fear memory. Physiol Rev. 2016;96:695–750. https://doi.org/10.1152/physrev.00018.2015.

25. de Vasconcelos Pereira. A, Cassel J-C. The nonspecific thalamus: a place in a wedding bed for making memories last? Neurosci Biobehav Rev. 2015;54:175–96. https://doi.org/10.1016/j.neubiorev.2014.10.021.

26. Clark BJ, Harvey RE. Do the anterior and lateral thalamic nuclei make distinct contributions to spatial representation and memory? Neurobiol Learn Mem. 2016;133:69–78. https://doi.org/10.1016/j.nlm.2016.06.002.

27. Mitchell AS. The mediodorsal thalamus as a higher order thalamic relay nucleus important for learning and decision-making. Neurosci Biobehav Rev. 2015;54:76–88. https://doi.org/10.1016/j.neubiorev.2015.03.001.

28. Lecourtier L, Deschaux O, Arnaud C, Chessel A, Kelly PH, Garcia R. Habenula lesions alter synaptic plasticity within the fimbria–accumbens pathway in the rat. Neuroscience. 2006;141:1025–32. https://doi.org/10.1016/j.neuroscience.2006.04.018.

29. Lecourtier L, DeFrancesco A, Moghaddam B. Differential tonic influence of lateral habenula on prefrontal cortex and nucleus accumbens dopamine release. Eur J Neurosci. 2008;27:1755–62. https://doi.org/10.1111/j.1460-9568.2008.06130.x.

30. Nishikawa T, Fage D, Scatton B. Evidence for, and nature of, the tonic inhibitory influence of habenulointerpeduncular pathways upon cerebral dopaminergic transmission in the rat. Brain Res. 1986;373:324–36. http://www.ncbi.nlm.nih.gov/pubmed/2424555. Accessed 15 Mar 2017.

31. Paxinos, G Watson C. The rat brain in stereotaxic coordinates. Sixth edit. Elsevier Academic Press; 2007.

32. Segura-Torres P, Capdevila-Ortis L, Marti-Nicolovius M, Morgado-Bernal I. Improvement of shuttle-box learning with pre- and post-trial intracranial self-stimulation in rats. Behav Brain Res. 1988;29:111–7.

33. Aldavert-Vera L, Segura-Torres P, Costa-Miserachs D, Morgado-Bernal I. Shuttle-box memory facilitation by posttraining intracranial self-stimulation: differential effects in rats with high and low basic conditioning levels. Behav Neurosci. 1996;110:346–52.

34. Aldavert-Vera L, Huguet G, Costa-Miserachs D, Ortiz SPD, Kádár E, Morgado-Bernal I, et al. Intracranial self-stimulation facilitates active-avoidance retention and induces expression of c-Fos and Nurr1 in rat brain memory systems. Behav Brain Res. 2013;250:46–57.

35. Ruiz-Medina J, Redolar-Ripoll D, Morgado-Bernal I, Aldavert-Vera L, Segura-Torres P. Intracranial self-stimulation improves memory consolidation in rats with little training. Neurobiol Learn Mem. 2008;89:574–81.

36. Lee I, Kesner RP. Differential contributions of dorsal hippocampal subregions to memory acquisition and retrieval in contextual fear-conditioning. Hippocampus. 2004;14:301–10. https://doi.org/10.1002/hipo.10177.

37. Holloway CM, McIntyre CK. Post-training disruption of Arc protein expression in the anterior cingulate cortex impairs long-term memory for inhibitory avoidance training. Neurobiol Learn Mem. 2011;95:425–32. https://doi.org/10.1016/j.nlm.2011.02.002.

38. Korb E, Wilkinson CL, Delgado RN, Lovero KL, Finkbeiner S. Arc in the nucleus regulates PML-dependent GluA1 transcription and homeostatic plasticity. Nat Neurosci. 2013;16:874–83. https://doi.org/10.1038/nn.3429.

39. Shinohara Y, Hirase H, Watanabe M, Itakura M, Takahashi M, Shigemoto R. Left-right asymmetry of the hippocampal synapses with differential subunit allocation of glutamate receptors. Proc Natl Acad Sci USA. 2008;105:19498–503. https://doi.org/10.1073/pnas.0807461105.

40. Shipton OA, El-Gaby M, Apergis-Schoute J, Deisseroth K, Bannerman DM, Paulsen O, et al. Left-right dissociation of hippocampal memory processes in mice. Proc Natl Acad Sci U S A. 2014;111:15238–43. https://doi.org/10.1073/pnas.1405648111.

41. Zirlinger M, Kreiman G, Anderson DJ. Amygdala-enriched genes identified by microarray technology are restricted to specific amygdaloid subnuclei. Proc Natl Acad Sci USA. 2001;98:5270.

42. Partin AC, Hosek MP, Luong JA, Lella SK, Sharma SAR, Ploski JE. Amygdala nuclei critical for emotional learning exhibit unique gene expression patterns. Neurobiol Learn Mem. 2013;104:110–21. https://doi.org/10.1016/j.nlm.2013.06.015.

43. Choi J-S, Cain CK, LeDoux JE. The role of amygdala nuclei in the expression of auditory signaled two-way active avoidance in rats. Learn Mem. 2010;17:139–47. http://www.pubmedcentral.nih.gov/articlerender.fcgi?artid=2832923&tool=pmcentrez&rendertype=abstract. Accessed 16 Mar 2016.

44. Gouty-Colomer LA, Hosseini B, Marcelo IM, Schreiber J, Slump DE, Yamaguchi S, et al. Arc expression identifies the lateral amygdala fear memory trace. Mol Psychiatry. 2016;21:364–75. http://www.ncbi.nlm.nih.gov/pubmed/25802982. Accessed 13 Mar 2017.

45. Tsanov M, Vann SD, Erichsen JT, Wright N, Aggleton JP, O'Mara SM. Differential regulation of synaptic plasticity of the hippocampal and the hypothalamic inputs to the anterior thalamus. Hippocampus. 2011;21:1–8. http://www.pubmedcentral.nih.gov/articlerender.fcgi?artid=3928917&tool=pmcentrez&rendertype=abstract. Accessed 16 Mar 2016.

46. Khodadad A, Adelson PD, Lifshitz J, Thomas TC. The time course of activity-regulated cytoskeletal (ARC) gene and protein expression in the whisker-barrel circuit using two paradigms of whisker stimulation. Behav Brain Res. 2015;284:249–56. https://doi.org/10.1016/j.bbr.2015.01.032.

47. Ota KT, Monsey MS, Wu MS, Young GJ, Schafe GE. Synaptic plasticity and NO-cGMP-PKG signaling coordinately regulate ERK-driven gene expression in the lateral amygdala and in the auditory thalamus following Pavlovian fear conditioning. Learn Mem. 2010;17:221–35. https://doi.org/10.1101/lm.1592510.

48. Aggleton JP, Nelson AJD. Why do lesions in the rodent anterior thalamic nuclei cause such severe spatial deficits? Neurosci Biobehav Rev. 2015;54:131–44. https://doi.org/10.1016/j.neubiorev.2014.08.013.

49. Mizumori SJ, Williams JD. Directionally selective mnemonic properties of neurons in the lateral dorsal nucleus of the thalamus of rats. J Neurosci. 1993;13:4015–28. http://www.ncbi.nlm.nih.gov/pubmed/8366357.

50. van Groen T, Kadish I, Wyss JM. The role of the laterodorsal nucleus of the thalamus in spatial learning and memory in the rat. Behav Brain Res. 2002;136:329–37. https://doi.org/10.1016/S0166-4328(02)00199-7.

51. Mair RG, Hembrook JR. Memory Enhancement with Event-Related Stimulation of the Rostral Intralaminar Thalamic Nuclei. J Neurosci. 2008;28:14293–300. https://doi.org/10.1523/JNEUROSCI.3301-08.2008.

52. Mitchell AS, Sherman SM, Sommer MA, Mair RG, Vertes RP, Chudasama Y. Advances in understanding mechanisms of thalamic relays in cognition and behavior. J Neurosci. 2014;34:15340–6. https://doi.org/10.1523/JNEUROSCI.3289-14.2014.

53. Kirouac GJ. Placing the paraventricular nucleus of the thalamus within the brain circuits that control behavior. Neurosci Biobehav Rev. 2015;56:315–29. https://doi.org/10.1016/j.neubiorev.2015.08.005.

54. Penzo MA, Robert V, Tucciarone J, De Bundel D, Wang M, Van Aelst L, et al. The paraventricular thalamus controls a central amygdala fear circuit. Nature. 2015;519:455–9. https://doi.org/10.1038/nature13978.

55. Lin H-C, Pan H-C, Lin S-H, Lo Y-C, Shen ET-H, Liao L-D, et al. Central thalamic deep-brain stimulation alters striatal-thalamic connectivity in cognitive neural behavior. Front Neural Circuits. 2015;9:87. http://www.

pubmedcentral.nih.gov/articlerender.fcgi?artid=4710746&tool=pmcen trez&rendertype=abstract. Accessed 16 Mar 2016.

56. Katz IK, Lamprecht R. Fear conditioning leads to alteration in specific genes expression in cortical and thalamic neurons that project to the lateral amygdala. J Neurochem. 2015;132:313–26. https://doi.org/10.1111/jnc.12983.

57. Aggleton JP. Understanding retrosplenial amnesia: insights from animal studies. Neuropsychologia. 2010;48:2328–38. https://doi.org/10.1016/j.neuropsychologia.2009.09.030.

58. Van der Werf Yd, Witter MP, Uylings HB, Jolles J. Neuropsycology of infarctions in the thalamus: a review. Neuropsychologia. 2000;38:613–27.

59. Morissette MC, Boye SM. Electrolytic lesions of the habenula attenuate brain stimulation reward. Behav Brain Res. 2008;187:17–26.

60. Gifuni AJ, Jozaghi S, Gauthier-Lamer AC, Boye SM. Lesions of the lateral habenula dissociate the reward-enhancing and locomotor-stimulant effects of amphetamine. Neuropharmacology. 2012;63:945–57. https://doi.org/10.1016/j.neuropharm.2012.07.032.

61. Duchesne V, Boye SM. Differential contribution of mesoaccumbens and mesohabenular dopamine to intracranial self-stimulation. Neuropharmacology. 2013;70:43–50. https://doi.org/10.1016/j.neuropharm.2013.01.005.

62. Goutagny R, Loureiro M, Jackson J, Chaumont J, Williams S, Isope P, et al. Interactions between the lateral habenula and the hippocampus: implication for spatial memory processes. Neuropsychopharmacology. 2013;38:1–9. https://doi.org/10.1038/npp.2013.142.

63. Hunt GE, McGregor IS. Rewarding brain stimulation induces only sparse Fos-like immunoreactivity in dopaminergic neurons. Neuroscience. 1998;83:501–15.

64. Chergui K, Nomikos GG, Mathe JM, Gonon F, Svensson TH. Burst stimulation of the medial forebrain bundle selectively increase Fos-like immunoreactivity in the limbic forebrain of the rat. Neuroscience. 1996;72:141–56.

65. White N, Major R. Facilitation of retention by self-stimulation and by experimenter-administered stimulation. Can J Psychol. 1978;32:116–23.

66. Segura-Torres P, Portell-Cortes I, Morgado-Bernal I. Improvement of shuttle-box avoidance with post-training intracranial self-stimulation, in rats: a parametric study. Behav Brain Res. 1991;42:161–7.

3

Extremely low frequency electromagnetic field exposure and restraint stress induce changes on the brain lipid profile of Wistar rats

Jesús Martínez-Sámano[1], Alan Flores-Poblano[1], Leticia Verdugo-Díaz[2], Marco Antonio Juárez-Oropeza[1] and Patricia V. Torres-Durán[1*]

Abstract

Background: Exposure to electromagnetic fields can affect human health, damaging tissues and cell homeostasis. Stress modulates neuronal responses and composition of brain lipids. The aim of this study was to evaluate the effects of chronic extremely low frequency electromagnetic field (ELF-EMF) exposure, restraint stress (RS) or both (RS + ELF-EMF) on lipid profile and lipid peroxidation in Wistar rat brain.

Methods: Twenty-four young male Wistar rats were allocated into four groups: control, RS, ELF-EMF exposure, and RS + ELF-EMF for 21 days. After treatment, rats were euthanized, the blood was obtained for quantitate plasma corticosterone concentration and their brains were dissected in cortex, cerebellum and subcortical structures for cholesterol, triacylglycerols, total free fatty acids, and thiobarbituric acid reactive substances (TBARS) analysis. In addition, fatty acid methyl esters (FAMEs) were identified by gas chromatography.

Results: Increased values of plasma corticosterone were found in RS and ELF-EMF exposed groups (p < 0.05), this effect was higher in RS + ELF-EMF group (p < 0.05, vs. control group). Chronic ELF-EMF exposure increased total lipids in cerebellum, and total cholesterol in cortex, but decreased polar lipids in cortex. In subcortical structures, increased concentrations of non-esterified fatty acids were observed in RS + ELF-EMF group. FAMEs analysis revealed a decrease of polyunsaturated fatty acids of cerebellum and increases of subcortical structures in the ELF-EMF exposed rats. TBARS concentration in lipids was increased in all treated groups compared to control group, particularly in cortex and cerebellum regions.

Conclusions: These findings suggest that chronic exposure to ELF-EMF is similar to physiological stress, and induce changes on brain lipid profile.

Keywords: ELF-EMF, Corticosterone, Cholesterol, Fatty acids

Background

Brain lipids have different roles such as structural, functional and metabolic. Brain lipids constitute about one-half of brain-tissue dry weight. The brain has fatty acids that are long-chain monocarboxylic acids, either saturated or unsaturated, and cholesterol; the most prevalent families of unsaturated fatty acids are n-3, n-6, and n-9 series and contains some unusual fatty acids, such as very long chain fatty acids [1]. However, fatty acids are associated to other compounds to form glycerophospholipids and sphingolipids. These lipids play important roles in the brain physiology, e.g. in signal transduction across membranes, formation of lipid rafts, and anchoring the cell membranes to the extracellular matrix; furthermore, lipids covalently coupled to proteins play a major role in anchoring marker proteins within membranes [2].

Cholesterol and phospholipids are the main constituents of biomembranes. Changes in membrane lipid content are usually associated to imbalance in lipid

---
*Correspondence: pavitodu@yahoo.com.mx
[1] Departamento de Bioquímica, Facultad de Medicina, Universidad Nacional Autónoma de México, Circuito Escolar s/n, Ciudad Universitaria, C.P. 04510 Mexico City, Mexico
Full list of author information is available at the end of the article

homeostasis. In central nervous system (CNS) the lipid imbalance could lead to functional alterations that could result in several pathologies [1] as Alzheimer, Huntington and Parkinson diseases [3].

Stress could be defined as a condition in which homeostasis is modified by several responses, physiological and adaptive, induced by stressing factors. Hypothalamic–pituitary–adrenal (HPA) axis and the autonomic nervous system enhance the stress hormones in plasma, glucocorticoids and catecholamines, respectively [4, 5]. Stress exposure also induces deep changes in brain functions. Chronic stress has been related to increase in oxidative parameters for instance, increase in protein and lipid peroxidation, increased activity of antioxidant enzymes in the cortex, hippocampus and cerebellum [6]. However, the stress effects on brain lipids have not been extensively characterized.

Nowadays, the presence of electromagnetic fields in daily life it has resulted in an increase concerns regarding to the potential adverse effects of exposure to non-ionizing radiation; particularly to extremely low frequency electromagnetic fields (ELF-EMF). The effects induced by ELF-EMF exposure on biological systems are unclear. However, some effects are reported in epidemiological studies due to the incidence of certain types of brain cancer, and mood disorders [7]. Recent studies have reported the possible oxidant effect of ELF-EMF in brain, through the actions of reactive oxygen species [8]. Some authors have considered ELF-EMF as a mild stressor, and the effects related to its exposure have been reviewed [9]. In a previous study, carried out in Wistar rats acutely exposed to ELF-EMF, we have shown that they increase serum non-esterified fatty acids (NEFAs) concentration at 24 h post exposure [10] and impairs the antioxidant status of rat brain [11]. There are reports that show changes on the levels of Thiobarbituric Acid Reactive Substances (TBARS) of rats exposed to ELF-EMF in the cerebral cortex [12] or in various brain areas [13]. However, the effects of ELF-EMF on brain lipids and their metabolism have not been elucidated extensively. The aim of the present study was to evaluate the effects of chronic extremely low frequency electromagnetic field (ELF-EMF) exposure, restraint stress (RS), and both (RS+ELF-EMF) on lipid profile and lipoperoxidation status in cortex, cerebellum, and subcortical structures of Wistar rat brain.

Methods

Reagents
All reagents and chemicals used for the buffers and solution preparation were of analytical grade. Chloroform and methanol were purchased from Merck (Mexico City, Mexico). Kits for the assessment of Total cholesterol (TC) and triacylglycerols (TAG) were purchased from

Spinreact (Mexico City, Mexico), and kits for Non Esterified Fatty Acids from Roche (Mexico City, Mexico).

Animals and treatments
Male Wistar rats (aged 8 weeks) were bred in Faculty of Medicine, UNAM. A total of 24 young rats were used in the experiments (weight 180–200 g); the rats were acclimated to the room and light conditions by 3 days before the experimental period. The animals had free access to water and food in a room with controlled temperature of 23 °C ± 2 and 12 h light–dark cycles. The animals were placed in acrylic homecages of $47 \times 21 \times 25$ cm. All procedures involving animal care were conducted in compliance with the guidelines of animal care, and previously approved by the ethics and research committee of UNAM School of Medicine. All efforts were made to minimize the number of animals used and their suffering. Rats were randomly assigned to four groups of 6 rats each: Control (C), intact animals (nonstressed, 21 days); Restraint stress (RS), (positive control for stress, 2 h/day for 21 days); Extremely low frequency electromagnetic field exposure (ELF-EMF, unrestrained, 2 h/day for 21 days); Restraint stress plus ELF-EMF exposure (RS+ELF-EMF, 2 h/day for 21 days).

After 21 days of treatment and immediately after last exposure, rats were euthanized by cervical dislocation and their blood was collected into heparinized tubes. Right away the brain was dissected in cortex, cerebellum and subcortical structures and stored at −70 °C until analysis.

Restraint stress model (RS)
The model of movement restraint was used as a positive control for physical and psychological stress [14]. Movement restraint was performed by placing the animals into acrylic cylinders (18 cm in length × 7 cm in diameter) for 120 min/day during 21 days from 12:00 to 14:00 h. Unrestrained rats were individually placed in acrylic homecages during the same period into the same experimental room.

Extremely low frequency electromagnetic field exposure
ELF-EMF exposure was applied with a device previously used in our laboratory [15]. The electromagnetic field was generated with a pair of Helmholtz coils (30 cm internal diameter) composed of 18 gauge copper wire in 350 turns. When electrical current pass through the coils in the same direction, it creates a highly uniform magnetic field in a 3-dimension region of space inside the coils. Helmholtz coil is a device for producing a region of nearly uniform magnetic field. The coils were connected in parallel to a 120 V adjustable transformer (Staco Energy Products, Dayton, OH). An oscilloscope

(Tecktronix 5103N, Beaverton, OR) was coupled to the system to monitor a 60 Hz sinusoidal magnetic waveform. The amplitude of the magnetic flux density was 2.4 mT, which was measured using a hand-held Gauss/Tesla meter (Alpha Lab, Salt Lake City, UT). Helmholtz coils were in an isolated room containing also the control animals out of the electromagnetic exposure area. Background static magnetic field value was about < 0.4 µT in the room where all animals were kept and in the central area of the switched off coils. The temperature inside the exposure chambers was 23.4 ± 0.4 °C. The temperature between the coils was monitored using a Hygrothermometer (Extech instruments, Waltham, MA), this parameter remained constant during the 2 h of stimulation. The coils were separated 15 cm from the upper and lower surfaces of the animal cage [11, 15]. ELF-EMF exposure was applied during the same time (from 12:00 to 14:00 h) to the corresponding groups [15].

Plasma corticosterone determination
Plasma corticosterone concentration was quantitated using an ELISA kit (Enzo Life Sciences, Farmingdale, NY, USA), and microplate reader Stat Fax 3200 (Awareness Technology Inc. Palm City, FL, USA) according to the manufacturer´s instructions.

Brain lipid analysis
Total lipids of cortex, cerebellum and subcortical structures were extracted [16] with a chloroform/methanol mixture by a modified Folch's method and gravimetrically evaluated: for cortex, cerebellum and subcortical structures samples, 0.5 g of fresh tissue was homogenized in 4 volumes of 0.05 M phosphate buffer, pH 7.2, containing 0.025% butylated hydroxytoluene as antioxidant. Then, the pH was adjusted to 6.0 by the addition of HCl dissolution, and this suspension was extracted three times with 3 volumes each of the chloroform/methanol mixture (Folch´s dissolvent). The extract was washed with 10 mL of water, the organic fraction was evaporated under a nitrogen stream, then weighed (for total lipids), and stored at − 70 °C prior to TC, TAG, NEFAs, and gas chromatography (GC) of fatty acid methyl esters (FAMEs) analyses were performed [17, 18]. The polar lipids (POL) were calculated as follows: $POL = TL - (TC + TAG + NEFAs)$. All results were adjusted per mg total lipids (TL) and for measuring the absorbance it was performed with Genesis 10 UV spectrophotometer (Thermo Electron Corporation, Louisville, KY, USA).

Gas chromatography–mass spectrometry analysis
FAMEs from brain lipid extract were analyzed according to Torres-Durán [18] by GC in a Hewlett Packard gas chromatograph (HP 5890; Hewlett Packard, Mexico City) coupled to a mass selective detector (HP model 5972), with helium as gas carrier; temperature program starts at 200 °C for 3 min, then increased to 260 °C at a ramp velocity of 4 °C/min during 15 min and then maintained at 260 °C for 7 min. Spectra were obtained at 70 eV ionizing energy and mass range scanned was 50–700 a.m.u. at 1.5 scan/s. Fatty acid methyl esters were identified by comparing retention times of authentic fatty acids (Supelco) and by their mass spectra. Column, fused silica capillary column (25 m × 0.2 mm, 0.2 mm i.d.) coated with dimethylpolysiloxane (0.33 µm film) Hewlett Packard, Ultra 1 HP.

Lipoperoxides determination
Thiobarbituric acid reactive substances were determined according to Torres-Duran et al. [18]. Absorbance of the samples was interpolated in curves for concentration of malondialdehyde (MDA, ng/mg TL).

Statistical analyses
Frequency distribution for variables was determined by Kolgomorov–Smirnov test. Comparisons between groups were done using ANOVA (corticosterone, MDA, total cholesterol and, polar lipids) using Bonferroni post hoc test for contrasts among groups or Kruskal–Wallis test (NEFAs and saturated/unsaturated fatty acid ratio).

Results
Effects of RS and ELF-EMF exposure on plasma corticosterone
In order to visualize the effect of ELF-EMF on the stress status, we quantified the plasma corticosterone concentration. Increased values of plasma corticosterone were found in all the experimental groups ($p < 0.05$), this effect was higher in RS + ELF-EMF group compared to control group (C vs. RS + ELF-EMF and RS vs. RS + ELF-EMF, $p < 0.05$) (Fig. 1).

RS and ELF-EMF effects on TL, TC, TAG, and POL
Total lipids concentration in all the experimental groups shows a tendency to decrease in cortex and subcortical structures (Table 1), the lowest value was observed in subcortical structures of the RS + ELF-EMF group. However, TL in the cerebellum shows an increase only in ELF-EMF group that was statistically significant.

Regarding with TC, the same table shows a significant increase on TC content in the cortex of ELF-EMF and RS + ELF-EMF groups, and in subcortical structures of RS + ELF-EMF group ($p < 0.05$), but without changes in the cerebellum. A decrease on POL content was found only in the cortex of ELF-EMF, and RS + ELF-EMF groups ($p < 0.05$ vs. C group). Subcortical structures in

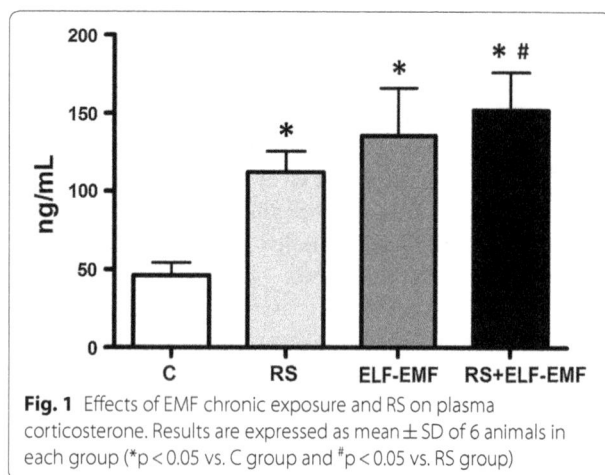

Fig. 1 Effects of EMF chronic exposure and RS on plasma corticosterone. Results are expressed as mean ± SD of 6 animals in each group (*$p < 0.05$ vs. C group and #$p < 0.05$ vs. RS group)

RS + ELF-EMF group showed lower POL values than in control and RS groups ($p < 0.05$). No statistical differences were found in cerebellum.

Triacylglycerol concentration was not different neither in the analyzed brain tissue (cortex, cerebellum, subcortical structures), nor in the four groups (C, RS, ELF-EMF, and RS + ELF-EMF). Their values were, in the range of 49.22–79.24 μg/mg TL.

The NEFAs content in cortex, cerebellum and subcortical structures are shown on Table 1. No statistically

significant differences were found between groups and cerebral regions analysed, except in subcortical structures, where the exposure to RS + ELF-EMF induced a slight NEFAs increase compared to the RS and C groups, causing 1.6 and 2.0-fold increases, respectively ($p < 0.05$).

Effects of RS and ELF-EMF exposure on FAMEs relative content in brain regions

The FAMEs profile showed that palmitic acid was the most abundant, with a range 33–51% in relative abundance in all analysed tissues (data not shown). For stearic acid, a 23–28% relative abundance was found in cortex and cerebellum and 32–36% in subcortical structures. In addition, the percentage of total unsaturated fatty acids was 15–40% in the studied brain regions. Stress induced by RS or ELF-EMF caused an increase in the saturated/unsaturated fatty acid ratio in the cortex ($p < 0.05$ vs. control group), but not in other analyzed brain regions (Fig. 2). This increase was due to palmitic acid in RS group ($51 ± 8.5$ vs. $39.4 ± 4.4$, $p < 0.05$ vs. C group). Finally, a significant increase of stearic acid was found in the cerebellum when the rats were exposed to ELF-EMF ($27.4 ± 2.0$ vs. $23.5 ± 1.9$ $p < 0.05$ vs. control group), but not in other groups (data not shown).

The following unsaturated fatty acids were identified in the brain regions studied: eicosatetraenoic, docosahexaenoic, docosatetraenoic, octadecenoic and eicosenoic

Table 1 Effects of ELF-EMF chronic exposure and RS on total lipids, total cholesterol, polar lipids and NEFAS in brain regions

Parameter	Group	Brain region		
		Cortex	Cerebellum	Subcortical structures
Total lipids (TL, mg/g wet weight)	C	60.5 ± 9.6	59.6 ± 3.7	70.5 ± 10.0
	RS	46.6 ± 8.7**	47.6 ± 5.7	47.4 ± 5.9*
	ELF-EMF	53.4 ± 7.3	71.4 ± 10.3&	59.3 ± 4.7*
	RS + ELF-EMF	42.3 ± 7.5**	55.6 ± 10.2	33.6 ± 5.6$,#
Total cholesterol (TC, μg/mg TL)	C	159.7 ± 1.0	188.3 ± 27.5	99.0 ± 18.6
	RS	169.6 ± 9.7	182.0 ± 25.4	101.8 ± 13.3
	ELF-EMF	194.3 ± 10.6*,&	148.5 ± 42.7	144.3 ± 35.0
	RS + ELF-EMF	198.6 ± 24.8*,&	173.0 ± 34.4	194.3 ± 67.6*,&
Polar lipids (POL, μg/mg TL)	C	753.5 ± 10.4	763.6 ± 73.6	831.2 ± 23.7
	RS	745.2 ± 14.0	714.0 ± 39.4	839.5 ± 14.2
	ELF-EMF	716.5 ± 22.5*	771.7 ± 56.6	786.9 ± 50.8
	RS + ELF-EMF	720.5 ± 26.0*	731.7 ± 48.2	729.4 ± 74.5*,&
NEFAs (μg/mg TL)	C	10.6 ± 1.9	16.5 ± 7.6	7.6 ± 2.2
	RS	9.3 ± 1.3	25.8 ± 9.4	9.5 ± 3.2
	ELF-EMF	9.9 ± 2.7	15.1 ± 3.8	10.4 ± 2.5
	RS + ELF-EMF	9.4 ± 3.5	15.0 ± 6.3	15.7 ± 4.3*,#

Results are expressed as mean ± SD of 6 animals in each group. For total lipids: **$p < 0.01$ versus control group, *$p < 0.05$ versus RS and RS + EMF groups, $$p < 0.05$ versus C group, and #$p < 0.05$ versus RS and EMF groups; for total cholesterol and polar lipids: *$p < 0.05$ versus control group and &$p < 0.05$ versus RS group; and NEFAS: *$p < 0.01$ versus control group and, #$p < 0.05$ versus RS and EMF groups

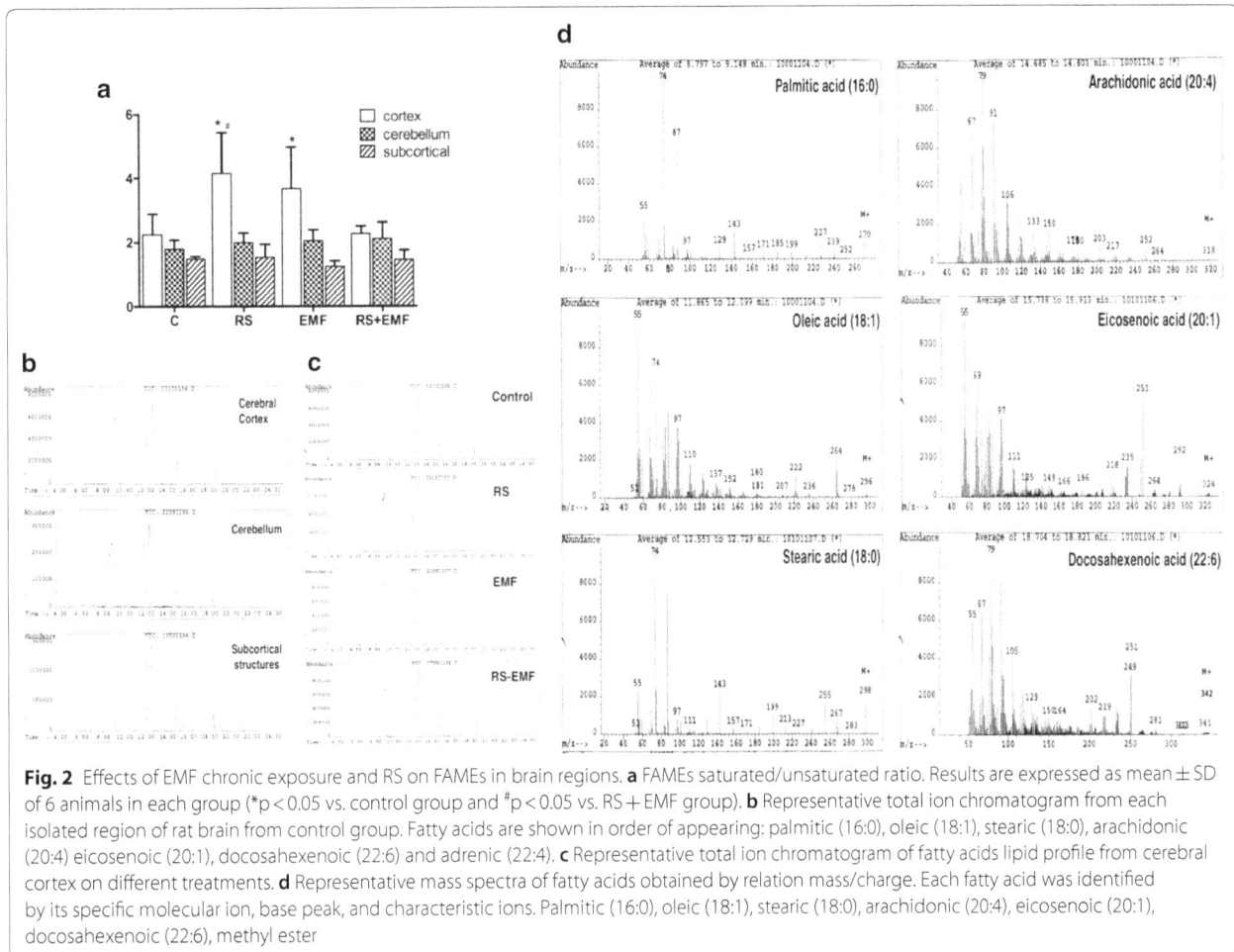

Fig. 2 Effects of EMF chronic exposure and RS on FAMEs in brain regions. **a** FAMEs saturated/unsaturated ratio. Results are expressed as mean ± SD of 6 animals in each group (*p < 0.05 vs. control group and #p < 0.05 vs. RS + EMF group). **b** Representative total ion chromatogram from each isolated region of rat brain from control group. Fatty acids are shown in order of appearing: palmitic (16:0), oleic (18:1), stearic (18:0), arachidonic (20:4) eicosenoic (20:1), docosahexenoic (22:6) and adrenic (22:4). **c** Representative total ion chromatogram of fatty acids lipid profile from cerebral cortex on different treatments. **d** Representative mass spectra of fatty acids obtained by relation mass/charge. Each fatty acid was identified by its specific molecular ion, base peak, and characteristic ions. Palmitic (16:0), oleic (18:1), stearic (18:0), arachidonic (20:4), eicosenoic (20:1), docosahexenoic (22:6), methyl ester

acids; however, only three unsaturated fatty acids (20:4, 22:4, and 22:6) showed differences among the treatments (Table 2). In brain cortex RS induced a decrease of eicosatetraenoic and docosahexaenoic acids percentages (p < 0.05 vs. C group), a decrease in docosatetraenoic acid was found in ELF-EMF group compared to C group (p < 0.05). In the cerebellum, we found a decrease of eicosatetraenoic and docosahexaenoic acids in ELF-EMF, and RS + ELF-EMF groups (p < 0.05 vs. C group). Cerebellum's docosatetraenoic acid was only detected in control group. Finally, in subcortical structures it was found an increase of all unsaturated fatty acids in ELF-EMF group (p < 0.05) when compared to control group, and to other treatments.

Effects of RS and ELF-EMF exposure on TBARS concentration in lipids of brain regions

TBARS (MDA concentration) in lipids was increased in all the treated groups compared to control group (p < 0.05), in cortical and cerebellar regions (Fig. 3). No

statistical differences were found among the groups in subcortical structures.

Discussion

The magnetic flux density used in this work was half the limit recommended for occupational exposures to 50/60 Hz magnetic fields, which is 5 mT for short term exposure (maximum exposure duration is 2 h per workday) [19]. Our results demonstrate that ELF-EMF exposure induces a significant increase in plasma corticosterone levels, indicating a chronic stress status similar to induced by RS. Although major stress was found in RS + ELF + EMF group, there isn't statistical difference between ELF + EMF and RS + ELF + EMF treatments. Nevertheless, this finding suggests a possible interaction, synergic or additive, that deserves further studies.

The RS model can induce deep changes in rat physiology; Hennebelle found an increment of 30-times basal corticosterone concentration when RS was applied 6 h/day for 21 days [20]. Buynitsky and Mostofsky [21] reported that a daily 3-week period of RS is used in

Table 2 Effects of ELF-EMF and RS exposure on FAMEs in brain regions

Relative abundance	% Eicosatetraenoic (20:4)	% Docosahexaenoic (22:6)	% Docosatetraenoic (22:4)
Cortex			
C	4.9 ± 1.2	2.2 ± 1.1	0.8 ± 0.4
RS	1.9 ± 1.0*	0.7 ± 0.1*	0.5 ± 0.3
ELF-EMF	2.7 ± 1.4*	0.8 ± 0.5*	0.3 ± 0.2*
RS + ELF-EMF	5.4 ± 0.8#	2.8 ± 0.8#	0.7 ± 0.2
Cerebellum			
C	2.8 ± 0.8	1.5 ± 0.8	0.3 ± 0.2
RS	1.9 ± 0.7	0.8 ± 0.5	ND
ELF-EMF	1.3 ± 0.6*	0.6 ± 0.4*	ND
RS + ELF-EMF	1.3 ± 0.5*	0.3 ± 0.2*	ND
Subcortical			
C	4.8 ± 0.7	2.5 ± 0.5	0.8 ± 0.2
RS	3.1 ± 1.5&	1.5 ± 0.9&	0.4 ± 0.3&
ELF-EMF	6.5 ± 0.6*	4.1 ± 1.3*	1.5 ± 0.5*
RS + ELF-EMF	4.4 ± 1.0&	2.4 ± 0.8&	0.6 ± 0.3&

Octadecenoic (18:1) and eicosaenoic (20:1) acids were found in all regions, average 20–30 and 0.8–2%, respectively, without differences versus control group. Results are expressed as mean ± SD of 6 animals in each group (*p < 0.05 vs. control group, &p < 0.05 vs. ELF-EMF group, and #p < 0.05 vs. RS and EMF groups)

ND no detected

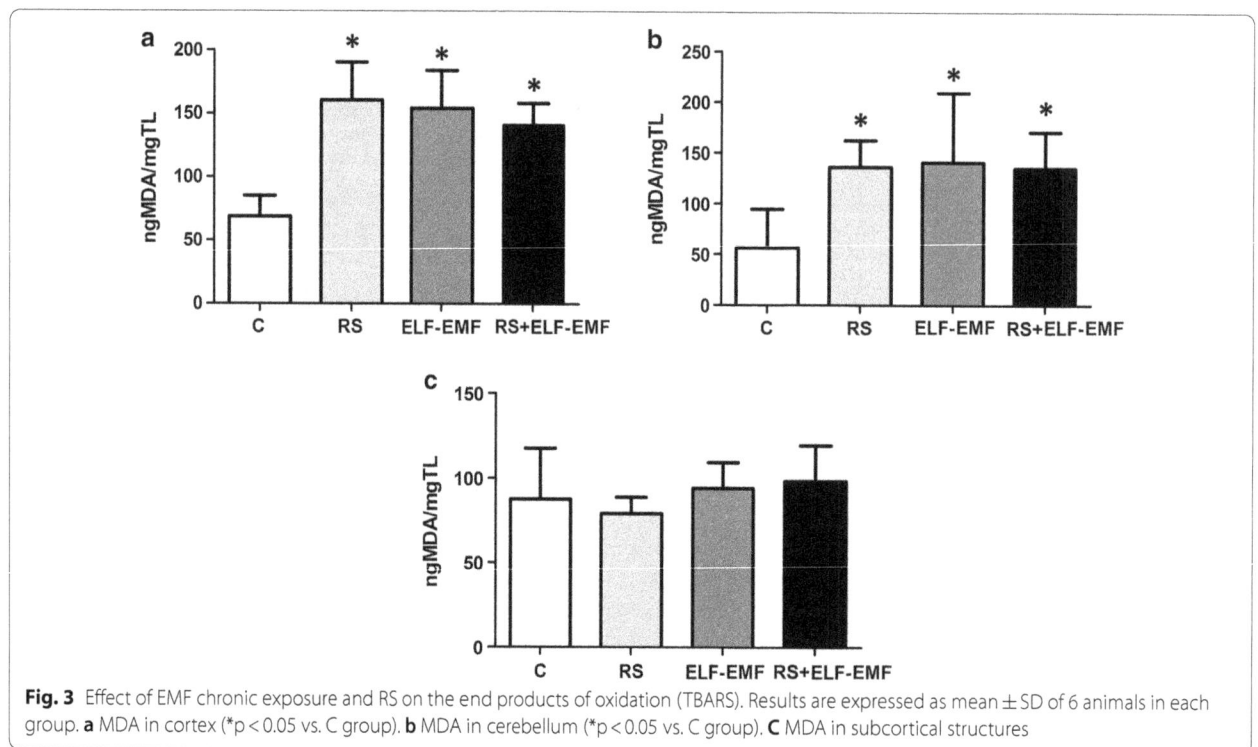

Fig. 3 Effect of EMF chronic exposure and RS on the end products of oxidation (TBARS). Results are expressed as mean ± SD of 6 animals in each group. **a** MDA in cortex (*p < 0.05 vs. C group). **b** MDA in cerebellum (*p < 0.05 vs. C group). **C** MDA in subcortical structures

rodents like a chronic stress physiological model, with an increase of corticosterone levels and metabolic perturbations that affects the function of the nervous system. In the present study, the three times increased corticosterone concentration on the exposure protocol supports the statement that RS and ELF-EMF alone, can act as a mild stress condition. These results are in accordance with previous studies, showing that plasma corticosterone levels are one of the most important indicators of stress [22, 23]. Some reports suggest that long-term ELF-EMF exposure may elevate the plasma corticosterone levels in rodents [23]. Taken together, RS + ELF-EMF may count as the addition of two stress situations, whose effects can be added. In the present study, an increase on corticosterone levels was found in RS, ELF-EMF, and RS + ELF-EMF groups, supporting the proposal that ELF-EMF exposure is like a mild stressor.

Lipids play a critical role in structure and function of the nervous system; glucocorticoids may alter lipid metabolism in brain and other tissues; as reported previously, where the administration of glucocorticoids can induce a shift in arachidonic acid metabolism in brain [24]. In the present study, we found changes on TC (increase), and POL (decrease) in the brain cortex of rats exposed to RS + ELF-EMF and ELF-EMF groups, and in subcortical structures in RS + ELF-EMF group, this finding corroborates previous reports in which movement/synthesis of cholesterol is brain are area-dependent. Segatto, found a differential activity pattern of 3-hydroxy-3-methylglutaryl coenzyme A reductase in different brain regions with the highest activity in brain cortex and the lowest activity in brainstem [25]. Cholesterol is essential for membrane structure and stability, it decreases during stress and depressive-like behaviour in rats [26], and in neuronal diseases in human beings [27, 28]. Oliveira found that free cholesterol was the most abundant of the lipids in all brain regions analyzed, showing higher levels in cerebellum [29]. Results of the present work confirm the observation of highest cholesterol levels in cerebellum, and extend the finding of resistance to mild stressor conditions at this brain area.

Increased cholesterol levels found in cortex and subcortical structures in response to ELF-EMF exposure or RS + ELF-EMF could be an adaptive response for cellular protection, as observed in cerebellum. On the contrary, reduced cholesterol levels could affect the animal behaviour [26], suggesting a decrease in brain function. The increasing CT observed in the present study suggest that brain cortex CT turnover increases in response to ELF-EMF exposure, as seen in neuroinflammation and in other pathologic conditions, according to different reports [27, 28, 30]. On the other hand, we found a decrease in POL content of the cortex in the groups exposed to ELF-EMF, and RS + ELF-EMF groups, this finding is in accordance with previous reports in which some noxious conditions as maternal deprivation, RS, and ELF-EMF stimulation have effects on phospholipids and phospholipid-dependent pathways [20, 31].

According to our results, Oliveira [29] found POL changes in cortex and cerebellum after deep chronic stress, sphingolipid and phospholipid metabolism were deeply affected, showing a decrease in: phosphatidylethanolamine, ether phosphatidylcholine, and an increase in lysophosphatidylethanolamine levels similar to Lee et al. [32].

It has been observed that stress modifies the profile of mainly POL and fatty acid in different brain regions; in our results, we found a decrease of POL in cortex and in subcortical structures of ELF-EMF and RS + ELF-EMF groups, suggesting an association of this effect to ELF-EMF stimulation.

Fatty acids are usually bound to complex lipids in the cell membrane, and many stimulus can induce the breakdown of these complex lipids, which can be converted to signalling molecules, second messengers, and other molecules involved in neuronal metabolism and survival [33]. In the present study, we found an increase of NEFAs (as breakdown index for fatty acid released from complex lipids) in subcortical structures of rats exposed to RS + ELF-EMF, but not in other brain regions studied. We suggest that this increase in NEFAs could be through phospholipase activation by ELF-EMF, as described by Piacentini et al. [34]; nevertheless, the regional effects in NEFAs composition remains unclear [31, 35].

In further analysis, we found changes in total FAMEs composition in cortex, cerebellum and subcortical structures. According to our chromatographic method, eicosatetraenoic, docosahexaenoic, docosatetranoic, octadecanoic, and eicosenoic acids were found with major abundance in the tissues analyzed. Under physiologic conditions, the balance of membrane lipid metabolism, particularly of arachidonic and docosahexaenoic acids, lead a very small and tightly controlled cellular pool of free arachidonic acid, but their levels increase very quickly upon cell activation, cerebral ischemia, seizures or other types of brain stress [30, 35, 36]. However, in the present study a decrease in the relative abundance of FAMEs was found, especially in brain cortex in RS group. This effect could be due to membrane-bound fatty acids transformation into other metabolites as suggested by Malcher-Lopes et al. [24]; similar findings were observed in the cerebellum, with a decrease in eicosatetraenoic and docosahexaenoic acids in rats exposed to ELF-EMF, but not in the RS group, this may suggest that an ELF-EMF-mediated mechanism is involved in metabolism of these lipids, this mechanism could be through phospholipase activation as suggested by some authors [30, 37, 38]. We also observed a differential effect on the subcortical structures; RS induces a decrease in eicosatetraenoic and docosahexaenoic acids, while ELF-EMF stimulation induces an increase in these lipids. These findings agree with those reported by Clejan et al. [39], who found a differential effect of ELF-EMF on phospholipases and their patterns in second messengers in hematopoietic cell lines.

The cellular effects of extremely low frequency electromagnetic fields remain unknown, but several hypothesis about the mechanism of action have been proposed; one is the lifetime extension of free radicals, and radical-mediated damages on macromolecules [8, 40]. Some authors have hypothesized that ELF-EMF can act on living organisms in a similar way to other stressors, like heat and RS, by inducing the neuroendocrine stress response [41, 42]. According to that proposal, the findings that cortex and cerebellum of experimental groups showed higher lipoperoxide levels than control group, but without differences in subcortical structures, could be explained because these areas were the closest and most exposed to ELF-EMF, so producing free radicals that induce lipid damage and increase of saturated-/unsaturated-fatty acids ratio. In a previous report we observed that acute exposure to EMF induces reduction in catalase and superoxide dismutase activities, without changes in lipoperoxidation [11]. In the present study, lipid damage could be by induction of oxidative imbalance due to chronic exposure, suggesting that chronic ELF-EMF exposure could be like a mild-stressor; this finding is supported by the increase levels in plasma corticosterone concentration and brain lipid peroxidation. Changes in lipid composition, could have deep effects on membrane function by affecting membrane-associated enzymes, receptors and ion channels [43]. In the present study, different effects of RS and ELF-EMF were found in different brain regions, we speculate that these effects may be mediated by specific mechanisms, like phospholipase [30] activation by ELF-EMF and genomic and non-genomic effects of glucocorticoids, but these observations deserve further research as has been suggested previously in clinical trials [44].

Conclusions

Changes found in the present study are in accordance with previous reports indicating the effects of chronic stress on brain lipid metabolism and suggest that the actions of extremely low frequency electromagnetic fields are similar to physiological stress. The effects found in different brain regions indicate that the extremely low frequency electromagnetic fields could be distance-dependent from the source of exposure due to findings in the analyzed brain regions. The effects in EMF versus RS were found differences on total cholesterol and polar lipids in cortex. In addition, in subcortical zone was found differences on total lipids. Although cerebellum's lipid peroxidation induced by any stressor

was similar to the found in cortex, minor changes in lipid profile were found in cerebellum and subcortical structures were more susceptible to increase NEFAs content in response to RS + ELF-EMF exposure.

Abbreviations

ANOVA: analysis of variance; C: control; CNS: central nervous system; ELF-EMF: extremely low frequency electromagnetic field; ELISA: enzyme-linked immune sorbent assay; FAMEs: fatty acid methyl esters; GC: gas chromatography; HPA: hypothalamic–pituitary–adrenal; MDA: malondialdehyde; mT: milliTesla; NEFAs: non-esterified fatty acids; POL: polar lipids; RS: restraint stress; TAG: triacylglycerols; TBARS: thiobarbituric acid reactive substances; TC: total cholesterol; TL: total lipids; UNAM: Universidad Nacional Autónoma de México.

Authors' contributions

All listed authors developed different substantial activities. JMS performed the main techniques of the experiment, and interpretation of data. AFP identified fatty acids and performed the experiments, he performed the mass spectrometry analyses and he was involved in drafting the manuscript. LVD contributed substantially to the experiment design. She participated in drafting and writing the manuscript. MAJO done statistical analysis of the results, he participated in drafting and writing the manuscript. PVTD contributed substantially on the lipid analysis and performed the experiments, drafting and writing the manuscript. Each author participated sufficiently in writing and reviewing the manuscript. All authors read and approved the final manuscript.

Author details

[1] Departamento de Bioquímica, Facultad de Medicina, Universidad Nacional Autónoma de México, Circuito Escolar s/n, Ciudad Universitaria, C.P. 04510 Mexico City, Mexico. [2] Departamento de Fisiología, Facultad de Medicina, Universidad Nacional Autónoma de México, Circuito Escolar s/n, Ciudad Universitaria, C.P. 04510 Mexico City, Mexico.

Acknowledgements

None.

Competing interests

The authors declare that they have no competing interests.

Funding

This work was supported by PAPIIT grants IN217812 to LVD and Faculty of Medicine, Universidad Nacional Autónoma de México.

References

1. Brady ST, Siegel GJ, Albers RW, Price DL, Benjamins J. Basic neurochemistry: principles of molecular, cellular, and medical neurobiology. 8th ed. Amsterdam; Boston: Elsevier/Academic Press; 2012. http://www.loc.gov/catdir/enhancements/fy1606/2012382367-d.html.
2. Adibhatla RM, Hatcher JF. Role of lipids in brain injury and diseases. Future Lipidol. 2007;2:403–22.
3. Farooqui T, Farooqui AA. Lipid-mediated oxidative stress and inflammation in the pathogenesis of Parkinson's disease. Park Dis. 2011;2011:247467.
4. Rostamkhani F, Zardooz H, Zahediasl S, Farrokhi B. Comparison of the effects of acute and chronic psychological stress on metabolic features in rats. J Zhejiang Univ Sci B. 2012;13:904–12.
5. Rabasa C, Pastor-Ciurana J, Delgado-Morales R, Gomez-Roman A, Carrasco J, Gagliano H, et al. Evidence against a critical role of CB1 receptors in adaptation of the hypothalamic-pituitary-adrenal axis and other consequences of daily repeated stress. Eur Neuropsychopharmacol. 2015;25:1248–59.

6. Wang Chao, He-ming Wu, Jing Xiao-rong, Meng Qiang, Liu Bei, Zhang Hua, et al. Oxidative parameters in the rat brain of chronic mild stress model for depression: relation to anhedonia-like response. J Membr Biol. 2012;245:675–81.

7. Feychting M, Ahlbom A, Kheifets L. EMF and health. Annu Rev Public Health. 2005;26:165–89.

8. Simko M. Cell type specific redox status is responsible for diverse electromagnetic field effects. Curr Med Chem. 2007;14:1141–52.

9. Consales C, Merla C, Marino C, Benassi B. Electromagnetic fields, oxidative stress, and neurodegeneration. Int J Cell Biol. 2012;2012:683897.

10. Torres-Duran PV, Ferreira-Hermosillo A, Juarez-Oropeza MA, Elias-Vinas D, Verdugo-Diaz L. Effects of whole body exposure to extremely low frequency electromagnetic fields (ELF-EMF) on serum and liver lipid levels, in the rat. Lipids Health Dis. 2007;6:31.

11. Martinez-Samano J, Torres-Duran PV, Juarez-Oropeza MA, Verdugo-Diaz L. Effect of acute extremely low frequency electromagnetic field exposure on the antioxidant status and lipid levels in rat brain. Arch Med Res. 2012;43:183–9.

12. Jelenkovic A, Janac B, Pesic V, Jovanovic DM, Vasiljevic I, Prolic Z. Effects of extremely low-frequency magnetic field in the brain of rats. Brain Res Bull. 2006;68:355–60.

13. Falone S, Mirabilio A, Carbone MC, Zimmitti V, Di Loreto S, Mariggio MA, et al. Chronic exposure to 50 Hz magnetic fields causes a significant weakening of antioxidant defence systems in aged rat brain. Int J Biochem Cell Biol. 2008;40:2762–70.

14. Sahin E, Gumuslu S. Stress-dependent induction of protein oxidation, lipid peroxidation and anti-oxidants in peripheral tissues of rats: comparison of three stress models (immobilization, cold and immobilization-cold). Clin Exp Pharmacol Physiol. 2007;34:425–31.

15. Vazquez-Garcia M, Elias-Vinas D, Reyes-Guerrero G, Dominguez-Gonzalez A, Verdugo-Diaz L, Guevara-Guzman R. Exposure to extremely low-frequency electromagnetic fields improves social recognition in male rats. Physiol Behav. 2004;82:685–90.

16. Heffner TG, Hartman JA, Seiden LS. A rapid method for the regional dissection of the rat brain. Pharmacol Biochem Behav. 1980;13:453–6.

17. Folch J, Lees M, Sloane Stanley GH. A simple method for the isolation and purification of total lipids from animal tissues. J Biol Chem. 1957;226:497–509.

18. Torres-Duran PV, Paredes-Carbajal MC, Mascher D, Zamora-Gonzalez J, Diaz-Zagoya JC, Juarez-Oropeza MA. Protective effect of *Arthrospira maxima* on fatty acid composition in fatty liver. Arch Med Res. 2006;37:479–83.

19. Interim guidelines on limits of exposure to 50/60 Hz electric and magnetic fields. International Non-ionizing Radiation Committee of the International Radiation Protection Association. Health Phys. 1990;58:113–22.

20. Hennebelle M, Balasse L, Latour A, Champeil-Potokar G, Denis S, Lavialle M, et al. Influence of omega-3 fatty acid status on the way rats adapt to chronic restraint stress. PLoS ONE. 2012;7:e42142.

21. Buynitsky T, Mostofsky DI. Restraint stress in biobehavioral research: recent developments. Neurosci Biobehav Rev. 2009;33:1089–98.

22. Lightman SL. The neuroendocrinology of stress: a never ending story. J Neuroendocr. 2008;20:880–4.

23. Mostafa RM, Mostafa YM, Ennaceur A. Effects of exposure to extremely low-frequency magnetic field of 2 G intensity on memory and corticosterone level in rats. Physiol Behav. 2002;76:589–95.

24. Malcher-Lopes R, Franco A, Tasker JG. Glucocorticoids shift arachidonic acid metabolism toward endocannabinoid synthesis: a non-genomic anti-inflammatory switch. Eur J Pharmacol. 2008;583:322–39.

25. Segatto M, Trapani L, Lecis C, Pallottini V. Regulation of cholesterol biosynthetic pathway in different regions of the rat central nervous system. Acta Physiol. 2012;206:62–71.

26. Sun S, Yang S, Mao Y, Jia X, Zhang Z. Reduced cholesterol is associated with the depressive-like behavior in rats through modulation of the brain 5-HT1A receptor. Lipids Health Dis. 2015;14:22.

27. Block RC, Dorsey ER, Beck CA, Brenna JT, Shoulson I. Altered cholesterol and fatty acid metabolism in Huntington disease. J Clin Lipidol. 2010;4:17–23.

28. Valenza M, Rigamonti D, Goffredo D, Zuccato C, Fenu S, Jamot L, et al. Dysfunction of the cholesterol biosynthetic pathway in Huntington's disease. J Neurosci. 2005;25:9932–9.

29. Oliveira TG, Chan RB, Bravo FV, Miranda A, Silva RR, Zhou B, et al. The impact of chronic stress on the rat brain lipidome. Mol Psychiatry. 2016;21:80–8.

30. Sun GY, Xu J, Jensen MD, Simonyi A. Phospholipase A2 in the central nervous system: implications for neurodegenerative diseases. J Lipid Res. 2004;45:205–13.

31. Mathieu G, Denis S, Lavialle M, Vancassel S. Synergistic effects of stress and omega-3 fatty acid deprivation on emotional response and brain lipid composition in adult rats. Prostaglandins Leukot Essent Fat Acids. 2008;78:391–401.

32. Lee LHW, Tan CH, Lo YL, Farooqui AA, Shui GH, Wenk MR, et al. Brain lipid changes after repetitive transcranial magnetic stimulation: potential links to therapeutic effects? Metabolomics. 2012;8:19–33.

33. Hayashi H, Karten B, Vance DE, Campenot RB, Maue RA, Vance JE. Methods for the study of lipid metabolism in neurons. Anal Biochem. 2004;331:1–16.

34. Piacentini MP, Piatti E, Fraternale D, Ricci D, Albertini MC, Accorsi A. Phospholipase C-dependent phosphoinositide breakdown induced by ELF-EMF in Peganum harmala calli. Biochimie. 2004;86:343–9.

35. Farooqui AA, Horrocks LA. Excitotoxity and neurological disorders: involvement of membrane phospholipids. Int Rev Neurobiol. 1994;36:267–323.

36. Martín Municio A, Miras-Portugal MT. Cell signal transduction, second messengers, and protein phosphorylation in health and disease. New York: Plenum Press; 1994. http://www.loc.gov/catdir/enhancements/fy100 6/94038606-t.html.

37. Dibirdik I, Bofenkamp M, Skeben P, Uckun F. Stimulation of Bruton's tyrosine kinase (BTK) and inositol 1,4,5-trisphosphate production in leukemia and lymphoma cells exposed to low energy electromagnetic fields. Leuk Lymphoma. 2000;40:149–56.

38. Kim SS, Shin HJ, Eom DW, Huh JR, Woo Y, Kim H, et al. Enhanced expression of neuronal nitric oxide synthase and phospholipase C-gamma1 in regenerating murine neuronal cells by pulsed electromagnetic field. Exp Mol Med. 2002;34:53–9.

39. Clejan S, Ide C, Walker C, Wolf E, Corb M, Beckman B. Electromagnetic field induced changes in lipid second messengers. J Lipid Mediat Cell Signal. 1996;13:301–24.

40. Patruno A, Tabrez S, Pesce M, Shakil S, Kamal MA, Reale M. Effects of extremely low frequency electromagnetic field (ELF-EMF) on catalase, cytochrome P450 and nitric oxide synthase in erythro-leukemic cells. Life Sci. 2015;121:117–23.

41. Sandyk R, Tsagas N, Anninos PA, Derpapas K. Magnetic fields mimic the behavioral effects of REM sleep deprivation in humans. Int J Neurosci. 1992;65:61–8.

42. Szemerszky R, Zelena D, Barna I, Bardos G. Stress-related endocrinological and psychopathological effects of short- and long-term 50 Hz electromagnetic field exposure in rats. Brain Res Bull. 2010;81:92–9.

43. Hong I, Garrett A, Maker G, Mullaney I, Rodger J, Etherington SJ. Repetitive low intensity magnetic field stimulation in a neuronal cell line: a metabolomics study. PeerJ. 2018;6:e4501.

44. Martinez D, Urban N, Grassetti A, Chang D, Hu MC, Zangen A, et al. Transcranial magnetic stimulation of medial prefrontal and cingulate cortices reduces cocaine self-administration: a pilot study. Front Psychiatry. 2018;9:80.

4

Neural correlates of free recall of "famous events" in a "hypermnestic" individual as compared to an age- and education-matched reference group

Thorsten Fehr[1,2,3]* , Angelica Staniloiu[4,6], Hans J. Markowitsch[4,6], Peter Erhard[1,3,5] and Manfred Herrmann[1,2,3]

Abstract

Background: Memory performance of an individual (within the age range: 50–55 years old) showing superior memory abilities (protagonist PR) was compared to an age- and education-matched reference group in a historical facts ("famous events") retrieval task.

Results: Contrasting task versus baseline performance both PR and the reference group showed fMRI activation patterns in parietal and occipital brain regions. The reference group additionally demonstrated activation patterns in cingulate gyrus, whereas PR showed additional widespread activation patterns comprising frontal and cerebellar brain regions. The direct comparison between PR and the reference group revealed larger fMRI contrasts for PR in right frontal, superior temporal and cerebellar brain regions.

Conclusions: It was concluded that PR generally recruits brain regions as normal memory performers do, but in a more elaborate way, and furthermore, that he applied a memory-strategy that potentially includes executively driven multi-modal transcoding of information and recruitment of implicit memory resources.

Keywords: Memory, fMRI, Superior memory, Memory strategy, Experts, Complex cognition

Background

Aside from the time-based distinction into short-term/working and long-term memory [1], memory is nowadays partitioned into content-based systems [2, 3]. Long term memory (LTM) has been discussed to be distinguished into episodic-autobiographical memory (memory for personal events or experiences), semantic memory (conscious knowledge of facts, including factual self-knowledge), perceptual memory (conscious familiarity judgments), procedural memory (mechanical, motor-related skills) and priming (higher likelihood of re-identifying previously perceived stimuli) [4–6]. Superior LTM performance has been described to tap into different memory systems. There are reports of individuals with highly superior autobiographical memory [7, 8], of semantic memory experts [9–11], and descriptions of specific types of hypermnesia [12, 13].

In general, LTM performance might be facilitated by the application of optimal learning strategies [14, 15] and/or the existence of elaborated, domain-specific expert knowledge networks [16], to which new information can be both efficiently associated to and recalled from. Parker et al. [7] proposed a specific form of superior memory performance, the hyperthymestic syndrome (HS), which is characterized by superior memory that is assumed to be automatically organized, and not based on explicit mnemonic strategies. It addresses idiosyncratic memory domains; these particular individuals do not necessarily score higher than average on standard memory tests tapping on information that is irrelevant for them. In a similar way, Norman Brown [17] put forth a model of "historical memory" elaboration that assumes

*Correspondence: fehr@uni-bremen.de
[2] University of Bremen, Hochschulring 18, 28359 Bremen, Germany
Full list of author information is available at the end of the article

an association of historical facts of public interest to individually relevant episodic information, which might be related to both the template theory proposed by Gobet and Clarkson [16] and, in case of superior performance, to the HS advanced by Parker et al. [7].

The neural mechanisms for memory encoding and retrieval are still under debate, and especially for superior memory performance, they are still largely unknown. In particular, since the prominent patient H.M. showed selective impairment in consciously encoding and consolidating new facts and events long-term [18–20], these processes were assumed to be mediated by the hippocampus and its adjacent medial temporal brain regions [21–23]. However, other regions of the limbic system situated in medial diencephalon and basal forebrain, equally contribute to these processes [5]. There are also theories suggesting that LTM networks can be associated with highly integrated networks distributed all over the neural system [24–26] and that the hippocampal formation is involved in both conscious and unconscious information processing [27, 28].

Functional neuroimaging and clinical studies involving patients with different forms of amnesia as a result of regional brain damage, however, support the idea that different memory systems might recruit at least partially "distinct" brain networks [5, 20, 29]. Aside from limbic structures involved in processes of binding and associating information to LTM, further cortical structures—sometimes referred to as expanded or greater limbic system [30, 31]—such as the retrosplenial cortex and the precuneus were related to processes of imagination, of the representation of memories, and to familiarity [32–34]. These structures might play an important role in both normal, but in particular, in superior LTM performance.

In the present study, we carried out a comprehensive neuropsychological assessment and additionally conducted a functional magnetic resonance imaging (fMRI) study that focussed on a memory retrieval task in an individual (PR) with superior historical facts knowledge ("famous events memory"). The present experimental design was specifically designed to examine the neural correlates of recalling memories related to historical facts. FMRI-contrast included the conditions 'recall of declarative memory content WITH reference to historical facts' and 'recall of declarative memory content WITHOUT reference to historical facts'. It was assumed that PR should show less pronounced activation patterns in frontal (i.e., executive memory organization), but enhanced neural involvement of limbic brain regions (automatic and/or pre-attentive memory organisation) and precuneus (perceptual, imaginative, confidence judgments and/or familiarity based memory strategies) in

comparison to an age- and education-matched reference group.

Results
Behavioural data
Before applying parametric t-statistics, a Shapiro–Wilk-test (S–W-T) was performed in order to test, whether variables of interest were normal-distributed. In the reference group, the percentage of freely recalled correct answers (consistently shown for both scanner session and post hoc debriefing) was significantly higher in the BASE (test on normal distribution: S–W-T, $W = .93$, $p = .45$) compared to the TASK (test on normal distribution: S–W-T, $W = .88$, $p = .13$)-condition (TASK: $41.7 \pm 8.3\%$; BASE: $89.6 \pm 7.2\%$; t Test: $t = 15.2$, $p < .001$; see Fig. 1a), and reference group members performed better than chance level in both TASK- and BASE-conditions (TASK vs. 25%: $t = -1.9$, $p < .05$; BASE vs. 25%: $t = -8.6$, $p < .001$ [35, 36]). Compared to the reference group, PR showed a higher correct percentage rate in the TASK-condition ($t = 4.1$, $p < .01$ [35, 36]; see Fig. 1a) and comparable performance in the BASE-condition. All participants showed high performance in the BASE task. As, however, performance-values were normal-distributed (see above) and PR's performance ranged in the middle of the reference-group performances, we rather tend to disclose a ceiling effect. Participants in the reference group showed longer response times for correctly answered TASK-trials (test on normal distribution: S–W-T, $W = .87$, $p = .09$) compared to BASE-trials (test on normal distribution: S–W-T, $W = .90$, $p = .24$) during free recall (TASK: 3728 ± 733 ms; BASE: 3056 ± 429 ms; $t = 4.4$, $p < .01$; see Fig. 1b). According to Crawford and Howell [35], PR (TASK: 3599 ms; BASE: 3664 ms) did not differ in any response time value from the reference group.

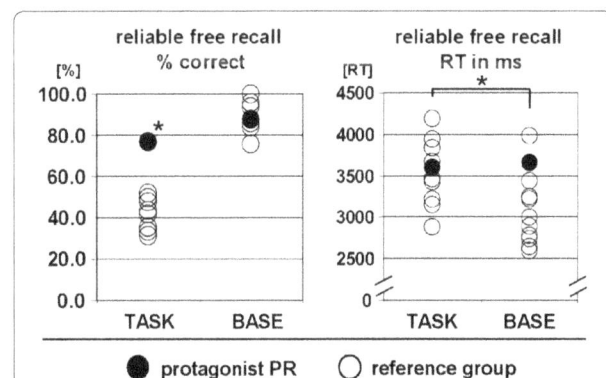

Fig. 1 Memory performance in percentage of correct freely recalled answers (left panel) and the respective mean response times (right panel); asterisks indicate significant differences ($p < .05$; details, see text) and whiskers indicate standard deviations

FMRI-data: TASK versus BASE-condition in PR and in reference participants

For the reference group, second level fMRI-analysis for TASK in contrast to BASE-condition revealed activation clusters in the right anterior and left posterior cingulate, bilateral precuneus, cuneus, and lingual gyrus (Fig. 2a; Table 1, column A). Protagonist PR showed activation clusters in widespread bilateral superior, medial, and middle frontal gyri, right postcentral gyrus, left precuneus, right middle and left inferior occipital gyri, left fusiform gyrus, and left cerebellar regions for the contrast TASK versus BASE-condition (Fig. 2b; Table 1, column B).

All PSC-value-distributions were tested for deviations from normal distribution via Shapiro–Wilk-Test: rPCG:

$W = .92$, $p = .33$; rSFG: $W = .86$, $p = .05$; lMFG: $W = .98$, $p = .96$; first cluster rMFG: $W = .94$, $p = .48$; second cluster rMFG: $.93$, $p = .42$; rSTG: $W = .94$, $p = .47$; rCUL: $W = .92$, $p = .29$. The direct comparison between PR and reference group yielded larger contrasts between TASK- and BASE-conditions distributed over precentral gyrus, right superior and bilateral middle frontal gyri, right superior temporal gyrus, and the left culmen (Fig. 2c; Table 1, column C). Reference group versus PR showed larger contrasts in left paracentral lobule, right precuneus, and left cuneus (Fig. 2d; Table 1, column D).

In Fig. 3, distributions of difference-values between PSC-values for TASK and BASE-conditions for several ROIs were illustrated for the reference group and

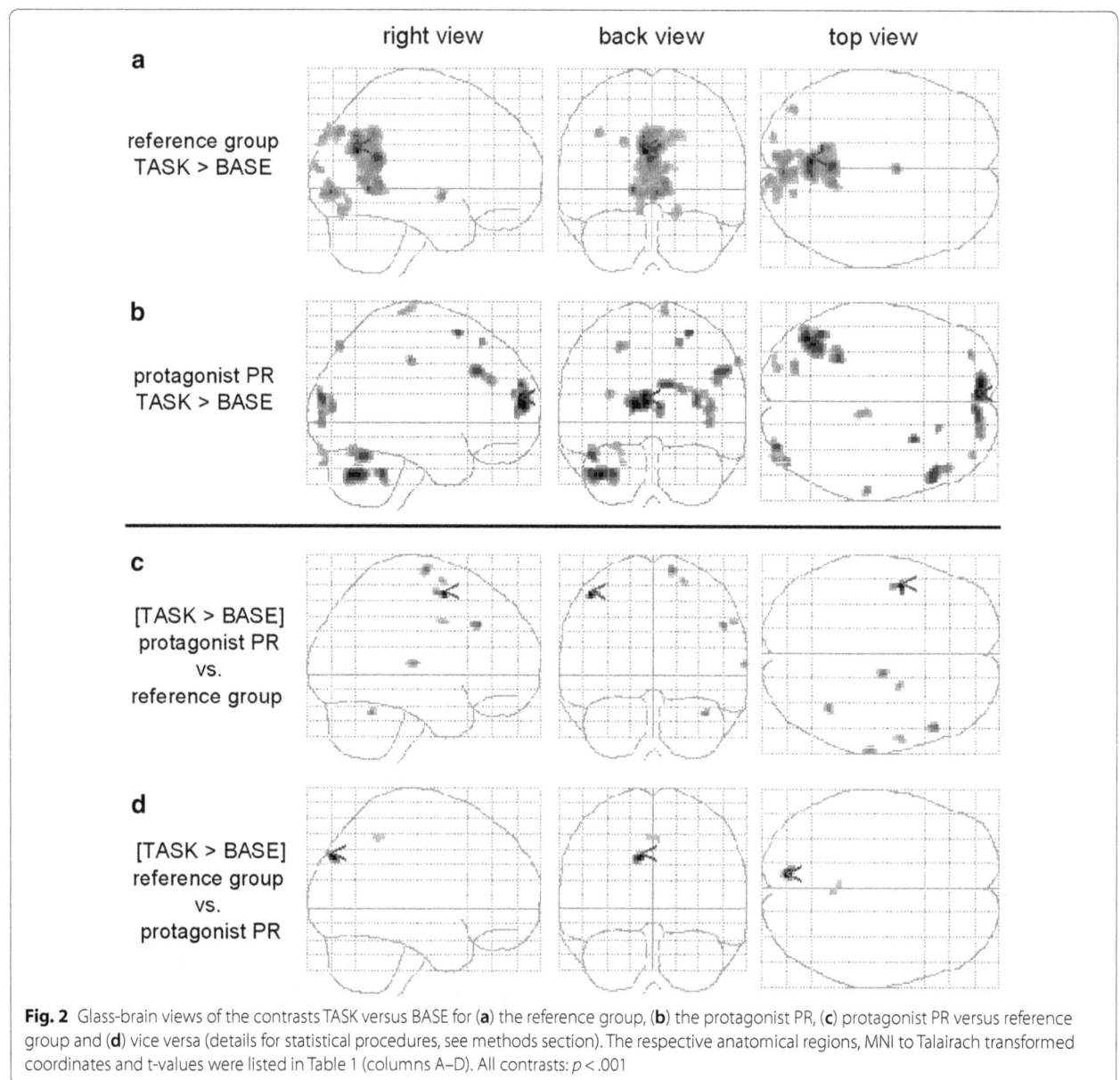

Fig. 2 Glass-brain views of the contrasts TASK versus BASE for (**a**) the reference group, (**b**) the protagonist PR, (**c**) protagonist PR versus reference group and (**d**) vice versa (details for statistical procedures, see methods section). The respective anatomical regions, MNI to Talairach transformed coordinates and t-values were listed in Table 1 (columns A–D). All contrasts: $p < .001$

Table 1 Anatomical regions, peak activation t-values, and Talairach-coordinates for contrasts between TASK- and BASE-conditions (arranged in columns A–D) separately for (column A) the reference group (RG, one-sample t-test), (column B) the protagonist (PR, first level contrast), (column C) PR versus RG, and (column D) RG versus PR (latter two comparisons according to Crawford and Garthwaite [42, 43]

Anatomical region	H	A Ref. group TASK>BASE				B Protagonist TASK>BASE				C TASK>BASE PR>RG				D TASK>BASE RG>PR			
		t	x	y	z	t	x	y	z	t	x	y	z	t	x	y	z
Peak activations: TASK versus BASE conditions																	
Precentral Gyrus	R									5.7	57	2	33				
Superior Frontal Gyrus	L					4.3	−12	59	8	7.4	14	−8	67				
	L					3.6	−32	51	16								
	R					4.2	10	57	21								
	R					3.8	22	59	17								
	R					3.7	20	30	48								
	R					3.4	38	53	16								
Medial Frontal Gyrus	L					4.4	−4	57	12								
	R					3.9	6	55	6								
	R					3.5	8	−22	70								
Middle Frontal Gyrus	L					4.2	50	27	30	9.9	−46	5	51				
	R					3.7	46	36	24	7.1	50	27	30				
	R					4.0	26	14	55	5.9	22	3	59				
Paracentral Lobule	L													4.7	−4	−40	48
Anterior Cingulate	R	8.2	2	−2	−5												
Posterior Cingulate	L	10.3	−2	−47	23												
Postcentral Gyrus	R					3.6	61	−21	40								
Precuneus	L	12.1	−6	−61	29	3.6	−24	−71	51					5.1	4	−46	47
	L	6.3	−40	−74	41												
	L	5.3	−6	−80	41												
	R	7.0	4	−72	40												
	R	4.6	2	−81	41												
Middle Occipital Gyrus	R					4.0	32	−85	19								
	R					3.7	42	−79	13								
	R					3.7	42	−87	6								

Table 1 (continued)

Anatomical region	H	A Ref. group TASK>BASE				B Protagonist TASK>BASE				C TASK>BASE PR>RG				D TASK>BASE RG>PR			
		t	x	y	z	t	x	y	z	t	x	y	z	t	x	y	z
Inferior Occipital Gyrus	L					3.3	−24	−88	−12								
Cuneus	L	6.3	−20	−88	36									11.0	−8	−78	37
	R	6.2	10	−90	17												
	R	6.1	16	−84	37												
Lingual Gyrus	L	9.6	−14	−54	3												
	L	7.2	−8	−85	1												
	L	6.9	−6	−78	1												
	R	8.3	4	−81	2												
	R	6.0	18	−76	−8												
Fusiform Gyrus	L					4.0	−44	−57	−17								
Superior Temporal Gyrus	R									6.1	65	−21	8				
Cerebellum/ Tuber	L					4.2	−38	−62	−27								
Cerebellum/ Culmen	L					3.9	−30	−44	−28	6.3	38	−51	−19				
Cerebellum/ Declive	L					3.4	−22	−86	−19								

H = hemisphere: L = left, R = right, all statistics *p* < .001, uncorrected, minimum voxel cluster size k = 10 voxels

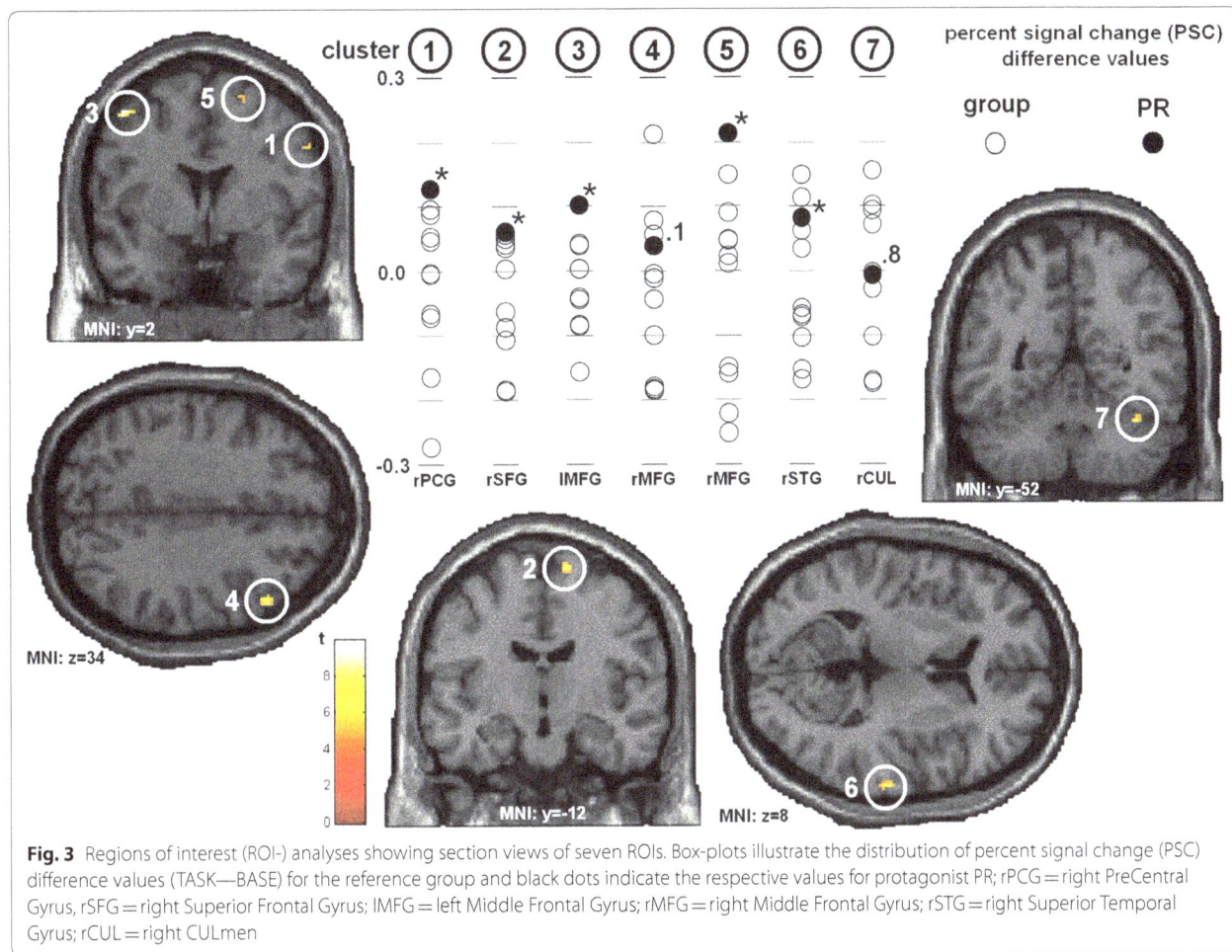

Fig. 3 Regions of interest (ROI-) analyses showing section views of seven ROIs. Box-plots illustrate the distribution of percent signal change (PSC) difference values (TASK—BASE) for the reference group and black dots indicate the respective values for protagonist PR; rPCG = right PreCentral Gyrus, rSFG = right Superior Frontal Gyrus; lMFG = left Middle Frontal Gyrus; rMFG = right Middle Frontal Gyrus; rSTG = right Superior Temporal Gyrus; rCUL = right CULmen

separately for PR. T-Test for single means yielded to individual versus group differences in right precentral gyrus, right superior frontal gyrus, left and right middle frontal gyri, and right superior temporal gyrus.

Discussion

In the present study, functional neuroimaging was used to compare a protagonist's (PR) superior memory performance in a famous events free retrieval task (contrasted with a semantic non-historical facts free retrieval task serving as baseline) with the performance of a reference group. PR performed significantly better than the reference group and showed activation patterns predominantly distributed over frontal and cerebellar, but also in parietal, occipital and occipito-temporal brain regions. The reference group demonstrated activation patterns in the cingulate cortex, parietal, and occipital brain regions. The direct comparison between PR and the reference group confirmed larger contrasts for frontal and cerebellar regions in PR and for parietal and occipital brain areas in the reference group. It appears that PR predominantly

recruited right hemispheric frontal resources potentially related to his superior memory retrieval performance [44, 45].

Which type of expert is PR?

First, PR showed superior memory performance for famous events retrieval, and he scored predominantly at average or above average in most retrograde and anterograde memory tests in the neuropsychological assessment. Only for complex anterograde non-verbal memory processing he scored below average. Incidentally, the case described by Parker et al. [7] also showed impairments in anterograde non-verbal memory tasks. Thus, while PR shares certain similitudes with HS (hyperthymestic syndrome [7]), he presents with unique features, which deviate from the HS prototype. He showed, beside superior historical facts memory, deviations from standards in non-idiosyncratically eminent memory domains. The mnemonic performance of PR can be at least partly understood within the model of Markowitsch and Tulving. Incidentally, Tulving [46] indirectly anticipated later models of mnemonic processing, which describe porous boundaries between memory systems [47]. In 1995, Tulving [46] proposed his SPI-model which states that encoding of information follows a regular sequence—that means it is serial in that way that first simple, implicitly functioning, memory systems are engaged and only at the end of the series explicit, episodic encoding occurs. Information then is stored in parallel memory systems in the brain and it can be retrieved independently from the systems used for the encoding process (SPI = Serial, Parallel, Independent). As PR describes his knowledge as "popping out automatically", it can be speculated that according to Tulving's [46] SPI-model, PR retrieves his knowledge "automatically", and therefore more independently from his initial encoding of it, than it likely is the case in most human beings.

In addition, PR showed sub-average performance on tests for executive functions. While this type of performance may be interpreted as a hint towards a savant-syndrome [48], there was no clear clinical, neuropsychological or anamnestic evidence in his case that he fell into this category. He showed a superior intelligence level comparable to the reference group as confirmed by a verbal intelligence test. Furthermore, he scored above average on standardized laboratory tests for assessing social cognition and emotional processing, although he reported some interpersonal difficulties in real-life, which were being addressed in psychotherapy. Incidentally, the case described by Parker et al. [7] also presented with some difficulties in the executive functioning domain. Furthermore, LePort et al. [8] found in a case series of patients with highly superior autobiographical memory abilities a psychological profile indicative of obsessive compulsive tendencies. These tendencies typically are accompanied by a reduction in cognitive flexibility, which gets translated in impaired performance on corresponding neuropsychological tasks. The deficient performance of PR on tasks tapping on cognitive flexibility and the anamnestic reports about PR may speak in favour of obsessive compulsive personality phenotypic traits. These traits may promote an automatic engagement in repetition of mnemonic material of special interest, with consequences for processes of encoding and consolidation. Conclusively, PR cannot be seen comparable to individuals with HS or to savants in the classical sense. It rather appears that he is an expert sharing some features of HS and savant people, but does not fully overlap with any of these prototypes, displaying unique features. In the following, characteristics in fMRI activation patterns are discussed to conclude about the individual mnemonic strategy that PR might have applied to score higher in free historical facts retrieval than the reference group.

Can the present functional neuroimaging data explain PR´s profile of superior memory performance?

The hypothesis that PR should show rather posterior and/or subcortical instead of frontal activation patterns when compared to the reference group, had to be rejected. The opposite was the case: PR showed predominantly right frontal patterns of larger contrasts between free historical and non-historical semantic facts retrieval. At first glance, this finding appears quite disillusioning in view of the hypotheses postulated in the introduction section, however, combined with the data that PR also showed remarkable cerebellar recruitment, a hybrid mental strategy of memory processing including both explicit and implicit components might be conceivable [10, 48]. And, this argument also goes with the hybrid classification (between savant and expert) concluded from the neuropsychological testing data as mentioned in the previous section.

Level of processing and multi-modal integration of memory

There were also exclusive activation patterns in PR not present in the reference group and vice versa, which could in part only be interpreted in an individual (PR) or group-internal (reference-group) way as the direct comparison between PR and the reference group did not reach statistical significance in the respective brain regions. In posterior brain regions, associated with perceptual information processing, PR showed activation patterns rather adjacent to primary (i.e., middle and inferior occipital gyrus, and postcentral gyrus) and less in hetero-modal, medial (i.e., cuneus and lingual gyrus) cortical brain regions as the reference group did. Rather medial activation patterns in the reference group might be related to a higher level complex or abstract memory processing [25]. This finding might also explain why PR scored above average in simple, but below average in complex recognition tasks that usually require a deeper associative memory strategy.

Transcoding and integration of information across processing modalities (i.e., implicit and explicit processing, and verbal, visual, and spatial modalities, etc.), as can be seen for example in synesthesia [49–51] was discussed as a potential feature of both superior expert and savant memory performance involving occipito-temporal regions such as the fusiform gyrus [9, 10]. The present data showed exclusive fusiform gyrus involvement in PR, but not in the reference group. It should however be mentioned that the direct comparison between groups via between-group t-test did not reveal differences in this region. Nevertheless, in combination with an exclusive cerebellar recruitment in PR, this data might point to an implicit-explicit (and vice versa) memory transcoding strategy facilitating superior memory performance in historical facts retrieval, but also in other simple memory processing domains as shown by the neuropsychological assessment.

The stronger involvement of superior temporal gyrus (STG) in PR additionally supports the idea of pronounced multi-modal integration of information in LTM potentially facilitating his retrieval performance. The multi-associative nature of STG has been documented by studies discussing the role of the STG in retrieving both autobiographical events [52–54] and semantic facts, such as public events or "long-established knowledge about the world" [52, 55, 56].

Furthermore, the right superior temporal cortex was thought to be engaged in spatial awareness and exploration [57]. Along this line of argumentation, the stronger recruitment of STG in PR may signify a strategy to navigate through personal past by making use of more elaborated spatial exploration strategies [53]. Recently, Manning and colleagues argued that public semantic memory is supported by both the semantic and episodic memory system [58]. The stronger involvement of the STG in PR in contrast to the reference group might again point to a particular engagement of the episodic memory system in public semantic knowledge processing in the case of PR and other individuals with highly superior autobiographical talents [8, 59–61].

Limitations of the present study

In future studies the number of tasks in the different task-condition should be perfectly matched.

For the present reference group there were 15–25 correct response trials in the TASK-condition left to be modeled for the respective fMRI-statistics. Despite normal distribution and despite numerous studies also reporting reliable data based on a quite low number of trials and/or individuals, this point should be carefully considered for an appropriate interpretation of the here presented data. In future studies additional measurement sessions should be taken into account to extend the number of valid trials. In the present study, we were however forced to balance the available time (PR was only available for a short time period) and test-statistical requirements.

Conclusions

Specific complex mental processes cannot be inferred directly from functional brain imaging data [62], however, there is evidence that regional brain activation can help to understand the underlying mental principles involved in a certain complex mental process such as the applied visual, verbal or spatial modality, or perceptual and/or executive processing types, and others more [63–65]. It appears that the utilization of individual mental strategies also plays an

important role in effective memory processing [61, 66–69]. And, these individual memory strategies can be modulated by executive mental processing as potentially reflected in the pronounced recruitment of frontal brain regions in PR. Furthermore, the present data support the idea that superior mental processing in experts can be facilitated by the conceptually driven recruitment of implicit/procedural memory resources (i.e., potentially reflected by the involvement of cerebellar brain areas [10]). A more detailed assessment of mental strategies in individuals with superior mental performance can provide insights into effective implicit memory usage potentially driven by explicit executive mental processing. Functional neuroimaging can help to evaluate the recruitment of implicit mental resources that are difficult to be assessed by explicit surveys.

Methods

Study participants

The individual protagonist PR (within the age range: 50–55 years old) was a healthy, right handed expert with superior memory abilities.

Applying a test-battery several months before the fMRI-measurement session provided a detailed neuropsychological performance-profile of PR (see Table 2 for details).

The reference group consisted of 10 male adults between 47 and 62 years (54.6 ± 4.3 years.; not differing in age from PR: $t = -.8$, $p = .445$; [35, 36]. All participants were right handed according to a modified version of the Edinburgh Handedness Questionnaire [37], and did not report psychiatric or neurological illness or psychotropic drug treatment. All participants were native German speakers holding a university degree. The participants were familiarized with the assessment environment and their participation was solely motivated by their interest in scientific investigations.

After the fMRI-session, verbal intelligence was examined in all participants with the MWT-B (Mehrfach–Wahl–Wortschatz-Test [38]), for which PR reached 130, and members of the reference group reached 126.0 ± 13.6 (test on normal distribution with Shapiro-Wilk-test: $W = .89$, $p = .18$). Here, PR did not differ from the group ($t = -.28$, $p = .79$ [35, 36]).

The study protocol was designed and performed according to the Helsinki Declaration (1964) and was approved by the Ethics Committee of Bremen University. All participants were informed about the procedure, and gave written consent to participate in the experiment.

Task and stimuli

The tasks were presented visually. The experimental set-up includes two task conditions, a baseline (BASE) and

Table 2 **Protagonist PR was examined with a battery of different test inventories**

Mental domains and tests	Score	Interpretation
Attention, concentration		
Trail making test A + B	A: 42 s, 1 error; B: 174 s, 0 errors	Below average
d2-R test	122 correct, 12 errors	Average
WMS-R, attention and concentration index	96	Average
Intelligence		
Mehrfach–Wahl–Wortschatz-test B	34 of 37 (IQ 130)	Above average
Wechsler intelligence test raw scores	24, 23, 15, 34 (IQ > 125)	
Visuo-constructive abilities		
Rey–Osterrieth figure (ROF), copy	36	Normal
Interference		
Color-word-interference test (CWIT)	12, 22, 37 s	Above average
Anterograde memory		
ROF, by heart after ½ h	21	Average
WMS-R, general memory	94	Average
Verbal learning memory test (VLMT)	63 learning, 7 interference; 15 + 15 in Trials 6 + 7, 50/0 in recognition	Above average
Doors test	simple recognition: A = 12; complex recognition: B = 5	Above average Below average
Retrograde memory		
Semantic: Famous Faces Test (38 pictures)	30 directly identified, 2 with cues	Above average
Episodic-autobiographical old memory (EAMT)	Gives per epoch well-described examples	Very good
Semantic old famous events (1970s–1990s)	22 named, 1 recognized, 2 unknown	Very good
Emotion		
Mind in the Eyes Test	19/24 correct	Above average
Florida Affect Battery	Facial Identity Discrimination: 20 of 20 Facial Affect Discrimination: 20 of 20	Above average Above average
Problem solving ability, cognitive flexibility, executive functions, risk taking behavior		
Cronin–Golomb concept formation task	15–16 of 17	Good average
Category test	4, 5, 5 categories	Below average
Tower of Hanoi (4 discs)	49 moves, 5 min, 21 s	Below average
Word fluency (COWAT Test)	17 + 10 + 14	Average
Wisconsin card sorting test (WCST)	20 correct, 12 errors 16 perseveration errors	Below average
Game of dice test (with 12 moves)	+800 € at finish	Thoughtful strategy
Tendencies for malingering		
Rey 15-Item Test	All correct	Inconspicuous
Test of memory malingering (TOMM)	Fist trial: 48 of 50	Inconspicuous
Test battery for forensic neuropsychology (TBFN)	13 correct, 2 false	Inconspicuous
Amsterdam short term memory test	Two errors in the first 15 trials	Inconspicuous

See details and references to the test battery listed in the Additional file 1: Supplementary online document S1

a task of interest (TASK). Both task conditions included questions in order to test semantic memory performance. BASE-condition tested semantic memory about common knowledge such as for example "How is the head of the Catholic church called?", and the TASK-condition tested semantic memory about public historical facts from contemporary history, for example "Which city hosted the Olympic Summer Games in 1996?".

The respective questions were presented via a digital projector on a mirror in the scanner tube in the center of the display as a centered text-block (see Fig. 4 for illustration). There was no time limit to think about the correct answer. Responses consisted of pressing the answer button with the right index finger. Individuals, however, were encouraged not to ruminate too long about the answer and they were asked to press a button

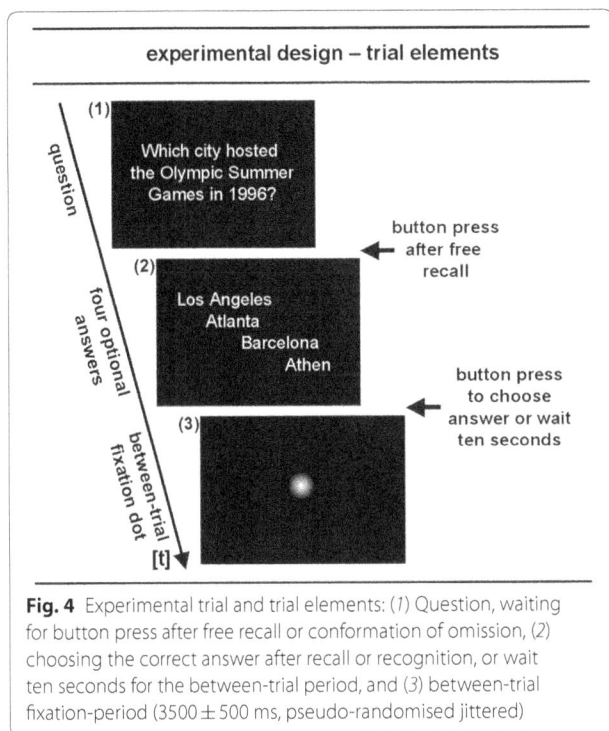

Fig. 4 Experimental trial and trial elements: (1) Question, waiting for button press after free recall or conformation of omission, (2) choosing the correct answer after recall or recognition, or wait ten seconds for the between-trial period, and (3) between-trial fixation-period (3500 ± 500 ms, pseudo-randomised jittered)

with the right index finger, if they either believed to know the correct answer or when they were sure not to know the answer. This procedure was applied to ensure that participants produced free recall and not recognition performance. After pressing the button, four alternative answers (one correct solution) were presented slightly shifted one below the other in the center of the display (see Fig. 4 for illustration). If participants freely recalled the correct answer, they were asked to choose it from the four alternatives. If however, they did not recall the correct answer, but recognized it among the four alternatives, they were allowed to choose the correct one. If they neither recalled nor recognized the correct answer, participants were asked to wait (ten seconds) for the next trial. Between trials a fixation dot was presented for a pseudo-randomly jittered interval ranging between 3000 and 4000 ms.

After the MRI-scanner session, all questions were again presented by a paper–pencil-test. The participants were asked again to answer correctly to all BASE- and TASK-questions and to further provide detailed information about whether they freely recalled, recognized or did not know the correct answers during the fMRI-measurement. BASE- and TASK-trials were only included in behavioural and fMRI-data-analyses, if they were consistently answered correctly during both the fMRI-measurement and the paper–pencil-test, and furthermore, if they were labeled to be freely recalled and not just recognized.

All other trials were neglected in behavioural data analyses and modeled as dummy-trials in the fMRI-analyses (see below).

50 BASE- and 48 TASK-trials were presented in a pseudo-randomized non-stationary probabilistic weighted sequence [39] during one experimental run of 17 ± 2 min.

FMRI data acquisition and analyses
FMRI-data acquisition
Functional magnetic resonance imaging (fMRI) data were collected on a SIEMENS MAGNETOM scanner (Skyra syngo MR D13, 3 Tesla). The images were acquired using a BOLD weighted gradient echo echoplanar imaging (EPI) sequence (TE 30 ms). Forty four slices were acquired in interleaved order with no gap in axial orientation parallel to AC-PC with a GRAPPA accelleration factor of two leading to a TR of 2500 ms. The image volume covered the entire cerebrum and cerebellum. The in plane resolution was 3×3 mm^2, the corresponding matrix 64×64, 411 ± 44 volumes were obtained during the functional run. Structural whole head T1 weighted images were acquired (TR/TE/TI/flip angle = 2400 m s/2.43 ms/900 ms/8°; matrix 256×256; slice thickness 1.0 mm; FOV 256 mm; 176 slices) for all participants.

FMRI-data analysis
Image analysis was performed using additional algorithms for the comparison of single individuals with group-related data (see below), which were implemented in SPM (http://www.fil.ion.ucl.ac.uk/spm/). For each session and participant, images were realigned to the first image in the time series to correct for head motion. The realigned images were spatially normalized into a standard stereotaxic space (Montreal Neurological Institute template) using a 12 parameter affine model. Dimensions after normalising procedures were $79(x) \times 95(y) \times 69(z)$ and resulting voxel size was 2 mm^3. These spatially normalized images were smoothed to minimize noise and residual differences in gyral anatomy with a Gaussian filter set at 8.0 mm. Prior to the statistical analysis, a temporal high pass filter (250 s) was applied and global effects were removed. Pre-processed data sets were analysed using second-level random effects models [40] on the individual parameter estimates.

FMRI data were modelled for different trial element phases (see Fig. 4 for illustration): (1) from the start of task presentation until the first button press (separately for correct, incorrect, and omitted trials), (2) from the display of the four response alternatives to the second button press or until the trial time runs out (separately for correct, incorrect, and omitted trials), and (3) the fixation dot period between task trials resulting in 13 regressors in the design matrices. At the single-individual level, a t-contrast at each voxel for each participant was computed to produce statistical images for the contrast TASK- versus BASE-condition for the free recall trial element. At the second level, the resulting contrast images were used to identify the main task effect TASK versus BASE-condition by means of a one sample t-test ($p < .001$, uncorrected). For PR, TASK versus BASE-conditions were contrasted using t-statistics ($p < .001$, uncorrected). Percent signal change values for several regions of interest (ROIs) were extracted applying the software package Marsbar (Version 4.2 [41]). ROIs were extracted according to activation clusters resulting from the contrast "PR vs. reference group" related to "TASK vs. BASE"-condition contrasts. This was done to comprehensibly illustrate core aspects of the present data.

In order to inferentially compare brain activation patterns between PR and the reference group, we decided to follow the methods suggested by Crawford and colleagues [35, 42, 43]. The respective algorithms were implemented as an SPM compliant function that reads the specified individual contrast images and their respective design matrices (SPM.mat files). The appropriate beta images are then loaded as scores for the respective tasks and the calculus is performed. The resulting images were written to disk as spmT image files for use in the result function of SPM ($p < .001$, uncorrected) (see Fehr et al. [10] for further methodological details).

Abbreviations

FMRI: functional magnetic resonance imaging; HS: hyperthymestic syndrome; LTM: long term memory; PR: protagonist; SPM: statistical parametric mapping; S–W-T: Shapiro–Wilk-test.

Authors' contributions

TF contributed to the experimental design, data acquisition, data analyses and manuscript writing. AS contributed to the neuropsychological testing of PR and manuscript writing. HJM contributed to the experimental design and manuscript writing. PE contributed to fMRI-data acquisition and manuscript writing. MH contributed to the experimental design and manuscript writing. All authors read and approved the final manuscript.

Author details

[1] Center for Cognitive Sciences, University of Bremen, Bremen, Germany. [2] University of Bremen, Hochschulring 18, 28359 Bremen, Germany. [3] Center for Advanced Imaging, Universities of Bremen and Magdeburg, Bremen, Germany. [4] Physiological Psychology, University of Bielefeld, Bielefeld, Germany. [5] AG in vivo MR, University of Bremen, Bremen, Germany. [6] Hanse Institute for Advanced Study (HWK), Delmenhorst, Germany.

Acknowledgements

Not applicable.

Competing interests

The authors declare that they have no competing interests.

Funding

Not applicable.

References

1. Baddeley A. Working memory: theories, models, and controversies. Annu Rev Psychol. 2012;63:1–29.
2. Tulving E. Episodic memory: from mind to brain. Annu Rev Psychol. 2002;53:1–25.
3. Tulving E. Episodic memory and autonoesis: uniquely human? In: Terrace HS, Metcalfe J, editors. The missing link in cognition: Self-knowing consciousness in man and animals. New York: Oxford University Press; 2005. p. 3–56.
4. Markowitsch HJ. Psychogenic amnesia. Neuroimage. 2003;20:132–8.
5. Markowitsch HJ, Staniloiu A. Amnestic disorders. Lancet. 2012;380:1429–40. https://doi.org/10.1016/s0140-6736(11)61304-4.
6. Staniloiu A, Markowitsch HJ. Dissociative amnesia. Lancet Psychiatry. 2014;1:226–41.
7. Parker ES, Cahill L, McGaugh JL. A case of unusual autobiographical remembering. Neurocase. 2006;12:35–49.
8. LePort AKR, Mattfeld AT, Dickinson-Anson H, Fallon JH, Craig EL, Stark CEL, Kruggel F, Cahill L, McGaugh JL. Behavioral and neuroanatomical investigation of Highly Superior Autobiographical Memory (HSAM). Neurobiol Learn Mem. 2012;98:78–92.
9. Amidzic O, Riehle HJ, Fehr T, Elbert T. Focal gamma band activity: the signature of chunks in the expert memory of chess players. Nature. 2001;412:603.
10. Fehr T, Weber J, Willmes K, Herrmann M. Neural correlates in exceptional mental arithmetic—About the neural architecture of prodigious skills. Neuropsychologia. 2010;48:1407–16.
11. Fehr T, Wallace G, Erhard P, Herrmann M. The functional neuroanatomy of expert calendar calculation: a matter of strategy? Neurocase. 2011;17:360–71.
12. Erdelyi MH, Becker J. Hypermnesia for pictures: incremental memory for pictures but not for words in multiple recall trials. Cogn Psychol. 1974;6:159–71.
13. Bluck S, Levine LJ, Laulhere TM. Autobiographical remembering and hypermnesia: a comparison of older and younger adults. Psychol Aging. 1999;14:671–82.
14. Bor D, Duncan J, Wisemann RJ, Owen AM. Encoding strategies dissociate prefrontal activity from working memory demand. Neuron. 2003;37:361–7.
15. Kuo MCC, Liu KPY, Chan CCH. Factors involved in memory encoding and their implications for the memory performance of older adults and people with mild cognitive impairment. World J Neurosci. 2012;2:103–12.
16. Gobet F, Clarkson G. Chunks in expert memory: evidence for the magical number four … or is it two? Memory. 2004;12:732–47.
17. Brown NR. Organization of public events in long-term memory. J Exp Psychol Gen. 1990;119:297–314.
18. Scoville WB, Milner B. Loss of recent memory after bilateral hippocampal lesions. J Neurol Neurosur Psychiatry. 1957;20:11–21.
19. Squire LR. The legacy of patient H.M. for neuroscience. Neuron. 2009;61:6–9.
20. Squire LR, Wixted JT. The cognitive neuroscience of human memory since H.M. Annu Rev Neurosci. 2011;34:259–88.
21. Wang S-H, Morris GM. Hippocampal-neocortical interactions in memory formation, consolidation, and reconsolidation. Annu Rev Psychol. 2010;61:49–79.
22. Rugg MD, Vilberg KL, Mattson JT, Yu SS, Johnson JD, Suzuki M. Item memory, context memory and the hippocampus; fMRI evidence. Neuropsychologia. 2012;50:3070–9.
23. Rugg MD, Vilberg K. Brain networks underlying episodic memory retrieval. Curr Opin Neurobiol. 2013;23:255–60.

Neural correlates of free recall of "famous events" in a "hypermnestic" individual as compared to an age...

43

24. Fuster JM. The cognit: a network model of cortical representation. Int J Psychophysiol. 2006;60:125–32.

25. Fuster JM. Cortex and memory: emergence of a new paradigm. J Cogn Neurosci. 2009;21:2047–72.

26. Basar E. The theory of the whole-brain-work. Int J Psychophysiol. 2006;60:133–8.

27. Henke K. A model for memory systems based on processing modes rather than consciousness. Nat Rev Neurosci. 2010;11:523–32.

28. Shohamy D, Turk-Browne NB. Mechanisms for widespread hippocampal involvement in cognition. J Exp Psychol Gen. 2013;142:1159–70.

29. Squire LR. Memory systems of the brain: a brief history and current perspective. Neurobiol Learn Mem. 2004;82:171–7.

30. Nauta WJH. Expanding border of the limbic system concept. In: Rasmussen T, Marino R, editors. Functional neurosurgery. New York: Raven Press; 1979. p. 7–23.

31. Nieuwenhuys R. The greater limbic system, the emotional motor system and the brain. Prog Brain Res. 1996;107:551–80.

32. Shah NJ, Marshall JC, Zafiris O, Schwab A, Zilles K, Markowitsch HJ, Fink GR. The neural correlates of person familiarity. A functional magnetic resonance imaging study with clinical implications. Brain. 2001;124:804–15.

33. Tulving E, Markowitsch HJ, Craik FIM, Habib R, Houle S. Novelty and familiarity activations in PET studies of memory encoding and retrieval. Cereb Cortex. 1996;6:71–9.

34. Herholz K, Kessler J, Ehlen P, Lenz O, Kalbe E, Markowitsch HJ. The role of prefrontal cortex, precuneus, and cerebellum during face-name association learning. Neuropsychologia. 2001;39:643–50.

35. Crawford JR, Howell DC. Comparing an individual's test score against norms derived from small samples. Clin Neuropsychol. 1998;12:482–6.

36. Crawford JR, Garthwaite PH. Investigation of the single case in neuropsychology: confidence limits on the abnormality of test scores and test score differences. Neuropsychologia. 2002;40:1196–208.

37. Oldfield R. The assessment and analysis of handedness. The Edinburgh Inventory. Neuropsychologia. 1971;9:97–113.

38. Lehrl S. Mehrfachwahl-Wortschatz-Intelligenztest (MWT-B) [Multiple choice lexis intelligence test]. Balingen: Spitta Verlag; 2005.

39. Friston KJ. Experimental design and statistical issues. In: Mazziotta JC, Toga AW, editors. Brain mapping: the disorders. San Diego: Academic Press; 2000. p. 33–58.

40. Holmes AP, Friston KJ. Generalisability, random effects, and population inference. Neuroimage. 1998;7:754.

41. Brett M, Anton J-L, Valabregue R, Poline J-B. Region of interest analysis using an SPM toolbox [abstract] Presented at the 8th International Conference on Functional Mapping of the Human Brain, June 2–6, 2002, Sendai, Japan. Available on CD-ROM in Neuroimage, 16, No 2; 2002.

42. Crawford JR, Garthwaite PH. Testing for suspected impairments and dissociations in single-case studies in neuropsychology: evaluation of alternatives using Monte Carlo simulations and revised tests for dissociations. Neuropsychology. 2005;19:318–31.

43. Crawford JR, Garthwaite PH. Evaluation of criteria for classical dissociations in single-case studies by Monte Carlo simulation. Neuropsychology. 2005;19:664–78.

44. Tulving E, Kapur S, Markowitsch HJ, Craik G, Habib R, Houle S. Neuroanatomical correlates of retrieval in episodic memory: auditory sentence recognition. Proc Natl Acad Sci USA. 1994;91:2012–5.

45. Lepage M, Ghaffar O, Nyberg L, Tulving E. Prefrontal cortex and episodic memory retrieval mode. Proc Natl Acad Sci USA. 2000;97:506–11.

46. Tulving E. Organization of memory: quo vadis? In: Gazzaniga MS, editor. The cognitive neurosciences. Cambridge: MIT Press; 1995. p. 839–47.

47. Dew ITZ, Cabeza R. The porous boundaries between explicit and implicit memory: behavioral and neural evidence. Ann NY Acad Sci. 2011;1224:174–90.

48. Treffert DA. The savant syndrome: an extraordinary condition. A synopsis: past, present, future. Philos Trans R Soc B. 2009;364:1351–7.

49. Marks LE. On colored-hearing synesthesia: cross-modal translations of sensory dimensions. Psychol Bull. 1975;82:303–31.

50. Marks LE, Mulvenna CM. Synesthesia, at and near its borders. Front Psychol. 2013. https://doi.org/10.3389/fpsyg.2013.00651.

51. Rouw R, Scholte HS, Colizoli O. Brain areas involved in synaesthesia: a review. J Neuropsychol. 2011;5:214–42.

52. Svoboda E, McKinnon M, Levine B. The functional neuroanatomy of autobiographical memory: a meta-analysis. Neuropsychologia. 2006;44:2189–208.

53. Piefke M, Weiss PH, Markowitsch HJ, Fink GR. Gender differences in the functional neuroanatomy of emotional episodic autobiographical memory. Hum Brain Mapp. 2005;24:313–24.

54. Fink GR, Markowitsch HJ, Reinkemeier M, Bruckbauer T, Kessler J, Heiss W-D. Cerebral representation of one's own past: neural networks involved in autobiographical memory. J Neurosci. 1996;16:4275–82.

55. Insausti R, Annese J, Amaral DG, Squire LR. Human amnesia and the medial temporal lobe illuminated by neuropsychological and neurohistological findings for patient E.P. Proc Natl Acad Sci USA. 2013;110:E1953–62. https://doi.org/10.1073/pnas.1306244110.

56. Maguire EA, Mummery CJ, Büchel C. Patterns of hippocampal–cortical interaction dissociate temporal lobe memory subsystems. Hippocampus. 2000;10:475–82.

57. Karnath HO. New insights into the functions of the superior temporal cortex. Nat Rev Neurosci. 2001;2:568–76. https://doi.org/10.1038/35086057.

58. Manning L, Denkova E, Unterberger L. Autobiographical significance in past and future public semantic memory: a case-study. Cortex. 2013;49:2007–20. https://doi.org/10.1016/j.cortex.2012.11.007.

59. De Renzi E, Liotti M, Nichelli P. Semantic amnesia with preservation of autobiographic memory, A case report. Cortex. 1987;23:575–97.

60. Yasuda K, Watanabe O, Ono Y. Dissociation between semantic and autobiographic memory: a case report. Cortex. 1997;33:623–38.

61. Maguire EA, Valentie ER, Wilding JM, Kapur N. Routes to remembering: the brains behind superior memory. Nat Neurosci. 2003;6:90–5.

62. Poldrack RA. Can cognitive processes be inferred from neuroimaging data? Trends Cogn Sci. 2006;10:59–63.

63. Houdé O, Zago L, Mellet E, Moutier S, Pineau A, Mazoyer B, Tzourio-Mazoyer N. Shifting from the perceptual brain to the logical brain: the neural impact of cognitive inhibition training. J Cogn Neurosci. 2000;12:721–8.

64. Houdé O, Tzourio-Mazoyer N. Neural foundations of logical and mathematical cognition. Nat Rev Neurosci. 2003;4:507–14.

65. Fehr T. A hybrid model for the neural representation of complex mental processing in the human brain. Cogn Neurodyn. 2013;7:89–103.

66. Addis DR, Knapp K, Roberts RP, Schacter DL. Routes to the past: neural substrates of direct and generative autobiographical memory retrieval. Neuroimage. 2012;59:2908–22. https://doi.org/10.1016/j.neuroimage.2011.09.066.

67. Raz A, Packard MG, Alexander GM, Buhle JT, Zhu H, Yu S, Peterson BS. A slice of π: an exploratory neuroimaging study of digit encoding and retrieval in a superior memorist. Neurocase. 2009;15:361–72.

68. Yin L-J, Lu Y-T, Fan M-X, Wang Z-X, Hu Y. Neural evidence for the use of digit-image mnemonic in a superior memorist: an fMRI study. Front Human Neurosci. 2015. https://doi.org/10.3389/fnhum.2015.00109.

69. Patihis L, Frenda SJ, LePort AKR, Petersen N, Nichols RM, Stark CEL, McGaugh JL, Loftus EF. False memories in highly autobiographical memory individuals. Proc Natl Acad Sci USA. 2013;110:20947–52.

5

Juvenile stress induces behavioral change and affects perineuronal net formation in juvenile mice

Hiroshi Ueno[1,2]* ⓘ, Shunsuke Suemitsu[3], Shinji Murakami[3], Naoya Kitamura[3], Kenta Wani[3], Yosuke Matsumoto[4], Motoi Okamoto[2], Shozo Aoki[3] and Takeshi Ishihara[3]

Abstract

Background: Many neuropsychiatric disorders develop in early life. Although the mechanisms involved have not been elucidated, it is possible that functional abnormalities of parvalbumin-positive interneurons (PV neurons) are present. Several previous studies have shown that juvenile stress is implicated in the development of neuropsychiatric disorders. We aimed to clarify the effects of juvenile stress on behavior and on the central nervous system. We investigated behavioral abnormalities of chronically-stressed mice during juvenilehood and the effect of juvenile stress on PV neurons and WFA-positive perineuronal nets (PNNs), which are associated with vulnerability and plasticity in the mouse brain.

Results: Due to juvenile stress, mice showed neurodevelopmental disorder-like behavior. Juvenile stressed mice did not show depressive-like behaviors, but on the contrary, they showed increased activity and decreased anxiety-like behavior. In the central nervous system of juvenile stressed mice, the fluorescence intensity of WFA-positive PNNs decreased, which may signify increased vulnerability.

Conclusion: This study suggested that juvenile stressed mice showed behavioral abnormalities, resembling those seen in neuropsychiatric disorders, and increased brain vulnerability.

Keywords: Behavior, Juvenile, Mouse, Perineuronal nets, Parvalbumin, Stress

Background

Many neuropsychiatric disorders are diagnosed at puberty [1]. Approximately half of adult neuropsychiatric disorders begin in adolescence [2, 3]. However, the cause of the onset remains unclear. It has been reported that the onset of neuropsychiatric disorders such as anxiety, neurosis, depression, post-traumatic stress disorder (PTSD), and schizophrenia are associated with stress exposure during juvenilehood [4, 5]. In recent years, many children worldwide are experiencing stress [6]. Chronic stress is known as a major risk factor for the onset of numerous neuropsychiatric disorders including depression [7–9].

Human behavior is greatly affected by the environment both during childhood and adolescence [10–12]. The maturing brain is very sensitive to stress [13–15]. At this period, stressful events are related to later social and emotional maladjusted behaviors [16]. In animal experiment models, animals stressed in early childhood show increased anxiety-like behavior [17], decreased spatial memory [18], increased corticosterone secretion [19], and altered hippocampal size after maturation [18, 20].

Many common early-stage stress experiment models have focused on the period during lactation through maternal deprivation and separation. However, the development of the pup brain continues after weaning, and brain development is affected by environmental factors. In this study, we focused on mice after weaning. At this time, mice already act independently, and some areas of the central nervous system have matured, but many other

*Correspondence: dhe422007@s.okayama-u.ac.jp
[1] Department of Medical Technology, Kawasaki University of Medical Welfare, 288, Matsushima, Kurashiki, Okayama 701-0193, Japan
Full list of author information is available at the end of the article

brain areas have not [21–23]. Mice at postnatal week 4 are considered to be in the state before human juvenile-hood, and their brain is still in the developmental stage [14]. Although the mechanisms involved in stress-related neuropsychiatric disorder development during juvenile-hood and adolescence have not been elucidated, it seems that environment, physiology, and heredity are all impli-cated in a complicatedly interrelated manner [24]. Using animal experiment models, we are just beginning to understand how juvenile organs react to stress [25].

It has been suggested that functional abnormalities in parvalbumin-positive interneurons (PV neurons) are one cause of anxiety, neurosis, depression, and schizo-phrenia [26–32]. PV neurons are GABAergic interneu-rons [33–35]. In the central nervous system, GABAergic interneurons mature after birth, and abnormalities in GABAergic interneurons have been reported in numer-ous neuropsychiatric disorders [36–40]. PV neurons mature depending on environmental inputs around juve-nilehood [41–43]. PV neurons form inhibitory synapses at the cell body and axon initial segments of pyramidal cells, and regulate the synchronous firing of pyramidal cells [44, 45]. Dysfunction of PV neurons causes mental disease-like behavior in mice [46, 47].

After birth, the cell bodies, proximal dendrites, and axon initial segments of many PV neurons are covered with special extracellular matrix molecules [48, 49]. This extracellular matrix molecules are called the perineu-ronal net (PNN). The PNN consists of hyaluronic acid, link proteins, tenascin, and aggrecan, versican, brevican, and neurocan, which are lecticans belonging to the fam-ily of chondroitin sulfate proteoglycans [50–53]. Lectin *Wisteria floribunda* agglutinin (WFA), which binds to *N*-acetylgalactosamine residues, is widely used to visual-ize PNNs [54]. Although the function of PNNs has not been clarified, it has been shown that they exert neuro-plasticity control and have neuroprotective effects [55]. It is thought that the critical period ends by the forma-tion of PNNs around PV neurons [56, 57]. Loss of PNNs around PV neurons restores plasticity, and reduces the excitability of PV neurons [58–60]. PNNs also protect PV neurons from oxidative stress [61, 62]. Altered PNNs have been reported postmortem in the brains of patients with schizophrenia and depression [63, 64], and mice with PNN dysfunction show behavioral abnormalities, such as those seen in neuropsychiatric disorders [65–67].

Behavioral abnormalities after maturation due to early life stress have been examined in detail, but behavioral anomalies in juvenilehoods under stress have not been clearly defined. If functional and structural anomalies are maintained until maturity, it is necessary to diag-nose young people who are experiencing stress as soon as possible. Therefore, we aimed to clarify behavioral

abnormalities in mice that had experienced stress during juvenilehood. In addition, we investigated the influence of stress on both PV neurons and PNNs in each brain region (frontal cortex, motor cortex, and the hippocam-pus) in juvenile mice.

The PV immunostaining-delineated CA2 neurons have not distinguishable differences in cell morphol-ogy compared with CA1 and CA3 regions. Hippocam-pal area CA2 is excluded from present study. Studies of neuropsychiatric disorders have implicated PV neuronal abnormalities in region-specific dysfunction and not in the sensory cortex. These reports indicate that there is region-specific vulnerability of PV neurons to neu-ropsychiatric conditions in the cortex. The motor cortex on the same section as the frontal cortex was examined simultaneously.

We physically and socially stressed mice for 10 days, which were at different developmental periods: early childhood (from postnatal day 21–30) and maturation phase (from postnatal day 81–90) on the same stress schedule. Therefore, in this study, we aimed to clarify the influence of stress on juvenile behaviors and on the for-mation of developing PV neurons and PNNs.

Methods
Animals
All animal experiments were performed in accordance with the U.S. National Institutes of Health (NIH) Guide for the Care and Use of Laboratory Animals (NIH Pub-lication No. 80-23, revised in 1996) and were approved by the Committee for Animal Experiments at Kawasaki Medical School Advanced Research Center. All efforts were made to minimize the number of animals used and their suffering. The day of birth was designated as postna-tal day (P0). Animals were purchased from Charles River Laboratories (Kanagawa, Japan) and housed in cages (5 animals/cage) with food and water provided ad libi-tum under a 12 h light/dark cycle at 23–26 °C. We used C57BL/6N male mice aged P21 (juvenile) and P71 (adult). Mice between the age of P0 and P28 are termed juvenile and mice between P28 and P56 should be termed adoles-cence. Since the adolescent period is quite ambiguity in rodents, we chose to start stress during what is consid-ered to be the juvenile period (P21–30). Adult mice were exposed to stress from P71 to P80. The animals were ran-domly assigned to either the control (n = 10) or stress groups (n = 10). All behavioral tests were conducted in behavioral testing rooms between 08.00 and 18.00 h dur-ing the light phase of the circadian cycle. Similar to previ-ous reports, we performed behavioral tests [68, 69]. After the tests, all equipment was cleaned with 70% ethanol and super hypochlorous water to prevent bias based on olfactory cues. Behavioral tests were performed two tests

each day (Fig. 1). It takes 3 h between tests. Mice are back in their home cage in the colony.

Stress

Animals in the stress groups were subjected to stress once a day according to a protocol similar to that used in previous studies [70–73]. Animals were subjected to stress using the following procedures: (1) tail-pinch for 10 min; (2) forced restraint in a plastic tube for 3 h without access to food or water; (3) hot air (approx. 38 °C) blown using a hair dryer for 10 min; (4) overnight illumination; (5) food and water deprivation for 8 h; (6) damp sawdust (200 mL water absorbed in sawdust bedding). One stressor was applied daily (Fig. 1). Control mice were housed in a separate room, having no contact with the stressed mice.

General health and neurological screening

Physical characteristics, including body weight, rectal temperature, and presence of whiskers or bald hair patches, were recorded. The righting, whisker twitch, and ear twitch reflexes were also evaluated. Neuromuscular strength was examined using the grip strength and wire hang tests according to a previous study [74]. A grip strength meter was used to assess forelimb grip strength. Mice were lifted and held by the tail so that their forepaws could grasp a wire grid; they then were pulled backward gently until they released the grid. The peak force applied by the mouse forelimbs was recorded in Newtons (N). We performed this test at both P21 and P30.

Elevated plus maze test

The apparatus consisted of two open arms (8×25 cm) and two closed arms of the same size with 30-cm high transparent walls. The arms were constructed of white plastic plates and were elevated to a height of 40 cm

above the floor. Arms of the same type were located opposite each other. Each mouse was placed in the central square of the maze, facing one of the closed arms, and was allowed to move freely between the two arms for 10 min. The number of arms entries, distance traveled (m), and percentage of time spent in the open arms were recorded on video and analyzed using video tracking software (ANY-MAZE, Stoelting Co., Wood Dale, IL).

Social interaction test

The apparatus consisted of a rectangular parallelepiped ($30 \times 60 \times 40$ cm). Each mouse was placed in the box for 10 min and allowed to freely explore for habituation. In the sociability test, an unfamiliar C57BL/6N male mouse (stranger mouse) that had no previous contact with the subject mouse was placed into one of the transparent cages ($7.5 \times 7.5 \times 10$ cm, which had several holes with a diameter of 1 cm) located at the corners of each lateral compartment. The stranger mouse was enclosed in the transparent cage, which allowed nose contact between the bars but prevented fighting. The subject mouse was placed in the center and allowed to explore the entire box for a 10-min session. One side of the rectangular area was identified as the stranger area and the other as the empty area. The amount of time spent in each area and around each cage during the 10-min sessions was measured. Data were recorded on video and analyzed using the ANY-MAZE software.

Porsolt forced swim test

The apparatus for the Porsolt forced swim test consisted of four Plexiglas cylinders (20 cm height × 10 cm diameter). The cylinders were filled with water (23 °C) up to a height of 7.5 cm. Mice were placed into the cylinders, and their behavior was recorded over a 6-min test period. In this test, we detect 'immobile period' when the animals stop struggling for one second or more. Immobility lasting for less than 1.5 s was not included in the analysis. Data acquisition and analysis were performed automatically using the ANY-MAZE software.

Tail suspension test

Each mouse was suspended 60 cm above the floor by the tail in a white plastic chamber by an adhesive tape placed < 1 cm from the tip of the tail. Its behavior was recorded for 6 min. Images were captured through a video camera, and immobility was measured. Similar to the Porsolt forced swim test, immobility was evaluated using the ANY-MAZE software.

Locomotor activity test

For measurements of locomotor activity, the mice were acclimated to the single housing environment for 2.5 h.

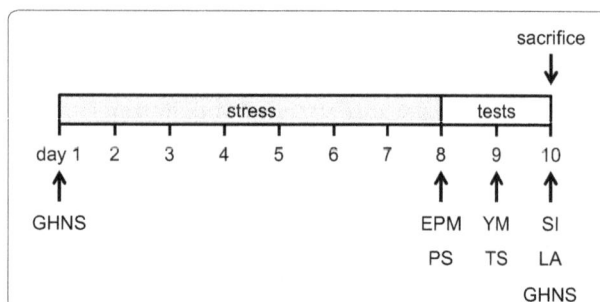

Fig. 1 Experimental time schedule. Animals in the stress groups were subjected to stress once a day from P21 (juvenile) or P71 (adult). Animals were subjected to two behavioral tests per day. *EPM* elevated plus maze, *PS* Porsolt forced swim, *YM* Y-maze, *TS* tail-suspension, *SI* social interaction, *LA* locomotor activity, *GHNS* general health and neurological screening

Locomotor activity data were measured using a photobeam activity system (ACTIMO-100; BRC Co., Nagoya, Aichi, Japan), and activity counts were recorded at 10-min intervals.

Y-maze test

Spatial working memory was measured using a Y-maze apparatus (arm length: 40 cm, arm bottom width: 3 cm, arm upper width: 10 cm, height of wall: 12 cm). Each subject was placed at the center of the Y-maze field. Visual cues were placed around the maze in the testing room and kept constant throughout the testing sessions. Mice were examined with no learning prior. The number of entries and alterations was recorded and analyzed automatically using the ANY-MAZE software. Data were collected for 10 min [75, 76].

Statistical analysis of behavioral tests

Data were analyzed with one-way analysis of variance (ANOVA) followed by Tukey's test, two-way repeated measures ANOVA followed by Fisher's LSD test, Student's t test, or paired t test. A p value < 0.05 was regarded as statistically significant. Data are shown as box plots.

Tissue preparation

Following behavioral experiments, we deeply anesthetized the animals with a lethal dose of sodium pentobarbital (120 mg/kg, i.p.) and transcardially perfused them with ice-cold phosphate-buffered saline (PBS) for 2 min and then 4% paraformaldehyde in PBS (pH 7.4) for 10 min (10 mL/min). In all cases, we dissected the brains and post-fixed them overnight with 4% paraformaldehyde in PBS at 4 °C and cryoprotected them by immersion in 15% sucrose for 12 h followed by 30% sucrose for 20 h at 4 °C. To cut sections, we froze the brains in O.C.T. Compound (Tissue-Tek; Sakuma Finetek, Tokyo, Japan) using dry ice-cold normal hexane and we prepared serial coronal sections of 40-μm thickness using a cryostat (CM3050S; Leica Wetzlar, Germany) at − 20 °C. We collected sections in ice-cold PBS containing 0.05% sodium azide.

Immunohistochemistry

The cryostat sections were treated with 0.1% triton X-100 in PBS for 15 min at 20 °C. After three washes in PBS, the sections were incubated with 10% normal donkey serum (ImmunoBioScience Co., WA) in PBS for 1 h at 20 °C. Sections were again washed three times in PBS and incubated with biotinylated WFA (B-1355, Vector Laboratories, Funakoshi Co., Tokyo, Japan; 1:200) and a primary antibodies in PBS overnight at 4 °C. After washing in PBS, the sections were incubated with streptavidin-conjugated to Alexa Fluor 594 (S11227, Thermo Fisher

Scientific, Tokyo, Japan; 1:1000) and secondary antibodies in PBS at 20 °C for 2 h. The sections were rinsed with PBS and mounted onto glass slides using Vectashield mounting medium (H-1400, Vector Laboratories). The prepared slides were stored at 4 °C until imaging.

Antibodies

The following primary antibodies were used: mouse anti-parvalbumin (clone PARV-19, P3088, Sigma-Aldrich Japan, Tokyo, Japan, 1:1000), mouse anti-NeuN (MAB377, Millipore, 1:1000), rabbit anti-Iba-1 (019-19741, Wako, Osaka, Japan, 1:1000), and mouse anti-Cat-315 (MAB1581, Millipore, Tokyo, Japan, 1:1000). The following secondary antibodies were used: Alexa Fluor 488-conjugated goat anti-mouse IgG (ab150113, Abcam, Tokyo, Japan; 1:1000), FITC-conjugated anti-mouse IgM (sc-2082, Santa Cruz, Texas, USA, 1:1000), and Texas Red-conjugated goat anti-rabbit IgG (TI-1000, Vector laboratories, 1:500).

Microscopic imaging and quantification of labeled neurons

To quantify the number of PV- WFA-, and Cat-315$^+$-positive neurons, confocal laser scanning microscopy of the stained sections was used according to a similar protocol [77]. Images (1024 × 1024 pixels) were saved as TIFF files using the ZEN software (Carl Zeiss Oberkochen, Germany). A 10 ×, or 20 × objective lens and a pinhole setting corresponding to a focal plane thickness of less than 1 μm were used. Data were quantified and presented according to the cortical layer profiles (L2/3 and L5/6) based on fluorescence Nissl staining (NeuroTrace 435/455 blue, N-21479, Molecular Probes, Eugene, OR). All confocal images were converted to TIFF files and analyzed with the Image J software (National Institutes of Health, Bethesda, MD; http://rsb.info.nih.gov/nih-image /). The number of neurons was quantified for at least three coronal sections per animal. The stained neurons or PNNs (defined as neurons with a soma size over 60 μm^2) were manually tagged and counted within the area of interest. Neuronal density estimates (cells/mm^2) were also calculated. The data were averaged per mouse. For analyzing PV-, WFA-, and Cat-315$^+$-positive PNN morphologies, samples were randomly selected, and high-magnification images using a 100 × objective lens were acquired.

Both fluorescent intensity and soma rea of PV neurons were quantified using at least three coronal sections per animal. Eight-bit grayscale images were captured using a digital camera. The ellipse circumscribing the PV-positive soma and WFA-positive PNNs was traced manually, and the gray levels for PV and WFA labeling were measured using the ImageJ software. We avoided fluorescence saturation by adjusting the exposure time and gain. The same capture conditions were used for all sections. Background intensity was subtracted using the unstained portions of each section. Data are presented as mean ± SEM. The slides were coded and quantified by a blinded independent observer.

Data analysis of histological quantifications

Data are expressed as the mean ± SEM of five animals per group. Statistical significance was determined by a two-way ANOVA followed by the Bonferroni t test. The statistical significance threshold was set at $p < 0.05$.

Results

Juvenile stress induces changes in body weight gain

We compared the general health and neurological characteristics of the juvenile-stressed and control groups. We found significant decreases in body weight and grip strength between juvenile-stressed and control group mice on P30 (Fig. 2a, stress × time: $F_{1,32} = 16.185$, $p = 0.003$; time in control: $F = 398.249$, $p < 0.0001$; time in stress group: $F = 219.906$, $p < 0.0001$; stress on P30: $F = 29.248$, $p < 0.0001$, Fig. 2c, stress × time: $F_{1,32} = 16.046$, $p = 0.0003$; time in control: $F = 51.697$, $p < 0.0001$; time in stress group: $F = 12.371$, $p = 0.0013$; stress on P30: $F = 21.798$, $p = 0.0001$). There were no significant differences in body temperature between

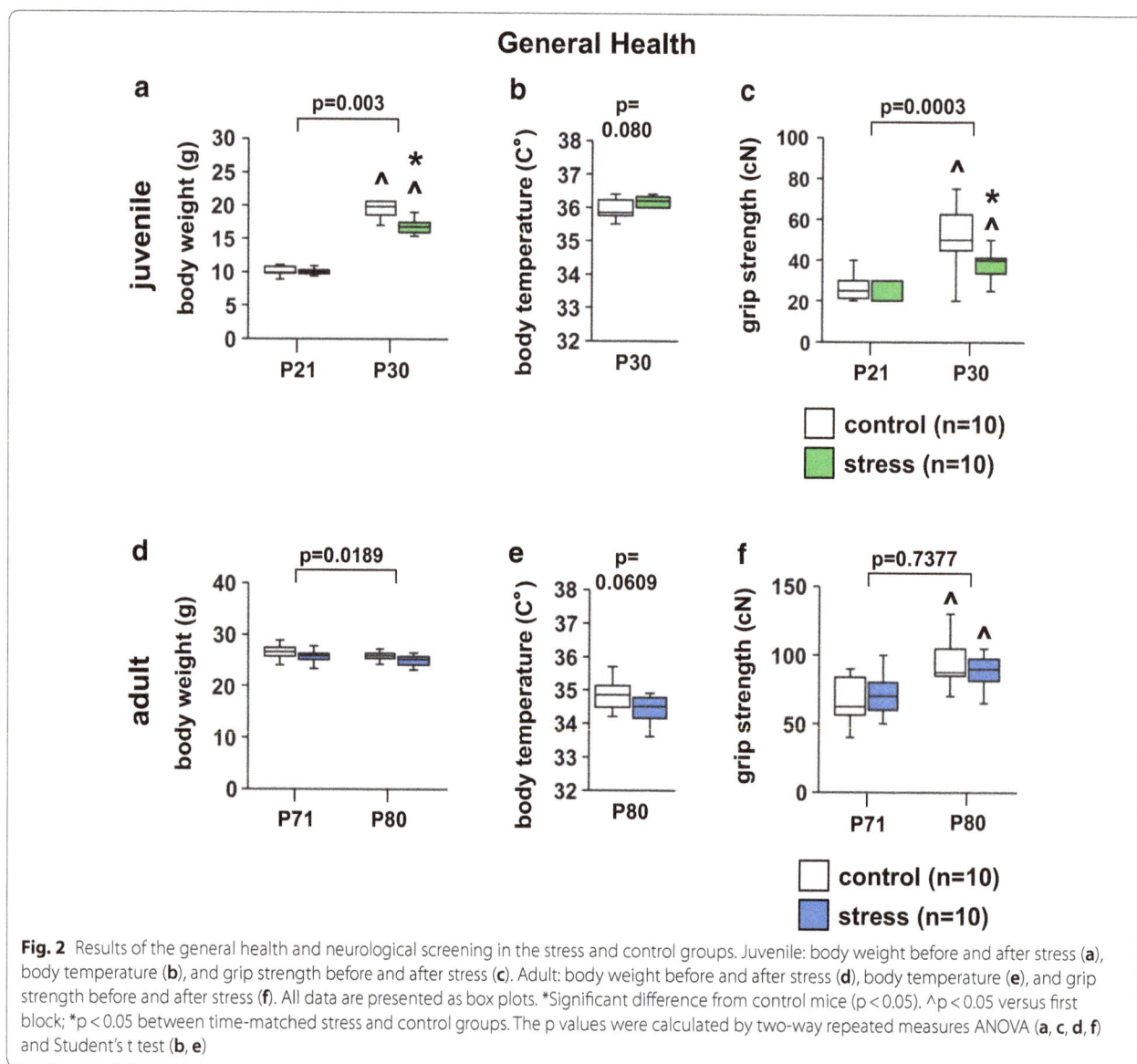

Fig. 2 Results of the general health and neurological screening in the stress and control groups. Juvenile: body weight before and after stress (**a**), body temperature (**b**), and grip strength before and after stress (**c**). Adult: body weight before and after stress (**d**), body temperature (**e**), and grip strength before and after stress (**f**). All data are presented as box plots. *Significant difference from control mice ($p < 0.05$). ^$p < 0.05$ versus first block; *$p < 0.05$ between time-matched stress and control groups. The p values were calculated by two-way repeated measures ANOVA (**a, c, d, f**) and Student's t test (**b, e**)

juvenile-stressed and control group mice on P30 (Fig. 2b, $t_{14} = 2.1448$, p = 0.080).

There were no significant differences in body weight, body temperature, and grip strength between adult-stressed and control group mice on P80 (Fig. 2d, stress × time: $F_{1,36} = 6.046$, p = 0.0189; time in control: $F = 1.303$, p = 0.2613; time in stress group: $F = 1.886$, p = 0.1782; stress on P80: $F = 3.440$, p = 0.0719, Fig. 2e, $t_{18} = 2.1009$, p = 0.0609; Fig. 2f, stress × time: $F_{1,36} = 0.114$, p = 0.7377; time in control: $F = 14.059$, p = 0.0006; time in stress group: $F = 4.183$, p = 0.0482; stress on P80: $F = 1.190$, p = 0.2826).

Juvenile stress did not change anxiety-like behaviors

We evaluated anxiety-like behavior in juvenile stressed mice. In the elevated plus maze test, we observed a significant increase in the total distance traveled in the juvenile-stressed compared with the control group mice (Fig. 3a, $t_{18} = 2.1009$, p = 0.0344). There were no significant differences in the number of total entries into the arms, and the percentage of time spent in the open arms between the juvenile-stressed and control group mice (Fig. 3b, $t_{18} = 2.1009$, p = 0.4545; Fig. 3c, $t_{18} = 2.1009$, p = 0.6605).

Next, we evaluated anxiety-like behavior in adult stressed mice. there were no significant differences in

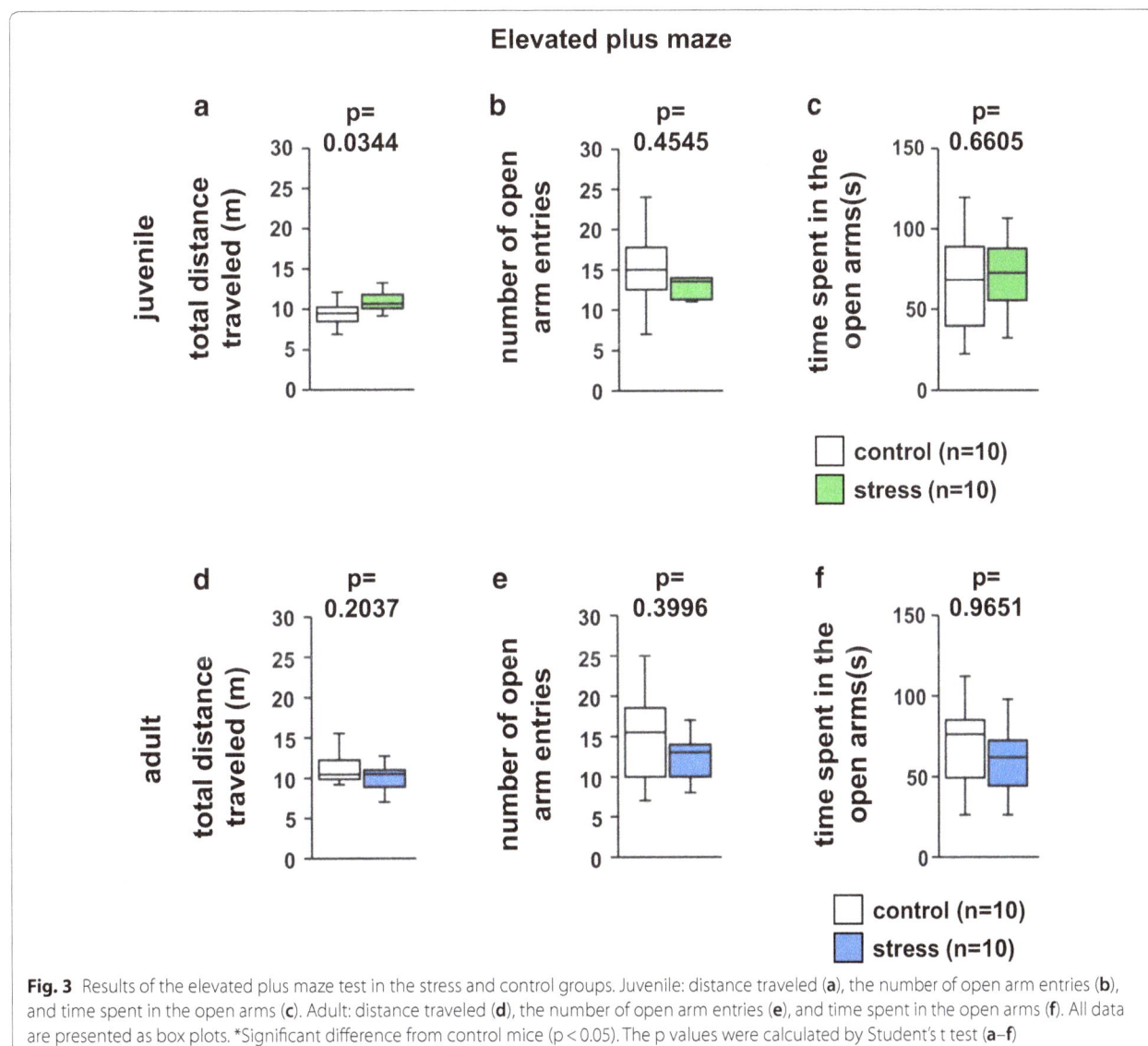

Fig. 3 Results of the elevated plus maze test in the stress and control groups. Juvenile: distance traveled (**a**), the number of open arm entries (**b**), and time spent in the open arms (**c**). Adult: distance traveled (**d**), the number of open arm entries (**e**), and time spent in the open arms (**f**). All data are presented as box plots. *Significant difference from control mice (p < 0.05). The p values were calculated by Student's t test (**a–f**)

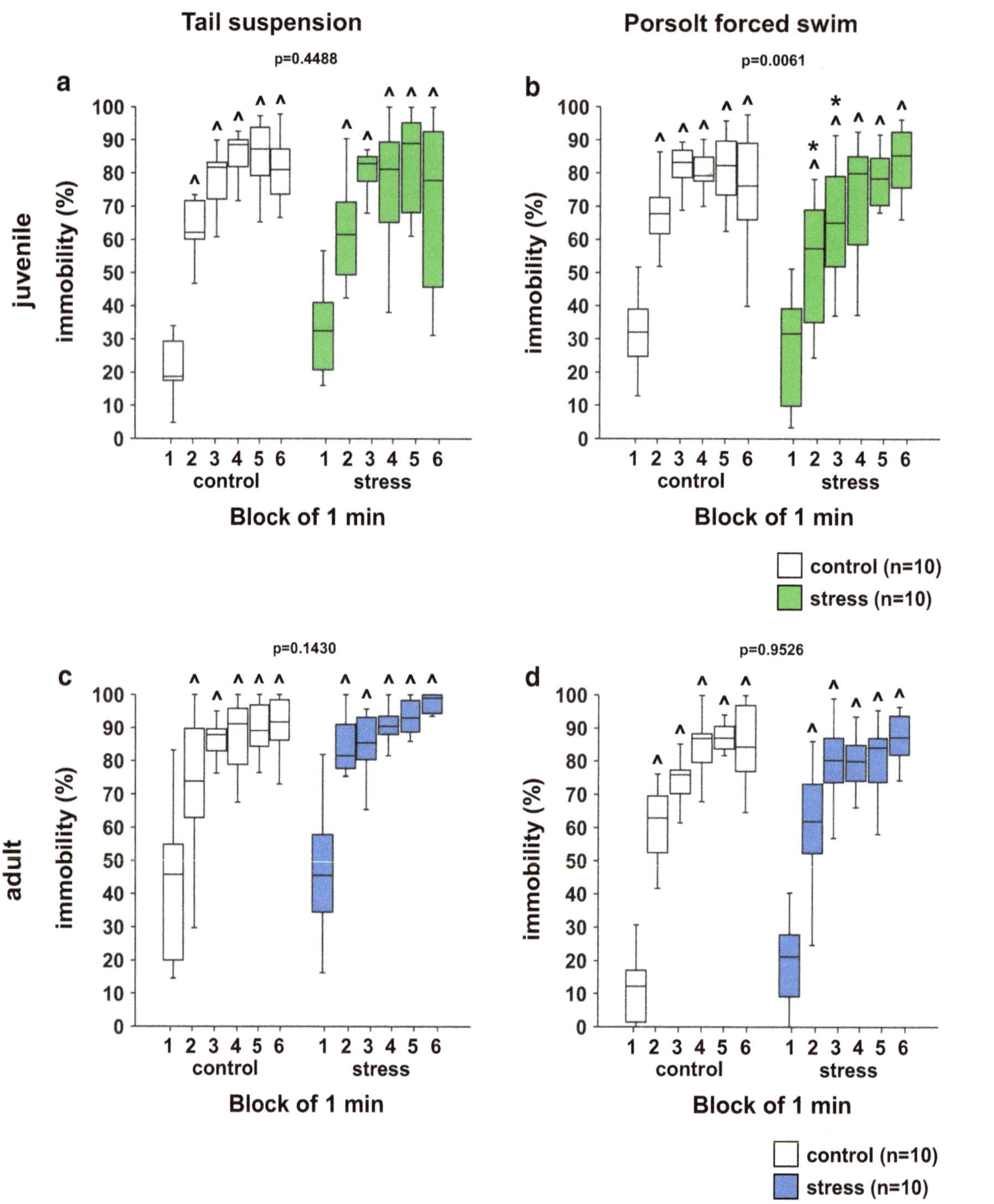

Fig. 4 Results of the tail-suspension test and Porsolt forced swim test in the stress and control groups. Juvenile: percentage of immobility time in each 1-min period (**a**) in the tail-suspension test. percentage of immobility time in each 1-min period (**b**) in the Porsolt forced swim test. Adult: percentage of immobility time in each 1-min period (**c**) in the tail-suspension test. Percentage of immobility time in each 1-min period (**d**) in the Porsolt forced swim test. All data are presented as box plots. *Significant difference from control mice ($p < 0.05$). ^$p < 0.05$ versus first block; *$p < 0.05$ between time-matched stress and control groups. The p values were calculated by two-way repeated measures ANOVA (**a**–**d**)

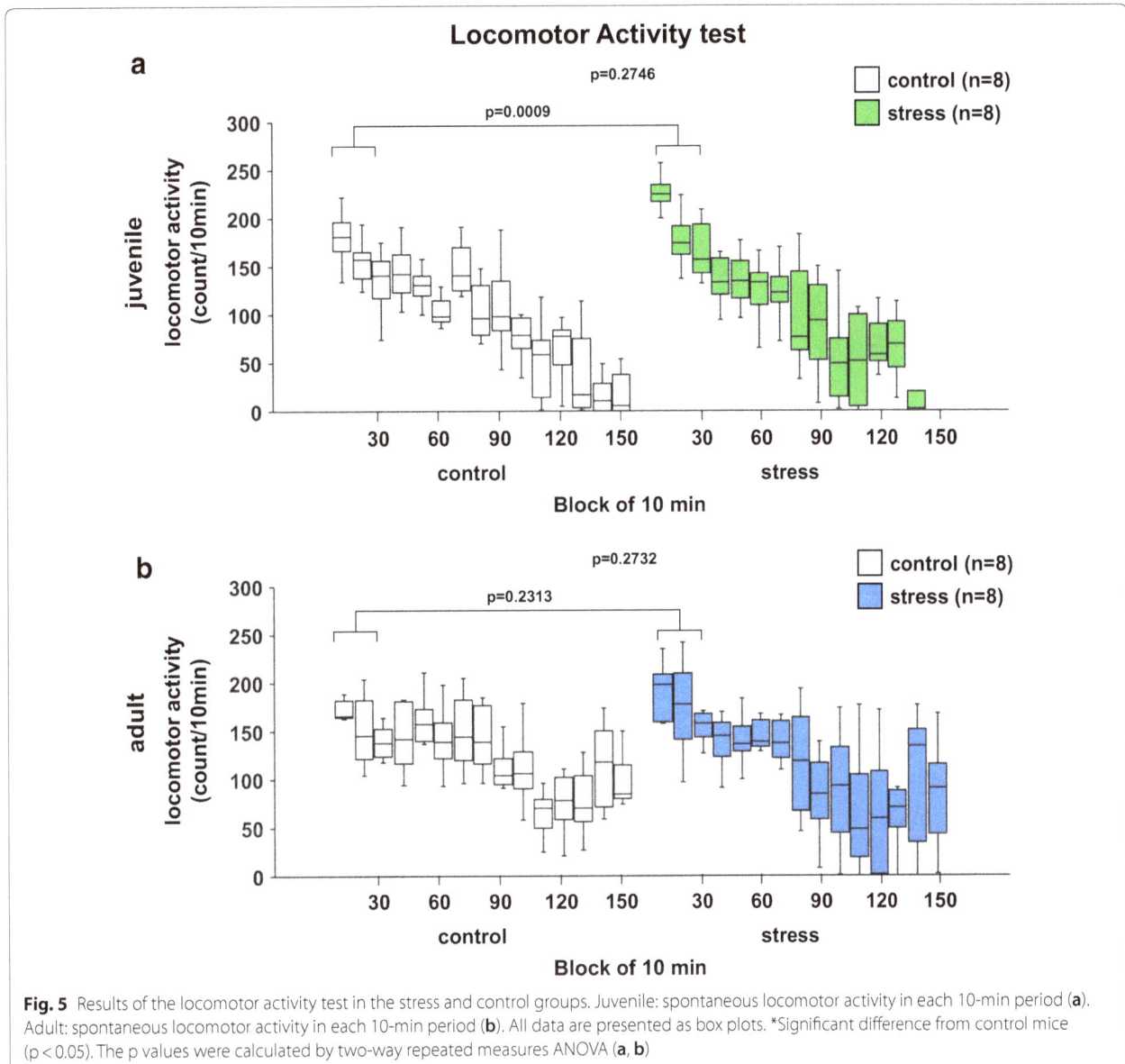

Fig. 5 Results of the locomotor activity test in the stress and control groups. Juvenile: spontaneous locomotor activity in each 10-min period (**a**). Adult: spontaneous locomotor activity in each 10-min period (**b**). All data are presented as box plots. *Significant difference from control mice (p < 0.05). The p values were calculated by two-way repeated measures ANOVA (**a**, **b**)

the number of total entries, total distance traveled, and percentage of time spent in the open arms between the adult-stressed and control group mice (Fig. 3d, $t_{18} = 2.1098$, p = 0.2037; Fig. 3e, $t_{18} = 2.1098$, p = 0.3996; Fig. 3f, $t_{18} = 2.1098$, p = 0.9651).

Juvenile stress reduced depressive-like behaviors

We evaluated depressive-like behavior in juvenile stressed mice. In the tail-suspension test, there were no significant differences in the percentage of immobility time in each 1-min period during the 6-min test period between the juvenile-stressed and control group mice

(See figure on next page.)
Fig. 6 Results of the Social interaction test in the stress and control groups. Juvenile: time spent in the area (**a**), total distance traveled (**b**), number of entries around the cage (**c**), and time spent around the cage (**d**). Adult: time spent in the area (**e**), total distance traveled (**f**), number of entries around the cage (**g**), and time spent around the cage (**h**). All data are presented as box plots. *Significant difference from control mice (p < 0.05). The p values were calculated by two-way ANOVA (**a**, **c**, **d**, **e**, **g**, **h**), one-way ANOVA (**b**, **f**), and paired t test (between the same group in **a**, **c**, **d**, **e**, **g**, **h**)

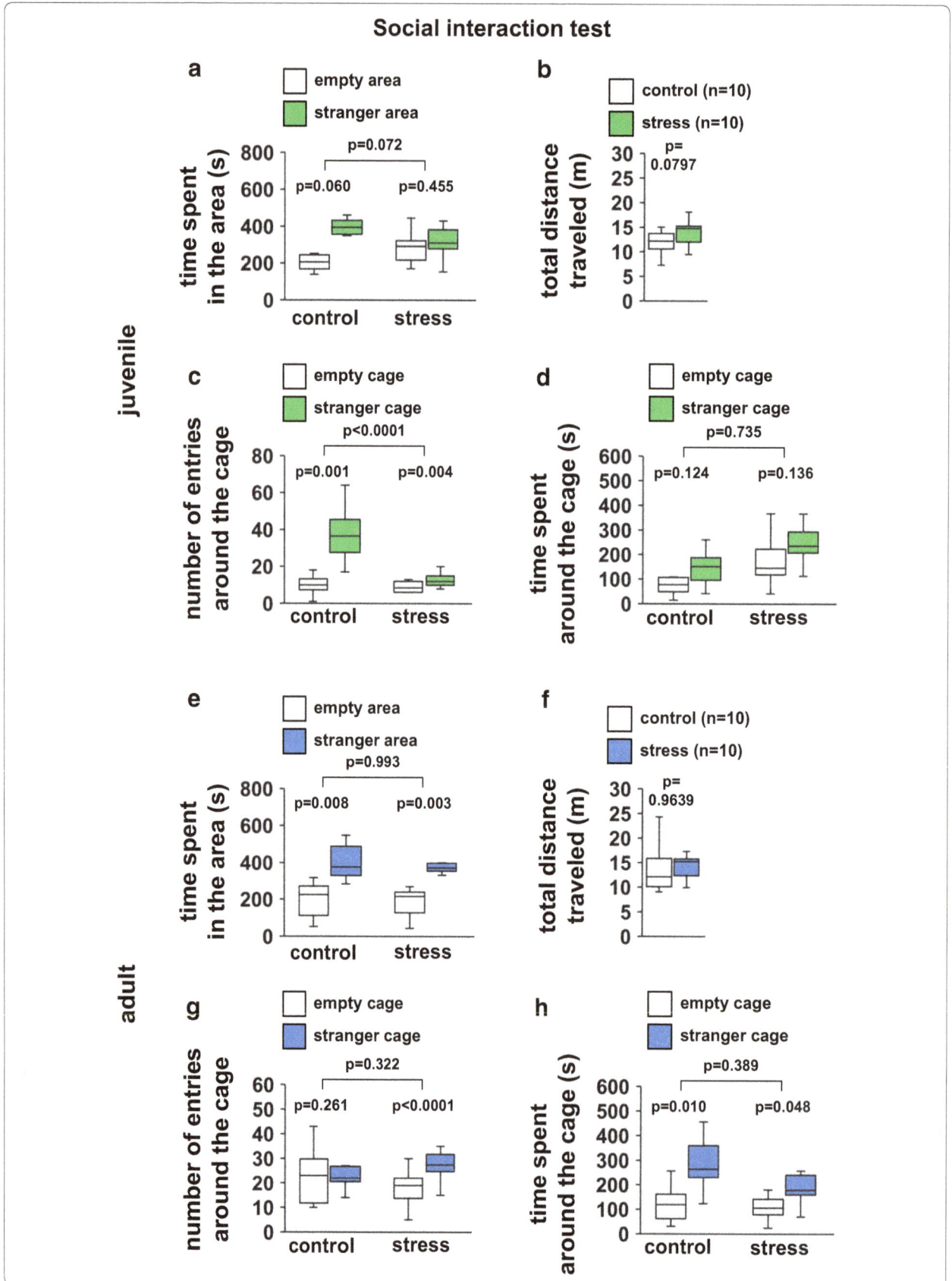

Social interaction test

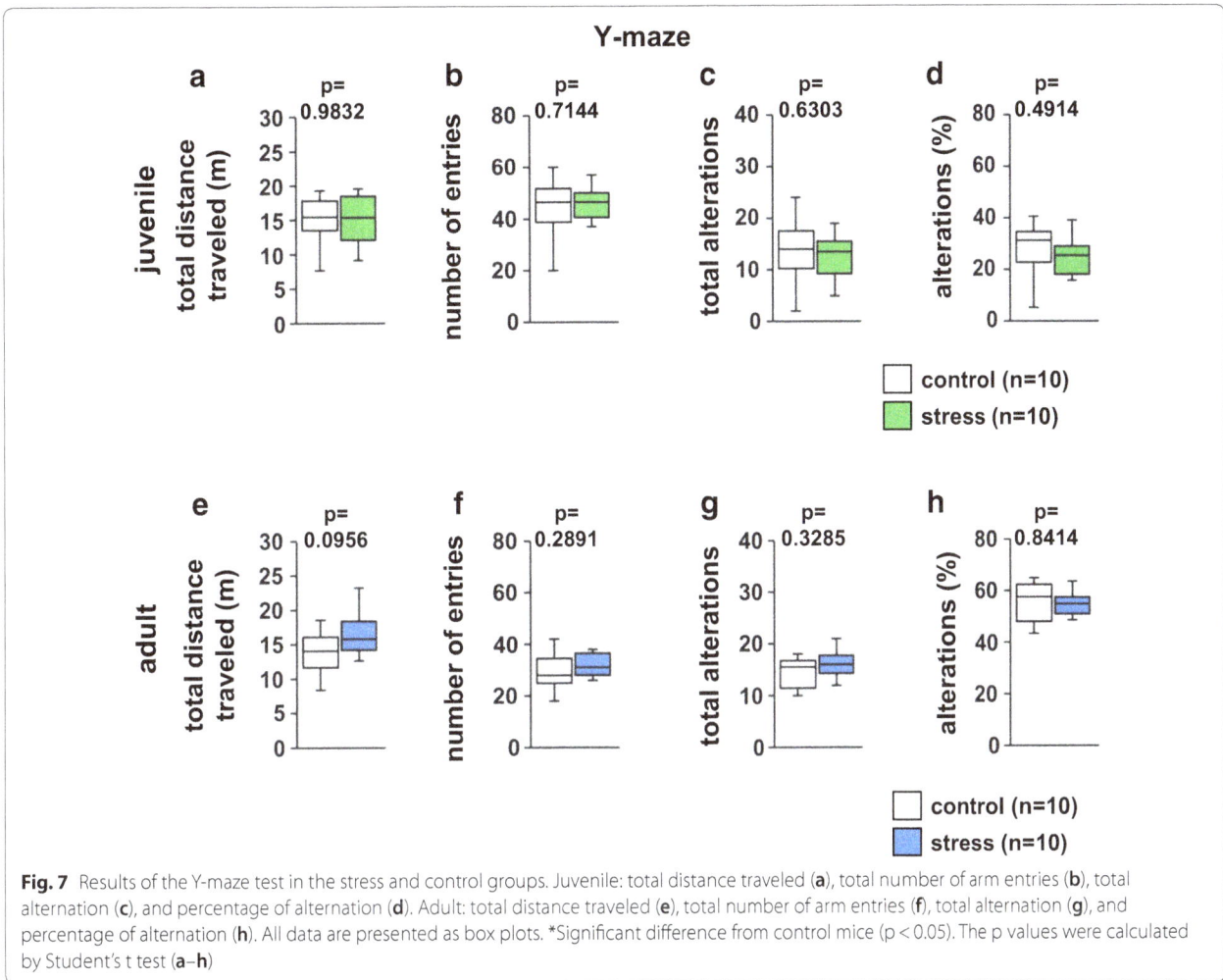

Fig. 7 Results of the Y-maze test in the stress and control groups. Juvenile: total distance traveled (**a**), total number of arm entries (**b**), total alternation (**c**), and percentage of alternation (**d**). Adult: total distance traveled (**e**), total number of arm entries (**f**), total alternation (**g**), and percentage of alternation (**h**). All data are presented as box plots. *Significant difference from control mice (p < 0.05). The p values were calculated by Student's t test (**a**–**h**)

(Fig. 4a, stress × time: $F_{1,102} = 0.578$, p = 0.4488; time in control: $F = 22.813$, p < 0.0001; time in stress group: $F = 13.792$, p < 0.0001). In the Porsolt forced swim test, the juvenile stressed mice spent significantly less time immobile in each 1-min period during the 6-min test period than did the control mice (Fig. 4b, stress × time: $F_{1,108} = 7.830$, p = 0.0061; time in control: $F = 16.349$, p < 0.0001; time in stress group: $F = 16.883$, p < 0.0001).

In the tail-suspension test, we found no significant differences between adult stressed and control mice (Fig. 4c, stress × time: $F_{1,108} = 2.176$, p = 0.1430; time in control: $F = 66.558$, p < 0.0001; time in stress group: $F = 50.135$, p < 0.0001). In the Porsolt forced swim test, during the 6-min test period, there were no significant differences in the percentage of immobility time in each 1-min period in the adult stressed than in the control mice (Fig. 4d, stress × time: $F_{1,108} = 0.004$, p = 0.9526; time in control: $F = 11.520$, p < 0.0001; time in stress group: $F = 12.582$, p < 0.0001).

Juvenile stress increased activity in a new environment

There were no significant differences in locomotor activity during the 150-min period between the adult juvenile stressed and control mice (Fig. 5a, $F_{1,210} = 1.200$, p = 0.2746; Fig. 5b, $F_{1,210} = 1.207$, p = 0.2732). For the first 30-min, we observed a significant increase in the locomotor activity in the juvenile-stressed compared with the control group mice (Fig. 5a, for the first 30-min; stress effect, $F_{1,42} = 12.750$, p = 0.0009; Fig. 5b, for the first 30-min; stress effect, $F_{1,42} = 1.476$, p = 0.2313).

Juvenile stress showed abnormal social behavior

In the social interaction test, we found several differences between juvenile stressed and control mice (Fig. 6a, $F_{1,36} = 3.434$, p = 0.072; Fig. 6c, $F_{1,36} = 20.774$, p < 0.0001; Fig. 6d, $F_{1,36} = 0.116$, p = 0.735). Control mice spent a significantly longer time in the area containing the novel (stranger) mouse in a transparent cage than in the area containing the empty cage (Fig. 6a, $t_9 = -2.147$, p = 0.060), but a similar amount of time in both around

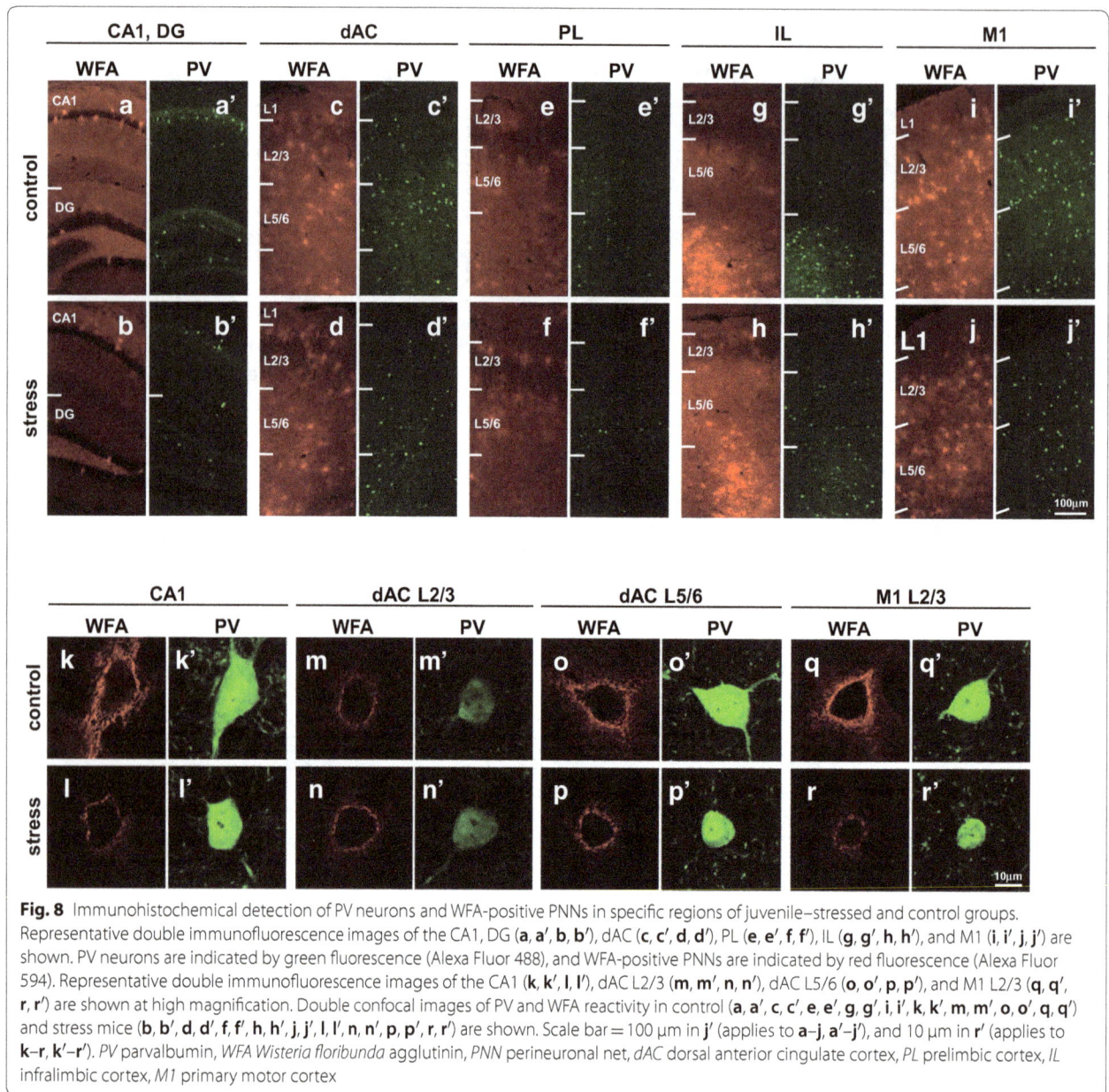

Fig. 8 Immunohistochemical detection of PV neurons and WFA-positive PNNs in specific regions of juvenile–stressed and control groups. Representative double immunofluorescence images of the CA1, DG (**a**, **a′**, **b**, **b′**), dAC (**c**, **c′**, **d**, **d′**), PL (**e**, **e′**, **f**, **f′**), IL (**g**, **g′**, **h**, **h′**), and M1 (**i**, **i′**, **j**, **j′**) are shown. PV neurons are indicated by green fluorescence (Alexa Fluor 488), and WFA-positive PNNs are indicated by red fluorescence (Alexa Fluor 594). Representative double immunofluorescence images of the CA1 (**k**, **k′**, **l**, **l′**), dAC L2/3 (**m**, **m′**, **n**, **n′**), dAC L5/6 (**o**, **o′**, **p**, **p′**), and M1 L2/3 (**q**, **q′**, **r**, **r′**) are shown at high magnification. Double confocal images of PV and WFA reactivity in control (**a**, **a′**, **c**, **c′**, **e**, **e′**, **g**, **g′**, **i**, **i′**, **k**, **k′**, **m**, **m′**, **o**, **o′**, **q**, **q′**) and stress mice (**b**, **b′**, **d**, **d′**, **f**, **f′**, **h**, **h′**, **j**, **j′**, **l**, **l′**, **n**, **n′**, **p**, **p′**, **r**, **r′**) are shown. Scale bar = 100 μm in **j′** (applies to **a–j**, **a′–j′**), and 10 μm in **r′** (applies to **k–r**, **k′–r′**). *PV* parvalbumin, *WFA* Wisteria floribunda agglutinin, *PNN* perineuronal net, *dAC* dorsal anterior cingulate cortex, *PL* prelimbic cortex, *IL* infralimbic cortex, *M1* primary motor cortex

cages (Fig. 6d, $t_9 = -1.695$, p = 0.124). Control mice increased the number of entries around the cage containing the stranger mouse than around empty cage (Fig. 6c, $t_9 = -4.839$, p = 0.001). In contrast, juvenile stressed mice spent a similar amount of time in both areas (Fig. 6a, $t_9 = -0.781$, p = 0.455), and had similar contact time with both cages (Fig. 6c, $t_9 = -3.783$, p = 0.004). During the 10-min period, juvenile stressed mice spent significantly more time around the cage containing the stranger mouse than around the empty cage (Fig. 6d, $t_9 = -1.638$, p = 0.136). There were no significant differences in the total distance traveled between juvenile stressed and control mice (Fig. 6b, $t_{18} = 2.1009$, p = 0.0797). Both control

and adult stressed mice spent a significantly longer time in the area containing the stranger mouse than in the area with the empty cage (Fig. 6e, $F_{1,36} = 0.0001$, p = 0.993, empty area versus stranger area: control, $t_9 = -3.408$, p = 0.008, stress, $t_9 = -3.950$, p = 0.003), and spent significantly more time around the cage containing the stranger mouse than around the empty cage (Fig. 6h, $F_{1,36} = 0.760$, p = 0.389, empty area versus stranger area: control, $t_9 = -3.244$, p = 0.010, stress, $t_9 = -2.281$, p = 0.048). Control mice had a similar number of contacts with both cages (Fig. 6g, $F_{1,36} = 1.010$, p = 0.322, empty area versus stranger area: control, $t_9 = -1.200$, p = 0.261). Adult stressed mice had an increased number of entries around the cage containing the stranger mouse than around the empty cage (Fig. 6g, $t_9 = -5.485$, p < 0.0001). During the 10-min period, there were no significant differences in the total distance traveled between adult stressed and control mice (Fig. 6f, $t_{18} = 2.1009$, p = 0.9639).

Juvenile stress did not change short-term spatial working memory

Short-term spatial working memory was examined by monitoring spontaneous alternation behavior in a Y-maze. There were no significant differences in these measures between the juvenile-stressed and control groups in the number of arm entries (Fig. 7b, $t_{18} = 2.1009$, p = 0.7144), in total alternations (Fig. 7c, $t_{18} = 2.1009$, p = 0.6303), alternation percentage (Fig. 7d, $t_{18} = 2.1009$, p = 0.4914), or total distance (Fig. 7a, $t_{18} = 2.1009$, p = 0.9832), indicating that juvenile stress did not affect short-term memory. The results for adult mice were similar (Fig. 7e, $t_{18} = 2.1009$, p = 0.0956; Fig. 7f, $t_{18} = 2.1009$, p = 0.2891; Fig. 7g, $t_{18} = 2.1009$, p = 0.3285; Fig. 7h, $t_{18} = 2.1009$, p = 0.8414).

Juvenile stress did not change the number of WFA-positive PNNs and PV neurons

We examined the effect of juvenile stress on the number of PV neurons and WFA-positive PNNs in several brain regions in juvenile stressed and control mice. Both PV neurons and WFA-positive PNNs were observed in all brain regions analyzed in this study (Fig. 8a–j, a'–j').

In all brain regions analyzed in this study, there was no difference in the density of both PV neurons and WFA-positive PNNs between the juvenile stressed and control mice (Fig. 9a–f). There was no difference in the percentage of PV neurons enveloped by WFA-positive PNNs in

the hippocampus, prefrontal cortex, and primary motor cortex between the control and the juvenile stressed mice groups (Fig. 9g–i). In all brain regions analyzed in this study, the percentage of WFA-positive PNNs was similar between the juvenile stressed and control mice (Fig. 9j–l).

Juvenile stress reduces WFA-positive fluorescence intensity but does not change PV-positive fluorescence intensity

An enlarged image of PV neurons and WFA-positive PNNs under the same conditions is shown in Fig. 8, revealing that PV fluorescence intensity and WFA fluorescence intensity differed in each brain region (Fig. 8k–r, k'–r'). In addition, WFA fluorescence intensity differed between the control and juvenile stressed mice.

Analysis of fluorescence intensity revealed that both PV and WFA fluorescence intensities differed in each region and each cortical layer of the mouse brain (Fig. 10a–f). There were no differences in PV fluorescence intensity in the hippocampus, prefrontal cortex, and primary motor cortex between control and juvenile stressed mice (Fig. 10a–c). In the CA1 region of the hippocampus, WFA fluorescence intensity was lower in juvenile stressed than in control mice (Fig. 10d). In the dorsal anterior cingulate cortex (dAC) and infralimbic cortex (IL) parts of the prefrontal cortex in juvenile stressed mice, WFA fluorescence intensity was lower than in the same region in control mice (Fig. 10e). In the L2/3 of the primary motor cortex, WFA fluorescence intensity was lower in juvenile stressed than in control mice (Fig. 10f).

Juvenile stress reduces the soma of PV neurons

We also analyzed the soma of PV neurons in several brain regions of the juvenile stressed and control mice (Fig. 11). We analyzed 575 cells (dAC: L2/3 = 72; L5/6 = 72; PL:

(See figure on next page.)

Fig. 9 Densities of PV neurons and WFA-positive PNNs in juvenile-stressed or control mice. The region-specific patterns of PV neuron density (**a–c**) and WFA-positive PNN density (**d–f**) in individual regions are shown. The region-specific pattern of the percentage of PV neurons enveloped by WFA-positive PNNs (**g–i**) and the percentage of WFA-positive PNNs that contain PV (**j–l**) are shown in the individual regions, hippocampus (CA1, CA3, and DG) (**a, d, g, j**), prefrontal cortex (dAC, PL, and IL) (**b, e, h, k**), motor cortex (**c, f, i, l**) of control or stress mice. All data are presented as the mean ± SEM. *Significant difference from control mice (p < 0.05). The p values indicate two-way ANOVA by Bonferroni t test. Abbreviations are the same as those in Fig. 8. **a** Hippocampus; group: $F_{1,66} = 0.086$, region: $F_{2,66} = 6.449$, group × region: $F_{2,66} = 0.111$. CA1: p = 0.6254. CA3: p = 0.8485. DG: p = 0.8626, **b** prefrontal cortex; group: $F_{1,132} = 0.126$, region: $F_{5,132} = 48.755$, group × region: $F_{5,132} = 0.966$. dAC L2/3: p = 0.3783. dAC L5/6: p = 0.4354. PL L2/3: p = 0.9115. PL L5/6: p = 0.2392. IL L2/3: p = 0.9986. IL L5/6: p = 0.1444, **c** M1; group: $F_{1,44} = 1.140$, region: $F_{1,44} = 0.997$, group × region: $F_{1,44} = 0.002$. M1 L2/3: p = 0.4744. M1 L5/6: p = 0.4345, **d** hippocampus; group: $F_{1,66} = 0.134$, region: $F_{2,66} = 11.937$, group × region: $F_{2,66} = 0.618$. CA1: p = 0.09717. CA3: p = 0.2794. DG: p = 0.6745, **e** prefrontal cortex; group: $F_{1,132} = 0.895$, region: $F_{5,132} = 16.458$, group × region: $F_{5,132} = 0.476$. dAC L2/3: p = 0.4839. dAC L5/6: p = 0.3845. PL L2/3: p = 0.9320. PL L5/6: p = 0.3263. IL L2/3: p = 0.4270. IL L5/6: p = 0.5232, **f** M1; group: $F_{1,44} = 3.048$, region: $F_{1,44} = 0.636$, group × region: $F_{1,44} = 0.144$. M1 L2/3: p = 0.3391. M1 L5/6: p = 0.1401, **g** hippocampus; group: $F_{1,66} = 0.145$, region: $F_{2,66} = 1.550$, group × region: $F_{2,66} = 0.730$. CA1: p = 0.6958. CA3: p = 0.2359. DG: p = 0.8866, **h** prefrontal cortex; group: $F_{1,114} = 0.132$, region: $F_{5,114} = 9.911$, group × region: $F_{5,114} = 6.183$. dAC L2/3: p = 0.9590. dAC L5/6: p = 0.2913. PL L2/3: p = 0.3957. PL L5/6: p = 0.1294. IL L5/6: p = 0.4050, **i** M1; group: $F_{1,44} = 3.446$, region: $F_{1,44} = 0.060$, group × region: $F_{1,44} = 0.6514$. M1 L2/3: p = 0.1093. M1 L5/6: p = 0.3271, **j** hippocampus; group: $F_{1,66} = 0.012$, region: $F_{2,66} = 3.619$, group × region: $F_{2,66} = 0.617$. CA1: p = 0.4328. CA3: p = 0.8622. DG: p = 0.4441, **k** prefrontal cortex; group: $F_{1,116} = 0.886$, region: $F_{5,116} = 17.793$, group × region: $F_{5,116} = 0.905$. dAC L2/3: p = 0.9922. dAC L5/6: p = 0.2344. PL L2/3: p = 0.9398. PL L5/6: p = 0.1568. IL L2/3: p = 0.3948. IL L5/6: p = 0.2722, **l** M1; group: $F_{1,44} = 6.832$, region: $F_{1,44} = 3.364$, group × region: $F_{1,44} = 0.049$. M1 L2/3: p = 0.0977. M1 L5/6: p = 0.0512

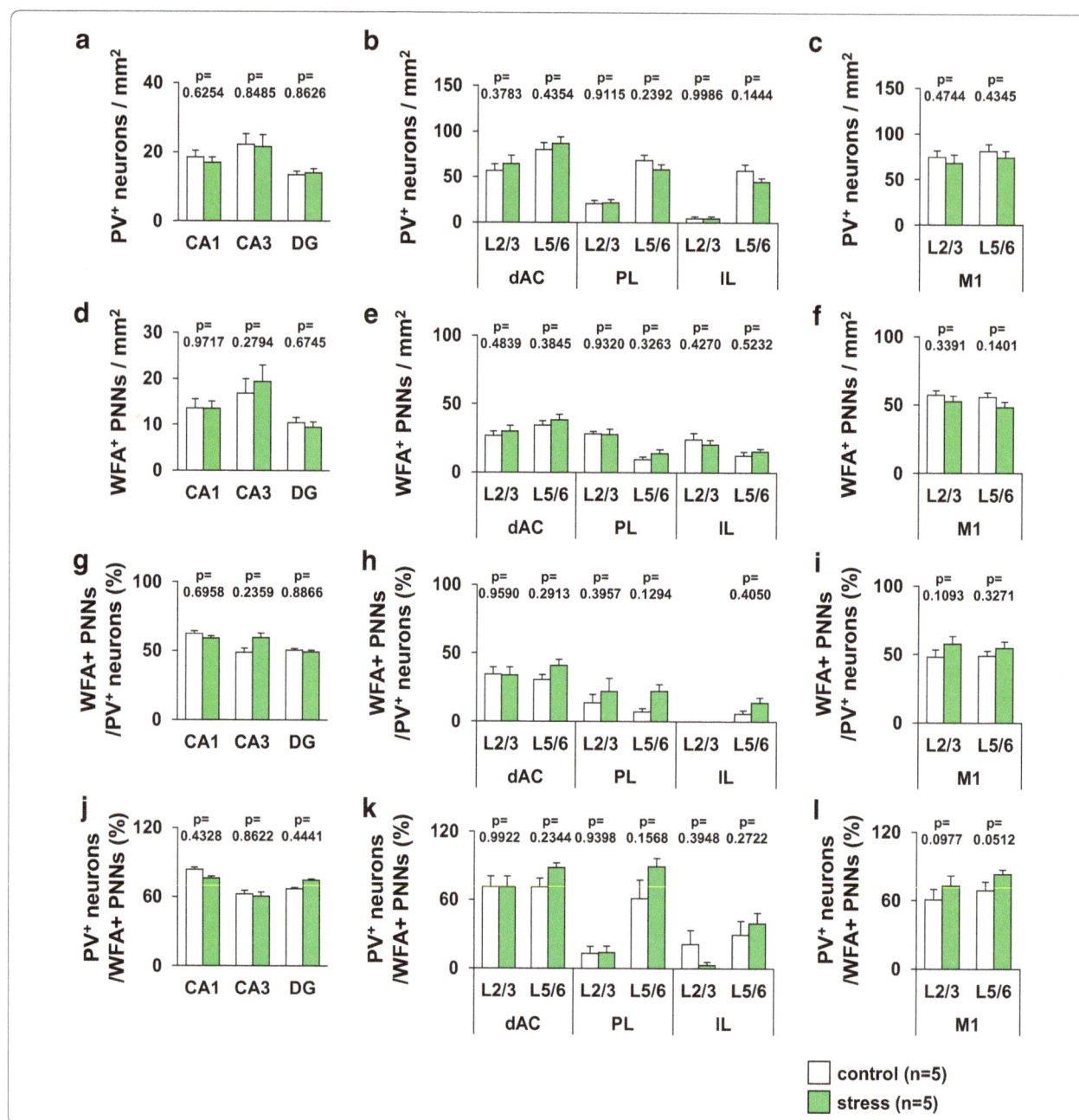

L2/3 = 40, L5/6 = 57; IL: L2/3 = 17, L5/6 = 65; M1: L2/3 = 71, L5/6 = 73; CA = 36; CA3 = 36; DG = 36) from control mice, and 567 cells (dAC: L2/3 = 66; L5/6 = 73; PL: L2/3 = 30, L5/6 = 65; IL: L2/3 = 14, L5/6 = 67; M1: L2/3 = 72, L5/6 = 72; CA = 36; CA3 = 36; DG = 36) from juvenile stressed mice. In the CA3 of the hippocampus and L2/3 of the dAC, the area of the soma of PV neurons was smaller in juvenile stressed than in control mice (Fig. 11a, b). No significant differences in soma size were found in the PV neurons of the primary motor

cortex between the control and the juvenile stressed mice groups (Fig. 11c).

Juvenile stress did not change the number of Cat-315-positive PNNs

We examined the effect of juvenile stress on the expression of aggrecan in several brain regions of the juvenile stressed and control mice. The anti-aggrecan antibody Cat-315 is frequently used as a marker of aggrecan-expression on PNNs. We observed more WFA-positive

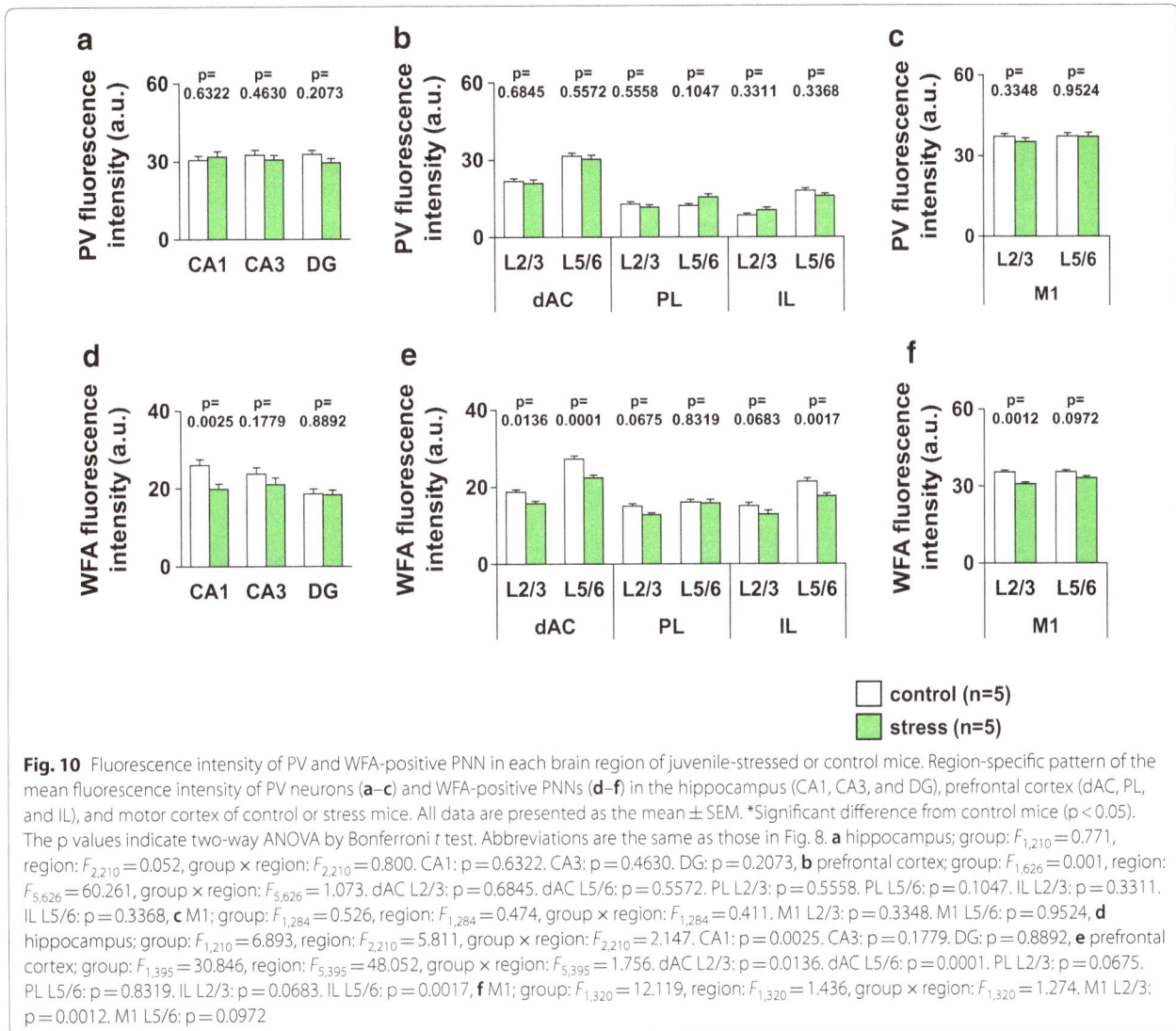

Fig. 10 Fluorescence intensity of PV and WFA-positive PNN in each brain region of juvenile-stressed or control mice. Region-specific pattern of the mean fluorescence intensity of PV neurons (**a–c**) and WFA-positive PNNs (**d–f**) in the hippocampus (CA1, CA3, and DG), prefrontal cortex (dAC, PL, and IL), and motor cortex of control or stress mice. All data are presented as the mean ± SEM. *Significant difference from control mice (p < 0.05). The p values indicate two-way ANOVA by Bonferroni t test. Abbreviations are the same as those in Fig. 8. **a** hippocampus; group: $F_{1,210} = 0.771$, region: $F_{2,210} = 0.052$, group × region: $F_{2,210} = 0.800$. CA1: p = 0.6322. CA3: p = 0.4630. DG: p = 0.2073, **b** prefrontal cortex; group: $F_{1,626} = 0.001$, region: $F_{5,626} = 60.261$, group × region: $F_{5,626} = 1.073$. dAC L2/3: p = 0.6845. dAC L5/6: p = 0.5572. PL L2/3: p = 0.5558. PL L5/6: p = 0.1047. IL L2/3: p = 0.3311. IL L5/6: p = 0.3368, **c** M1; group: $F_{1,284} = 0.526$, region: $F_{1,284} = 0.474$, group × region: $F_{1,284} = 0.411$. M1 L2/3: p = 0.3348. M1 L5/6: p = 0.9524, **d** hippocampus; group: $F_{1,210} = 6.893$, region: $F_{2,210} = 5.811$, group × region: $F_{2,210} = 2.147$. CA1: p = 0.0025. CA3: p = 0.1779. DG: p = 0.8892, **e** prefrontal cortex; group: $F_{1,395} = 30.846$, region: $F_{5,395} = 48.052$, group × region: $F_{5,395} = 1.756$. dAC L2/3: p = 0.0136. dAC L5/6: p = 0.0001. PL L2/3: p = 0.0675. PL L5/6: p = 0.8319. IL L2/3: p = 0.0683. IL L5/6: p = 0.0017, **f** M1; group: $F_{1,320} = 12.119$, region: $F_{1,320} = 1.436$, group × region: $F_{1,320} = 1.274$. M1 L2/3: p = 0.0012. M1 L5/6: p = 0.0972

PNNs in the mouse cerebral cortex at P30, while in some brain regions, Cat-315-positive PNN was not yet expressed at P30 (Fig. 12a–d, a′–d′). We did not observe Cat-315-positive PNNs in the mouse prefrontal cortex.

Further, we quantified the number of Cat-315-positive PNNs in the hippocampus and primary motor cortex of the juvenile stressed and control mice (Fig. 12e, f). There was no difference in the density of Cat-315-positive PNNs between juvenile stressed and control mice (Fig. 12e, f). To examine whether juvenile stress affects Cat-315-positive PNN component expression on WFA-positive PNNs in the hippocampus and primary motor cortex of juvenile stressed mice, we quantified the percentage of WFA-positive PNNs co-localized with Cat-315-positive PNNs, and it was similar between the juvenile stressed and control mice (Fig. 12g, h).

Juvenile stress did not affect immune activation in the central nervous system

To examine whether juvenile stress affects immune activation in the central nervous system of juvenile stressed mice, we observed the morphology of Iba-1-positive microglia in the hippocampus, prefrontal cortex, and primary motor cortex (Fig. 13). Monoclonal antibody Iba-1 is frequently used as a comprehensive marker of microglia. There was no significant difference in the morphology of Iba-1-positive microglia between the control and juvenile stressed mice in the hippocampus, prefrontal cortex, and primary motor cortex (Fig. 13).

Discussion

In this study, we investigated the influence of stress on behavioral abnormalities and on the development of PV neurons and WFA-positive PNNs in juvenile and adult

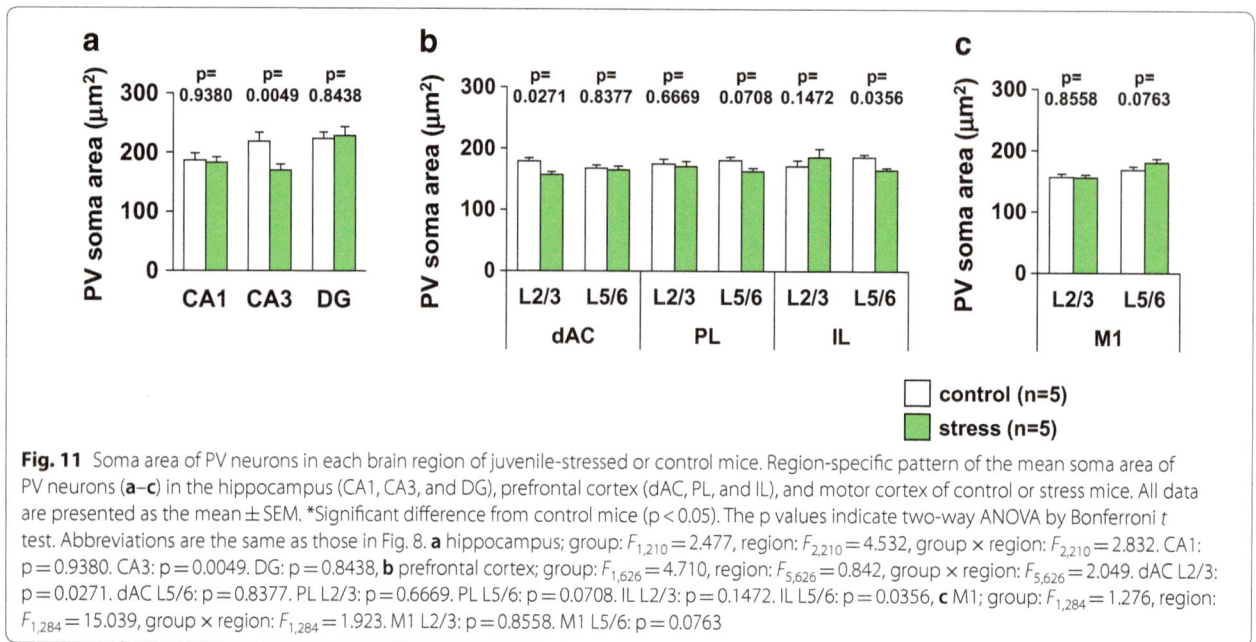

Fig. 11 Soma area of PV neurons in each brain region of juvenile-stressed or control mice. Region-specific pattern of the mean soma area of PV neurons (**a–c**) in the hippocampus (CA1, CA3, and DG), prefrontal cortex (dAC, PL, and IL), and motor cortex of control or stress mice. All data are presented as the mean ± SEM. *Significant difference from control mice ($p < 0.05$). The p values indicate two-way ANOVA by Bonferroni t test. Abbreviations are the same as those in Fig. 8. **a** hippocampus; group: $F_{1,210} = 2.477$, region: $F_{2,210} = 4.532$, group × region: $F_{2,210} = 2.832$. CA1: $p = 0.9380$. CA3: $p = 0.0049$. DG: $p = 0.8438$, **b** prefrontal cortex; group: $F_{1,626} = 4.710$, region: $F_{5,626} = 0.842$, group × region: $F_{5,626} = 2.049$. dAC L2/3: $p = 0.0271$. dAC L5/6: $p = 0.8377$. PL L2/3: $p = 0.6669$. PL L5/6: $p = 0.0708$. IL L2/3: $p = 0.1472$. IL L5/6: $p = 0.0356$, **c** M1; group: $F_{1,284} = 1.276$, region: $F_{1,284} = 15.039$, group × region: $F_{1,284} = 1.923$. M1 L2/3: $p = 0.8558$. M1 L5/6: $p = 0.0763$

mice. We discovered that juvenile stress causes increased activity, decreased depressive-like behavior, and social deficits in mice. Furthermore, we revealed that the fluorescence intensity of WFA-positive PNNs decreased in the central nervous system of juvenile stressed mice. These results suggest that juvenile stress affects the development of the mouse brain and causes behavioral abnormalities different from those seen in the case of stressed mature mice.

Juvenile stressed mice had lower body weight and decreased grip strength than control mice. Using the present stress program, mature mice did not show physical changes. Previous studies using juvenile rats and mice also reported that body weight decreases owing to juvenile stress [70, 78]. Decreased essential enzyme secretion for normal cell growth, decreased DNA synthesis, and reduced growth hormone have been implicated as the underlying mechanisms [79, 80]. Indeed, in human studies, it has been reported that the weight of stressed adolescents is lower than that of healthy children [81]. Decreased body weight during the developmental stage may be an indication that the individual is experiencing stress [82].

In the new home cage, juvenile stressed mice showed excessive activity in the first 30 min compared to control mice. In the case of mature mice, such hyperactive behaviors were not observed. In mature mice, the activity level decreases or does not change owing to chronic stress [83–86]. Hyperactivity is a symptom of neuropsychiatric disorders, such as autism spectrum disorder (ASD), and attention deficit hyperactivity disorder (ADHD) [87–90].

Juvenile stressed mice had increased total distance traveled in the elevated plus maze test compared to control mice. An increased total distance seen in the elevated plus maze test may indicate increased locomotor activity or maladaptive-like behavior to the new environment [91]. However, in juvenile stressed mice, increased activity was not observed in all behavioral tests. There were no significant differences in the percentage of time spent in the open arms between the juvenile-stressed and control group mice in the elevated plus maze test. In studies using rats, decreased anxiety-like behavior caused by juvenile stress has been reported [92, 93]. Further studies are needed to elucidate the detailed mechanism.

In this study, depressive-like behavior was decreased in juvenile stressed mice in the Porsolt forced swim test, compared to control mice. Previous studies reported that depressive-like behaviors increase when the animals are exposed to chronic stress [94–98]. In this study, stressed mature mice did not show depressive-like behavior. This result may be due to a shorter stress period than that used in other chronically stressed models [78, 99]. Differences between juvenile stressed and adult stressed mice have also been reported in other studies [78]. It is suggested that these are due to differences in released corticosterone, hypothalamic–pituitary–adrenal depressive-like behavior function, and brain developmental stage [14, 100]. Further studies are needed to elucidate the detailed mechanism; however, based on our results, it is suggested that juvenile mice are more sensitive to stress than adult mice.

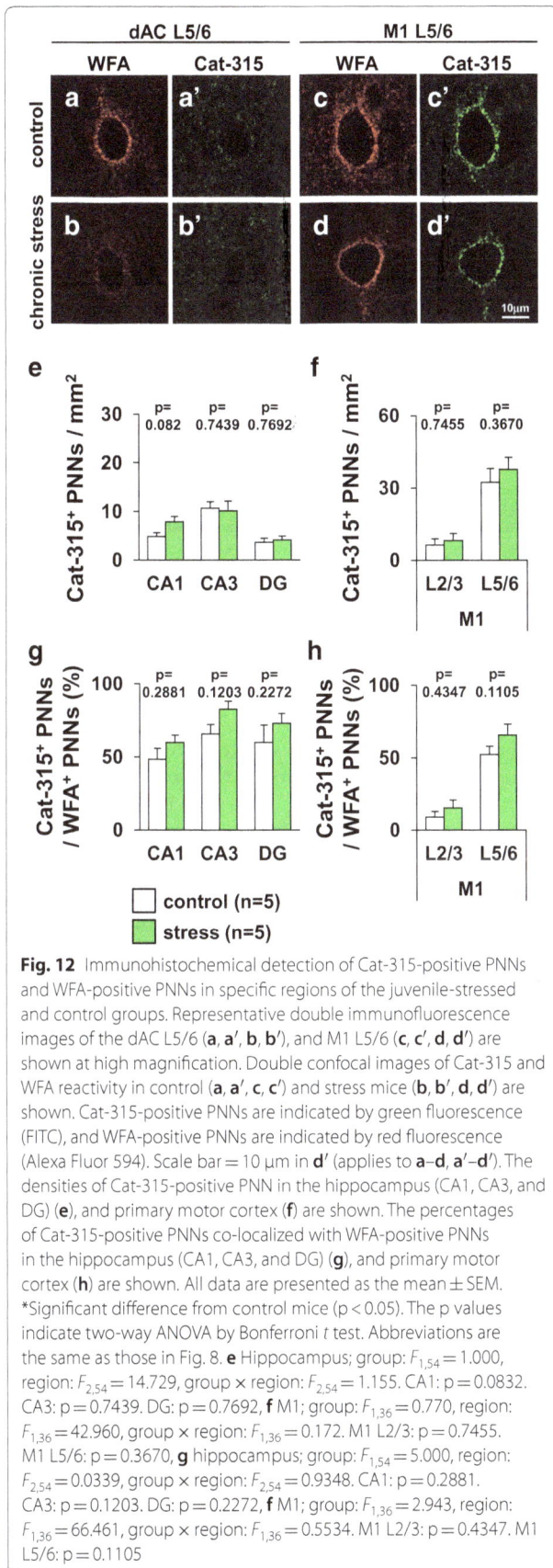

Fig. 12 Immunohistochemical detection of Cat-315-positive PNNs and WFA-positive PNNs in specific regions of the juvenile-stressed and control groups. Representative double immunofluorescence images of the dAC L5/6 (**a**, **a'**, **b**, **b'**), and M1 L5/6 (**c**, **c'**, **d**, **d'**) are shown at high magnification. Double confocal images of Cat-315 and WFA reactivity in control (**a**, **a'**, **c**, **c'**) and stress mice (**b**, **b'**, **d**, **d'**) are shown. Cat-315-positive PNNs are indicated by green fluorescence (FITC), and WFA-positive PNNs are indicated by red fluorescence (Alexa Fluor 594). Scale bar = 10 μm in **d'** (applies to **a–d**, **a'–d'**). The densities of Cat-315-positive PNN in the hippocampus (CA1, CA3, and DG) (**e**), and primary motor cortex (**f**) are shown. The percentages of Cat-315-positive PNNs co-localized with WFA-positive PNNs in the hippocampus (CA1, CA3, and DG) (**g**), and primary motor cortex (**h**) are shown. All data are presented as the mean ± SEM. *Significant difference from control mice (p < 0.05). The p values indicate two-way ANOVA by Bonferroni t test. Abbreviations are the same as those in Fig. 8. **e** Hippocampus; group: $F_{1,54} = 1.000$, region: $F_{2,54} = 14.729$, group × region: $F_{2,54} = 1.155$. CA1: p = 0.0832. CA3: p = 0.7439. DG: p = 0.7692. **f** M1; group: $F_{1,36} = 0.770$, region: $F_{1,36} = 42.960$, group × region: $F_{1,36} = 0.172$. M1 L2/3: p = 0.7455. M1 L5/6: p = 0.3670. **g** hippocampus; group: $F_{1,54} = 5.000$, region: $F_{2,54} = 0.0339$, group × region: $F_{2,54} = 0.9348$. CA1: p = 0.2881. CA3: p = 0.1203. DG: p = 0.2272. **f** M1; group: $F_{1,36} = 2.943$, region: $F_{1,36} = 66.461$, group × region: $F_{1,36} = 0.5534$. M1 L2/3: p = 0.4347. M1 L5/6: p = 0.1105

In juvenile stressed mice, social preference to stranger mice was reduced compared with control mice. When adult mice were exposed to chronic stress, there was no reduction in sociability [101, 102]. When genetic abnormality occurs in the energy metabolism of PV neurons, social ability is altered in mice [103]. In mice deficient in PV protein, abnormal social behavior and decreased memory ability, such as those seen in ASD-like behavioral abnormalities was observed [46]. In this study, we found WFA-positive PNNs reduced fluorescence intensity around PV neurons in juvenile stressed mice, and it is possible that PV neurons were functioning abnormally. Therefore, in juvenile stressed mice, social preference to stranger mice was altered compared with control mice. Chronic stress affects social interaction and function of paraventricular nucleus [104, 105]. Even in juvenile stressed mice, there may be abnormality in paraventricular nucleus. Further research is necessary to elucidate this mechanism. Abnormal social behavior is a symptom of neuropsychiatric disorders, such as ASD, ADHD, and schizophrenia [106–108].

Adult mice showed an alternation percentage statistically above chance level (50% of alternation) whereas juvenile mice did not in a Y-maze. This indicates that this test is not reliable for juvenile mice.

Juvenile stressed mice showed decreased depressive-like behavior, increased locomotor activity, and abnormal social behavior compared to control mice. It was revealed that chronically stressed juvenile mice showed ADHD- and ASD-like behavioral abnormalities. As described below, there is a possibility that this behavior was caused by PV neuron dysfunction due to decreased PNN condense.

In recent years, it has been shown that the balance between excitation and inhibition in the central nervous system is important for normal brain activity, and any imbalance is believed to cause neuropsychiatric disorder-like behaviors [109, 110]. Abnormalities in the PV neurons have been shown postmortem in the brains of patients with neuropsychiatric disorders, such as schizophrenia and depression [26, 111]. In experimental models, pups born to dams stressed during pregnancy show behavioral abnormalities, indicating decrease in the number of cortical PV neurons and WFA-positive PNNs [112]. The development of PV neurons in the sensory cortex is dependent on sensory inputs, and the development of PV neurons is delayed when sensory inputs are deprived [113–116]. In this study, stress was applied to juvenile mice, but there was no change in both the number of PV neurons and the number of WFA-positive PNNs in the hippocampus, prefrontal cortex, and primary motor cortex. It has been reported that *Vicia villosa* agglutinin (VVA)-positive PNNs increase in the

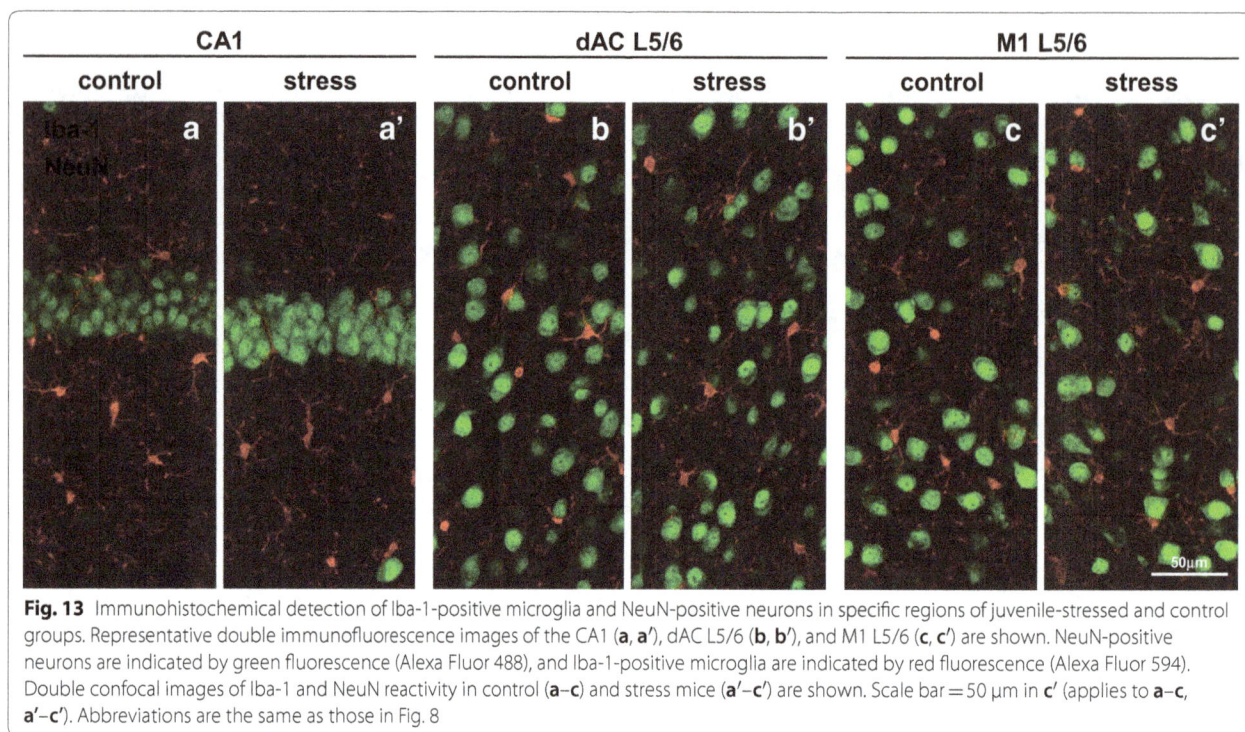

Fig. 13 Immunohistochemical detection of Iba-1-positive microglia and NeuN-positive neurons in specific regions of juvenile-stressed and control groups. Representative double immunofluorescence images of the CA1 (**a**, **a'**), dAC L5/6 (**b**, **b'**), and M1 L5/6 (**c**, **c'**) are shown. NeuN-positive neurons are indicated by green fluorescence (Alexa Fluor 488), and Iba-1-positive microglia are indicated by red fluorescence (Alexa Fluor 594). Double confocal images of Iba-1 and NeuN reactivity in control (**a–c**) and stress mice (**a'–c'**) are shown. Scale bar = 50 μm in **c'** (applies to **a–c**, **a'–c'**). Abbreviations are the same as those in Fig. 8

prefrontal cortex of juvenilehood stressed rats within a few weeks [93]. This study showed that stress applied to juvenile mice for approximately 1 week had no obvious influence on the development of PV neurons.

In this study, it was revealed that the fluorescence intensity of WFA-positive PNN in juvenile stressed mice was decreased in the hippocampus, prefrontal cortex, and primary motor cortex compared to control mice. The PNN is a structure enriched with a special extracellular matrix molecule, and a decreased fluorescence intensity is presumed to signify decreased concentration or change in PNN components [115, 116]. Therefore, it is suggested that there was increased synaptic plasticity and increased vulnerability in the brains of juvenile stressed mice compared with control mice. When genetic abnormality occurs in the PNNs formation, social ability is altered in mice [117–119]. It has been reported that stress at a young age changes the hippocampus structurally and functionally [120, 121]. Juvenile stress causes structural and functional changes in the hippocampus [120, 121]. Both the hippocampus and prefrontal cortex are areas vulnerable to stress [62, 122, 123]. In particular, these areas are sensitive to stress during early childhood and adolescence [124, 125]. It has been reported that experiences in early life dramatically alter the structure and function of the brain after maturation [13, 122], and the alterations in PNN extracellular matrix molecules observed in this

study could be maintained until maturity [91]. Epidemiological studies have shown that juvenile stress is associated with depression, anxiety, PTSD, and suicide development in adulthood [126, 127]. Chronic stress activates microglia in the central nervous system [128]. However, in this study we have not confirm the activated microglia image. Further studies are needed to elucidate the mechanism of PNN abnormality obtained in this study.

Conclusions

The present results indicate that juvenile stress affects brain development and causes behavioral abnormalities resembling behaviors linked to developmental disorders in mice. Juvenile individuals are more sensitive and respond differently to stress than mature individuals. The study results may help establish a method to prevent the onset of neuropsychiatric disorders in both juvenilehood and adolescence.

Abbreviations
ADHD: attention deficit hyperactivity disorder; ASD: autism spectrum disorder; PNN: perineuronal net; PTSD: post-traumatic stress disorder; PV: parvalbumin; WFA: *Wisteria floribunda* agglutinin.

Authors' contributions
All authors had full access to all the study data and take full responsibility for the integrity of the data and the accuracy of the data analysis. HU, MO, TI:

Study concept and design. HU, SS: Acquisition of data. HU, SS: Analysis and interpretation of data. HU, MO: Drafting of the manuscript. SM, NK, KW, YM, SA, TI: Critical revision of the manuscript for important intellectual content. HU, SS: Statistical analysis. MO, SA, TI: Study supervision. All authors read and approved the final manuscript.

Author details

[1] Department of Medical Technology, Kawasaki University of Medical Welfare, 288, Matsushima, Kurashiki, Okayama 701-0193, Japan. [2] Department of Medical Technology, Graduate School of Health Sciences, Okayama University, Okayama 700-8558, Japan. [3] Department of Psychiatry, Kawasaki Medical School, Kurashiki 701-0192, Japan. [4] Department of Neuropsychiatry, Graduate School of Medicine, Dentistry and Pharmaceutical Sciences, Okayama University, Okayama 700-8558, Japan.

Acknowledgements

We thank Y. Nakadoi and M. Masatsugu for technical assistance. We thank the Kawasaki Medical School Central Research Institute for providing the instruments that supported this work. The authors would like to thank Editage (www.editage.jp) for the English language review.

Competing interests

The authors declare that they have no competing interests.

Funding

This research did not receive any specific grant from funding agencies in the public commercial or not-for-profit sectors.

References

1. Costello EJ, Mustillo S, Erkanli A, Keeler G, Angold A. Prevalence and development of psychiatric disorders in childhood and adolescence. Arch Gen Psychiatry. 2003;60:837–44.
2. Jones PB. Adult mental health disorders and their age at onset. Br J Psychiatry Suppl. 2013;54:5–10.
3. Kessler RC, Berglund P, Demler O, Jin R, Merikangas KR, Walters EE. Lifetime prevalence and age-of-onset distributions of DSM-IV disorders in the National Comorbidity Survey Replication. Arch Gen Psychiatry. 2005;62:593–602.
4. Turner RJ, Lloyd DA. Stress burden and the lifetime incidence of psychiatric disorder in young adults: racial and ethnic contrasts. Arch Gen Psychiatry. 2004;61:481–8.
5. Pelcovitz D, Kaplan S, Goldenberg B, Mandel F, Lehane J, Guarrera J. Post-traumatic stress disorder in physically abused adolescents. J Am Acad Child Adolesc Psychiatry. 1994;33:305–12.
6. Finkelhor D, Cross TP, Cantor EN. The justice system for juvenile victims: a comprehensive model of case flow. Trauma Violence Abuse. 2005;6:83–102.
7. Dunn VJ, Abbott RA, Croudace TJ, Wilkinson P, Jones PB, Herbert J, Goodyer IM. Profiles of family-focused adverse experiences through childhood and early adolescence: the ROOTS project a community investigation of adolescent mental health. BMC Psychiatry. 2011;11:109.
8. Shanahan L, Copeland WE, Costello EJ, Angold A. Child-, adolescent- and young adult-onset depressions: differential risk factors in development? Psychol Med. 2011;41:2265–74.
9. Kendler KS, Karkowski LM, Prescott CA. Causal relationship between stressful life events and the onset of major depression. Am J Psychiatry. 1999;156:837–41.
10. Blakemore SJ. Development of the social brain during adolescence. Q J Exp Psychol (Hove). 2008;61:40–9.
11. Caspi A, Roberts BW, Shiner RL. Personality development: stability and change. Annu Rev Psychol. 2005;56:453–84.
12. Gunnar M, Quevedo K. The neurobiology of stress and development. Annu Rev Psychol. 2007;58:145–73.
13. Romeo RD, McEwen BS. Stress and the adolescent brain. Ann N Y Acad Sci. 1094;2006:202–14.
14. Spear LP. The adolescent brain and age-related behavioral manifestations. Neurosci Biobehav Rev. 2000;24:417–63.
15. Casey BJ, Jones RM. Neurobiology of the adolescent brain and behavior: implications for substance use disorders. J Am Acad Child Adolesc Psychiatry. 2010;49:1189–201.
16. Avital A, Richter-Levin G. Exposure to juvenile stress exacerbates the behavioural consequences of exposure to stress in the adult rat. Int J Neuropsychopharmacol. 2005;8:163–73.
17. Pohl J, Olmstead MC, Wynne-Edwards KE, Harkness K, Menard JL. Repeated exposure to stress across the childhood-adolescent period alters rats' anxiety- and depression-like behaviors in adulthood: the importance of stressor type and gender. Behav Neurosci. 2007;121:462–74.
18. Isgor C, Kabbaj M, Akil H, Watson SJ. Delayed effects of chronic variable stress during peripubertal-juvenile period on hippocampal morphology and on cognitive and stress axis functions in rats. Hippocampus. 2004;14:636–48.
19. Barha CK, Brummelte S, Lieblich SE, Galea LA. Chronic restraint stress in adolescence differentially influences hypothalamic–pituitary–adrenal axis function and adult hippocampal neurogenesis in male and female rats. Hippocampus. 2011;21:1216–27.
20. McEwen BS. The neurobiology of stress: from serendipity to clinical relevance. Brain Res. 2000;886:172–89.
21. Agoglia AE, Holstein SE, Small AT, Spanos M, Burrus BM, Hodge CW. Comparison of the adolescent and adult mouse prefrontal cortex proteome. PLoS ONE. 2017;12:e0178391.
22. Semple BD, Blomgren K, Gimlin K, Ferriero DM, Noble-Haeusslein LJ. Brain development in rodents and humans: identifying benchmarks of maturation and vulnerability to injury across species. Prog Neurobiol. 2013;106–107:1–16.
23. Bernheim A, Halfon O, Boutrel B. Controversies about the enhanced vulnerability of the adolescent brain to develop addiction. Front Pharmacol. 2013;4:118.
24. Rice F, Harold GT, Thapar A. Negative life events as an account of age-related differences in the genetic aetiology of depression in childhood and adolescence. J Child Psychol Psychiatry. 2003;44:977–87.
25. Romeo RD. Adolescence: a central event in shaping stress reactivity. Dev Psychobiol. 2010;52:244–53.
26. Lewis DA, Curley AA, Glausier JR, Volk DW. Cortical parvalbumin interneurons and cognitive dysfunction in schizophrenia. Trends Neurosci. 2012;35:57–67.
27. Beasley CL, Reynolds GP. Parvalbumin-immunoreactive neurons are reduced in the prefrontal cortex of schizophrenics. Schizophr Res. 1997;24:349–55.
28. Khundakar A, Morris C, Thomas AJ. The immunohistochemical examination of GABAergic interneuron markers in the dorsolateral prefrontal cortex of patients with late-life depression. Int Psychogeriatr. 2011;23:644–53.
29. Sauer JF, Strüber M, Bartos M. Impaired fast-spiking interneuron function in a genetic mouse model of depression. Elife. 2015;4:e04979.
30. Liang D, Li G, Liao X, Yu D, Wu J, Zhang M. Developmental loss of parvalbumin-positive cells in the prefrontal cortex and psychiatric

anxiety after intermittent hypoxia exposures in neonatal rats might be mediated by NADPH oxidase-2. Behav Brain Res. 2016;296:134–40.

31. Tovote P, Fadok JP, Lüthi A. Neuronal circuits for fear and anxiety. Nat Rev Neurosci. 2015;16:317–31.

32. Zou D, Chen L, Deng D, Jiang D, Dong F, McSweeney C, Zhou Y, Liu L, Chen G, Wu Y, Mao Y. DREADD in parvalbumin interneurons of the dentate gyrus modulates anxiety, social interaction and memory extinction. Curr Mol Med. 2016;16:91–102.

33. Butt SJ, Stacey JA, Teramoto Y, Vagnoni C. A role for GABAergic interneuron diversity in circuit development and plasticity of the neonatal cerebral cortex. Curr Opin Neurobiol. 2017;43:149–55.

34. Sultan KT, Shi SH. Generation of diverse cortical inhibitory interneurons. Wiley Interdiscip Rev Dev Biol. 2018. https://doi.org/10.1002/wdev.306.

35. Wood KC, Blackwell JM, Geffen MN. Cortical inhibitory interneurons control sensory processing. Curr Opin Neurobiol. 2017;46:200–7.

36. Chu J, Anderson SA. Development of cortical interneurons. Neuropsychopharmacology. 2015;40:16–23.

37. Gonzalez-Burgos G, Cho RY, Lewis DA. Alterations in cortical network oscillations and parvalbumin neurons in schizophrenia. Biol Psychiatry. 2015;77:1031–40.

38. Takano T. Interneuron dysfunction in syndromic autism: recent advances. Dev Neurosci. 2015;37:467–75.

39. Jacob J. Cortical interneuron dysfunction in epilepsy associated with autism spectrum disorders. Epilepsia. 2016;57:182–93.

40. Konradi C, Yang CK, Zimmerman EI, Lohmann KM, Gresch P, Pantazopoulos H, Berretta S, Heckers S. Hippocampal interneurons are abnormal in schizophrenia. Schizophr Res. 2011;131:165–73.

41. Urakawa S, Takamoto K, Hori E, Sakai N, Ono T, Nishijo H. Rearing in enriched environment increases parvalbumin-positive small neurons in the amygdala and decreases anxiety-like behavior of male rats. BMC Neurosci. 2013;14:13.

42. Le Magueresse C, Monyer H. GABAergic interneurons shape the functional maturation of the cortex. Neuron. 2013;77:388–405.

43. Patz S, Grabert J, Gorba T, Wirth MJ, Wahle P. Parvalbumin expression in visual cortical interneurons depends on neuronal activity and TrkB ligands during an Early period of postnatal development. Cereb Cortex. 2004;14:342–51.

44. Sohal VS, Zhang F, Yizhar O, Deisseroth K. Parvalbumin neurons and gamma rhythms enhance cortical circuit performance. Nature. 2009;459:698–702.

45. Massi L, Lagler M, Hartwich K, Borhegyi Z, Somogyi P, Klausberger T. Temporal dynamics of parvalbumin-expressing axo-axonic and basket cells in the rat medial prefrontal cortex in vivo. J Neurosci. 2012;32:16496–502.

46. Wöhr M, Orduz D, Gregory P, Moreno H, Khan U, Vörckel KJ, Wolfer DP, Welzl H, Gall D, Schiffmann SN, Schwaller B. Lack of parvalbumin in mice leads to behavioral deficits relevant to all human autism core symptoms and related neural morphofunctional abnormalities. Transl Psychiatry. 2015;5:e525.

47. Xenos D, Kamceva M, Tomasi S, Cardin JA, Schwartz ML, Vaccarino FM. Loss of TrkB signaling in parvalbumin-expressing basket cells results in network activity disruption and abnormal behavior. Cereb Cortex. 2017;18:1–15.

48. Song I, Dityatev A. Crosstalk between glia, extracellular matrix and neurons. Brain Res Bull. 2018;136:101–8.

49. Slaker M, Blacktop JM, Sorg BA. Caught in the net: perineuronal nets and addiction. Neural Plast. 2016;2016:7538208.

50. Giamanco KA, Matthews RT. Deconstructing the perineuronal net: cellular contributions and molecular composition of the neuronal extracellular matrix. Neuroscience. 2012;218:367–84.

51. Kwok JC, Carulli D, Fawcett JW. In vitro modeling of perineuronal nets: hyaluronan synthase and link protein are necessary for their formation and integrity. J Neurochem. 2010;114:1447–59.

52. Bandtlow CE, Zimmermann DR. Proteoglycans in the developing brain: new conceptual insights for old proteins. Physiol Rev. 2000;80:1267–90.

53. Yamaguchi Y. Lecticans: organizers of the brain extracellular matrix. Cell Mol Life Sci. 2000;57:276–89.

54. Seeger G, Lüth HJ, Winkelmann E, Brauer K. Distribution patterns of *Wisteria floribunda* agglutinin binding sites and parvalbumin-immunoreactive neurons in the human visual cortex: a double-labelling study. J Hirnforsch. 1996;37:351–66.

55. Slaker M, Blacktop JM, Sorg BA. Caught in the net: perineuronal nets and addiction. Neural Plast. 2016;2016:7538208.

56. Hensch TK. Critical period plasticity in local cortical circuits. Nat Rev Neurosci. 2005;6:877–88.

57. Lensjø KK, Lepperød ME, Dick G, Hafting T, Fyhn M. Removal of perineuronal nets unlocks juvenile plasticity through network mechanisms of decreased inhibition and increased gamma activity. J Neurosci. 2017;37:1269–83.

58. Pizzorusso T, Medini P, Berardi N, Chierzi S, Fawcett JW, Maffei L. Reactivation of ocular dominance plasticity in the adult visual cortex. Science. 2002;298:1248–51.

59. Balmer TS. Perineuronal nets enhance the excitability of fast-spiking neurons. eNeuro. 2016;3:4.

60. Fawcett JW. The extracellular matrix in plasticity and regeneration after CNS injury and neurodegenerative disease. Prog Brain Res. 2015;218:213–26.

61. Cabungcal JH, Steullet P, Morishita H, Kraftsik R, Cuenod M, Hensch TK, Do KQ. Perineuronal nets protect fast-spiking interneurons against oxidative stress. Proc Natl Acad Sci USA. 2013;110:9130–5.

62. Ueno H, Suemitsu S, Murakami S, Kitamura N, Wani K, Okamoto M, Matsumoto Y, Ishihara T. Region-specific impairments in parvalbumin interneurons in social isolation-reared mice. Neuroscience. 2017;359:196–208.

63. De Luca C, Papa M. Looking inside the matrix: perineuronal nets in plasticity, maladaptive plasticity and neurological disorders. Neurochem Res. 2016;41:1507–15.

64. Pantazopoulos H, Berretta S. In sickness and in health: perineuronal nets and synaptic plasticity in psychiatric disorders. Neural Plast. 2016;2016:9847696.

65. Yoshioka N, Miyata S, Tamada A, Watanabe Y, Kawasaki A, Kitagawa H, Takao K, Miyakawa T, Takeuchi K, Igarashi M. Abnormalities in perineuronal nets and behavior in mice lacking CSGalNAcT1, a key enzyme in chondroitin sulfate synthesis. Mol Brain. 2017;10:47.

66. Banerjee SB, Gutzeit VA, Baman J, Aoued HS, Doshi NK, Liu RC, Ressler KJ. Perineuronal nets in the adult sensory cortex are necessary for fear learning. Neuron. 2017;95:169–79.

67. Popelář J, Díaz Gómez M, Lindovský J, Rybalko N, Burianová J, Oohashi T, Syka J. The absence of brain-specific link protein Bral2 in perineuronal nets hampers auditory temporal resolution and neural adaptation in mice. Physiol Res. 2017;66:867–80.

68. Umemori J, Takao K, Koshimizu H, Hattori S, Furuse T, Wakana S, Miyakawa T. ENU-mutagenesis mice with a non-synonymous mutation in Grin1 exhibit abnormal anxiety-like behaviors, impaired fear memory, and decreased acoustic startle response. BMC Res Notes. 2013;6:203.

69. Watanabe Y, Tsujimura A, Takao K, Nishi K, Ito Y, Yasuhara Y, Nakatomi Y, Yokoyama C, Fukui K, Miyakawa T, Tanaka M. Relaxin-3-deficient mice showed slight alteration in anxiety-related behavior. Front Behav Neurosci. 2011;5:50.

70. Brydges NM, Hall L, Nicolson R, Holmes MC, Hall J. The effects of juvenile stress on anxiety, cognitive bias and decision making in adulthood: a rat model. PLoS ONE. 2012;7:e48143.

71. Ducottet C, Griebel G, Belzung C. Effects of the selective nonpeptide corticotropin-releasing factor receptor 1 antagonist antalarmin in the chronic mild stress model of depression in mice. Prog Neuropsychopharmacol Biol Psychiatry. 2003;27:625–31.

72. Willner P, Towell A, Sampson D, Sophokleous S, Muscat R. Reduction of sucrose preference by chronic unpredictable mild stress, and its restoration by a tricyclic antidepressant. Psychopharmacology. 1987;93:358–64.

73. Li YF, Chen HX, Liu Y, Zhang YZ, Liu YQ, Li J. Agmatine increases proliferation of cultured hippocampal progenitor cells and hippocampal neurogenesis in chronically stressed mice. Acta Pharmacol Sin. 2006;27:1395–400.

74. Nakatani J, Tamada K, Hatanaka F, Ise S, Ohta H, Inoue K, Tomonaga S, Watanabe Y, Chung YJ, Banerjee R, Iwamoto K, Kato T, Okazawa M, Yamauchi K, Tanda K, Takao K, Miyakawa T, Bradley A, Takumi T. Abnormal behavior in a chromosome-engineered mouse model for human 15q11-13 duplication seen in autism. Cell. 2009;137:1235–46.

75. Tamada K, Tomonaga S, Hatanaka F, Nakai N, Takao K, Miyakawa T, Nakatani J, Takumi T. Decreased exploratory activity in a mouse model

of 15q duplication syndrome; implications for disturbance of serotonin signaling. PLoS ONE. 2010;15:e15126.

76. Kouzu Y, Moriya T, Takeshima H, Yoshioka T, Shibata S. Mutant mice lacking ryanodine receptor type 3 exhibit deficits of contextual fear conditioning and activation of calcium/calmodulin-dependent protein kinase II in the hippocampus. Brain Res Mol Brain Res. 2000;76:142–50.

77. Ueno H, Suemitsu S, Matsumoto Y, Okamoto M. Sensory deprivation during early postnatal period alters the density of interneurons in the mouse prefrontal cortex. Neural Plast. 2015;2015:753179.

78. Sadler AM, Bailey SJ. Repeated daily restraint stress induces adaptive behavioural changes in both adult and juvenile mice. Physiol Behav. 2016;167:313–23.

79. Chapillon P, Patin V, Roy V, Vincent A, Caston J. Effects of pre- and postnatal stimulation on developmental, emotional, and cognitive aspects in rodents: a review. Dev Psychobiol. 2002;41:373–87.

80. Viveros MP, Llorente R, Díaz F, Romero-Zerbo SY, Bermudez-Silva FJ, Rodríguez de Fonseca F, Argente J, Chowen JA. Maternal deprivation has sexually dimorphic long-term effects on hypothalamic cell-turnover, body weight and circulating hormone levels. Horm Behav. 2010;58:808–19.

81. van Jaarsveld CH, Fidler JA, Steptoe A, Boniface D, Wardle J. Perceived stress and weight gain in adolescence: a longitudinal analysis. Obesity (Silver Spring). 2009;17:2155–61.

82. Jeong JY, Lee DH, Kang SS. Effects of chronic restraint stress on body weight, food intake, and hypothalamic gene expressions in mice. Endocrinol Metab. 2013;28:288–96.

83. Litteljohn D, Nelson E, Hayley S. IFN-γ differentially modulates memory-related processes under basal and chronic stressor conditions. Front Cell Neurosci. 2014;8:391.

84. DeVallance E, Riggs D, Jackson B, Parkulo T, Zaslau S, Chantler PD, Olfert IM, Bryner RW. Effect of chronic stress on running wheel activity in mice. PLoS ONE. 2017;12:e0184829.

85. Yu H, Wang DD, Wang Y, Liu T, Lee FS, Chen ZY. Variant brain-derived neurotrophic factor Val66Met polymorphism alters vulnerability to stress and response to antidepressants. J Neurosci. 2012;32:4092–101.

86. Yoon SH, Kim BH, Ye SK, Kim MH. Chronic non-social stress affects depressive behaviors but not anxiety in mice. Korean J Physiol Pharmacol. 2014;18:263–8.

87. Velligan DI, Diamond P, Glahn DC, Ritch J, Maples N, Castillo D, Miller AL. The reliability and validity of the Test of Adaptive Behavior in Schizophrenia (TABS). Psychiatry Res. 2007;151:55–66.

88. Pugliese CE, Anthony L, Strang JF, Dudley K, Wallace GL, Kenworthy L. Increasing adaptive behavior skill deficits from childhood to adolescence in autism spectrum disorder: role of executive function. J Autism Dev Disord. 2015;45:1579–87.

89. Matejcek Z. Is ADHD adaptive or non-adaptive behavior? Neuro Endocrinol Lett. 2003;24:148–50.

90. Stein MA, Szumowski E, Blondis TA, Roizen NJ. Adaptive skills dysfunction in ADD and ADHD children. J Child Psychol Psychiatry. 1995;36:663–70.

91. Matsumoto Y, Katayama K, Okamoto T, Yamada K, Takashima N, Nagao S, Aruga J. Impaired auditory-vestibular functions and behavioral abnormalities of Slitrk6-deficient mice. PLoS ONE. 2011;6:e16497.

92. Komada M, Takao K, Miyakawa T. Elevated plus maze for mice. J Vis Exp. 2008;22:22.

93. de Araújo Costa Folha OA, Bahia CP, de Aguiar GPS, Herculano AM, Coelho NLG, de Sousa MBC, Shiramizu VKM, de Menezes Galvão AC, de Carvalho WA, Pereira A. Effect of chronic stress during adolescence in prefrontal cortex structure and function. Behav Brain Res. 2017;326:44–51.

94. Burokas A, Martín-García E, Gutiérrez-Cuesta J, Rojas S, Herance JR, Gispert JD, Serra MÁ, Maldonado R. Relationships between serotonergic and cannabinoid system in depressive-like behavior: a PET study with [11C]-DASB. J Neurochem. 2014;130:126–35.

95. Yao B, Cheng Y, Wang Z, Li Y, Chen L, Huang L, Zhang W, Chen D, Wu H, Tang B, Jin P. DNA N6-methyladenine is dynamically regulated in the mouse brain following environmental stress. Nat Commun. 2017;8:1122.

96. Monteiro S, Roque S, de Sá-Calçada D, Sousa N, Correia-Neves M, Cerqueira JJ. An efficient chronic unpredictable stress protocol to induce stress-related responses in C57BL/6 mice. Front Psychiatry. 2015;6:6.

97. Miyata S, Koyama Y, Takemoto K, Yoshikawa K, Ishikawa T, Taniguchi M, Inoue K, Aoki M, Hori O, Katayama T, Tohyama M. Plasma corticosterone activates SGK1 and induces morphological changes in oligodendrocytes in corpus callosum. PLoS ONE. 2011;6:e19859.

98. Chu X, Zhou Y, Hu Z, Lou J, Song W, Li J, Liang X, Chen C, Wang S, Yang B, Chen L, Zhang X, Song J, Dong Y, Chen S, He L, Xie Q, Chen X, Li W. 24-hour-restraint stress induces long-term depressive-like phenotypes in mice. Sci Rep. 2016;6:32935.

99. Jeong JY, Lee DH, Kang SS. Effects of chronic restraint stress on body weight, food intake, and hypothalamic gene expressions in mice. Endocrinol Metab (Seoul). 2013;28:288–96.

100. Lyons DM, Parker KJ, Schatzberg AF. Animal models of early life stress: implications for understanding resilience. Dev Psychobiol. 2010;52:616–24.

101. Trainor BC, Pride MC, Villalon Landeros R, Knoblauch NW, Takahashi EY, Silva AL, Crean KK. Sex differences in social interaction behavior following social defeat stress in the monogamous California mouse (Peromyscus californicus). PLoS ONE. 2011;6:e17405.

102. Greenberg GD, Laman-Maharg A, Campi KL, Voigt H, Orr VN, Schaal L, Trainor BC. Sex differences in stress-induced social withdrawal: role of brain derived neurotrophic factor in the bed nucleus of the stria terminalis. Front Behav Neurosci. 2014;7:223.

103. Inan M, Zhao M, Manuszak M, Karakaya C, Rajadhyaksha AM, Pickel VM, Schwartz TH, Goldstein PA, Manfredi G. Energy deficit in parvalbumin neurons leads to circuit dysfunction, impaired sensory gating and social disability. Neurobiol Dis. 2016;93:35–46.

104. Li J, Li HX, Shou XJ, Xu XJ, Song TJ, Han SP, Zhang R, Han JS. Effects of chronic restraint stress on social behaviors and the number of hypothalamic oxytocin neurons in male rats. Neuropeptides. 2016;60:21–8.

105. Herman JP, Flak J, Jankord R. Chronic stress plasticity in the hypothalamic paraventricular nucleus. Prog Brain Res. 2008;170:353–64.

106. Brüne M, Schaub D, Juckel G, Langdon R. Social skills and behavioral problems in schizophrenia: the role of mental state attribution, neuro-cognition and clinical symptomatology. Psychiatry Res. 2011;190:9–17.

107. O'Haire ME, McKenzie SJ, Beck AM, Slaughter V. Social behaviors increase in children with autism in the presence of animals compared to toys. PLoS ONE. 2013;8:e57010.

108. Alessandri SM. Attention, play, and social behavior in ADHD preschoolers. J Abnorm Child Psychol. 1992;20:289–302.

109. Marín O. Interneuron dysfunction in psychiatric disorders. Nat Rev Neurosci. 2012;13:107–20.

110. Rossignol E. Genetics and function of neocortical GABAergic interneurons in neurodevelopmental disorders. Neural Plast. 2011;2011:649325.

111. Enwright JF III, Huo Z, Arion D, Corradi JP, Tseng G, Lewis DA. Transcriptome alterations of prefrontal cortical parvalbumin neurons in schizophrenia. Mol Psychiatry. 2017. https://doi.org/10.1038/mp.2017.216.

112. Paylor JW, Lins BR, Greba Q, Moen N, Moraes RS, Howland JG, Winship IR. Developmental disruption of perineuronal nets in the medial prefrontal cortex after maternal immune activation. Sci Rep. 2016;6:37580.

113. Jiao Y, Zhang Z, Zhang C, Wang X, Sakata K, Lu B, Sun QQ. A key mechanism underlying sensory experience-dependent maturation of neocortical GABAergic circuits in vivo. Proc Natl Acad Sci USA. 2011;108:12131–6.

114. Koh DX, Sng JC. HDAC1 negatively regulates Bdnf and Pvalb required for parvalbumin interneuron maturation in an experience-dependent manner. J Neurochem. 2016;139:369–80.

115. Chattopadhyaya B, Di Cristo G, Higashiyama H, Knott GW, Kuhlman SJ, Welker E, Huang ZJ. Experience and activity-dependent maturation of perisomatic GABAergic innervation in primary visual cortex during a postnatal critical period. J Neurosci. 2004;24:9598–611.

116. Ueno H, Suemitsu S, Okamoto M, Matsumoto Y, Ishihara T. Sensory experience-dependent formation of perineuronal nets and expression of Cat-315 immunoreactive components in the mouse somatosensory cortex. Neuroscience. 2017;355:161–74.

117. McRae PA, Porter BE. The perineuronal net component of the extracellular matrix in plasticity and epilepsy. Neurochem Int. 2012;61:963–72.

118. Yamada J, Ohgomori T, Jinno S. Perineuronal nets affect parvalbumin expression in GABAergic neurons of the mouse hippocampus. Eur J Neurosci. 2015;41:368–78.

119. Yoshioka N, Miyata S, Tamada A, Watanabe Y, Kawasaki A, Kitagawa H, Takao K, Miyakawa T, Takeuchi K, Igarashi M. Abnormalities in

perineuronal nets and behavior in mice lacking CSGalNAcT1, a key enzyme in chondroitin sulfate synthesis. Mol. Brain. 2017;10:47.

120. Tottenham N, Sheridan MA. A review of adversity, the amygdala and the hippocampus: a consideration of developmental timing. Front Hum Neurosci. 2010;3:68.

121. Fenoglio KA, Brunson KL, Baram TZ. Hippocampal neuroplasticity induced by early-life stress: functional and molecular aspects. Front Neuroendocrinol. 2006;27:180–92.

122. Andersen SL, Teicher MH. Delayed effects of early stress on hippocampal development. Neuropsychopharmacology. 2004;29:1988–93.

123. Benes FM, Turtle M, Khan Y, Farol P. Myelination of a key relay zone in the hippocampal formation occurs in the human brain during childhood, adolescence, and adulthood. Arch Gen Psychiatry. 1994;51:477–84.

124. McEwen BS, Morrison JH. The brain on stress: vulnerability and plasticity of the prefrontal cortex over the life course. Neuron. 2013;79:16–29.

125. McEwen BS, Nasca C, Gray JD. Stress effects on neuronal structure: hippocampus, amygdala, and prefrontal cortex. Neuropsychopharmacology. 2016;41:3–23.

126. Weich S, Patterson J, Shaw R, Stewart-Brown S. Family relationships in childhood and common psychiatric disorders in later life: systematic review of prospective studies. Br J Psychiatry. 2009;194:392–8.

127. Kausch O, Rugle L, Rowland DY. Lifetime histories of trauma among pathological gamblers. Am J Addict. 2006;15:35–43.

128. de Pablos RM, Herrera AJ, Espinosa-Oliva AM, Sarmiento M, Muñoz MF, Machado A, Venero JL. Chronic stress enhances microglia activation and exacerbates death of nigral dopaminergic neurons under conditions of inflammation. J Neuroinflammation. 2014;11:34.

6

The spatio-temporal dynamics of deviance and target detection in the passive and active auditory oddball paradigm: a sLORETA study

Christoph Justen[1,2] and Cornelia Herbert[2*]

Abstract

Background: Numerous studies have investigated the neural underpinnings of passive and active deviance and target detection in the well-known auditory *oddball paradigm* by means of event-related potentials (ERPs) or functional magnetic resonance imaging (fMRI). The present auditory oddball study investigates the spatio-temporal dynamics of passive versus active deviance and target detection by analyzing amplitude modulations of early and late ERPs while at the same time exploring the neural sources underling this modulation with standardized low-resolution brain electromagnetic tomography (sLORETA).

Methods: A 64-channel EEG was recorded from twelve healthy right-handed participants while listening to 'standards' and 'deviants' (500 vs. 1000 Hz pure tones) during a passive (block 1) and an active (block 2) listening condition. During passive listening, participants had to simply listen to the tones. During active listening they had to attend and press a key in response to the deviant tones.

Results: Passive and active listening elicited an N1 component, a mismatch negativity (MMN) as difference potential (whose amplitudes were temporally overlapping with the N1) and a P3 component. N1/MMN and P3 amplitudes were significantly more pronounced for deviants as compared to standards during both listening conditions. Active listening augmented P3 modulation to deviants significantly compared to passive listening, whereas deviance detection as indexed by N1/MMN modulation was unaffected by the task. During passive listening, sLORETA contrasts (deviants > standards) revealed significant activations in the right superior temporal gyrus (STG) and the lingual gyri bilaterally (N1/MMN) as well as in the left and right insulae (P3). During active listening, significant activations were found for the N1/MMN in the right inferior parietal lobule (IPL) and for the P3 in multiple cortical regions (e.g., precuneus).

Discussion: The results provide evidence for the hypothesis that passive as well as active deviance and target detection elicit cortical activations in spatially distributed brain regions and neural networks including the ventral attention network (VAN), dorsal attention network (DAN) and salience network (SN). Based on the temporal activation of the neural sources underlying ERP modulations, a neurophysiological model of passive and active deviance and target detection is proposed which can be tested in future studies.

Keywords: EEG, Source localization, N1, Mismatch negativity, MMN, P3, Attention, Salience, Attention networks

*Correspondence: cornelia.herbert@uni-ulm.de
[2] Institute of Psychology and Education, Applied Emotion and Motivation Research, University of Ulm, Ulm, Germany
Full list of author information is available at the end of the article

Background

Rapid orientation of selective attention towards changes in the acoustic environment is essential for successful interaction with our environment. Remarkably, the deviance of a perceived stimulus determines to what extent attention is captured by this stimulus. In other words, the more deviant a stimulus is, the more attention is allocated towards this particular stimulus [1]. In the auditory domain, the essential ability of deviance detection has been studied mostly in the so-called *oddball paradigm* [2]. In this experimental paradigm two auditory stimuli (e.g., pure tones) are presented as targets (*deviants*) or as non-targets (*standards*). Deviants are usually embedded in a continuous stream of standards and differ from standards in at least one perceptual dimension (for instance, a difference in frequency, pitch or loudness). This difference in stimulus presentation frequency and in physical stimulus properties between deviants and standards seems sufficient to prioritize processing of deviants over standards during passive and hence, involuntary (*bottom-up*) stimulus processing. In addition, detection of deviant stimuli may benefit from active, i.e., voluntary (*top-down*) controlled stimulus processing, for instance, when deviants are actively attended by the participants as targets for task-related voluntary discrimination of deviants and standards [3].

Due to its simplicity, the auditory oddball paradigm constitutes an ideal research paradigm for cognitive neuroscience to investigate the neural mechanisms of auditory deviance and target detection during passive and active listening conditions. So far, several event-related potential (ERP) and functional magnetic resonance imaging (fMRI) studies have been conducted to determine on the one hand the time course and on the other hand the brain regions underlying auditory deviance and target detection in this paradigm (for meta-analytic research e.g., [4]). Effects have been investigated during task conditions of passive or active listening (for ERP studies see e.g., [5–8]; for fMRI see e.g., [9–13]). In general, this body of research provided important insight into auditory processing under unattended (passive) and attended (active) task conditions while at the same time raising questions about the temporal activation of specific brain regions and brain networks involved in auditory deviance and target processing during passive versus active listening conditions.

According to influential theoretical models of attention allocation proposed by Corbetta and Shulman [14] and data from a recent meta-analysis based on functional imaging studies [4], processing of deviant stimuli (in contrast to standard stimuli) is associated with bottom-up as well as top-down stimulus processing and activation of two distinct fronto-parietal networks, namely the 'dorsal attention network' (DAN) and the 'ventral attention network' (VAN) [4, 14, 15]. The DAN comprises the superior parietal lobule/precuneus (SPL; Brodmann area (BA7)), the intraparietal sulcus (IPS; BA 6/7), parts of the middle temporal cortex (BA 21) and the inferior frontal junction (IFJ; BA 6/9/44). The VAN comprises the temporoparietal junction (TPJ; BAs 39/40), the supramarginal gyrus (SMG; BA 39), the superior temporal gyrus (STG; BAs 22/41/42), the frontal operculum (FO; BA 44/45/47), the inferior frontal gyrus (IFG; BAs 44/45/47), the anterior cingulate cortex (ACC; BAs 24/32/33) and the anterior insula (AI, BA 13) [4, 14, 15]. According to recent meta-analytic research, putting together the results of 75 neuroimaging studies using either auditory or visual oddball paradigms, processing of deviants versus standards activates the DAN and the VAN differently during passive versus active stimulus processing [4]. Parts of the DAN seem to be activated during the processing of deviants and standards, and specifically its frontal parts seem to be involved in voluntary target detection in line with the idea of the dorsolateral prefrontal cortex (DLPFC; BAs 8/9/10/46) playing a central role in top-down selective attentional control [4, 16]. In contrast to the DAN, the VAN seems to be exclusively involved in the detection of deviant stimuli and brain regions belonging to the VAN seem to be more active when deviants are voluntarily attended as compared to conditions in which they are not attended (e.g., during passive listening). The VAN is therefore supposed to enable 'attentional shifting' to deviant stimuli, probably to initiate an appropriate behavioral response when deviants are important for the task [17].

However, this raises questions about which brain networks and brain regions might be involved in auditory deviance processing when there is no task at hand. Theoretically, some brain structures of the VAN such as the insula and ACC but also brain regions of the DAN (e.g., precuneus) form part of the 'salience network' (SN) [18, 19]. Amongst these brain regions in particular the insular cortex is considered to be involved in bottom-up detection of salient events and the selection of these for additional processing [20]. In addition, it has been shown that in the oddball paradigm, attentional processing (e.g., attention orientation) to auditory stimuli can activate visual processing regions (e.g., lateral and medial occipital areas) and hence, processing regions typically engaged in object recognition and in the perception of visual objects [21, 22] in tasks requiring spatial attention (e.g., see [23]). Thus, specific brain regions in the visual cortex (such as the lateral occipital cortex (LOC) or the lingual gyrus (LG) in the medial visual cortex) may also be activated during attentive processing of acoustic stimuli [24]. However, whether the aforementioned visual processing areas are also activated during task conditions of passive and thus, unattended listening to deviant and standard pure tones in the oddball paradigm needs to be investigated further [25–27].

So far, the above outlined assumptions about the activation of the DAN and VAN during auditory processing have been derived mainly from meta-analytic research [4] including functional neuroimaging studies. Thus, it has not been investigated whether activation of the DAN and VAN could be modeled by source imaging techniques that rely on EEG activity such as sLORETA. Crucially, exploring the time course of auditory deviance and target detection through electroencephalography (EEG) and event-related brain potentials (ERPs) and simultaneous targeting the brain regions of the VAN and DAN by means of sLORETA could be especially fruitful in situations where fMRI is not available or too costly. Moreover, due to its high temporal resolution in the millisecond time-range, EEG and EEG based source imaging offers the possibility to investigate the time course of deviance and target detection in the auditory oddball paradigm (e.g., be investigating modulation of ERPs) while at the same time the neural sources underlying ERP modulation can be estimated within the same temporal resolution of milliseconds. Akin to functional imaging, in EEG-ERP source imaging studies, effects can be investigated during passive listening conditions, during which intentional discrimination between deviants and standards via explicit instructions is not required. In addition, investigation of effects associated with active listening conditions (e.g., explicit instruction to attend to deviant stimuli) is also possible, thus allowing direct comparisons of ERPs, their neural sources and their modulation during deviance and target detection in a within-subject design including task conditions of passive and active listening.

Regarding the time course of auditory deviance and target detection, ERP components most consistently elicited during the auditory oddball paradigm are the N1, the N2a or auditory mismatch negativity (N2a/MMN; e.g., see [28]), and the late P3 (e.g., see [29–31]).Whereas the N1 and MMN are brain potentials whose amplitudes are significantly influenced by differences in physical stimulus properties, the magnitude of the P3 amplitude is significantly influenced by cognitive and task demands (e.g., see [32]). The N1 and the MMN have been found during passive listening as well as during active processing of deviant stimuli [33]. In contrast to the N1, the MMN is computed by subtracting the averaged ERP waveform of standard stimuli from the averaged ERP waveform of deviant stimuli. The resulting negative deflection is peaking between 100 and 250 ms after stimulus onset [34]; amplitudes of the MMN being often more pronounced at fronto-central electrode sites [35]. Regarding its latency,

the MMN can overlap with the auditory N1 component (e.g., see [36]) peaking between 80 and 120 ms post-stimulus [37], especially if deviant and standard stimuli are clearly perceptually distinct from each other. The auditory MMN has been proposed to indicate mostly pre-attentive sensory stimulus discrimination [38] as well as automatic, and thus involuntary auditory change detection [39, 40]. Hence, the modulation of the MMN is assumed to be driven by involuntary mechanisms of the brain's sensory processing system matching the incoming stimulus to its internally stored representation (or template). This matching is considered to occur "unconsciously" and temporally prior to stimulus categorization [41].

Amplitudes of the P3, temporally following early brain potentials such as the N1 and N2a/MMN, are most pronounced between 300 and 450 ms after stimulus-onset at central-parietal as well as parietal electrode sites [30]. Previous auditory oddball studies suggest that the P3 is elicited only by sufficiently deviant stimuli [42] with P3 amplitudes being larger in response to voluntarily attended than unattended deviant stimuli (e.g., see [5]). Accordingly, the P3 is thought to reflect voluntary switch of attention [39, 40, 43] and in depth-processing of a stimulus signaling stimulus evaluation based on memory [44] and context updating [29, 45].

Taken together, one might expect N1, N2a/MMN and P3 modulation to be differentially sensitive to task effects. Moreover, one could speculate that different neural sources may underlie N1, MMN and P3 modulation during deviance and target detection in passive and active listening conditions. Compared to the huge amount of EEG–ERP studies or fMRI studies investigating either the time course or the brain regions involved in auditory deviant and target detection only few studies investigated both, the time course and the neural sources of auditory deviance and target detection in the oddball paradigm, for instance with combined EEG–fMRI methodology [13]). Although combining fMRI and EEG/ERP methodology is beneficial, localization of neural generators of ERP components might still be affected by the relatively poor temporal resolution of conventional functional neuroimaging techniques [46]. To this end, (standardized) low-resolution brain electromagnetic tomography (LORETA and sLORETA, respectively) have been developed to make assumptions about the location of neural generators of brain electrical activity derived from multi-channel EEG recordings with high temporal resolution [47–49]. The validity of (s)LORETA has been confirmed in a number of combined fMRI-EEG studies (e.g., see [48]). More specifically, Mulert et al. compared brain activations in an active auditory oddball paradigm as measured by fMRI with brain activations derived from

EEG and LORETA [50]. The comparison between fMRI and LORETA activation patterns contrasting deviants versus standards during active and hence, attended processing of deviants versus standards showed concurrent activations in brain regions associated with the VAN, namely the TPJ (BAs 39/40), the supplementary motor area (SMA; BA 6), the ACC (BAs 24/32/33), the middle frontal gyrus (MFG; BA 46) and the anterior insula (AI, BA 13). Interestingly, neural generators of the P3 partially overlapping with the VAN, including TPJ (BAs 39/40), DLPFC (BAs 8/9/10/46), ACC (BAs 24/32/33) and parts of the parietal and temporal cortices could be already confirmed in recent EEG-sLORETA studies (e.g., see [50–52]). Thus, source localization with sLORETA can be a means to successfully estimate neural sources underlying target detection in the oddball paradigm without losing information about the time course.

Aim and objectives of the present study

Building upon the previous findings outlined above, the aims of the present auditory oddball study were to methodologically combine EEG–ERP methodology with sLORETA in the oddball task in order to (a) investigate the time course of auditory deviant and target detection by studying ERP modulation in active as well as in passive listening conditions and (b) examine the temporal activation of brain regions contributing to the observed ERP modulation patterns in the two different listening conditions. Thus, by taking advantage of the high temporal resolution of the sLORETA source imaging technique the present study allows to explore which brain regions belonging to the hypothesized brain networks (i.e., DAN, VAN and SN) might contribute to the modulation of early and late ERP components elicited by deviant and standard pure tones during active and passive listening. In line with previous research and the assumptions outlined above the present study aimed at testing the following hypotheses and open questions regarding the temporal activation of specific brain regions during auditory deviant and target detection: firstly, we were interested in whether passive listening of deviant compared to standard stimuli will be associated with activations in brain regions belonging to the VAN or the SN, indicating involuntary attentional orientation towards deviant stimuli when no behavioral response is required. Secondly, we were interested in whether during passive listening brain regions belonging to the VAN and, or the SN will contribute as neural sources to automatic deviant detection (MMN) or to later processing stages of deviance processing as indicated by modulation of the P3. Thirdly, during the attended oddball paradigm, activations in brain regions associated with the VAN and the DAN could be expected in the time window of the MMN and

the P3 component indicating (1) involuntary attentional orientation towards deviant stimuli and (2) voluntary modulation of attention in order to maintain attentional resources for responding behaviorally to deviant stimuli. Finally, previous fMRI studies found activation in the visual cortex during passive auditory processing in the oddball paradigm. Thus, cortical activations in lateral/medial occipital areas could also be expected to occur in the present study during passive listening and activation of these brain regions might be associated with the modulation of early and late ERPs.

Methods
Participants

Twelve right-handed university students (7 females, 5 males) aged between 19 and 26 years ($M = 21.3$ years, $SD = 2.15$) participated in the present study. All participants were in good health and reported no psychological or hearing disorders. The experiment (including EEG recordings) was conducted at the Institute of Psychology of the German Sport University Cologne, Germany and was part of a larger project of the authors (see funding sources, and [53]). The experimental protocol complied with the Declaration of Helsinki and was approved by the local ethics committee of the German Sport University Cologne, Germany. All participants gave written informed consent prior to the start of the experiment and received a momentary compensation for their participation.

General procedure

Prior to the start of the EEG session, participants had been seated in a comfortable chair and were informed about the general procedures of the experiment including EEG recordings. The experiment consisted of a passive and active auditory oddball paradigm; the passive condition (block 1) being always followed by the active condition (block 2). Block order was kept constant across participants as not to confound passive with active processing due to possible carry over effects. Particularly, the induction of an overt (behavioral) response to deviant pure tones during the active paradigm and hence active orientation of attention towards the deviant stimuli may have influenced deviance processing during passive listening if the active paradigm had been presented first (cf., [5]). Auditory stimuli were presented at constant sound pressure level of about 75 dB/SPL using Shure SHR440 on-ear headphones (Shure, Niles, IL, USA). During the *passive* oddball paradigm (block 1), participants were instructed to listen passively to the presented auditory stimuli. Accordingly, no behavioral response was required. For the active oddball paradigm (block 2), participants were told to respond to the deviant pure tones as quickly as possible by pressing the space bar on a keyboard with their right index finger. To avoid horizontal eye movements (saccades) while listening, participants were instructed to fixate their view on a fixation cross presented on the video screen. Additionally, participants were told to keep their eyes open during stimulus presentations (block 1 and block 2, respectively).

Passive and active tone oddball paradigm

The oddball paradigm consisted of two auditory stimuli, a low (500 Hz) pure tone which was presented as "standard" and a high (1000 Hz) pure tone which was presented as "deviant" stimulus (cf., [54]). Thus, both pure tones differed only in the frequency domain and both were perceptually sufficiently different from each other to be clearly recognized as standard and deviant during stimulus presentation. Both auditory stimuli had durations of 50 ms (including a 5 ms fade-in/out time). The experimental paradigm consisted of in total of 400 trials (325 standard trials and 75 deviant trials, respectively) with a fixed inter-stimulus-interval (ISI) of 950 ms duration. Stimulus presentation and recording of responses were controlled by the Inquisit 4.0 software package (Millisecond Software, Seattle, WA, USA). The experimental script was downloaded from the official Inquisit website ([55]).

EEG recordings

Continuous EEG data (sampling frequency: 2.048 Hz) were recorded from 64 Ag/AgCl sintered electrode using standardized EEG recording sites (Fp1, Fpz, Fp2, AF7, AF3, AF4, AF8, F7, F5, F3, F1, Fz, F2, F4, F6, F8, FT7, FC5, FC3, FC1, FCz, FC2, FC4, FC6, FT8, T7, C5, C3, C1, Cz, C2, C4, C6, T8, TP7, CP5, CP3, CP1, CPz, CP2, CP4, CP6, TP8, P7, P5, P3, P1, Pz, P2, P4, P6, P8, PO7, PO5, PO3, POz, PO4, PO6, PO8, O1, Oz, O2, M1 and M2). Electrodes were mounted on a Waveguard EEG cap (Advanced Neuro Technology B.V., Enschede, The Netherlands). The electrode sites of this montage were arranged according to the international 10/10-system [56] and all EEG channels were referenced to the common average of all scalp electrodes. Forehead electrode AFz was used as ground electrode. Blue Sensor N disc electrodes (Ambu, Ballerup, Denmark) were placed at the outer canthi of both eyes and additionally below the left eye for horizontal and vertical electrooculography (HEOG and VEOG, respectively). All electrode impedances were kept below 10 kΩ.

Preprocessing of EEG data

EEG data were preprocessed offline with the ASALAB (Version: 4.7.8) software package [57]. Preprocessing included down-sampling to 512 Hz, band-pass

filtering between 0.5 and 20 Hz (24 dB/oct) and band-stop (notch) filtering of 50 Hz (24 dB/oct). Eye blinks and saccade-related artifacts were corrected with an artifact correction feature based on principle component analysis (PCA), as introduced by [58]. Further data analysis of artifact-free EEG data involved re-referencing to linked mastoids/linked ears (M1 and M2), segmentation into epochs for each stimulus type and condition, resulting in epochs from 100 ms before and 700 ms after stimulus onset for each of the four different experimental conditions including "Deviants" and "Standards" during the passive listening condition as well as "Deviants" and "Standards" during the active listening condition. All epochs were scanned for artifacts using an automated artifact detection algorithm. The automatic artifact rejection threshold in all epochs (between − 100 and 700 ms after stimulus onset) was set to ± 100 μV within a 400 ms interval (between 0 and 400 ms after stimulus onset). Epochs exceeding this threshold were discarded. All extracted epochs were baseline corrected using the interval from 100 ms before stimulus onset. Referencing, segmentation and baseline correction as well as any further analysis step (e.g., averaging) were done in EEGLAB (Version: 13.4.4b; [59]) and MATLAB (Version: R2013a, 8.1.0.604; The MathWorks Inc., Natick, MA, USA). Grand averaged ERPs were generated for all four aforementioned experimental conditions.

ERP analysis and statistics

Detection of the time windows in which ERP amplitudes including the N1 and P3 were most pronounced was done with the built-in EEGLAB function "statcond" [60]. Averaged ERPs to deviant and standard stimuli (during both passive and active listening condition, respectively) were submitted to non-parametric paired t-tests with 5.000 permutations at all time points between 0 (stimulus onset) and 700 ms after stimulus onset with 62 electrode sites included. To control for multiple comparisons, the false discovery rate (FDR; for an introduction, see [61]) was used for all statistical analyses (as implemented in the EEGLAB function "FDR") with an FDR-level of 5% ($q = 0.05$). By maintaining reasonable limits on the likelihood of false discoveries (i.e., it is suitable for a reasonable correction on a large number of comparisons), the FDR procedure provides a much better spatial and temporal resolution as compared to parametric t-tests using the "classical" Bonferroni correction (for an introduction, see [62]).

Regarding analysis of the MMN and the P3, difference waves were calculated from the averaged ERP waveforms elicited by deviant and standard pure tones in both experimental conditions ("Deviants" and "Standards" during the passive listening condition and "Deviants" and

"Standards" during the active listening condition, respectively) using the Maas Univariate ERP Toolbox [63–65]. All time points in the MMN (50–150 ms) and the P3 time window (200–450 ms) as well all 62 scalp electrodes were included in the statistical tests (i.e., 3.224 and 9.610 total comparisons, respectively).

Difference waves were submitted to a repeated measures, two-tailed cluster-based permutation test based on the cluster mass statistic [66] using a family-wise alpha level of 0.05. Repeated measures t-tests were performed for each contrast ("Deviants" and "Standards" during the passive listening condition and "Deviants" and "Standards" during the active listening condition, respectively) using the original data and 2.500 random within-participant permutations of the data. For each permutation, all t-scores corresponding to uncorrected p-values of 0.01 or less were clustered: to this end, electrodes within a distance of approximately 5.44 cm were considered spatial neighbors and adjacent time points were considered temporal neighbors. The sum of the t-scores in each cluster is the "mass" of that cluster and the most extreme cluster mass in each of the 2.501 sets of tests was used to estimate the distribution of the null hypothesis (i.e., no difference between "Deviants" and "Standards" in the passive as well as "Deviants" and "Standards" in the active listening condition, respectively). More specifically, the assumption of the null hypothesis of the permutation test is that positive differences between conditions could have just as likely been negative differences and vice versa. Thus, the distribution of the null hypothesis is symmetric around a difference of 0. The permutation cluster mass percentile ranking of each cluster from the observed data was used to derive its p-value. The p-value of the cluster was assigned to each member of the cluster and t-scores that were not included in a cluster were given a p-value of 1. This permutation test analysis was used instead of the conventional testing of mean amplitude values because it provides much better spatial and temporal resolution while maintaining control of the family-wise alpha level (i.e., it corrects for a large number of comparisons). 2.500 permutations were used to estimate the distribution of the null hypothesis as it is over twice the number recommend by [67] for a family-wise alpha level of 0.01. For the cluster mass permutation test, all desired p-values, critical t-scores, and the corresponding family-wise alpha levels are reported (please see Results, "Passive tone oddball paradigm—ERPs (N1, MMN and P3)" and "Active tone oddball paradigm—ERPs (N1, MMN and P3)" sections).

EEG source localization analysis
Neural generators of the ERPs were analyzed with the sLORETA software (University Hospital of Psychiatry, Zürich, Switzerland; [68]). Source estimations were done on single participants' data and were restricted to the time windows showing significant differences in the ERP waveforms between the contrasted conditions (see EEG-ERP results, "Behavioral results—active tone oddball paradigm", "Passive tone oddball paradigm—ERPs (N1, MMN and P3)", "Active tone oddball paradigm—ERPs (N1, MMN and P3)", "Passive and active deviants—passive and active standards ERPs" sections). In sLORETA, computations are based on a realistic head model [69] using the MNI-152 template [70], with the three-dimensional solution space restricted to cortical gray matter, as determined by the probabilistic Talairach atlas [71, 72]. The standard electrode positions of the MNI-152 template were taken from [56] as well as [73]. The intracerebral volume is partitioned in 6.239 voxels with a spatial resolution of $5 \times 5 \times 5$ mm each. Thus, the obtained sLORETA images represent the standardized electric activity at each voxel in the neuroanatomic Montreal Neurological Institute (MNI) space as the exact magnitude of the estimated current density. Anatomical labels are reported in Brodmann areas (BA) in line with MNI space, with a correction to Talairach space [74]. For sLORETA no pre-registration of individual subjects is required. The matching or co-registration of the individual EEG data with the MNI-152 template is based on the scalp-recorded electric potential distribution and computed on the basis of the cortical three-dimensional distribution of current density. Thus, the software automatically co-registers the data according to the head surface points (electrode locations provided in the electrode configuration file). As introduced by Nichols and Holmes [75], statistical non-parametric mapping (SnPM) was used to compute the standardized intracerebral current density distribution at time intervals or time points showing significant differences based on non-parametric voxel-by-voxel paired samples t-tests (with 5.000 permutations) on the three-dimensional sLORETA images. Statistical significance was assessed by defining critical thresholds (t_{crit}) corrected for multiple comparisons ($p < 0.01$ and $p < 0.05$, respectively) for all tested voxels and time windows. The null hypotheses equaled the assumption that there were no differences between "Deviants" and "Standards" in both the passive and active listening condition, respectively.

Standardized current density values at each voxel have been computed in the solution space as a linear and weighted sum of the scalp electric potentials. Activation of a given voxel was based on the smoothness assumption, meaning that neighboring voxels show a highly synchronous activity [76]. Support comes from electro-physiological studies showing that electrical activity of neighboring neural populations is highly correlated [76, 77]. As proposed by [78], activated voxels exceeding t_{crit}

were considered as being regions of cortical activation. Finally, statistical analysis resulted in a three-dimensional intracerebral current density distribution and obtained cortical regions were classified in relation to their corresponding BA [79] and normalized coordinates (Talairach and MMI, respectively).

Results

Behavioral results—active tone oddball paradigm

Participants' reaction times (RTs) to deviant pure tones were between 223 and 379 ms ($M = 285.6$ ms, $SD = 38.5$). On average, participants responded to all trials with deviant pure tones with high accuracy ($M = 74.8$, $SD = 0.7$).

Passive tone oddball paradigm—ERPs (N1, MMN and P3)

Passive listening to deviant and standard pure tones elicited an N1 component as well as a P300 component. As shown in Fig. 1 and as revealed by the grand average of the ERP waveforms, N1 amplitudes were most pronounced between 67 and 129 ms (peak at about 95 ms) after stimulus onset; P3 amplitudes were most pronounced during 232–354 ms (peak at about 300 ms) post-stimulus. In addition, difference waves—subtracting

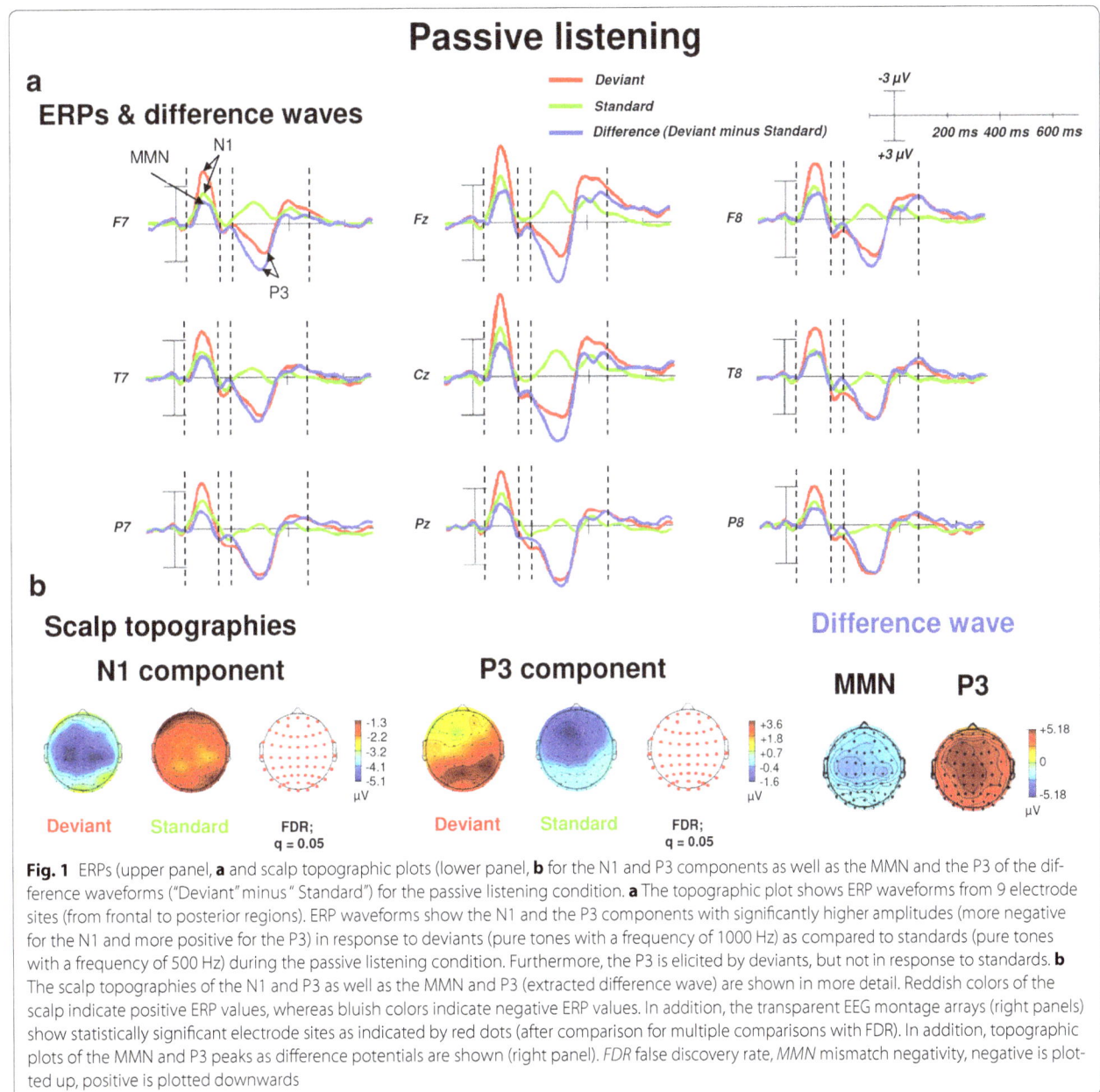

Fig. 1 ERPs (upper panel, **a** and scalp topographic plots (lower panel, **b** for the N1 and P3 components as well as the MMN and the P3 of the difference waveforms ("Deviant" minus " Standard") for the passive listening condition. **a** The topographic plot shows ERP waveforms from 9 electrode sites (from frontal to posterior regions). ERP waveforms show the N1 and the P3 components with significantly higher amplitudes (more negative for the N1 and more positive for the P3) in response to deviants (pure tones with a frequency of 1000 Hz) as compared to standards (pure tones with a frequency of 500 Hz) during the passive listening condition. Furthermore, the P3 is elicited by deviants, but not in response to standards. **b** The scalp topographies of the N1 and P3 as well as the MMN and P3 (extracted difference wave) are shown in more detail. Reddish colors of the scalp indicate positive ERP values, whereas bluish colors indicate negative ERP values. In addition, the transparent EEG montage arrays (right panels) show statistically significant electrode sites as indicated by red dots (after comparison for multiple comparisons with FDR). In addition, topographic plots of the MMN and P3 peaks as difference potentials are shown (right panel). *FDR* false discovery rate, *MMN* mismatch negativity, negative is plotted up, positive is plotted downwards

ERP waveforms elicited in response to "Deviants" from "Standards"—during the passive listening condition revealed an MMN component. As shown in Fig. 1, the amplitude of the MMN overlapped with the time window of the N1 component between 66 and 128 ms after stimulus onset. As also shown in Fig. 1, amplitudes of the N1, MMN and the P3 were significantly more pronounced for deviants as compared to standards.

Regarding early time windows, the maximum number of statistically significant differences between "Deviants" and "Standards" occurred in the N1/MMN time window between 82 and 103 ms post-stimulus (desired $p = .05$, critical t-score $= -2.20$ corresponding to a family-wise alpha-level of .05 and a Bonferroni test-wise alpha-level of .000004; see also "Passive tone oddball paradigm" section; electrodes: anterior-frontal and fronto-temporal: AF7, AF4, AF3, FT8, Fp1, Fp2, Fpz; frontal: F8, F7, F6, F5, F4, F3, F2, F1, Fz, FC6, FC5, FC4, FC3, FC2, FC1, FCz; central: C6, C4, C3, C2, C1, Cz; temporal: T8). This seems to be in line with previous findings of an 'early' MMN peaking at about 100 ms [32]. To ensure the validity of this interpretation, electrodes were re-referenced offline to a common average reference (CAR). According to the literature, CAR or a nose reference are recommended as these montages are known to be the best reference sites to robustly determine the MMN [80]. As expected, this procedure confirmed the characteristic polarity inversion of the extracted MMN at both mastoid electrodes sites (M1 and M2, respectively). Thus, the extracted MMN of the difference wave occurred in the averaged time window of the N1 component observed in the averaged ERP waveforms [36].

For the P3 component the maximum number of statistically significant differences between "Deviants" and "Standards" was observed between 269 and 322 ms post-stimulus (desired $p = .05$, critical t-score $= 2.20$ corresponding to a family-wise alpha-level of .05 and a Bonferroni test-wise alpha-level of .000008; see also "Passive tone oddball paradigm" section; electrodes: frontal: AF8, AF7, AF4, AF3, Fp1, Fp2, Fpz, F8, F7, F6, F5, F4, F3, F2, F1, Fz, FC6, FC5, FC4, FC3, FC2, FC1, FCz, FT8, FT7; central: C6, C5, C4, C3, C2, C1, Cz, CP6, CP5, CP4, CP3, CP2, CP1, CPz; temporal: T8, T7, TP8, TP7; parietal: P8, P7, P6, P5, P4, P3, P2, P1, Pz, PO8, PO7, PO6, PO5, PO4, PO3, POz; occipital: O2, O1, Oz).

Active tone oddball paradigm—ERPs (N1, MMN and P3)

Active listening to deviant and standard pure tones elicited an N1, an MMN as well as a P300 component. As shown in Fig. 2, the MMN component (obtained from the difference wave by subtracting "Deviants" from "Standards" during the active listening condition) was again overlapping with the time window of the N1

component elicited in response to "Deviants" and "Standards". N1 amplitudes were most pronounced in the time window from 60 to 114 ms (peak: at about 90 ms), the MMN amplitude was most pronounced between 56 and 117 ms post-stimulus and the P3 amplitudes were most pronounced during 232–378 ms (peak: at about 300 ms) post-stimulus. As also shown in Fig. 2, amplitudes of the N1, MMN and the P3 were more pronounced for deviants as compared to standards, i.e., amplitudes were more negative going for the N1 and MMN and more positive going for the P3 when listening to "Deviants" as compared to "Standards".

Regarding early time windows (N1, MMN), the maximum number of statistically significant differences between "Deviants" 3.5.2and "Standards" was observed between 83 and 95 ms post-stimulus (desired $p = .05$, critical t-score $= -2.21$ corresponding to a family-wise alpha-level of .05 and a Bonferroni test-wise alpha-level of .000016; see also "Active tone oddball paradigm" section; electrodes: frontal: AF8, F8, F7, F6, FC6, FC5, FC4, FC3, FC2, FC1; central: C6, C5, C4, C3,C2, C1, Cz, CP6, CP4, CP3, CP2, CP1, CPz; parietal: Pz). Again (see "Passive tone oddball paradigm—ERPs (N1, MMN and P3)" section), re-referencing to CAR confirmed the characteristic polarity inversion of the extracted MMN at the left and right mastoid electrodes sites (M1 and M2, respectively).

For the P3 component the maximum number of statistically significant differences between "Deviants" and "Standards" was observed between 253 and 351 ms after stimulus onset (desired $p = .05$, critical t-score $= 2.10$ corresponding to a family-wise alpha-level of .05 and a Bonferroni test-wise alpha-level of .000008; see also "Active tone oddball paradigm"; electrodes: frontal: AF8, AF7, AF4, AF3, Fp2, Fp1, Fpz, F8, F7, F6, F5, F4, F3, F2, F1, Fz, FC6, FC5, FC4, FC3, FC2, FC1, FCz, FT8, FT7; central: C6, C5, C4, C3, Cz, CP6, CP5, CP4, CP3, CP2, CP1, CPz, C6, C5, C4, C3, C2, C1, Cz, CP4, CP3, CPz; temporal: T8, T7, TP8, TP7; parietal: P8, P7, P6, P5, P4, P3, P2, P1, Pz, PO8, PO7, PO6, PO5, PO4, PO3, POz; occipital: O2, O1, Oz).

Passive and active deviants—passive and active standards ERPs

Contrasting ERP waveforms elicited by passive and active deviant pure tones during both oddball listening conditions revealed significant differences in ERP amplitudes between 228 and 456 ms post-stimulus onset, corresponding to the P3 component (see also "Passive and active deviants" section). In this time window, the amplitudes were more negative going during passive as compared to active listening (see Figs. 1 and 2). No amplitude differences were found in earlier time windows.

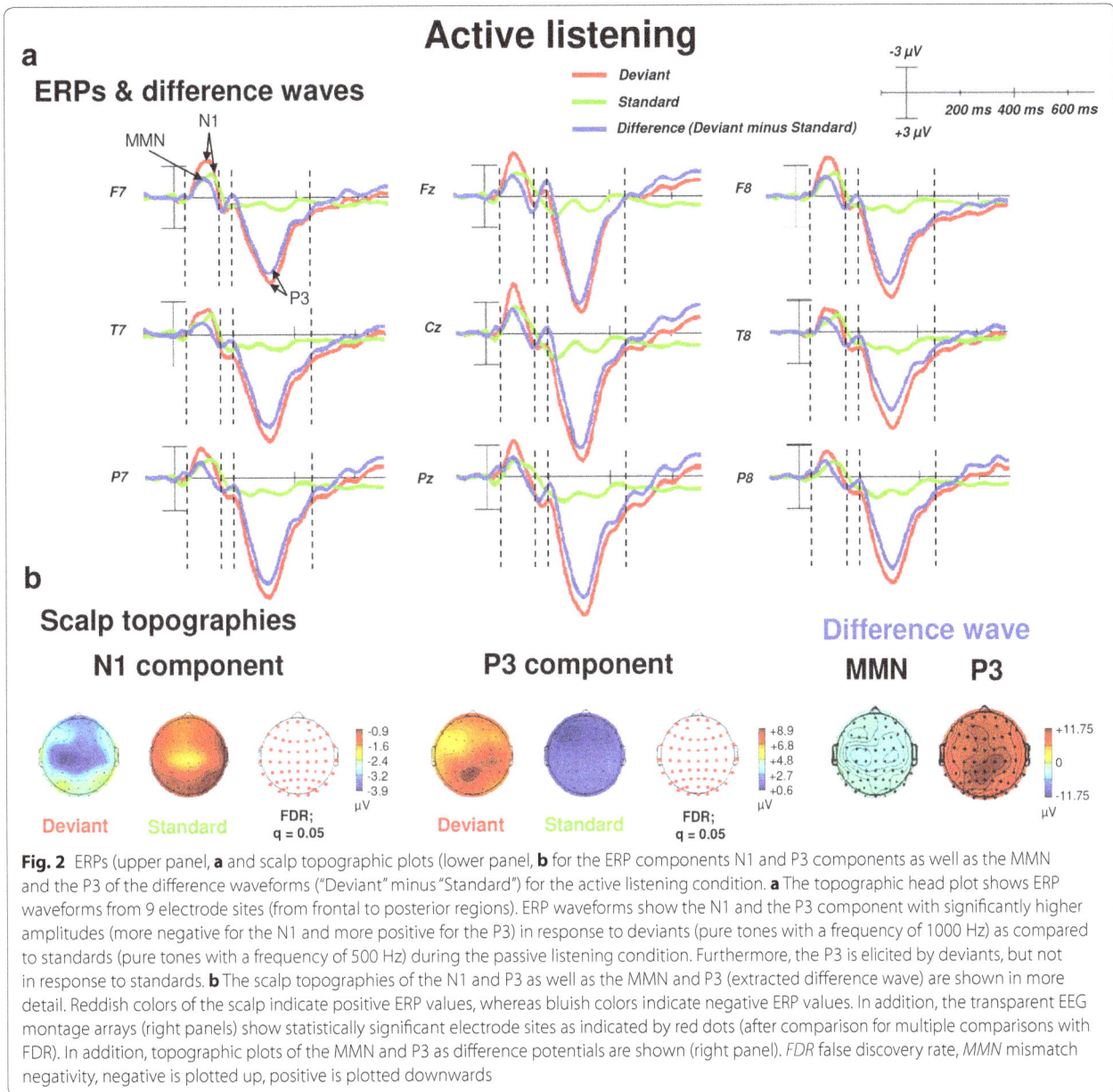

Fig. 2 ERPs (upper panel, **a** and scalp topographic plots (lower panel, **b** for the ERP components N1 and P3 components as well as the MMN and the P3 of the difference waveforms ("Deviant" minus "Standard") for the active listening condition. **a** The topographic head plot shows ERP waveforms from 9 electrode sites (from frontal to posterior regions). ERP waveforms show the N1 and the P3 component with significantly higher amplitudes (more negative for the N1 and more positive for the P3) in response to deviants (pure tones with a frequency of 1000 Hz) as compared to standards (pure tones with a frequency of 500 Hz) during the passive listening condition. Furthermore, the P3 is elicited by deviants, but not in response to standards. **b** The scalp topographies of the N1 and P3 as well as the MMN and P3 (extracted difference wave) are shown in more detail. Reddish colors of the scalp indicate positive ERP values, whereas bluish colors indicate negative ERP values. In addition, the transparent EEG montage arrays (right panels) show statistically significant electrode sites as indicated by red dots (after comparison for multiple comparisons with FDR). In addition, topographic plots of the MMN and P3 as difference potentials are shown (right panel). *FDR* false discovery rate, *MMN* mismatch negativity, negative is plotted up, positive is plotted downwards

Contrasting ERP waveforms elicited by standard pure tones during active versus passive listening revealed a significant difference in ERP amplitudes between 190 and 418 ms after stimulus onset (see also "Passive and active standards" section). No significant differences were found in earlier time windows corresponding to the N1 or MMN component.

sLORETA source localization analysis
Passive tone oddball paradigm
As shown in Fig. 3, contrasting deviant against standard pure tones with sLORETA during the passive oddball listening condition (contrast: "Deviants" > "Standards")

revealed significant activations in the lingual gyri (bilaterally) (BAs 17/18/19; *t*-score 4.06; $p < 0.01$) as well as in the right superior temporal gyrus (STG; BAs 13/22/39/42; *t*-score 3.97; $p < 0.05$) between 82 and 103 ms after stimulus onset, which corresponds with the ERP analysis time window in which N1 and MMN amplitude differences were most pronounced, see "Passive tone oddball paradigm—ERPs (N1, MMN and P3)").

In addition, between 269 and 322 ms (P3 component) significant electrocortical activations included the insular cortex bilaterally (BA 13; *t*-score 4.80; $p < 0.01$) and the right lingual gyrus (LG; BA 18; *t*-score 4.78; $p < 0.01$), see Fig. 3. For a complete overview of all retrieved

Passive listening

a   MMN: Deviants > Standards

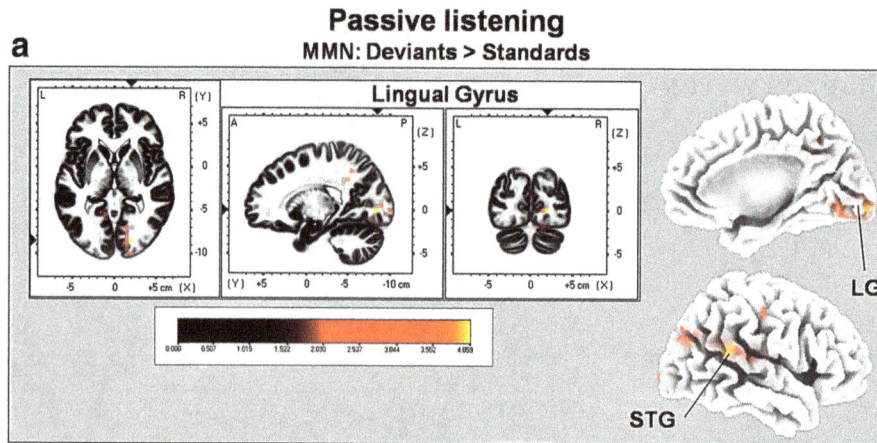

b   P3: Deviants > Standards

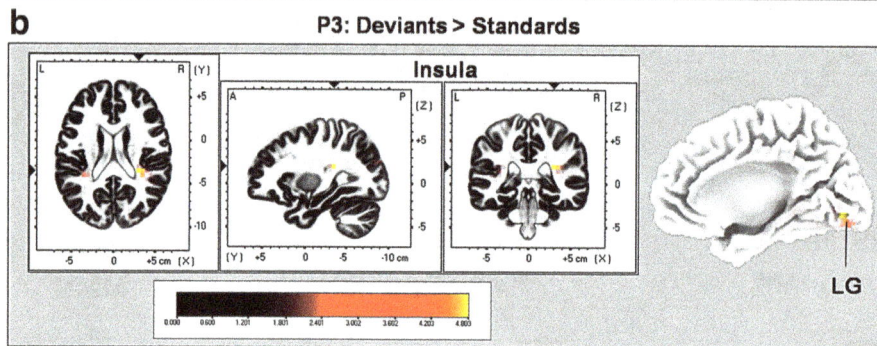

Active listening

c   MMN: Deviants > Standards

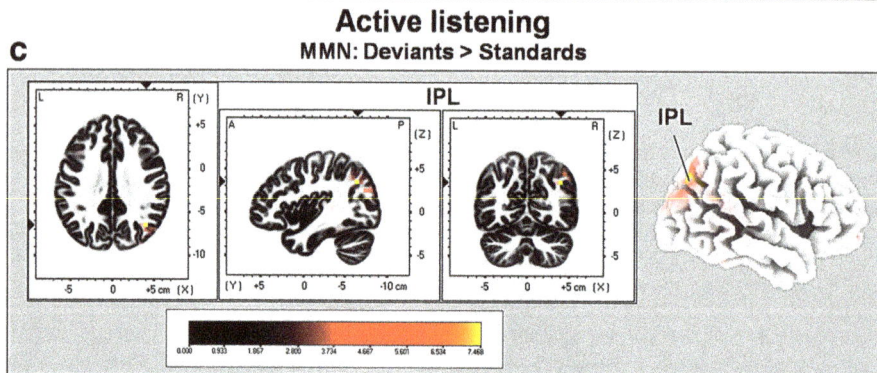

d   P3: Deviants > Standards

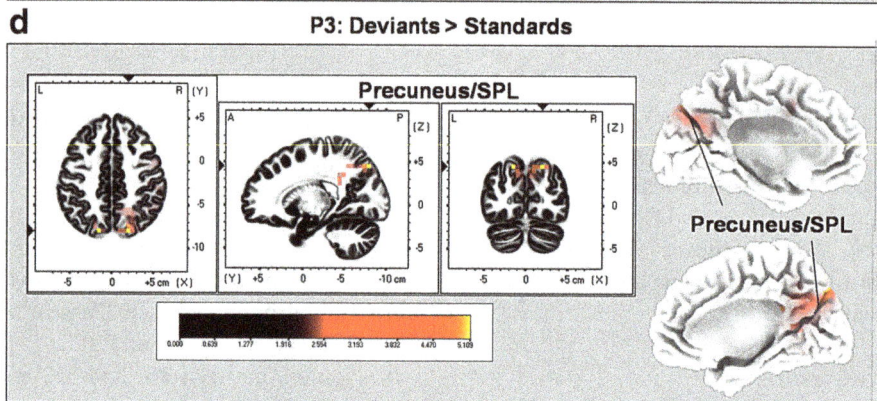

(See figure on previous page.)

Fig. 3 Results of the standardized low-resolution brain electrotomography (sLORETA) source localization analysis in the 'passive' and 'active' pure tone oddball paradigm. Images have been obtained after statistical non-parametric mapping (SnPM) and co-registration to the stereotaxic Talairach space based on the Co-Planar Stereotaxic Atlas of the Human Brain [72] and the probabilistic MNI-152 template [70]. Activated voxels are indicated by yellowish and reddish colors [after correction for multiple comparisons ($p < 0.01$ and $p < 0.05$, respectively)]. **a** In the averaged time windows of the 'unattended' MMN component (80–123 ms), the peak of highest cortical activity has been found in the right LG (BAs 17/18/19) and right STG (BAs 13/22/39/42). **b** In the averaged time windows of the 'attended' MMN component (83–95 ms), the peak of highest cortical activity has been found in the right IPL (BAs 7/39/40). **c** In the averaged time windows of the 'unattended' P3 component (269–322 ms), the peak of highest cortical activity has been found in both insulae bilaterally (BA 13) and the right LG (BA 18). **d** In the averaged time windows of the 'attended' P3 component (253–351 ms), the peak of highest cortical activity has been found in the precuneus/SPL bilaterally (BAs 7/19/23/21). *L* left, *R* right, *LG* lingual gyrus, *STG* superior temporal gyrus, *IPL* inferior parietal lobule, *SPL* superior parietal lobule, *MNI* Montreal Neurological Institute, *X, Y, Z* corresponding MNI coordinates, *BA* Brodmann area

statistically significant results including all anatomical regions and activated voxels, see Tables 1 and 2.

Active tone oddball paradigm

Contrasting deviant against standard pure tones in the active oddball listening condition (contrast: "Deviants" > "Standards") with sLORETA revealed significant activation in the right inferior parietal lobule (IPL; BAs 7/39/40; t-score $= 8.12$; $p < 0.01$) between 83 and 95 ms after stimulus onset and hence, in the time window of the N1 and MMN amplitude (see ERP results in 3.3). Furthermore, significant activations were found in the precuneus bilaterally (BAs 7/19/23/31; t-score 5.11; $p < 0.01$), the cingulate cortices bilaterally (BA 31; t-score 4.86; $p > 0.01$), the superior temporal gyri bilaterally (STG; BAs 13/22/39/41; t-score 4.79; $p < 0.01$), the left and right precentral gyri (BAs 4/6; t-score 4.81; $p < 0.01$),

the left and right postcentral gyri (BAs 2/3/7/40; t-score 4.64; $p < 0.01$), the right posterior cingulate cortex (BAs 23/30/31; t-score 4.59, $p < 0.01$) and the right intraparietal lobe (IPL, BAs 39/40; t-score 4.04; $p < 0.01$) in the time window between 253 and 351 ms (overlapping with the time window of the P3 component), see Fig. 3.

For a complete overview of all retrieved statistically significant results including all anatomical regions and activated voxels, see Tables 3 and 4.

Passive and active deviants

Contrasting "Deviants" elicited during active listening against "Deviants" elicited during passive listening (i.e., Deviants active > Deviants passive) revealed significant differences in activation in the right middle frontal gyrus (MTG; BAs 6/8/9/10/46; t-score 5.24, $p < 0.01$), the left precuneus (BAs 7/19; t-score 5.06, $p < 0.01$), the right

Table 1 sLORETA results from the contrast: "Deviant" versus "Standard" (1000 vs. 500 Hz pure tones) in the N1/MMN time window from 80 to 123 ms post stimulus-onset during passive listening

Brain region				Coordinates (X, Y, Z)						t-value		No. of voxels
Structure	BA	Hemisphere	Lobe	Talairach (max.)			MNI (max.)			Max.	Min.	
Lingual gyrus	*17*, 18, 19	R/L	Occipital	20	−82	4	20	−85	0	4.06**	3.30*	30
Superior Temporal Gyrus (STG)	13, *22*, 39, 42	R	Temporal	64	38	20	65	−40	20	3.97*	3.29*	9

Talairach/MNI coordinates and t-values are referred to the peak activity in each brain region. Italic numbers indicate maximal brain electrical activity in the corresponding BA. Only clusters of size ≥ 9 voxels are reported

**$p < 0.01$, *$p < 0.05$, *L* left, *R* right, *BA* Brodmann area, *MNI* Montreal Neurological Institute

Table 2 sLORETA results from the contrast: "Deviant" versus "Standard" (1000 vs. 500 Hz pure tones) in the N1/MMN time window from 83 to 95 ms post stimulus-onset during active listening

Brain region				Coordinates (X, Y, Z)						t-value		No. of voxels
Structure	BA	Hemisphere	Lobe	Talairach (max.)			MNI (max.)			Max.	Min.	
Inferior Parietal Lobule (IPL)	7, *39*, 40	R	Parietal/Temporal	45	−66	40	45	−70	40	8.12**	4.66**	10

Talairach/MNI coordinates and t-values are referred to the peak activity in each brain region. Italic numbers indicate maximal brain electrical activity in the corresponding BA. Only clusters of size ≥ 9 voxels are reported

**$p < 0.01$, *L* left, *R* right, *BA* Brodmann area, *MNI* Montreal Neurological Institute

Table 3 sLORETA results from the contrast: "Deviant" versus "Standard" (1000 vs. 500 Hz pure tones) in the P3 time window from 269 to 322 ms post stimulus-onset during passive listening

Brain region				Coordinates (X, Y, Z)						t-value		No. of voxels
Structure	BA	Hemisphere	Lobe	Talairach (max.)			MNI (max.)			Max.	Min.	
Insula	13	R/L	Sub-lobar	30	−33	20	30	−35	20	4.80**	3.59*	11
Lingual Gyrus	18	R	Occipital	10	−78	0	10	−80	−5	4.78**	3.59*	11

Talairach/MNI coordinates and t-values are referred to the peak activity in each brain region. Italic numbers indicate maximal brain electrical activity in the corresponding BA. Only clusters of size ≥ 9 voxels are reported

**p < 0.01, *p < 0.05, L left, R right, BA Brodmann area, MNI Montreal Neurological Institute

Table 4 sLORETA results from the contrast: "Deviant" versus "Standard" (1000 vs. 500 Hz pure tones) in the P3 time window from 253 to 351 ms post stimulus-onset during active listening

Brain region				Coordinates (X, Y, Z)						t-value		No. of voxels
Structure	BA	Hemisphere	Lobe	Talairach (max.)			MNI (max.)			Max.	Min.	
Precuneus	7, 19, 23, 31	R/L	Parietal/Occipital	20	−75	45	20	−80	45	5.11**	4.03**	132
Cingulate Gyrus	31	R/L	Limbic	15	−42	25	15	−45	25	4.86**	4.06**	20
Precentral Gyrus	4, 6	R	Frontal	45	−8	37	45	−10	40	4.81**	4.08**	13
Superior Temporal Gyrus (STG)	13, 22, 39, 41	R/L	Temporal	−50	−28	15	−50	−30	15	4.79**	4.04**	9
Postcentral Gyrus	2, 3, 7, 40	R/L	Parietal	−50	−24	15	−50	−25	15	4.64**	4.03**	11
Cuneus	7, 18, 19, 30	R/L	Occipital	−10	−76	36	−10	−80	35	4.62**	4.04**	35
Posterior Cingulate	23, 30, 31	R	Limbic	10	−53	16	10	−55	15	4.59**	4.05**	13
Inferior Parietal Lobule (IPL)	39, 40	R	Parietal	35	−47	39	35	−50	40	4.45**	4.04**	22

Talairach/MNI coordinates and t-values are referred to the peak activity in each brain region. Italic numbers indicate maximal brain electrical activity in the corresponding BA. Only clusters of size ≥ 9 voxels are reported

**p < 0.01, L left, R right, BA Brodmann area, MNI Montreal Neurological Institute

inferior frontal gyrus (IFG; BAs 9/13/45; t-score 4.86, p < 0.01), the left postcentral gyrus (BAs 2/5/7/40; t-score 4.80, p < 0.01), the left superior parietal lobule (SPL; BA 7; t-score 4.77, p < 0.01), the right precentral gyrus (BAs 6/9; t-score 4.36, p < 0.01), and the right inferior parietal lobule (IPL; BA 40; t-score 4.27, p < 0.01) in time window between 244 and 343 ms, corresponding to the time window in which amplitudes of the P3 component were most pronounced during passive and active listening conditions (see "Active tone oddball paradigm—ERPs (N1, MMN and P3)", "Passive and active deviants—passive and active standards ERPs" sections), see Table 5.

Table 5 sLORETA results from the contrast: "Deviant" during active listening versus "Deviant" during passive listening in the time window between 228 and 456 ms after stimulus onset

Brain region				Coordinates (X, Y, Z)						t-value		No. of voxels
Structure	BA	Hemisphere	Lobe	Talairach (max.)			MNI (max.)			max.	min.	
Middle frontal gyrus	6, 8, 9, 10, 46	R	Frontal	54	12	36	55	10	40	5.24**	4.00**	27
Precuneus	7, 19	L	Parietal	−10	−55	63	−10	−60	65	5.06**	3.81*	47
Inferior frontal gyrus	9, 13, 45	R/L	Frontal	54	11	32	55	10	35	4.86**	3.81*	16
Superior parietal lobule	7	R/L	Parietal	−15	−51	58	−15	−55	60	4.77**	3.81*	11
Precentral gyrus	6, 9	R	Frontal	45	21	36	45	20	40	4.42**	3.81*	9
Inferior parietal lobule	40	R	Parietal	50	−37	43	50	−40	45	4.27**	3.92**	12

Talairach/MNI coordinates and t-values are referred to the peak activity in each brain region. Itlaic numbers indicate maximal brain electrical activity in the corresponding BA. Only clusters of size ≥ 9 voxels are reported

**p < 0.01, *p < 0.05, L left, R right, BA Brodmann area, MNI Montreal Neurological Institute

Passive and active standards

Contrasting standards during both listening conditions (contrast: "Standards" active listening condition > "Standards" passive listening condition) revealed significant activation in the right middle frontal gyrus (BAs 10/11; 40, 53, − 11; *t*-score 4.39; *p* < 0.05) in the time window between 190 and 418 ms. As this contrast revealed only three significant voxels, no table is provided.

Discussion

The present study examined the spatio-temporal dynamics of auditory deviance and target detection in the auditory oddball paradigm by combining the advantages of the EEG–ERP methodology and the sLORETA source localization technique within the same experiment and subjects (i.e., within subject design). The design included both, passive as well as active listening conditions to specify and contrast the neural mechanisms underlying active and passive deviance and target detection. To this end, participants were instructed to listen (1) passively to pure tones without giving an overt behavioral response (experimental block 1) and (2) to listen to pure tones while being engaged in an active task (experimental block 2) which afforded to distinguish between the two presented pure tones by responding to the deviants by giving an overt behavioral response (button press).

Time course of passive and active deviance and target detection

Passive and active listening elicited an N1 and P3 component and additionally an MMN as difference potential when deviants were contrasted against standards. Amplitudes of the MMN which temporally overlapped with the amplitudes of the N1 were significantly more negative for deviant as compared to standard pure tones during passive and active listening conditions. This modulation pattern is in line with those reported in previous ERP studies using comparable auditory oddball paradigms with pure tones (e.g., see [81, 82]). Comparisons between deviants or standards during active versus passive listening (see "Passive and active deviants— passive and active standards ERPs", "Passive and active deviants" and Passive and active standards" sections) revealed no significant amplitude differences in the time window of the N1/MMN when passive and active listening conditions were compared against each other. Thus, voluntary guidance of selective attention to deviants may not facilitate deviance detection in early time windows of cortical stimulus processing (N1/MMN) beyond passive listening. This finding supports the assumption of particularly the MMN reflecting pre-attentive sensory stimulus discrimination [38] and automatic (involuntarily) auditory change detection [39, 40], i.e., processes that cannot be influenced by task-related attentive

processes. Regarding the overlap between amplitudes of the N1 and the MMN additional explanations for MMN modulation during auditory deviance processing have been proposed: as shown in Figs. 1 and 2, the time window of the N1 significantly overlapped with the MMN. In addition, N1 amplitudes were significantly reduced to standards during passive and active listening conditions. This may be explained by the observation that neurons reacting to standards only show a reduced electrical activity due to repeated stimulus presentation leading to habituation of these particular neurons. In contrast, neurons that fire in response to deviants show a much higher electrical activity. According to the literature, this phenomenon might be explained by the so-called refractoriness of certain neurons and thus by their selective sensitivity to different frequencies [36, 83, 84]. Hence, due to the amplitude overlap of the MMN and the N1, MMN modulation could also result from neural adaption in the auditory cortex [85]. However, whether this mechanism actually underlies N1/MMN overlap has not been sufficiently clarified yet and requires further neurophysiological testing.

Neural sources of passive and active deviance and target detection
Early time windows (N1/MMN)

When passive listening to "Deviants" vs. "Standards" was compared, source localization with sLORETA revealed activation in the left and right occipital cortex as well as in the right superior temporal gyrus (STG; BA 22) in the N1/MMN time window. Activation of the right STG included the auditory cortex (BA 42) and multisensory association areas (BAs 39/22). This is well in line with the idea of bottom-up and stimulus-driven deviance detection. During active processing of "Deviants" vs. "Standards" the largest voxel cluster was located in the right inferior parietal lobule (IPL; BAs 39/40). The right IPL is part of the ventral attention network (VAN) and plays an important role in visuospatial attention and attentive monitoring of stimuli for goal-directed eye or limb movements [86]. Thus, during active listening IPL activation during early stages of deviance processing (i.e., in the N1/MMN time window) may be a consequence of anticipatory control of attention in order to maintain current task goals (i.e., the voluntary selection of deviant stimuli). Altogether, this suggests that during passive and active listening early stages of deviance processing may be modulated by different brain regions and neural processes although, at a cortical level, with respect to ERPs, N1 and MMN amplitude modulation did not differ significantly between passive and active listening conditions.

Late time windows (P3)

For the time window corresponding to the P3 component the contrast "Deviants" > "Standards" revealed activation of the right and left insula during passive listening. Activation of the left and the right insula in the P3 window during passive listening is in line with previous studies reporting involvement of the insula (in particular the right insula) in auditory processing [87] and target detection (e.g., see [88]). More specifically, the insula is part of the VAN and also part of the so-called *salience network* (SN) [18, 19] that marks stimulus events as salient for additional processing and mediates activation of and between brain networks involved in bottom-up and top-down controlled attention. Crucially, during active listening, P3 modulation elicited by deviants as compared to standards was associated with activation in a distributed network including the precuneus and surrounding areas in the superior parietal lobule (SPL; BA 7), the posterior cingulate cortex (PPC; BAs 23/31) as well as motor-related areas. Most of the aforementioned brain regions form part of the dorsal attention networks (DAN). The present results therefore suggest that activation of brain regions belonging to the DAN network may occur only during active listening and during later time windows (P3) associated with voluntary guided target detection. Interestingly, the largest voxel cluster (size: 132 voxels) was located within the precuneus/SPL bilaterally. The precuneus is a cortical structure located in the superior parietal cortex. It is one of the core structures of the DAN [4, 14] and associated with voluntary attentional switching [89], but also modulated by saliency [90]. Activation of the precuneus/SPL (e.g., BA 7) was also observed in the contrast comparing processing of deviants during active > passive listening; again in the time P3 time window. In addition, P3 modulation was significantly larger for "Deviants" during active as compared to passive listening. Activation of the precuneus/SPL in the P3 time window during active listening may therefore indeed indicate the increase in attentional demands from passive to active, attentive and thus, voluntary and top-down controlled target detection.

Taken together, the sLORETA source localization analysis support the hypothesis that unattended (passive) as well as attended deviance and target detection elicit cortical activations in spatially distributed brain regions belonging to different brain networks including the VAN, DAN and SN.

A neurophysiolological model of passive and active auditory deviance and target detection

As illustrated in Fig. 4, based on the results of the present study a neurophysiological model of passive and active auditory deviance and target detection can be proposed that may act as a guide for future research. As shown in Fig. 4, this model illustrates that passive and active auditory deviance detection in the auditory oddball paradigm are associated with activation of brain regions belonging

to at least two different brain networks: these include on the one hand auditory processing regions in the STG (e.g., BA 22) and the insula (BA 13) as key region of the VAN and SN involved in passive auditory deviance detection, and on the other hand, parietal and frontal brain regions as key regions of the VAN and particularly of the DAN involved in task-related auditory deviance and target detection [18, 91]. Activation of the STG and insula during passive listening is in close agreement with previously conducted neuroimaging studies combining fMRI with multi-channel EEG recordings during an auditory oddball paradigm and a passive listening task [10, 12]. Results of these studies obtained from fMRI indicated comparable cortical activations in the right STG and the right superior temporal plane (BAs 41/42) and right anterior insula during passive listening of auditory deviant stimuli. Also, going beyond previous research, the present results suggest that during passive listening activation of the VAN and the SN in particular may occur at later stages of stimulus selection, i.e., when deviants in contrast to standards are selected for further processing and associated with the elicitation of a P3 component. Earlier processing stages associated with automatic deviance detection as reflected by N1/MMN modulation on the contrary seem to be related specifically with activation of sensory brain regions belonging to the VAN (superior temporal gyrus) as well as with visual cortical activation. Although brain regions in the visual cortex, such as the lateral occipital cortex are typically associated with the processing of visual information (e.g., visual objects) in visual spatial attention tasks [21–23], more recent functional imaging studies [9, 92] showed in line with our findings that specific regions in the visual cortex (such as the LOC or the lingual gyrus in the medial visual cortex) may be activated during the processing of salient acoustic stimuli [24] and as suggested by our study this may occur even or specifically if no task is at hand. Moreover, in contrast to passive listening, during active listening auditory processing may be fully taken over by the brain's attention networks including activation of brain regions belonging to the VAN during deviance detection in the N1/MMN time window and of the DAN during target detection in the P3 time window.

Limitations and future outlook

Although the results of the present study including the proposed model support a number of the hypotheses tested there are limitations that must be taken with caution. A major disadvantage of the present study may be the small sample size. However, effect sizes calculated for the t-tests reported under 3.2–3.5 revealed at least moderate effects (Cohen's $d \geq |0.6|$) resulting in a post hoc power estimation of at least 0.6. Nevertheless, due to the small

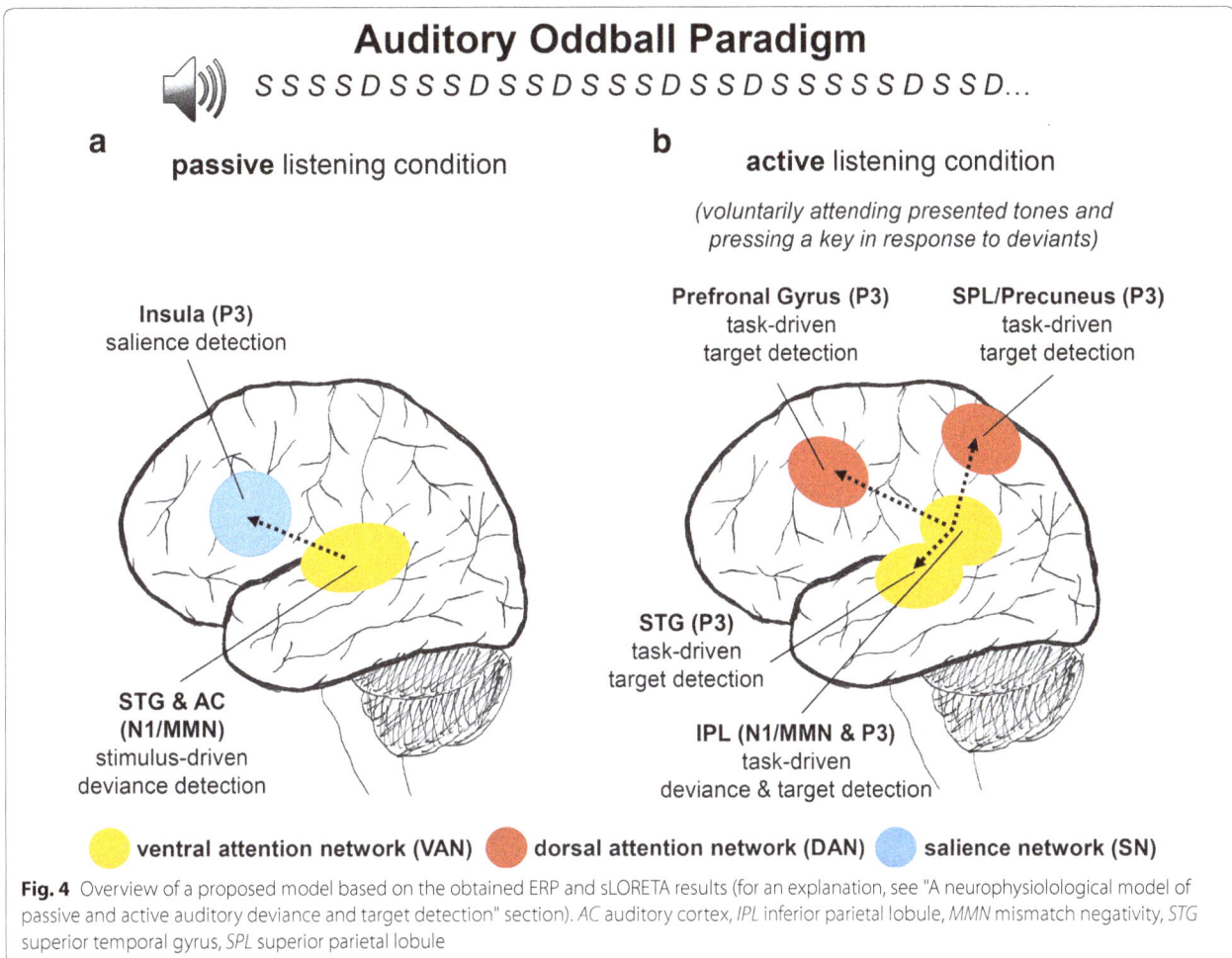

Fig. 4 Overview of a proposed model based on the obtained ERP and sLORETA results (for an explanation, see "A neurophysiolological model of passive and active auditory deviance and target detection" section). *AC* auditory cortex, *IPL* inferior parietal lobule, *MMN* mismatch negativity, *STG* superior temporal gyrus, *SPL* superior parietal lobule

sample size the generalizability of the reported effects and the proposed model may be limited (see Fig. 4).

Another confound in the present study might be the temporal overlap of the N1 and MMN component. This phenomenon may be observed when the perceptual difference between "Deviants" and "Standards" is particularly prominent in the frequency domain [93]. Regarding the question which and how many brain networks may be activated during passive versus active deviance and target detection further research may unravel the functional connectivity between the hypothesized networks. The present results suggest that besides the VAN and DAN, the SN may indeed play an important role in auditory deviance and target detection during passive listening. In contrast to the VAN, the SN is believed to be involved in the detection of stimulus saliency, expectancy and automatic selection of an adaptive and suitable (behavioral) response [18]. The core structure of the SN consists of the dorsal part of the ACC (dACC; BAs 24/32/33), subcortical and limbic structures (e.g. amygdala), as well as

both insulae bilaterally [91]. Given the high degree of functional and anatomical overlap between the SN and the VAN, some researchers see both networks as parts of the same system [94]. However, given that according to meta-analytic findings the VAN should be more active when stimuli are task-relevant which was confirmed in this study and the fact that, in this study activation of the insula was not found during active listening, the present results agree with the notion to conceptualize the SN and VAN as two distinct networks [95, 96] with distinct roles during auditory processing.

Yet, another restriction that needs to be mentioned is related to the mathematical algorithms implemented in sLORETA. These algorithms are mainly based on non-parametric voxel-by-voxel comparisons for why sLORETA results—like conventional fMRI results—should not be interpreted causally. To overcome some of these methodological limitations, the application of repetitive transcranial magnetic stimulation (rTMS) may offer a non-invasive and thus elegant way to selectively inhibit or facilitate cortical activity in superficial brain regions (e.g., IPL or SPL/precuneus) and even in deeper cortical structures such as the insula [97] by applying fast trains of electromagnetic pulses [98]. Hence, in future studies, rTMS would offer potential prove for the neurophysiological model derived from the present data regarding passive as well as active auditory deviance and target detection.

Conclusion

In summary, the present study investigated the temporal and spatial dynamics of auditory deviance and target detection in an auditory oddball paradigm by combining EEG–ERP and sLORETA methods. Despite abundant previous research investigating either the time course or the neural sources and brain structures of auditory processing in the auditory oddball paradigm the present study is one of the few studies so far that combined analysis of ERPs with sLORETA source imaging during passive and active listening conditions in a within subject design in an attempt to explore when and where in the brain auditory deviance and target detection takes place during passive and active listening conditions. The results of the present study as well as the neurophysiological model derived from the current findings may be tentative due to the small sample size but may bolster future studies validating the suggested temporal activation pattern in larger samples of participants.

Authors' contributions

Both authors contributed extensively to the work presented in this paper. Both authors made substantial contributions to the conception and design, the analysis and interpretation of the data. CJ and CH designed the experiment. CJ ran the experiment and collected the data. CJ analyzed the data with support of CH. CJ and CH interpreted the data and CJ and CH wrote the manuscript. Both authors read and approved the final manuscript.

Author details

[1] University of Tuebingen, Tuebingen, Germany. [2] Institute of Psychology and Education, Applied Emotion and Motivation Research, University of Ulm, Ulm, Germany.

Acknowledgements

We would like to thank Prof. Dr. Dr. Markus Raab for the opportunity to use the EEG laboratory located at the Institute of Psychology of the German Sport University Cologne, Germany.

Competing interests

The authors declare that they have no competing interests.

Funding

This study was supported by the German Research Foundation (DFG; HE5880-3/1), awarded to CH.

References

1. Watkins S, Dalton P, Lavie N, Rees G. Brain mechanisms mediating auditory attentional capture in humans. Cereb Cortex. 2007;17:1694–700.
2. Halgren E, Squires NK, Wilson CL, Rohrbaugh JW, Babb TL, Crandall PH. Endogenous potentials generated in the human hippocampal formation and amygdala by infrequent events. Science. 1980;210:803 LP–805LP.
3. Bledowski C, Prvulovic D, Goebel R, Zanella FE, Linden DEJ. Attentional systems in target and distractor processing: a combined ERP and fMRI study. Neuroimage. 2004;22:530–40.
4. Kim H. Involvement of the dorsal and ventral attention networks in oddball stimulus processing: a meta-analysis. Hum Brain Mapp. 2014;35:2265–84.
5. Bennington JY, Polich J. Comparison of P300 from passive and active tasks for auditory and visual stimuli. Int J Psychophysiol. 1999;34:171–7.
6. Gurtubay IG, Alegre M, Labarga A, Malanda A, Iriarte J, Artieda J. Gamma band activity in an auditory oddball paradigm studied with the wavelet transform. Clin Neurophysiol. 2001;112:1219–28.
7. Kennan RP, Horovitz SG, Maki A, Yamashita Y, Koizumi H, Gore JC. Simultaneous recording of event-related auditory oddball response using transcranial near infrared optical topography and surface EEG. Neuroimage. 2002;16:587–92.
8. Lee T-W, Yu YW-Y, Wu H-C, Chen T-J. Do resting brain dynamics predict oddball evoked-potential? BMC Neurosci. 2011;12:1–10.
9. Kiehl KA, Laurens KR, Duty TL, Forster BB, Liddle PF. Neural sources involved in auditory target detection and novelty processing: an event-related fMRI study. Psychophysiology. 2001;38:133–42.
10. Liebenthal E, Ellingson ML, Spanaki MV, Prieto TE, Ropella KM, Binder JR. Simultaneous ERP and fMRI of the auditory cortex in a passive oddball paradigm. Neuroimage. 2003;19:1395–404.
11. Linden DEJ, Prvulovic D, Formisano E, Völlinger M, Zanella FE, Goebel R, et al. The functional neuroanatomy of target detection: an fMRI study of visual and auditory oddball tasks. Cereb Cortex. 1999;9:815–23.
12. Müller BW, Stude P, Nebel K, Wiese H, Ladd ME, Forsting M, et al. Sparse imaging of the auditory oddball task with functional MRI. NeuroReport. 2003;14:1597–601.
13. Opitz B, Mecklinger A, von Cramon DY, Kruggel F. Combining electrophysiological and hemodynamic measures of the auditory oddball. Psychophysiology. 1999;36:142–7.
14. Corbetta M, Shulman GL. Control of goal-directed and stimulus-driven attention in the brain. Nat Rev Neurosci. 2002;3:215–29.
15. Vossel S, Geng JJ, Fink GR. Dorsal and ventral attention systems: distinct neural circuits but collaborative roles. Neurosci. 2014;20:150–9.
16. Rossi AF, Pessoa L, Desimone R, Ungerleider LG. The prefrontal cortex and the executive control of attention. Exp Brain Res. 2009;192:489–97.
17. Palaniyappan L, Liddle PF. Does the salience network play a cardinal role in psychosis? An emerging hypothesis of insular dysfunction. J Psychiatry Neurosci. 2012;37:17–27.
18. Menon V, Uddin LQ. Saliency, switching, attention and control: a network model of insula function. Brain Struct Funct. 2010;214:655–67.
19. Seeley WW, Menon V, Schatzberg AF, Keller J, Glover GH, Kenna H, et al. Dissociable intrinsic connectivity networks for salience processing and executive control. J Neurosci. 2007;27:2349–56.
20. Sridharan D, Levitin DJ, Menon V. A critical role for the right fronto-insular cortex in switching between central-executive and default-mode networks. Proc Natl Acad Sci. 2008;105:12569–74.
21. Grill-Spector K, Kushnir T, Edelman S, Avidan G, Itzchak Y, Malach R. Differential processing of objects under various viewing conditions in the human lateral occipital complex. Neuron. 1999;24:187–203.
22. Grill-Spector K, Kourtzi Z, Kanwisher N. The lateral occipital complex and its role in object recognition. Vis Res. 2001;41:1409–22.
23. Murray SO, Wojciulik E. Attention increases neural selectivity in the human lateral occipital complex. Nat Neurosci. 2004;7:70–4.
24. McDonald JJ, Störmer VS, Martinez A, Feng W, Hillyard SA. Salient sounds activate human visual cortex automatically. J Neurosci. 2013;33:9194–201.
25. Ji J, Porjesz B, Begleiter H, Chorlian D. P300: the similarities and differences in the scalp distribution of visual and auditory modality. Brain Topogr Kluwer Acad Publ Plenum Publ. 1999;11:315–27.
26. Kemner C, Verbaten MN, Cuperus JM, Camfferman G, van Engeland H. Auditory event-related brain potentials in autistic children and three different control groups. Biol Psychiatry. 1995;38:150–65.

27. Anderer P, Pascual-Marqui RD, Semlitsch HV, Saletu B. Differential effects of normal aging on sources of standard N1, target N1 and target P300 auditory event-related brain potentials revealed by low resolution electromagnetic tomography (LORETA). Electroencephalogr Clin Neurophysiol Potentials Sect. 1998;108:160–74.

28. Grimm S, Escera C. Auditory deviance detection revisited: evidence for a hierarchical novelty system. Int J Psychophysiol. 2012;85:88–92.

29. Polich J. Updating P300: an integrative theory of P3a and P3b. Clin Neurophysiol. 2007;118:2128–48.

30. Polich J, Kok A. Cognitive and biological determinants of P300: an integrative review. Biol Psychol. 1995;41:103–46.

31. Squires NK, Squires KC, Hillyard SA. Two varieties of long-latency positive waves evoked by unpredictable auditory stimuli in man. Electroencephalogr Clin Neurophysiol. 1975;38:387–401.

32. Luck SJ. An introduction to the event-related potential technique. Cambrigde: MIT Press; 2005.

33. Näätänen R, Paavilainen P, Rinne T, Alho K. The mismatch negativity (MMN) in basic research of central auditory processing: a review. Clin Neurophysiol. 2007;118:2544–90.

34. Garrido MI, Kilner JM, Stephan KE, Friston KJ. The mismatch negativity: a review of underlying mechanisms. Clin Neurophysiol Off J Int Fed Clin Neurophysiol. 2009;120:453–63.

35. Duncan CC, Barry RJ, Connolly JF, Fischer C, Michie PT, Näätänen R, et al. Event-related potentials in clinical research: guidelines for eliciting, recording, and quantifying mismatch negativity, P300, and N400. Clin Neurophysiol. 2009;120:1883–908.

36. Campbell T, Winkler I, Kujala T. N1 and the mismatch negativity are spatiotemporally distinct ERP components: disruption of immediate memory by auditory distraction can be related to N1. Psychophysiology. 2007;44:530–40.

37. Näätänen R, Picton T. The N1 wave of the human electric and magnetic response to sound: a review and an analysis of the component structure. Psychophysiology. 1987;24:375–425.

38. Näätänen R, Alho K. Mismatch negativity—a unique measure of sensory processing in audition. Int J Neurosci. 1995;80:317–37.

39. Escera C, Alho K, Schröger E, Winkler I. Involuntary attention and distractibility as evaluated with event-related brain potentials. Audiol Neuro Otol. 2000;5:151–66.

40. Escera C, Alho K, Winkler I, Näätänen R. Neural mechanisms of involuntary attention to acoustic novelty and change. J Cogn Neurosci. 1998;10:590–604.

41. Patel SH, Azzam PN. Characterization of N200 and P300: selected studies of the event-related potential. Int J Med Sci. 2005;2(4):147–54.

42. Picton TW. The P300 wave of the human event-related potential. J Clin Neurophysiol. 1992;9:456–79.

43. Debener S, Kranczioch C, Herrmann CS, Engel AK. Auditory novelty oddball allows reliable distinction of top-down and bottom-up processes of attention. Int J Psychophysiol. 2002;46:77–84.

44. Kok A. On the utility of P3 amplitude as a measure of processing capacity. Psychophysiology. 2001;38:557–77.

45. Donchin E, Coles M. Is the P300 component a manifestation of context updating? Behav Brain Sci. 1988;11:357–74.

46. Birn RM, Cox RW, Bandettini PA. Detection versus estimation in event-related fMRI: choosing the optimal stimulus timing. Neuroimage. 2002;15:252–64.

47. Pascual-Marqui RD. Review of methods for solving the EEG inverse problem. Int J Bioelectromagn. 1999;1:75–86.

48. Vitacco D, Brandeis D, Pascual-Marqui R, Martin E. Correspondence of event-related potential tomography and functional magnetic resonance imaging during language processing. Hum Brain Mapp. 2002;17:4–12.

49. Pascual-Marqui RD, Michel CM, Lehmann D. Low resolution electromagnetic tomography: a new method for localizing electrical activity in the brain. Int J Psychophysiol. 1994;18:49–65.

50. Mulert C, Jäger L, Schmitt R, Bussfeld P, Pogarell O, Möller H-J, et al. Integration of fMRI and simultaneous EEG: towards a comprehensive understanding of localization and time-course of brain activity in target detection. Neuroimage. 2004;22:83–94.

51. Mulert C, Pogarell O, Juckel G, Rujescu D, Giegling I, Rupp D, et al. The neural basis of the P300 potential. Eur Arch Psychiatry Clin Neurosci. 2004;254:190–8.

52. Volpe U, Mucci A, Bucci P, Merlotti E, Galderisi S, Maj M. The cortical generators of P3a and P3b: a LORETA study. Brain Res Bull. 2007;73:220–30.

53. Justen C, Herbert C. Snap your fingers! An ERP/sLORETA study investigating implicit processing of self- vs. other-related movement sounds using the passive oddball paradigm. Front Hum Neurosci. 2016;10:465.

54. Williams LM, Simms E, Clark CR, Paul RH, Rowe D, Gordon E. The test-retest reliability of a standardized neurocognitive and neurophysiological test battery: "Neuromarker". Int J Neurosci. 2005;115:1605–30.

55. Millisecond: Auditory Oddball Task [Internet]. 2017 [cited 2017 Jan 28]. http://www.millisecond.com/download/library/Oddball/.

56. Jurcak V, Tsuzuki D, Dan I. 10/20, 10/10, and 10/5 systems revisited: their validity as relative head-surface-based positioning systems. Neuroimage. 2007;34:1600–11.

57. Zanow F, Knösche TR. ASA—advanced source analysis of continuous and event-related EEG/MEG signals. Brain Topogr. 2004;16:287–90.

58. Ille N, Berg P, Scherg M. Artifact correction of the ongoing EEG ssing spatial filters based on artifact and brain signal topographies. J Clin Neurophysiol. 2002;19:113–24.

59. Delorme A, Makeig S. EEGLAB: an open source toolbox for analysis of single-trial EEG dynamics including independent component analysis. J Neurosci Methods. 2004;134:9–21.

60. Delorme A. Statistical methods. In: Webster JG, editor. Encyclopedia of medical devices and instrumentation. Hoboken: Wiley; 2004. p. 240–56.

61. Benjamini Y, Hochberg Y. Controlling the false discovery rate: a practical and powerful approach to multiple testing. J R Stat Soc Ser B. 1995;1:289–300.

62. Lage-Castellanos A, Martínez-Montes E, Hernández-Cabrera JA, Galán L. False discovery rate and permutation test: an evaluation in ERP data analysis. Stat Med. 2010;29:63–74.

63. Groppe DM, Urbach TP, Kutas M. Mass univariate analysis of event-related brain potentials/fields I: a critical tutorial review. Psychophysiology. 2011;48:1711–25.

64. Groppe DM, Urbach TP, Kutas M. Mass univariate analysis of event-related brain potentials/fields II: simulation studies. Psychophysiology. 2011;48:1726–37.

65. Mass Univariate ERP Toolbox [Internet]. 2017 [cited 2017 Jan 28]. http://openwetware.org/wiki/Mass_Univariate_ERP_Toolbox.

66. Bullmore ET, Suckling J, Overmeyer S, Rabe-Hesketh S, Taylor E, Brammer MJ. Global, voxel, and cluster tests, by theory and permutation, for a difference between two groups of structural MR images of the brain. IEEE Trans Med Imaging. 1999;18:32–42.

67. Manly BFJ. Randomization, bootstrap and Monte Carlo methods in biology texts in statistical science. 2nd ed. London: Chapman & Hall/CRC; 1997.

68. LORETA—Low Resolution Electromagnetic Tomography [Internet]. 2017 [cited 2017 Jan 28]. http://www.uzh.ch/keyinst/loreta.htm.

69. Fuchs M, Kastner J, Wagner M, Hawes S, Ebersole JS. A standardized boundary element method volume conductor model. Clin Neurophysiol. 2002;113:702–12.

70. Mazziotta J, Toga A, Evans A, Fox P, Lancaster J, Zilles K, et al. A probabilistic atlas and reference system for the human brain: International Consortium for Brain Mapping (ICBM). Philos Trans R Soc Lond B Biol Sci R. Soc. 2001;356:1293–322.

71. Lancaster JL, Woldorff MG, Parsons LM, Liotti M, Freitas CS, Rainey L, et al. Automated Talairach Atlas labels for functional brain mapping. Hum Brain Mapp. 2000;10:120–31.

72. Talairach J, Tournoux P. Co-planar stereotaxic atlas of the human brain. Stuttgart; New York: G. Thieme; 1988.

73. Oostenveld R, Praamstra P. The five percent electrode system for high-resolution EEG and ERP measurements. Clin Neurophysiol. 2001;112:713–9.

74. Brett M, Johnsrude IS, Owen AM. The problem of functional localization in the human brain. Nat Rev Neurosci. 2002;3:243–9.

75. Nichols TE, Holmes AP. Nonparametric permutation tests for functional neuroimaging: a primer with examples. Hum Brain Mapp. 2002;15:1–25.

76. Silva L, Amitai Y, Connors B. Intrinsic oscillations of neocortex generated by layer 5 pyramidal neurons. Science. 1991;251:433–5.

77. Haalman I, Vaadia E. Dynamics of neuronal interactions: relation to behavior, firing rates, and distance between neurons. Hum Brain Mapp. 1997;5:249–53.

78. Friston KJ. Statistical parametric mapping and other analysis of functional imaging data. In: Toga AW, Mazziotta JC, editors. Brain Mapp. 2nd. ed. Amsterdam; Boston: Academic Press; 2002. p. 363–85.

79. Brodmann K, Gary LJ. Brodmann's localization in the cerebral cortex. New York: Springer; 2006.

80. Koelsch S. Brain and Music. 1st ed. Chichester, West Sussex; Hoboken, NJ: Wiley-Blackwell: John Wiley & Sons, Inc; 2012.

81. Godey B, Schwartz D, de Graaf J, Chauvel P, Liégeois-Chauvel C. Neuromagnetic source localization of auditory evoked fields and intracerebral evoked potentials: a comparison of data in the same patients. Clin Neurophysiol. 2001;112:1850–9.

82. Zouridakis G, Simos PG, Papanicolaou AC. Multiple bilaterally asymmetric cortical sources account for the auditory N1 m component. Brain Topogr. 1998;10:183–9.

83. McEvoy L, Hari R, Imada T, Sams M. Human auditory cortical mechanisms of sound lateralization: II. Interaural time differences at sound onset. Hear Res. 1993;67:98–109.

84. Näätänen R, Sams M, Alho K, Paavilainen P, Reinikainen K, Sokolov EN. Frequency and location specificify of the human vertex N1 wave. Electroencephalogr Clin Neurophysiol. 1988;69:523–31.

85. Jääskeläinen IP, Ahveninen J, Bonmassar G, Dale AM, Ilmoniemi RJ, Levänen S, et al. Human posterior auditory cortex gates novel sounds to consciousness. Proc Natl Acad Sci USA. 2004;101:6809–14.

86. Singh-Curry V, Husain M. The functional role of the inferior parietal lobe in the dorsal and ventral stream dichotomy. Neuropsychologia. 2009;47:1434–48.

87. Bamiou D-E, Musiek FE, Luxon LM. The insula (Island of Reil) and its role in auditory processing. Brain Res Rev. 2003;42:143–54.

88. Müller BW, Achenbach C, Oades RD, Bender S, Schall U. Modulation of mismatch negativity by stimulus deviance and modality of attention. Neuroreport. 2002;13.

89. Le TH, Pardo JV, Hu X. 4 T-fMRI study of nonspatial shifting of selective attention: cerebellar and parietal contributions. J Neurophysiol. 1998;79:1535–48.

90. Indovina I, Macaluso E. Dissociation of stimulus relevance and saliency factors during shifts of visuospatial attention. Cereb Cortex. 2007;17:1701–11.

91. Uddin LQ. Salience processing and insular cortical function and dysfunction. Nat Rev Neurosci. 2014;16:55–61.

92. Goldman RI, Wei C-Y, Philiastides MG, Gerson AD, Friedman D, Brown TR, et al. Single-trial discrimination for integrating simultaneous EEG and fMRI: identifying cortical areas contributing to trial-to-trial variability in the auditory oddball task. Neuroimage. 2009;47:136–47.

93. Tiitinen H, May P, Reinikainen K, Näätänen R. Attentive novelty detection in humans is governed by pre-attentive sensory memory. Nature. 1994;372:90–2.

94. Kucyi A, Hodaie M, Davis KD. Lateralization in intrinsic functional connectivity of the temporoparietal junction with salience- and attention-related brain networks. J Neurophysiol. 2012;108:3382–92.

95. Cole MW, Reynolds JR, Power JD, Repovs G, Anticevic A, Braver TS. Multi-task connectivity reveals flexible hubs for adaptive task control. Nat Neurosci. 2013;16:1348–55.

96. Power JD, Cohen AL, Nelson SM, Wig GS, Barnes KA, Church JA, et al. Functional network organization of the human brain. Neuron. 2011;72:665–78.

97. Ciampi de Andrade D, Galhardoni R, Pinto LF, Lancelotti R, Rosi J Jr, Marcolin MA, et al. Into the Island: a new technique of non-invasive cortical stimulation of the insula. Neurophysiol Clin Neurophysiol. 2012;42:363–8.

98. Walsh V, Cowey A. Transcranial magnetic stimulation and cognitive neuroscience. Nat Rev Neurosci. 2000;1:73–9.

7

Amelioration of spinal cord injury in rats by blocking peroxynitrite/calpain activity

Mushfiquddin Khan[1]*●, Tajinder S. Dhammu[1], Inderjit Singh[1,2] and Avtar K. Singh[2,3]

Abstract

Background: Spinal cord injury (SCI) is one of the leading causes of disability and chronic pain. In SCI-induced pathology, homeostasis of the nitric oxide (NO) metabolome is lost. Major NO metabolites such as S-nitrosoglutathione (GSNO) and peroxynitrite are reported to play pivotal roles in regulating the activities of key cysteine proteases, calpains. While peroxynitrite (a metabolite of NO and superoxide) up regulates the activities of calpains leading to neurodegeneration, GSNO (a metabolite of NO and glutathione) down regulates the activities of calpains leading to neuroprotection. In this study, effect of GSNO on locomotor function and pain threshold and their relationship with the levels of peroxynitrite and the activity of calpain in the injured spinal cord were investigated using a 2-week rat model of contusion SCI.

Results: SCI animals were initially treated with GSNO at 2 h after the injury followed by a once daily dose of GSNO for 14 days. Locomotor function was evaluated by "Basso Beattie and Bresnahan (BBB) locomotor rating scale" and pain by mechanical allodynia. Peroxynitrite level, as expression of 3-nitrotyrosine (3-NT), calpain activity, as the degradation products of calpain substrate alpha II spectrin, and nNOS activity, as the expression phospho nNOS, were measured by western blot analysis. Treatment with GSNO improved locomotor function and mitigated pain. The treatment also reduced the levels of peroxynitrite (3-NT) and decreased activity of calpains. Reduced levels of peroxynitrite resulted from the GSNO-mediated inhibition of aberrant activity of neuronal nitric oxide synthase (nNOS).

Conclusions: The data indicates that higher levels of 3-NT and aberrant activities of nNOS and calpains correlated with SCI pathology and functional deficits. Treatment with GSNO improved locomotor function and mitigated mechanical allodynia acutely post-injury. Because GSNO shows potential to ameliorate experimental SCI, we discuss implications for GSNO therapy in clinical SCI research.

Keywords: BBB, Calpains, GSNO, nNOS, Peroxynitrite, SCI, Pain

Background

Spinal cord injury (SCI) results in locomotor deficits and pain due to the production of noxious metabolites which are held responsible for profound neurodegeneration [1, 2]. SCI is a major medical and socio-economic problem, and the rate of SCI is increasing every year [3]. The incidence of SCI is highest among young adults due to motor vehicle accidents, violence and sports accidents [4]. Other than critical care management, no current FDA-approved drug therapy exists for traumatic SCI

[1]. Several pharmacological therapies, including methylprednisolone, have been evaluated time and again in SCI [2] without clinical success. SCI is divided into two distinct types of injury: primary and secondary. Primary (immediate phase after SCI) injury includes physical damage as a direct result of the traumatic event. It cannot be reversed. Secondary injury follows the initial physical insult, resulting from mechanistic crosstalk between and among several deleterious pathways, including redox and excitotoxicity [1]. Secondary injury is therefore amenable to reversal and treatment. A critical examination of injury mechanisms shows a disturbed nitric oxide (NO) metabolome [5, 6]. We hypothesize this metabolome to be responsible for the production of neuronal nitric oxide synthase (nNOS)-dependent deleterious peroxynitrite.

*Correspondence: khanm@musc.edu
[1] Department of Pediatrics, 508 Children's Research Institute, Medical University of South Carolina, 173 Ashley Ave, Charleston, SC 29425, USA
Full list of author information is available at the end of the article

As a consequence, much less NO is available for S-nitrosoglutathione (GSNO) biosynthesis and thus GSNO-mediated regulation of enzymatic activities is lost. Reduced NO bioavailability and the consequent decrease in GSNO levels are associated with chronic neurovascular injuries, and exogenous GSNO supplementation is reported to ameliorate CNS injuries [7–11]. Therefore, the objective of this study was to investigate the efficacy of GSNO for functional recovery and its role in regulation of the nNOS/calpain system in a rat model of contusion SCI.

GSNO is an endogenous molecule of the human body, produced mainly in NOS expressing cells by the reaction of NO with glutathione (GSH) in the presence of oxygen [12]. GSNO's biosynthesis is also influenced by altered redox [13]. It is present in the brain and other organs [14]. GSNO reductase (GSNOR) is the major GSNO-degrading enzyme and thus GSNOR knock out mice store GSNO in excess [15]. GSNOR degrades GSNO to ammonia and oxidized glutathione (GSSG) without releasing free NO [16], indicating that the NO moiety of GSNO is not recycled by the enzymatic activity of GSNOR. GSNO is directly involved in cell signaling via S-nitrosylation of target proteins, including calpains, NF-κB, STAT3, neuronal NOS (nNOS) [8, 9, 17–21]. Several studies showing the efficacy of GSNO in human diseases have been listed by Hornyak et al. [22]. None of the studies reported significant side effects in humans associated with the use of exogenous GSNO. In animal studies, GSNO protects against cardiac ischemic injury [23], indicating the therapeutic potential of GSNO-mediated S-nitrosylation mechanism [9, 24]. S-nitrosylation of PTEN (a lipid phosphatase) has been shown to inhibit its activity, leading to the activation of Akt and thus the stimulation of neurorepair process in an animal model of stroke [25]. The Akt activation has been shown to be associated with stabilization of hypoxia-inducible factor-1 alpha (HIF-1α), which, in turn, induces the expression vascular endothelial growth factor (VEGF) leading to therapeutic angiogenesis/neurogenesis and consequent recovery of function [26].

In spite of the significant role of GSNO in cellular functions, neither GSNO nor its S-nitrosylation mechanism has been investigated for anti-neurodegenerative efficacy in SCI. Decreased synthesis of GSNO due to reduced levels of either GSH [19] or NO [27] or both in SCI, combined with increased degradation of GSNO by inflammation-induced enzyme activity of GSNO reductase (GSNOR) [24], will likely contribute to the reduced levels of GSNO in SCI. Deficient S-nitrosylation is considered to be a general neurodegenerative mechanism [28–30]. Via S-nitrosylation, GSNO protects against neurodegeneration by targeting multiple signaling pathways,

including anti-inflammatory, anti-oxidant and vascular effects [9, 31–33]. GSNO also stimulates production of neurotrophic factors [11, 34] and induces neuroregeneration [35]. On the other hand, peroxynitrite is formed by an instantaneous diffusion limited reaction between NO and superoxide under oxidative conditions. This reaction not only reduces NO bioavailability but also increases peroxynitrite-mediated tissue/cell damage. Peroxynitrite causes a sustained activation of calpains [36], leading to neurodegeneration and functional deficits [10, 21]. In SCI, the observed increased 3-nitrotyrosine (3NT) levels, a peroxynitrite adduct of tyrosine residue, in the injured cord [37, 38] suggest its pathological role in SCI. We observed that GSNO treatment of SCI decreased the levels of peroxynitrite via inhibition of nNOS activation, which paralleled with decreased calpain activity and improved Basso Beattie and Bresnahan (BBB) locomotor rating scale scores as well as the threshold for mechanical allodynia out to 2 weeks post-injury.

Methods

Experimental procedure

Reagents

GSNO (Item#: GSNO-100) was purchased from World Precision Instruments (Sarasota, FL, USA). All other chemicals and reagents used were purchased from Sigma-Aldrich (St. Louis, MO), unless stated otherwise.

Animals

Animals were young adult male Sprague–Dawley (SD) rats, obtained from Harlan Laboratory (Wilmington, MA), weighing 250–300 g at the time of surgery. All animals received humane care in compliance with the Medical University of South Carolina's (MUSC) guidance and the National Research Council's criteria for humane care. Animal procedures were approved by the institutional animal care and use committee (IACUC) of MUSC.

Experimental groups, drugs and dose

The animals (n = 21) were randomly divided into three groups: (1) SCI animals treated with vehicle (SCI; n = 7), (2) SCI animals treated with GSNO (GSNO; n = 7), and (3) sham-operated treated with vehicle (Sham; n = 7). In the SCI + GSNO treatment group, the rats were administered freshly prepared GSNO (0.05 mg/kg body weight), which was dissolved in sterile saline (~ 25 μl) and administered iv at 2 h after SCI. The dose of GSNO treatment was based on our previously reported dose response curve study, using 10 μg to 100 μg/kg body weight in a rat model of SCI and TBI [7, 10, 39]. The dose 50 μg/kg was found most effective in reducing contusion volume measured at 7 days after TBI [39]. Tests on uninjured sham rats did not produce alterations in physiologic parameters (blood pressure, heart rate, and body temperature) measured at 1 h following GSNO treatment [39]. Details of a GSNO study on physiologic parameters in rats have been previously described [10, 19].

Rat model of contusion SCI

Surgical anesthesia was induced by ketamine (90 mg/kg body weight) and xylazine (10 mg/kg body weight) administered intraperitoneally (ip). The animal was then placed onto a heated pad, and core body temperature was maintained at 37.0 ± 1 °C. The animals were secured in a stereotaxic frame. A dab of sterile ophthalmic ointment was placed on each eye to compensate for the decrease in lacrimation during anesthesia. SCI at the T9-T10 level was produced on the exposed spinal cord following a dorsal median incision and laminectomy. SCI was induced using a computer controlled impactor device described by Dr. Bilgen [40] and used in our studies [7, 41, 42] under aseptic conditions. SCI was performed with 2 mm tissue deformation and an impact velocity of 1.5 m/s and contusion time 85 ms. These parameters and conditions produced reproducible moderate spinal cord injury as described in our publications [7, 41]. Sham animals had the same procedures, with the exception of the impact. The impact tip was wiped clean with sterile alcohol after each impact and cleaned/disinfected further with cidex after surgery. During impact, body temperature was maintained at 37 °C by a heating pad. Immediately after injury, the incision was closed with nylon suture, and 2% lidocaine jelly was applied to the lesion site to minimize any possible discomfort. Post-surgical care: the bladders of all animals were expressed two to three times per day initially and later as needed. The body weight and humane endpoints were regularly monitored. Analgesic treatment was avoided after surgery because pain is also a target of this investigation. Antibiotic treatment was used in the event of persistent infection, which occurred rarely. The animals were sacrificed after the specified period of time with an overdose of ketamine/xylazine (90/10 mg/kg body weight) administered ip, as approved by the IACUC of MUSC.

Evaluation of locomotor function

All 7 rats were assessed at the indicated time points using the "Basso Beattie Bresnahan (BBB) locomotor rating scale" [43]. The BBB rating was described with a 21-point scale to measure hind limb function at various time points after injury. The scale assesses several different categories, including limb movement and tail position [43]. In our experiments, sham operated animals scored 21 (normal) on the BBB rating scale, whereas the SCI animals at day 0 had complete hind limb paralysis, thus scoring 0. Two investigators blinded to the experimental groups evaluated rats using the BBB scale as previously described from our laboratory [7]. All rats in both SCI and GSNO (SCI + GSNO) had significantly lower BBB score evaluated on day 1 after SCI.

Evaluation of mechanical allodynia

Before the testing of mechanical allodynia, all rats were habituated for at least 2 h on a metal mesh inside a *von Frey* plastic chamber. Nociception was measured by the paw pressure threshold using anesthesiometer (AM) (Ugo Basile, Italy), which applies a linearly increasing mechanical force to the dorsum of the rat's hind paw. The test was performed as previously described from our laboratory [44, 45]. The nociceptive threshold was defined as the force in grams at which the rat withdrew its paw. Continuously increasing pressure was applied to the dorsal surface of the hind paws. The time the animal withdrew its paw was recorded. Three trials were made on each paw with 5 min inter-test intervals. Testing was performed once per day until the end of the experiment. All rats in both SCI and GSNO (SCI + GSNO) developed significant pain when evaluated on day 3 after SCI.

Western blot analysis

At the endpoint, the animals were euthanized by decapitation under deep anesthesia and spinal cord was harvested for biochemical experiments. The spinal cords were snap frozen and stored at -70 °C for subsequent assays, if needed.

In the traumatic penumbra area (8 mm segment consists of 2 mm epicenter, 3 mm caudal from epicenter, 3 mm rostral from epicenter) from the injured cord tissue, western blot was performed as described earlier [9, 46] using following antibodies. nNOS (Abcam Cat# ab1376, RRID:AB_300614, 0.2 µg/ml concentration), phospho nNOS Ser^{1417}, equivalent to human Ser^{1412} (Abcam Cat# ab90443, RRID:AB_2049208, 1.0 µg/ml concentration), 3-NT (Abcam Cat# ab7048, RRID:AB_305725, 0.1 µg/ml concentration), alpha II spectrin (Cell Signaling Cat# SC-46696, RRID:AB_671135, 0.2 µg/ml concentration) and β-actin (Sigma-Aldrich Cat# A3853, RRID:AB_262137, 0.2 µg/ml concentration), followed by horseradish peroxidase-conjugated, goat anti-rabbit secondary antibody (Jackson ImmunoResearch Lab Cat# 111-035-045, RRID:AB_2337938, 1:4000 dilution). All non-phospho antibodies were diluted with 1XTBS-T with 2% non-fat dry milk. The pnNOS antibody was diluted using 1X TBS-T with 2% bovine serum albumin. Protein concentrations were determined using protein assay dye from Bio-Rad Laboratories (Hercules, CA). Twenty microgram protein was used for western analysis. Densitometry of protein expression was performed using a GS800 calibrated densitometer from Bio-Rad laboratories (Hercules, CA).

Statistical evaluation

Statistical analysis was performed using software Graph pad Prism 5.01 as described previously [35]. The results are presented as the mean $\pm$ SD. Statistical significance was analyzed by one-way or two-way (ANOVA) with repeated measures with time, and Bonferroni post hoc test was used for multiple comparisons. A p value < 0.05 was considered significant.

Results

Effects of exogenous GSNO treatment on locomotor function

Evaluation of locomotor functions using BBB score in rats is the standard method [43, 47, 48] to determine the efficacy of a preclinical/test drug in SCI. BBB scoring at 1, 3, 7 and 14 days shows that SCI rats had significantly greater impaired motor function compared with sham animals (Fig. 1). GSNO treatment significantly improved the recovery of locomotor function on day 14 ($p < 0.001$) compared with the SCI group animals (Fig. 1). The data showed slow but steady recovery with time, supporting the efficacy of GSNO for functional improvement following SCI.

Effects of exogenous GSNO treatment on neuropathic pain

Chronic neuropathic pain is associated with SCI, with substantial impact on quality of life in humans [49, 50]. Significant mechanical sensitivity differences were observed in both SCI and GSNO-treated SCI (GSNO) groups after SCI compared with the sham group. From day 7 onward, the GSNO group had a significantly improved/increased mechanical withdrawal latency compared with the SCI group (Fig. 2), indicating an improved pain threshold.

Effects of exogenous GSNO treatment on the levels of peroxynitrite (3-NT) and the activation of nNOS (Ser^{1412} phosphorylation)

We and others have identified neuronal peroxynitrite as a major causative factor in SCI pathology [37, 38, 46, 51], and decreasing peroxynitrite levels by GSNO is a major mechanism in GSNO-mediated neuroprotection and functional recovery in TBI [8, 10, 39]. Neuronal peroxynitrite is produced by the aberrant activity of nNOS after CNS trauma. Peroxynitrite levels, measured by the expression of 3-NT, were significantly higher in the SCI compared with the sham group (Fig. 3a, b, $p < 0.001$). Treatment with GSNO significantly decreased these elevations (Fig. 3a, b). The levels of 3-NT in SCI correlated well with the activation of nNOS (increased phosphorylation at Ser^{1412}) compared with the sham group (Fig. 3c, d, $p < 0.001$). GSNO treatment of SCI significantly down regulated nNOS activation compared with SCI (Fig. 3c, d, $p < 0.001$). The parallel between the levels of 3-NT and the activation of nNOS (pnNOS) indicates that SCI-induced peroxynitrite may have originated mainly from

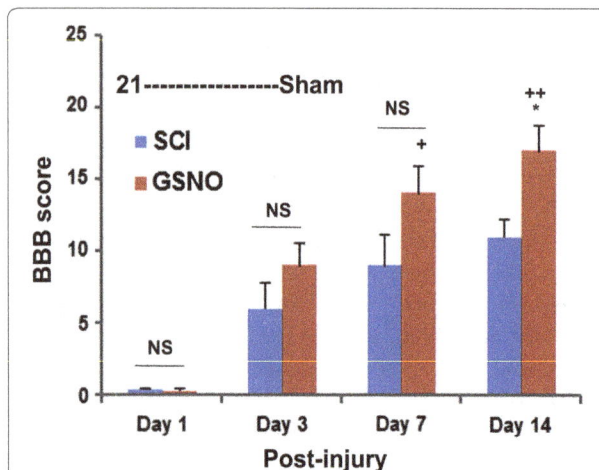

Fig. 1 Effect of GSNO on locomotor function. Studies on locomotor function using BBB locomotor rating scale were performed at days 1, 3, 7 and 14. BBB rating was evaluated by a blinded observer. Score of 21 (BBB) was assigned to sham animals displaying coordinated gait, consistent toe clearance, lifted tail, steady trunk, and parallel paw position throughout their stance. Data are presented as mean $\pm$ standard deviation (n $=$ 7). $^+p < 0.05$ versus GSNO day 1, 3, $^{++}p < 0.01$ versus GSNO day 1, 3, $^*p < 0.05$ versus SCI day 14. *NS* non-significant

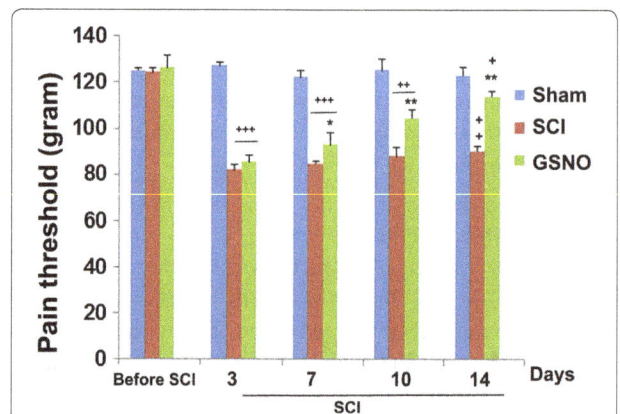

Fig. 2 Effect of GSNO on nociception. Pain threshold was measured with aesthesiometer (AM) for 14 days following SCI. GSNO treatment significantly improved the hyperalgesia associated with SCI. Data are presented as mean $\pm$ standard deviation (n $=$ 7). $^{+++}p < 0.001$; $^{++}p < 0.01$; $^+p < 0.05$ versus Sham, $^{**}p < 0.01$; $^*p < 0.05$ versus SCI

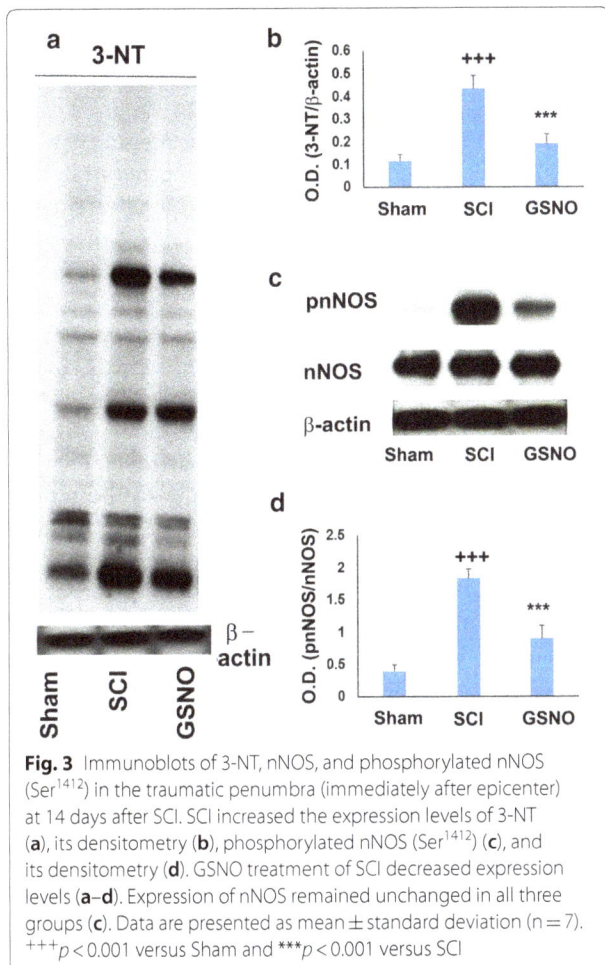

Fig. 3 Immunoblots of 3-NT, nNOS, and phosphorylated nNOS (Ser^{1412}) in the traumatic penumbra (immediately after epicenter) at 14 days after SCI. SCI increased the expression levels of 3-NT (**a**), its densitometry (**b**), phosphorylated nNOS (Ser^{1412}) (**c**), and its densitometry (**d**). GSNO treatment of SCI decreased expression levels (**a–d**). Expression of nNOS remained unchanged in all three groups (**c**). Data are presented as mean ± standard deviation (n = 7). $^{+++}p < 0.001$ versus Sham and $^{***}p < 0.001$ versus SCI

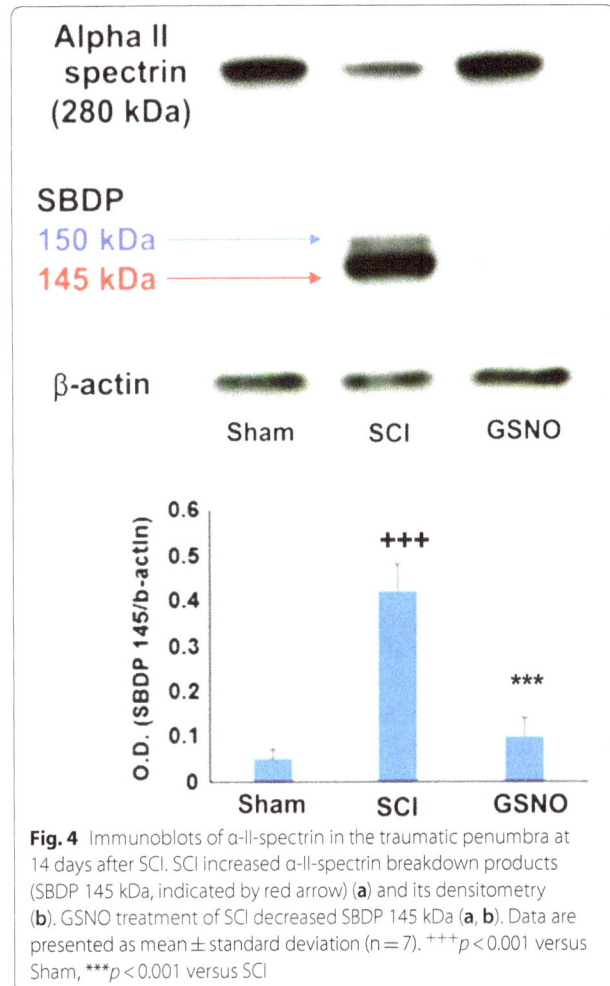

Fig. 4 Immunoblots of α-II-spectrin in the traumatic penumbra at 14 days after SCI. SCI increased α-II-spectrin breakdown products (SBDP 145 kDa, indicated by red arrow) (**a**) and its densitometry (**b**). GSNO treatment of SCI decreased SBDP 145 kDa (**a**, **b**). Data are presented as mean ± standard deviation (n = 7). $^{+++}p < 0.001$ versus Sham, $^{***}p < 0.001$ versus SCI

nNOS, and the activity of nNOS is regulated/inhibited by GSNO, likely via S-nitrosylation.

Effects of exogenous GSNO treatment on the activity of calpains measured as α-II-spectrin breakdown products

Neuronal alpha-II-spectrin (280 kDa) is one of the major substrates of calpains [52]. The calpain-specific alpha II spectrin breakdown product (SBDP)145 kDa fragment is used as a marker of calpain activity [53]. The band at 150 kDa is also a cleavage product of calpain activity; however, it is not specific to calpain activity [54]. The intensity of the 150 kDa band was significantly less than the 145 kDa band. Calpain activity, measured via α-II-spectrin breakdown product (SBDP) 145 kDa, was significantly higher ($p < 0.001$) in the SCI group compared with the sham (Fig. 4a, b). GSNO treatment of SCI significantly ($p < 0.001$) decreased the levels of SBDP 145 kDa, indicating that GSNO decreased the activity of calpains (Fig. 4a, b). The activity of calpains (Fig. 4) correlated well with levels of 3-NT and the activation of nNOS, as shown in Fig. 3.

Discussion

This is a preliminary mechanism-based study showing that SCI-induced functional deficits (Fig. 1), and neuropathic pain (Fig. 2) paralleled aberrant activation of nNOS, increased levels of peroxynitrite (Fig. 3) and high activity of calpains (Fig. 4) in a 2-week rat model of contusion SCI. The study further shows the therapeutic efficacy of GSNO. It improved functional deficits (Fig. 1) and increased the pain threshold (Fig. 2) by inhibiting the activities of both nNOS (Fig. 3) and calpains (Fig. 4) and reducing the levels of injurious peroxynitrite (Fig. 3).

Locomotor function deficits and pain are two major consequences intrinsic to SCI [49]. Deleterious metabolites, formed by the aberrant activities of otherwise regulatory enzymes such as nNOS, are primarily responsible for producing potent oxidizing/neurodegenerating agents, such as peroxynitrite, in neurons. Excessive accumulation of neuronal peroxynitrite is implicated in neuronal cell death and subsequent neurodegeneration [55]. In fact, scavenging peroxynitrite using peroxynitrite decomposition catalysts such as FeTPPS has been reported to ameliorate SCI [56], supporting this direct deleterious role of peroxynitrite. Inhibition of nNOS activity following SCI [57] has also been shown to provide neuroprotection, and nNOS KO mice show improved recovery after SCI [58], indicating a deleterious role of nNOS activity in SCI. An nNOS-based therapy for SCI therefore offers a logical approach. Reversible down regulation of nNOS activity, such as via-S-nitrosylation, is preferred because it maintains the required physiological activity of nNOS. The roles of other NOS enzymes (inducible and endothelial) in the chronic phase pathology, such as in neurodegeneration and pain, is not clear [59]. Peroxynitrite produced in neurons is a product of an instantaneous reaction between nNOS-derived NO and superoxide. Because NO is used for the formation of peroxynitrite (3-NT), the biosynthesis of GSNO, a product of a slow reaction between NO and GSH, and GSNO-mediated regulatory mechanisms are derailed. Because deleterious nNOS activity is down regulated by a GSNO-mediated S-nitrosylation mechanism [60], reduced NO/GSNO levels contribute to nNOS-dependent neurodegeneration and pain SCI pathology. Such a derailed NO/GSNO metabolism in SCI may also be responsible for functional deficits. Therefore, we tested the hypothesis that GSNO reduces the levels of peroxynitrite, inhibits the activity of nNOS, and improves behavioral function and cellular plasticity in young adult male rats.

Pain is one of the major issues in SCI for obvious reasons but also because it impairs recovery after SCI [61]. Both inflammatory and neuropathic pain (caused by a lesion or disease of somatosensory function) are present in the majority of SCI patients [50, 62]. Due to the lack of mechanistic understanding of pain, satisfactory pain-management therapy of SCI is not yet available. We observed that the GSNO treatment significantly increased the pain threshold and reduced calpain activity after 2 weeks of SCI (Fig. 2), indicating that GSNO possesses an analgesic property in addition to improving functional deficits (Fig. 1). Furthermore, significant increases in tissue peroxynitrite levels (Fig. 3) correlated well with calpain-mediated cytoskeleton degradation (Fig. 4), indicating peroxynitrite's contribution to neurodegeneration. Recently, we have shown that the activity of calpains is upregulated by peroxynitrite whereas GSNO, via S-nitrosylation, inhibits the activity of calpains in TBI [8], indicating a similar role of peroxynitrite versus GSNO in this SCI study. Peroxynitrite originating from nNOS [63] and NMDA receptor activity [64] is also recognized among the prominent causes of neuropathic pain following nerve injury. GSNO, likely via S-nitrosylation, down regulates the activity

of nNOS, thus reducing the levels of peroxynitrite and its associated pain. Decreased levels of peroxynitrite in brains and improved neurological functions have also been shown after GSNO treatment in rat models of stroke and TBI [34, 51], indicating that the mechanism of S-nitrosylation invokes anti-neurodegeneration and anti-pain activities in CNS trauma. These observations establish the therapeutic potential of GSNO-mediated mechanisms in simultaneously treating neurodegeneration and neuropathic pain following SCI.

Inflammation is another significant component of SCI, contributing to neurodegeneration and pain. Interestingly, GSNO-mediated mechanisms are also shown to down regulate the expression of pro-inflammatory cytokines and NF-κB [18, 39], as well as the activation of STAT3 [20]. These actions contribute to the reduction of inflammation-mediated neurodegeneration and pain. As an alternative mechanism to alleviate pain in SCI, IL-10 has been shown to be a potent anti-neuropathic pain molecule [65–67], and GSNO-mediated mechanisms are reported to upregulate the levels of IL-10 [68] as well as to reduce pain in a rat model of cauda equine compression [44]. We add one caveat that excessive accumulation of GSNO, as observed in GSNOR knock out mice, creates altered redox pathology, leading to sensitization to pain [15] and thus rendering GSNOR knock out mice 'not suitable' for pain related studies. A critical balance of NO/GSNO versus peroxynitrite is requisite to maintain the homeostasis of the NO metabolome, ameliorating SCI pathology. Low dose exogenous supplementation of GSNO seems to be an ideal approach to improve pain threshold and to provide neuroprotection. One advantage of using GSNO supplementation is that GSNO-mediated regulatory mechanisms are reversible, and thus the physiological levels of activity of targeted enzymes can be maintained. The improved BBB score (Fig. 1) and increased pain threshold (Fig. 2) reported here support the efficacy of GSNO in ameliorating SCI and provide a rationale to further investigate GSNO therapy in SCI. *Limitations* the most affected population from SCI is young adult males. Therefore, we used young adult male animals in this preliminary study; however, the exclusion of female rats demands further testing in these populations. We are also aware that a 2-week SCI study is relatively short to sufficiently characterize the injury course. Moreover, biochemical studies of the early acute phase are needed. Therefore, in follow-up study, the efficacy of GSNO therapy and the cause-and-effect relationship between GSNO and peroxynitrite/calpain system will be investigated for both acute and longer chronic periods of time, using both male and female young adult animals.

Conclusions

Under SCI pathology, superoxide reacts with NO and this reaction produces a large amount of injurious peroxynitrite. Increased levels of peroxynitrite cause an upregulation of calpain activity and thus neuronal cytoskeleton degradation. Peroxynitrite is also recognized as a mediator of pain. Under such pathological conditions, S-nitrosylation-mediated biological regulation (inhibition) of the activity of nNOS and calpain is lost due to its reduced bioavailability, and thus levels of NO/GSNO. Replenishment of exogenous GSNO was found to inhibit the activation of nNOS, thus blocking the production of peroxynitrite and reducing the activity of calpains, leading to improved locomotor function and decreased mechanical allodynia acutely post-injury in SCI animals. Furthermore GSNO's administration to humans is not associated with adverse effects [22]. Therefore, testing the efficacy of exogenous GSNO in humans may lead to an SCI therapy of clinical relevance.

Abbreviations
BBB: Basso Beattie and Bresnahan; GSNO: S-nitrosoglutathione; HIF-1α: hypoxia-inducible factor-1 alpha; IHC: immunohistochemistry; nNOS: neuronal nitric oxide synthase; NO: nitric oxide; 3-NT: 3-nitrotyrosine; PTEN: phosphatase with sequence homology to tensin; SCI: spinal cord injury; Sham: sham-operated animals; VEGF: vascular endothelial growth factor.

Authors' contributions
This study is based on an original idea of MK, AKS and IS. MK and AKS wrote the manuscript and all authors reviewed the manuscript. TS Dhammu carried out animal and biochemical studies. MK, AKS, TS Dhammu, and IS critically examined biochemical studies. TS Dhammu performed locomotor behavior and neuropathic pain studies. MK performed statistical analysis. All authors read and approved the final manuscript.

Author details
[1] Department of Pediatrics, 508 Children's Research Institute, Medical University of South Carolina, 173 Ashley Ave, Charleston, SC 29425, USA. [2] Ralph H Johnson VA Medical Center, Charleston, SC, USA. [3] Department of Pathology and Laboratory Medicine, Medical University of South Carolina, Charleston, SC, USA.

Acknowledgements
We would like to thank Ms. Danielle Lowe, a medical graduate student from the MUSC, for assistance with statistical analysis. We acknowledge Dr. Tom Smith from the MUSC Writing Center for his valuable editing of the manuscript.

Competing interests
The authors declare that they have no competing interests.

Funding
This study was made possible by the VA Office of Research and Development (VA merit awards; BX003401 and RX002090) and the South Carolina Spinal Cord Injury Research Fund (Grant# SCIRF2017 I-01). This work was also supported by the NIH, Grants C06 RR018823 and No. C06 RR015455 from the Extramural Research Facilities Program of the National Center for Research Resources.

References
1. Siddiqui AM, Khazaei M, Fehlings MG. Translating mechanisms of neuroprotection, regeneration, and repair to treatment of spinal cord injury. Prog Brain Res. 2015;218:15–54.
2. Varma AK, Das A, Wallace G, Barry J, Vertegel AA, Ray SK, Banik NL. Spinal cord injury: a review of current therapy, future treatments, and basic science frontiers. Neurochem Res. 2013;38(5):895–905.
3. Furlan JC, Sakakibara BM, Miller WC, Krassioukov AV. Global incidence and prevalence of traumatic spinal cord injury. Can J Neurol Sci. 2013;40(4):456–64.
4. Selvarajah S, Hammond ER, Haider AH, Abularrage CJ, Becker D, Dhiman N, Hyder O, Gupta D, Black JH 3rd, Schneider EB. The burden of acute traumatic spinal cord injury among adults in the united states: an update. J Neurotrauma. 2014;31(3):228–38.
5. Tardivo V, Crobeddu E, Pilloni G, Fontanella M, Spena G, Panciani PP, Berjano P, Ajello M, Bozzaro M, Agnoletti A, et al. Say "no" to spinal cord injury: is nitric oxide an option for therapeutic strategies? Int J Neurosci. 2015;125(2):81–90.
6. Liu D, Ling X, Wen J, Liu J. The role of reactive nitrogen species in secondary spinal cord injury: formation of nitric oxide, peroxynitrite, and nitrated protein. J Neurochem. 2000;75(5):2144–54.
7. Chou PC, Shunmugavel A, Sayed HE, Desouki MM, Nguyen SA, Khan M, Singh I, Bilgen M. Preclinical use of longitudinal MRI for screening the efficacy of s-nitrosoglutathione in treating spinal cord injury. J Magn Reson Imaging. 2011;33(6):1301–11.
8. Khan M, Dhammu TS, Matsuda F, Annamalai B, Dhindsa TS, Singh I, Singh AK. Targeting the nNOS/peroxynitrite/calpain system to confer neuroprotection and aid functional recovery in a mouse model of TBI. Brain Res. 2016;1630:159–70.
9. Khan M, Dhammu TS, Sakakima H, Shunmugavel A, Gilg AG, Singh AK, Singh I. The inhibitory effect of S-nitrosoglutathione on blood-brain barrier disruption and peroxynitrite formation in a rat model of experimental stroke. J Neurochem. 2012;123(Suppl 2):86–97.
10. Khan M, Sakakima H, Dhammu TS, Shunmugavel A, Im YB, Gilg AG, Singh AK, Singh I. S-nitrosoglutathione reduces oxidative injury and promotes mechanisms of neurorepair following traumatic brain injury in rats. J Neuroinflammation. 2011;8(1):78.
11. Sakakima H, Khan M, Dhammu TS, Shunmugavel A, Yoshida Y, Singh I, Singh AK. Stimulation of functional recovery via the mechanisms of neurorepair by S-nitrosoglutathione and motor exercise in a rat model of transient cerebral ischemia and reperfusion. Restor Neurol Neurosci. 2012;30(5):383–96.
12. Singh SP, Wishnok JS, Keshive M, Deen WM, Tannenbaum SR. The chemistry of the S-nitrosoglutathione/glutathione system. Proc Natl Acad Sci USA. 1996;93(25):14428–33.
13. Jourd'heuil D, Jourd'heuil FL, Feelisch M. Oxidation and nitrosation of thiols at low micromolar exposure to nitric oxide. Evidence for a free radical mechanism. J Biol Chem. 2003;278(18):15720–6.
14. Kluge I, Gutteck-Amsler U, Zollinger M, Do KQ. S-nitrosoglutathione in rat cerebellum: identification and quantification by liquid chromatography-mass spectrometry. J Neurochem. 1997;69(6):2599–607.
15. Montagna C, Di Giacomo G, Rizza S, Cardaci S, Ferraro E, Grumati P, De Zio D, Maiani E, Muscoli C, Lauro F, et al. S-nitrosoglutathione reductase deficiency-induced S-nitrosylation results in neuromuscular dysfunction. Antioxid Redox Signal. 2014;21(4):570–87.
16. Barnett SD, Buxton ILO. The role of S-nitrosoglutathione reductase (GSNOR) in human disease and therapy. Crit Rev Biochem Mol Biol. 2017;52(3):340–54.
17. Jaffrey SR, Erdjument-Bromage H, Ferris CD, Tempst P, Snyder SH. Protein S-nitrosylation: a physiological signal for neuronal nitric oxide. Nat Cell Biol. 2001;3(2):193–7.
18. Khan M, Sekhon B, Giri S, Jatana M, Gilg AG, Ayasolla K, Elango C, Singh AK, Singh I. S-nitrosoglutathione reduces inflammation and protects brain against focal cerebral ischemia in a rat model of experimental stroke. J Cereb Blood Flow Metab. 2005;25(2):177–92.
19. Khan M, Jatana M, Elango C, Paintlia AS, Singh AK, Singh I. Cerebrovascular protection by various nitric oxide donors in rats after experimental stroke. Nitric Oxide. 2006;15(2):114–24.
20. Kim J, Won JS, Singh AK, Sharma AK, Singh I. STAT3 regulation by S-nitrosylation: implication for inflammatory disease. Antioxid Redox Signal. 2014;20(16):2514–27.

21. Khan M, Dhammu TS, Baarine M, Kim J, Paintlia MK, Singh I, Singh AK. GSNO promotes functional recovery in experimental TBI by stabilizing HIF-1α. Behav Brain Res. 2018;340:63–70.

22. Hornyak I, Pankotai E, Kiss L, Lacza Z. Current developments in the therapeutic potential of S-nitrosoglutathione, an endogenous NO-donor molecule. Curr Pharm Biotechnol. 2011;12(9):1368–74.

23. Konorev EA, Tarpey MM, Joseph J, Baker JE, Kalyanaraman B. S-nitroso-glutathione improves functional recovery in the isolated rat heart after cardioplegic ischemic arrest-evidence for a cardioprotective effect of nitric oxide. J Pharmacol Exp Ther. 1995;274(1):200–6.

24. Que LG, Liu L, Yan Y, Whitehead GS, Gavett SH, Schwartz DA, Stamler JS. Protection from experimental asthma by an endogenous bronchodilator. Science. 2005;308(5728):1618–21.

25. Numajiri N, Takasawa K, Nishiya T, Tanaka H, Ohno K, Hayakawa W, Asada M, Matsuda H, Azumi K, Kamata H, et al. On-off system for PI3-kinase-Akt signaling through S-nitrosylation of phosphatase with sequence homology to tensin (PTEN). Proc Natl Acad Sci USA. 2011;108(25):10349–54.

26. Cheng XW, Kuzuya M, Kim W, Song H, Hu L, Inoue A, Nakamura K, Di Q, Sasaki T, Tsuzuki M, et al. Exercise training stimulates ischemia-induced neovascularization via phosphatidylinositol 3-kinase/Akt-dependent hypoxia-induced factor-1 alpha reactivation in mice of advanced age. Circulation. 2010;122(7):707–16.

27. Malinski T, Bailey F, Zhang ZG, Chopp M. Nitric oxide measured by a porphyrinic microsensor in rat brain after transient middle cerebral artery occlusion. J Cereb Blood Flow Metab. 1993;13(3):355–8.

28. Schonhoff CM, Matsuoka M, Tummala H, Johnson MA, Estevez AG, Wu R, Kamaid A, Ricart KC, Hashimoto Y, Gaston B, et al. S-nitrosothiol depletion in amyotrophic lateral sclerosis. Proc Natl Acad Sci USA. 2006;103(7):2404–9.

29. Ju TC, Chen SD, Liu CC, Yang DI. Protective effects of S-nitrosoglutathione against amyloid beta-peptide neurotoxicity. Free Radic Biol Med. 2005;38(7):938–49.

30. Rauhala P, Mohanakumar KP, Sziraki I, Lin AM, Chiueh CC. S-nitrosothiols and nitric oxide, but not sodium nitroprusside, protect nigrostriatal dopamine neurons against iron-induced oxidative stress in vivo. Synapse. 1996;23(1):58–60.

31. Prasad R, Giri S, Nath N, Singh I, Singh AK. GSNO attenuates EAE disease by S-nitrosylation-mediated modulation of endothelial-monocyte inter-actions. Glia. 2007;55(1):65–77.

32. Chiueh CC, Rauhala P. The redox pathway of S-nitrosoglutathione, glu-tathione and nitric oxide in cell to neuron communications. Free Radic Res. 1999;31(6):641–50.

33. Hess DT, Stamler JS. Regulation by S-nitrosylation of protein post-transla-tional modification. J Biol Chem. 2012;287(7):4411–8.

34. Paintlia MK, Paintlia AS, Singh AK, Singh I. S-nitrosoglutathione induces ciliary neurotrophic factor expression in astrocytes, which has implica-tions to protect the central nervous system under pathological condi-tions. J Biol Chem. 2013;288(6):3831–43.

35. Khan M, Dhammu TS, Matsuda F, Baarine M, Dhindsa TS, Singh I, Singh AK. Promoting endothelial function by S-nitrosoglutathione through the HIF-1alpha/VEGF pathway stimulates neurorepair and functional recovery following experimental stroke in rats. Drug Des Dev Ther. 2015;9:2233–47.

36. Whiteman M, Armstrong JS, Cheung NS, Siau JL, Rose P, Schantz JT, Jones DP, Halliwell B. Peroxynitrite mediates calcium-dependent mito-chondrial dysfunction and cell death via activation of calpains. FASEB J. 2004;18(12):1395–7.

37. Xiong Y, Hall ED. Pharmacological evidence for a role of perox-ynitrite in the pathophysiology of spinal cord injury. Exp Neurol. 2009;216(1):105–14.

38. Xiong Y, Rabchevsky AG, Hall ED. Role of peroxynitrite in second-ary oxidative damage after spinal cord injury. J Neurochem. 2007;100(3):639–49.

39. Khan M, Im YB, Shunmugavel A, Gilg AG, Dhindsa RK, Singh AK, Singh I. Administration of S-nitrosoglutathione after traumatic brain injury protects the neurovascular unit and reduces secondary injury in a rat model of controlled cortical impact. J Neuroinflammation. 2009;6:32.

40. Bilgen M. A new device for experimental modeling of central nervous system injuries. Neurorehabil Neural Repair. 2005;19(3):219–26.

41. Shunmugavel A, Khan M, Chou PC, Dhindsa RK, Marcus M, Copay AG, Subach BR, Schuler TC, Bilgen M, Orak JK, et al. Simvastatin protects bladder and renal functions following spinal cord injury in rats. J Inflamm. 2010;7(1):17.

42. Shunmugavel A, Khan M, Hughes FM Jr, Purves JT, Singh A, Singh I. S-nitrosoglutathione protects the spinal bladder: novel therapeutic approach to post-spinal cord injury bladder remodeling. Neurourol Urodyn. 2015;34(6):519–26.

43. Basso DM, Beattie MS, Bresnahan JC. A sensitive and reliable locomotor rating scale for open field testing in rats. J Neurotrauma. 1995;12(1):1–21.

44. Shunmugavel A, Khan M, Martin MM, Copay AG, Subach BR, Schuler TC, Singh I. S-nitrosoglutathione administration ameliorates cauda equina compression injury in rats. Neurosci Med. 2012;3(3):294–305.

45. Shunmugavel A, Martin MM, Khan M, Copay AG, Subach BR, Schuler TC, Singh I. Simvastatin ameliorates cauda equina compression injury in a rat model of lumbar spinal stenosis. J Neuroimmune Pharmacol. 2013;8(1):274–86.

46. Khan M, Dhammu TS, Matsuda F, Singh AK, Singh I. Blocking a vicious cycle nNOS/peroxynitrite/AMPK by S-nitrosoglutathione: implication for stroke therapy. BMC Neurosci. 2015;16:42.

47. Datto JP, Bastidas JC, Miller NL, Shah AK, Arheart KL, Marcillo AE, Dietrich WD, Pearse DD. Female rats demonstrate improved locomotor recovery and greater preservation of white and gray matter after traumatic spinal cord injury compared to males. J Neurotrauma. 2015;32(15):1146–57.

48. Sung JK, Miao L, Calvert JW, Huang L, Louis Harkey H, Zhang JH. A pos-sible role of RhoA/Rho-kinase in experimental spinal cord injury in rat. Brain Res. 2003;959(1):29–38.

49. Christensen MD, Hulsebosch CE. Chronic central pain after spinal cord injury. J Neurotrauma. 1997;14(8):517–37.

50. Finnerup NB. Pain in patients with spinal cord injury. Pain. 2013;154(Suppl 1):S71–6.

51. Carrico KM, Vaishnav R, Hall ED. Temporal and spatial dynamics of peroxynitrite-induced oxidative damage after spinal cord contusion injury. J Neurotrauma. 2009;26(8):1369–78.

52. Wang KK. Calpain and caspase: can you tell the difference? Trends Neuro-sci. 2000;23(1):20–6.

53. Yoon JS, Lee JH, Son TG, Mughal MR, Greig NH, Mattson MP. Pregabalin suppresses calcium-mediated proteolysis and improves stroke outcome. Neurobiol Dis. 2011;41(3):624–9.

54. Carragher NO. Calpain inhibition: a therapeutic strategy targeting multi-ple disease states. Curr Pharm Des. 2006;12(5):615–38.

55. Pacher P, Beckman JS, Liaudet L. Nitric oxide and peroxynitrite in health and disease. Physiol Rev. 2007;87(1):315–424.

56. Genovese T, Mazzon E, Esposito E, Muia C, Di Paola R, Bramanti P, Cuz-zocrea S. Beneficial effects of FeTSPP, a peroxynitrite decomposition catalyst, in a mouse model of spinal cord injury. Free Radic Biol Med. 2007;43(5):763–80.

57. Sharma HS, Badgaiyan RD, Alm P, Mohanty S, Wiklund L. Neuroprotective effects of nitric oxide synthase inhibitors in spinal cord injury-induced pathophysiology and motor functions: an experimental study in the rat. Ann NY Acad Sci. 2005;1053:422–34.

58. Farooque M, Isaksson J, Olsson Y. Improved recovery after spinal cord injury in neuronal nitric oxide synthase-deficient mice but not in TNF-alpha-deficient mice. J Neurotrauma. 2001;18(1):105–14.

59. Ahlawat A, Rana A, Goyal N, Sharma S. Potential role of nitric oxide synthase isoforms in pathophysiology of neuropathic pain. Inflammop-harmacology. 2014;22(5):269–78.

60. Qu ZW, Miao WY, Hu SQ, Li C, Zhuo XL, Zong YY, Wu YP, Zhang GY. N-methyl-D-aspartate receptor-dependent denitrosylation of neu-ronal nitric oxide synthase increase the enzyme activity. PLoS ONE. 2012;7(12):e52788.

61. Turtle JD, Strain MM, Aceves M, Huang YJ, Reynolds JA, Hook MA, Grau JW. Pain input impairs recovery after spinal cord injury: treatment with lidocaine. J Neurotrauma. 2017;34(6):1200–8.

62. Hagen EM, Rekand T. Management of neuropathic pain associated with spinal cord injury. Pain Ther. 2015;4(1):51–65.

63. Tanabe M, Nagatani Y, Saitoh K, Takasu K, Ono H. Pharmacological assess-ments of nitric oxide synthase isoforms and downstream diversity of NO signaling in the maintenance of thermal and mechanical hyper-sensitivity after peripheral nerve injury. Neuropharmacology. 2009;56(3):702–8.

64. Leem JW, Kim HK, Hulsebosch CE, Gwak YS. Ionotropic glutamate receptors contribute to maintained neuronal hyperexcitability following spinal cord injury in rats. Exp Neurol. 2010;224(1):321–4.

65. Milligan ED, Soderquist RG, Malone SM, Mahoney JH, Hughes TS, Langer SJ, Sloane EM, Maier SF, Leinwand LA, Watkins LR, et al. Intrathecal polymer-based interleukin-10 gene delivery for neuropathic pain. Neuron Glia Biol. 2006;2(4):293–308.

66. Milligan ED, Sloane EM, Langer SJ, Hughes TS, Jekich BM, Frank MG, Mahoney JH, Levkoff LH, Maier SF, Cruz PE, et al. Repeated intrathecal injections of plasmid DNA encoding interleukin-10 produce prolonged reversal of neuropathic pain. Pain. 2006;126(1–3):294–308.

67. Milligan ED, Penzkover KR, Soderquist RG, Mahoney MJ. Spinal interleukin-10 therapy to treat peripheral neuropathic pain. Neuromodulation. 2012;15(6):520–6 **(discussion 526)**.

68. Samuvel DJ, Shunmugavel A, Singh AK, Singh I, Khan M. S-Nitrosoglutathione ameliorates acute renal dysfunction in a rat model of lipopolysaccharide-induced sepsis. J Pharm Pharmacol. 2016;68(10):1310–9.

8

Melatonin ameliorates cognitive memory by regulation of cAMP-response element-binding protein expression and the anti-inflammatory response in a rat model of post-traumatic stress disorder

Bombi Lee[1,2]* ⓘ, Insop Shim[1,3], Hyejung Lee[1] and Dae-Hyun Hahm[1,2]*

Abstract

Background: Post-traumatic stress disorder (PTSD) is an important psychological disease that can develop following the physical experience or witnessing of traumatic events. The psychopathological response to traumatic stressors increases inflammation in the hippocampus and induces memory deficits. Melatonin (MTG) plays critical roles in circadian rhythm disorders, Alzheimer's disease, and other neurological disorders. However, the cognitive efficiency of MTG and its mechanisms of action in the treatment of PTSD remain unclear. Thus, the present study investigated the effects of MTG on spatial cognitive impairments stimulated by single prolonged stress (SPS) in rats, an animal model of PTSD. Male rats received intraperitoneal (i.p.) administration of various doses of MTG for 21 consecutive days after the SPS procedure.

Results: SPS-stimulated cognitive impairments in the object recognition task and Morris water maze were reversed by MTG treatment (25 mg/kg, i.p). Additionally, MTG significantly increased cognitive memory-related decreases in cAMP-response element-binding (CREB) protein and mRNA levels in the hippocampus. Our results also demonstrate that MTG significantly inhibited SPS-stimulated cognitive memory impairments by inhibiting the expression of proinflammatory cytokines, including tumor necrosis factor-α (TNF-α), and interleukin-6 (IL-6) in the rat brain.

Conclusion: The present results indicate that MTG can be beneficial for SPS-stimulated memory impairments via changes in CREB expression and proinflammatory mediators. Thus, MTG may be a prophylactic strategy for the prevention or mitigation of the progression of some features of the PTSD pathology.

Keywords: Melatonin, Memory, Post-traumatic stress disorder, cAMP-response element-binding protein, Proinflammatory cytokines

*Correspondence: bombi@khu.ac.kr; dhhahm@khu.ac.kr
[1] Acupuncture and Meridian Science Research Center, College of Korean Medicine, Kyung Hee University, 26, Kyungheedae-ro, Dongdaemun-gu, Seoul 02447, Republic of Korea
Full list of author information is available at the end of the article

Background

Declarative memory dysfunction is related to post-traumatic stress disorder (PTSD), which manifests following exposure to severe trauma [1]. In humans, early traumatic experiences and adversity significantly enhance one's vulnerability to various psychiatric disorders, including memory impairment and PTSD, in adulthood [2]. The psychopathological conditions in response to traumatic stressors are caused by intrusive memories in which individuals re-experience the original traumatic experience, avoid trauma-associated events, have unpleasant recollections, avoid associated events, and exhibit negative cognition/mood, hyperarousal, and marked social impairments [3, 4]. Moreover, the persistent occurrence of extremely repulsive memory associated with the trauma and an incapacity to dissipate these fear memory are major characteristics of this disease [5]. PTSD patients also exhibit significant cognitive deficits, including damaged declarative and working memory abilities and impairments in attention and concentration [6–8]. Furthermore, cognitive impairments and memory dysfunction continually appear in conjunction with the development of PTSD [5]. The cognitive deficits observed in PTSD patients have been hypothesized to be the result of unpleasant flashback memories that temporarily interfere with the capability to procedure new memories or information [9–11]. For instance, placing a rat in a context in which it has been shocked impairs memory on an entirely different test [7, 11], such as the localization of a hidden platform in a water maze.

Single prolonged stress (SPS) is a well-validated animal model of PTSD [12]. Several studies have suggest that animals exposed to SPS exhibit states that mimic human mental disorders, including enhanced anxiety, impaired fear extinction, changes in hypothalamic-pituitary-adrenal (HPA) axis function [13], and increased cytokines in the hippocampus [14]. The hippocampus, which plays an major role in cognition and memory, is particularly vulnerability to neuronal damage caused by SPS [5, 15]. Furthermore, this damage can subsequently result in impairments in spatial learning and memory and synaptic plasticity [15, 16].

A recent study discovered that hippocampal volume is reduced in patients with PTSD [17], which emphasizes the association between stress and the loss of hippocampus neurons. In hippocampus brain-derived neurotrophic factor (BDNF) and cAMP-response element-binding protein (CREB) play major roles in pathological responses of the central nervous system (CNS) and have been related to PTSD [5, 18]. Furthermore, the hippocampus is susceptible to the inflammatory response to traumatic stress, which disrupts neuronal circuitry [19, 20], is associated with the psychosocial stress of PTSD, and alters the protein and gene expression of inflammatory mediators [21].

Currently, selective serotonin reuptake inhibitors (SSRIs) are an important mediator of the progression of PTSD and are used as potential pharmacological interventions [22, 23]. However, the used of SSRIs is contentious due to their continually reported side effects and their associated poor patient compliance [24]. Thus, there is a critical need for a novel therapeutic strategy for the treatment of PTSD [25].

Melatonin (N-acetyl-5-methoxytryptamine, MTG) is the major hormone released by the pineal gland at night and is secreted into the cerebrospinal fluid and circulation [26]. This neurohormone plays a important role in the modulation of the biological clock, specifically the sleep-wake cycle and the induction of physiological sleep [26, 27]. MTG plays numerous physiological roles as a regulator of circadian rhythms, a protector of mitochondria, an anti-inflammatory, an antioxidant, and a neuroprotectant agent [28–32]. The beneficial effects of MTG on neurological diseases have been widely investigated. Additionally, MTG is also thought to be involved in the modulation of complex processes, such as learning and memory [33, 34], via its binding to receptors widely distributed throughout the brain [35]. For instance, MTG in rats promotes memory in the novel object recognition task [ORT; 36, 37] and the olfactory social memory test [38]. The exogenous administration of MTG results in neuroprotective effects [39, 40] and enhance cognitive capacity [41]. MTG may exert particular therapeutic effects in patients with Alzheimer disease (AD) and Parkinson's disease [PD; 42, 43] by protecting against neurotoxicity induced by beta-amyloid (Aβ) peptides [44, 45]. For example, MTG supplementation may weakens Aβ accumulation, inflammation, neurodegeneration, and memory impairments in AD patients and an animal model of AD [32, 41, 46]. Therefore, MTG and its receptor agonists are considered prospective therapeutic agents for AD treatment [32, 41, 46]. Additionally, some studies have shown that MTG attenuates pyramidal neuronal cell damage in the hippocampus in global cerebral ischemia [47–50]. The neuroprotective effects of MTG are related to inhibited oxidative stress and neuroinflammation [51, 52].

Based on such findings, MTG was hypothesized to alleviate SPS-stimulated memory impairment as measured by an ORT and the Morris water maze (MWM) test. Additionally, the possible mechanisms underlying the neuroprotective effects of MTG were assessed in a rat model of PTSD, and the relationships between stress-stimulated cognition and memory impairment and BDNF and CREB expressions and inflammation in the hippocampus region were evaluated. The present findings will contribute to the development of novel approaches to the treatment of trauma- and stress-related disorders, including PTSD.

Methods

Animals and MTG administration

Eight-week male SD rats weighing 200–230 g were obtained from Samtaco Animal Co. (Osan, South Korea). The vivarium room was kept on a 12-h light/dark cycle (lights on at 8:00, lights off at 20:00) under relative humidity of $55 \pm 15\%$ and a controlled temperature at 22 ± 2 °C. All rats were caged for 7 days to acclimatize before beginning the experimental protocol. Ethics approval was obtained from Kyung Hee University's Institutional Animal Care and Use Committee (KHUASP(SE)-15-115). All experimental procedures were performed according to the Guide for the Care and Use of Laboratory Animals.

MTG (5, 10 and 25 mg/kg, body weight, Sigma-Aldrich Chemical Co. St. Louise, MO, USA) and fluoxetine for positive drug (10 mg/kg, FLX, fluoxetine hydrochloride; Sigma) were applied by intraperitoneally (i.p.) after the exposure to SPS for 21 days. The standard doses and period of MTG used in the this study was applied on other study [53, 54]. MTG and FLX were liquefied in 0.9% saline before use.

The rats were randomly divided into six groups of six to seven individuals each as follows: the saline-treated group (CON group, n = 7), the SPS-stimulated plus saline-treated group (SPS group as a control, n = 7), the SPS-stimulated plus 5 mg/kg MTG-treated group (SPS+MTG5 group, n = 6), the SPS-stimulated plus 10 mg/kg MTG-treated group (SPS+MTG10 group, n = 6), the SPS-stimulated plus 20 mg/kg MTG-treated group (SPS + MTG20 group, n = 7) and the SPS-stimulated plus 10 mg/kg fluoxetine-treated group (SPS + FLX group, n = 7). The entire experimental schedules are shown in the Fig. 1.

Single prolonged stress

Rat were exposed to SPS for 14 successive days as described by Patki's group with a slight modification [55, 56]. Briefly, rats were restrained for 2 h on a holder and then promptly placed in a forced swimming condition for 20 min. The rats were allowed to dry and recuperate for 15 min and then exposed to ether vapor until loss of consciousness. Following the SPS procedure, rats were housed one per cage and left undisturbed for 14 days to allow PTSD-like symptoms to become apparent [55]. The other half of the rats for control group were momentarily placed in a separate area of the room during the SPS procedure. All rats were returned to the vivarium room and housed for 14 days without disturbance other.

Object recognition task

The novel ORT was used to estimate the cognitive capability of rats. This test was essentially the same as that described by Okuda et al. [57]. Briefly, the equipment was consists square wood box and painted with black $(45 \times 45 \times 45 \text{ cm}^3)$. The objects in the equipment is prepared a familiar objects and a novel object. The familiar objects (A1 and A2) to be discriminated were two similar toys as due to make objects enough heavy, so that rats could not be able to move objects. The novel object (B) was different shape and different color toy. On habituate, the rats were adapted to the object recognition box during 10 min. The test phase was started 24 h after the habituation. Rats were exposed inside the equipment with two familiar objects during 5 min. During the test phase, rats housed to the testing chamber, where rats were exposed to one novel object (B) and one of the familiar object during 5 min. The exploration (sniffing) time for the novel and familiar objects is measured. The discrimination index is calculated of discrimination between the familiar and the novel object accurate for exploration. It is expressed as: (time spent on novel object—time spent on familiar object)/(time spent on novel object + time spent on familiar object).

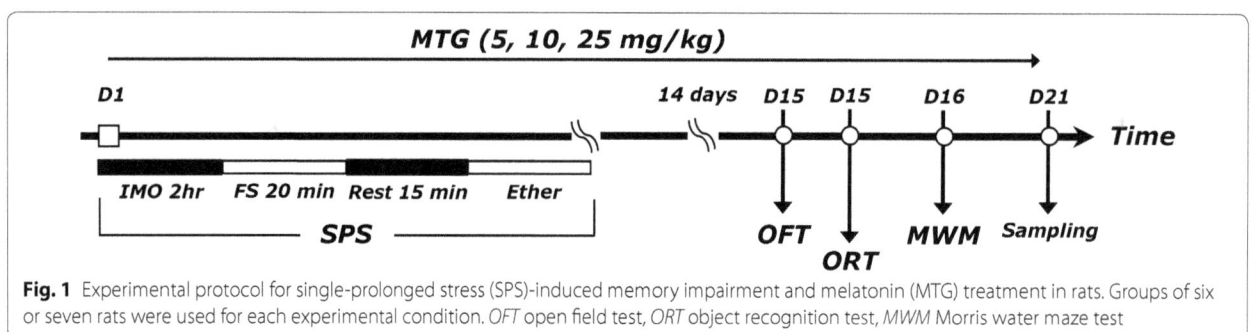

Fig. 1 Experimental protocol for single-prolonged stress (SPS)-induced memory impairment and melatonin (MTG) treatment in rats. Groups of six or seven rats were used for each experimental condition. *OFT* open field test, *ORT* object recognition test, *MWM* Morris water maze test

Morris water maze test

After the ORT, the MWM test was used to measure the time and distance spent swimming to reach a submerged platform in the MWM test, performed as previously described [58]. MWM test was made of a spatial probe test and a place navigation test. The MWM consisted of a circular pool (200 cm diameter and 50 cm deep). The pool contained water maintained at a temperature of 22 ± 2 °C. The escape platform (15 cm diameter) in diameter was located 1.5 cm below the water in one of four sections of the pool. The hidden platform trial for acquisition test and probe trails for retention test were monitored by a video camera mounted on the ceiling, and data were analyzed by using a tracking program (S-MART: PanLab Co., Barcelona, Spain). The rats performed three training trials per day for five successively days. Each trial was terminated when the rat found the platform or after 180 s. On day 6, the platform was removed. In this probe trial, the each trial was 1 min in duration. The swimming path length, swimming speed, and time spent in the target quadrant were analyzed.

Open field test (OFT)

Before the completion of the MWM test, the rats were exposed to the OFT. The OFT was carried out according to a previously described method [55]. In the dimly lit room, rats was exposed singly in a square black plexiglass apparatus ($60 \times 60 \times 30$ cm) and tracked by a video tracking system for 5 min. Locomotion were analyzed by the distance and speed of movements and observed by a computerized video-tracking analysis program S-MART (PanLab Co., Barcelona, Spain). The number of rearing was also manually scored by examining the records in the OFT.

Measurement of corticosterone (CORT), BDNF, CREB and proinflammatory markers

All rats were deeply anesthetized through inhalation of isoflurane (1.2%) and were humanely sacrificed 1 day after behavioral measurement. The concentration of CORT, tumor necrosis factor-α (TNF-α), and interleukin-6 (IL-6) in the blood, and BDNF and CREB in the brain 21 days after SPS have been described previously [58]. The blood (n = 4/group) was rapidly collected via the abdominal aorta. The hippocampus (n = 4/group) was quickly removed from the rat brain in a randomized order. The CORT, TNF-α, IL-6, BDNF and CREB concentrations were measured by a competitive enzyme-linked immunosorbent assay (ELISA) using a CORT antibody (Novus Biologicals, LLC., Littleton, CO, USA), a TNF-α antibody (Abcam, Cambridge, MA, USA), an IL-6 antibody (Abcam), a BDNF antibody (R&D Systems, Minneapolis, MN, USA), and a CREB antibody (Thermo

Fisher Scientific, Waltham, MA, USA) according to the manufacturer's protocol. Detectable CORT (46–304 ng/mL), BDNF (9–45 pg/mg), CREB (1–62 pg/mg), TNF-α (4–52 pg/mL), and IL-6 (1–54 pg/mL) concentrations ranged. Intra-assay and inter assay variation ranged from 1.35–10.31% CV and 4.73–16.59% CV, respectively. 100% specificity to rat CORT, BDNF, CREB, TNF-α and IL-6 were reported in manufacturer protocol.

Total RNA preparation and RT-PCR analysis

The expression of BDNF, CREB, TNF-α and IL-6 mRNA was evaluated by reverse transcription-polymerase chain reaction (RT-PCR) according to a previously described method [58]. In brief, total RNA was extracted from the hippocampus (n = 3/group) of each rat using TRIzol reagent (Life Technologies, Carlsbad, CA, USA) according to the manufacturer's instructions. cDNA was synthesized from 2 µg total RNA using reverse transcriptase (Takara Bio, Otsu, Japan) with random hexamers (COSMO Genetech, Seoul, Korea), and then amplified at 57 °C for 27 cycles in the BDNF reaction, at 51 °C for 27 cycles in the CREB reaction, at 58 °C for 30 cycles in the TNF-α reaction, and at 60 °C for 30 cycles in the IL-6 reaction by PCR using Taq DNA polymerase (Takara, Kyoto, Japan) on a thermal cycler. Data were normalized against GADPH expression in the corresponding sample.

Immunohistochemistry

The immunohistochemical analyses have been described previously [58]. The sections obtained from the brains were immunostained for CREB expression using the avidin-biotin-peroxidase complex (ABC) method. Briefly, the sections were incubated with a primary rabbit anti-CREB antibody (1:200 dilution, Cell Signaling, Boston, MA, USA) in PBS plus 0.3% Triton X-100 (PBST) for 72 h at 4 °C. Next, the sections were incubated for 120 min at room temperature with secondary antibodies (1:200 dilution, Vector Laboratories Co., Burlingame, CA, USA) in PBST containing 2% normal serum. To visualize immunoreactivity, the sections were incubated for 90 min in ABC reagent (Vectastain Elite ABC kit, Vector Labs. Co.), and then in a solution containing 3,3'-diaminobenzidine (DAB; Sigma-Aldrich) and 0.01% H_2O_2 for 1 min. The sections were viewed at 200× magnification, and the number of CREB-labeled cells was quantified in the hippocampus.

Statistical analysis

All data are expressed as mean $\pm$ SEM. The data were analyzed with SPSS 13.0 (Chicago, IL, USA). Data were analyzed by the multiple way of analysis of variance (ANOVA) and Tukey's post hoc tests. Between-subjects two-way ANOVA was used to analyze the effects of MTG treatment and time. In all of the analyses, differences were considered statistically significant at $p < 0.05$.

Results

Effect of MTG on SPS-stimulated changes in the plasma CORT level

ELISA analysis showed that rats who underwent SPS exposure had a significantly higher plasma CORT concentration (297.87%) than rats in the saline-treated (CON) group 21 days after SPS exposure ($p < 0.05$; Fig. 2). However, administration of MTG at 25 mg/kg decreased the SPS-stimulated increase in the plasma CORT level ($p < 0.05$). However, administration of MTG at 5 or 10 mg/kg did not alter plasma CORT levels in the SPS-pretreated rats. Thus, the SPS procedure caused memory impairments in rats and was utilized to develop the PTSD or traumatic stress model in rats. The increased plasma CORT concentration in the SPS group was significantly replaced to levels similar to those in the CON group by 10 mg FLX ($p < 0.05$). This reversal display that the CORT concentration in the plasma of rats treating 25 mg/kg MTG was similar to that of rats treating 10 mg/kg FLX. Suppression of the increase in plasma CORT level by

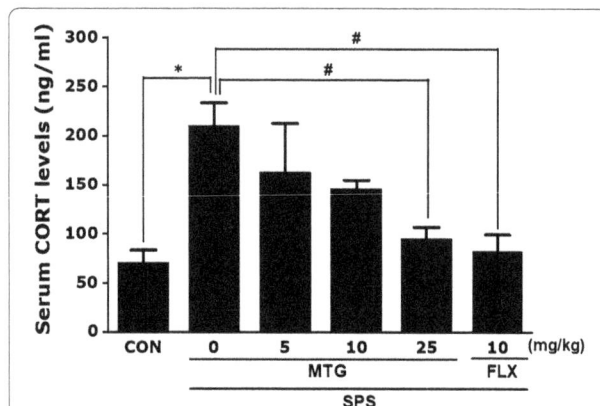

Fig. 2 Effects of MTG on plasma corticosterone (CORT) levels in rats with SPS-induced memory impairments: assessed with an enzyme-linked immunosorbent assay (ELISA). Parameters were determined at the end of the experiments. Data are expressed as the mean ± SEM of 4 animals in each group. *$p < 0.05$ versus the CON group; #$p < 0.05$ versus the SPS group

MTG also provided a base for the scientific inference that SPS-induces memory impairment in rats.

Effects of MTG on SPS-stimulated memory impairment

The novel object recognition for learning and memory function was indicated by means of the exploration (sniffing) times of familiar and novel objects and by computation of the discrimination indix by the ORT (Fig. 3a and b). Analyses of sniffing times for old objects by one-way ANOVA revealed no significant differences between the groups (F(5,39) = 1.857, $p = 0.128$). There was no significant difference among the groups in sniffing time for old objects. Analyses of sniffing times for novel objects by one-way ANOVA revealed significant differences between groups (F(5,39) = 37.059, $p < 0.001$), and *post hoc* comparisons using Tukey's test manifested a significant reduction in sniffing time for novel objects in all SPS-stimulated groups compared to the sniffing time in controls ($p < 0.001$; Fig. 3a). The negative effect of stress on recognition memory, indicated by sniffing time, was altered by MTG treatment (5 and 10 mg/kg). There were no statistically significant effects of MTG (5 and 10 mg/kg) treatment on the remaining parameters measured in the ORT. However, the rats in the SPS + MTG25 group indicated longer sniffing times for novel objects than the rats in the SPS group ($p < 0.001$). *Post-hoc* examination with Tukey test revealed that the discrimination index of PTSD group was significantly reduced compared to the CON group ($p < 0.05$; Fig. 3b). However, the rats in the SPS + MTG25 group indicated a higher discrimination index than the rats in the SPS group ($p < 0.05$). This difference also showed that the recovery of recognition memory after the SPS stimulated deficit was almost comparable in the SPS + MTG25 and the SPS + FLX groups.

In MWM test, SPS-stimulated rats were weak to learn during acquisition trial and retention trial. The effects of MTG treatment on swimming time to reach the submerged platform in the MWM test are shown in Fig. 3c–f. The SPS group indicated marked retardation in escape latency during all trial sessions, especially due to memory impairments resulting from SPS-stimulated learning and memory deficits.

PTSD influenced performance in the acquisition phase. More specifically, the SPS group indicated

---

(See figure on next page.)

Fig. 3 Effects of MTG on recognition memory assessed by the novel object recognition test (ORT) in which the time spent sniffing familiar and novel objects during a 3-min choice trial (**a**) and the ability to discriminate (**b**) between familiar and novel objects were measured. The Morris water maze (MWM) test was used to assess the effects of MTG on spatial learning and memory. Time to escape (latency) from the water onto a submerged platform during acquisition trials (**c**), percentages of time spent in the target quadrant (**d**), percentages of distance traversed in the target quadrant (**e**), and swimming speed (**f**) were used as outcome measures. The open field test (OFT) was used to assess the effect of MTG on locomotor activity (counts) and total number of rearing bouts (**g**). Six or seven rats were used per treatment group. Data are represented as the mean ± SEM. *$p < 0.05$, **$p < 0.01$, ***$p < 0.001$ versus the CON group; #$p < 0.05$, ##$p < 0.01$, ###$p < 0.001$ versus the SPS group

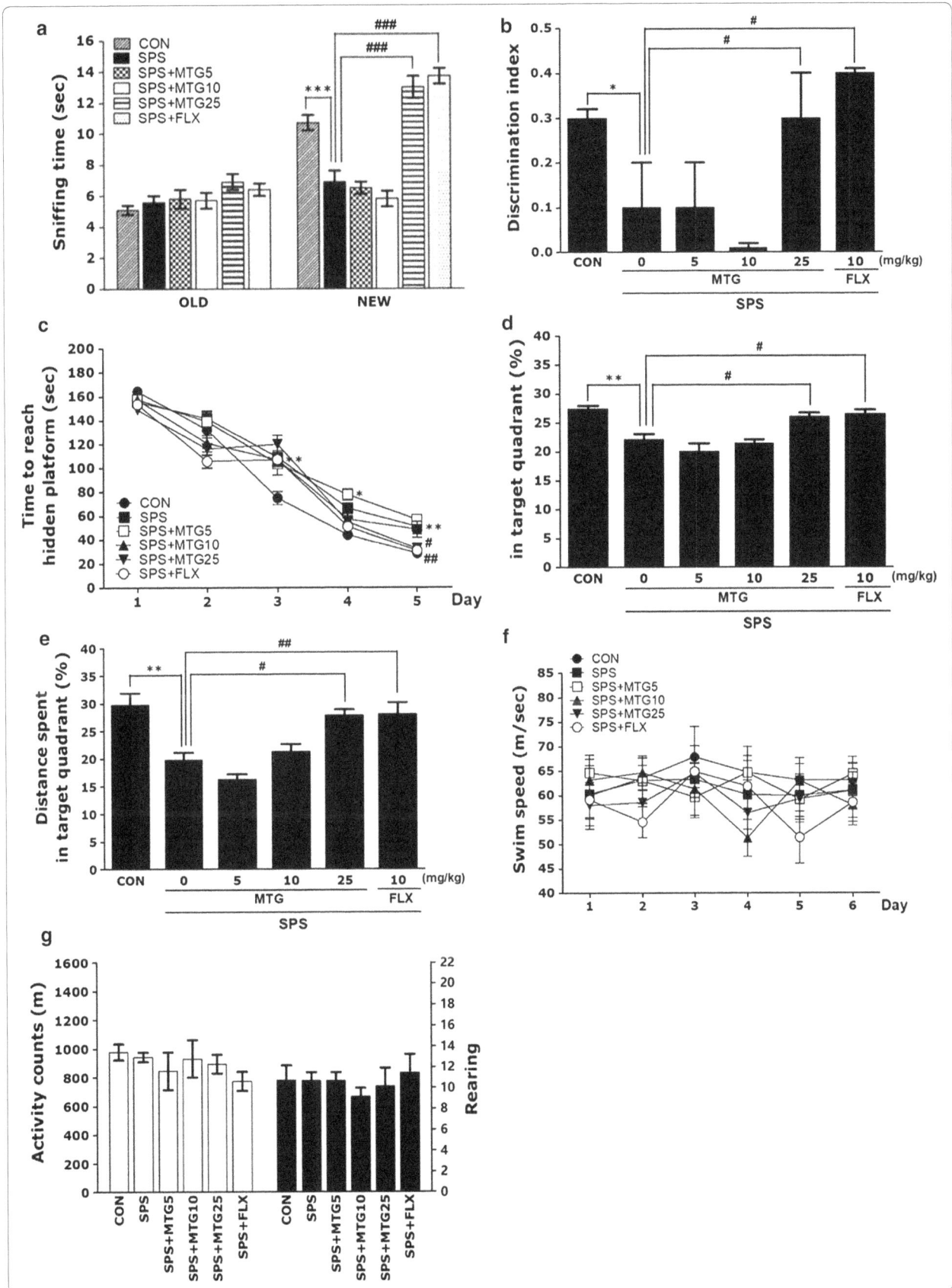

significantly enhanced latency compared with the CON group (Fig. 3c, d). ANOVA (6×5, treatment $\times$ time) disclosed a significant difference among groups ($F(5,34) = 16.240$, $p < 0.01$) and an effect of the day of training ($F(4136) = 351.639$, $p < 0.01$); however, a group $\times$ day interaction was not discovered ($F(20,136) = 1.588$, $p = 0.064$). The SPS group indicated worse performance than the CON group ($p < 0.05$ on the days 3 and 5, $p < 0.01$ on the day 4). Tukey's *post hoc* test showed that rats in the SPS+MTG25 group had significantly reduced swimming latency compared to those in the SPS group ($p < 0.01$ on day 5). Both the 5 and 10 mg/kg MTG treatment groups still exhibited longer swimming durations than the SPS group. To examine the effect of SPS and MTG on the spatial memory of rats, performance in the probe trial on day 6 was investigated by calculating the percentages of time spent swimming in the speculated position of the platform. The swimming times and distances were reduced in the rats that swam directly to the target area where the platform had been located. The rats exposed to SPS indicated serious deficits of spatial memory performance in the MWM test ($p < 0.01$; Fig. 3d, e). A reduction in distance traveled was observed when 10 mg/kg MTG was administered to rats exposed to SPS, although this result was only marginally significant. Therefore, 10 mg/kg MTG could not completely restore the impaired memory in SPS rats. The rats in the 25 mg/kg MTG-treated group spent more time around the platform area than those in the SPS group ($p < 0.05$). Furthermore, the swimming latency in rats that received MTG was higher than the latency in the SPS group, indicating a reversal of the SPS-stimulated impairment in memory. Thus, MTG-treated rats indicated a significant improvement in the memory retention test because they spent more time in the quadrant where the platform was previously located and swam over the previous location of the platform more continually. The SPS group was not significantly different from the other groups in mean swimming speed, as analyzed by dividing the total swim distance by latency ($p = 0.645$; Fig. 3f). Based on these results, rats treated with 25 mg/kg MTG indicated greater enhancement in acquisition during the hidden platform trial and, consequently, arrived the platform more quicker than the SPS-stimulated rats. Our results also showed that the swimming latency of the SPS-stimulated rats treating 25 mg/kg MTG was similar to that of rats treating 10 mg/kg of FLX.

A parametric one-way ANOVA was executed, and as shown in Fig. 3g, no PTSD-associated differences were discovered in locomotor activity (motor function) or total number of rearings (hyperactivity) in the OFT. There was no significant difference between saline-treated rats, SPS-exposed rats, and MTG-treated rats in remarked locomotor activity ($F(5,39) = 1.271$, $p = 0.322$) or total number of rearings ($F(5,39) = 0.337$, $p = 0.887$).

Because no significant difference in locomotor activity was remarked among groups in the OFT, the remarked deficits in learning and memory in the rats exposed to SPS were not attributable to differences in locomotor activity. Rats may also indicate water-avoidance behaviors when tackled with an MWM test. However, this results demonstrate that no rats presented anxiety-like behaviors in the OFT after a stress exposure in the MWM test.

Effects of MTG on SPS-stimulated changes in BDNF and CREB in the hippocampus

Figure 4 indicates that the hippocampal levels of BDNF and CREB were significantly different among the groups. One-way ANOVA of the concentrations of BDNF and CREB in the hippocampus disclosed a significant difference among the groups [($F(5,23) = 3.961$, $p < 0.05$) and (($F(5,23) = 6.133$, $p < 0.01$). The *post hoc* test results showed a significant decline in BDNF and CREB concentrations in the hippocampus of the SPS group compared with those in the CON group ($p < 0.05$; Fig. 4). Furthermore, 10 mg/kg MTG could not completely reverse the decreased concentration of hippocampal BDNF and CREB observed in the SPS group. Daily administration of 25 mg/kg MTG reversed the SPS-stimulated decrease in BDNF level in the hippocampus, although this result was only marginally significant. Daily administration of 25 mg/kg MTG significantly reversed the SPS-stimulated decrease in CREB concentration in the hippocampus ($p < 0.05$). Additionally, the CREB concentration in the hippocampus of rats treating 10 mg/kg FLX was similar to that in the hippocampus of rats treating 25 mg/kg MTG.

To further investigate the effects of MTG on the expression of neurotrophic factors in the hippocampus of rats exposed to SPS, BDNF and CREB mRNA expression was analyzed by RT-PCR. Although the mRNA level of BDBF in the SPS group was lower than that in the CON group, this result was only marginally significant. However, CREB mRNA expression in the SPS group was significantly lower than that in the CON group ($p < 0.01$). The decreased expression of CREB mRNA in the SPS group was significantly reinstated to levels similar to those in the CON group by 25 mg/kg MTG ($p < 0.01$). Furthermore, CREB mRNA expression in the hippocampus of rats treating 25 mg/kg MTG was similar to that of rats treating 10 mg/kg FLX.

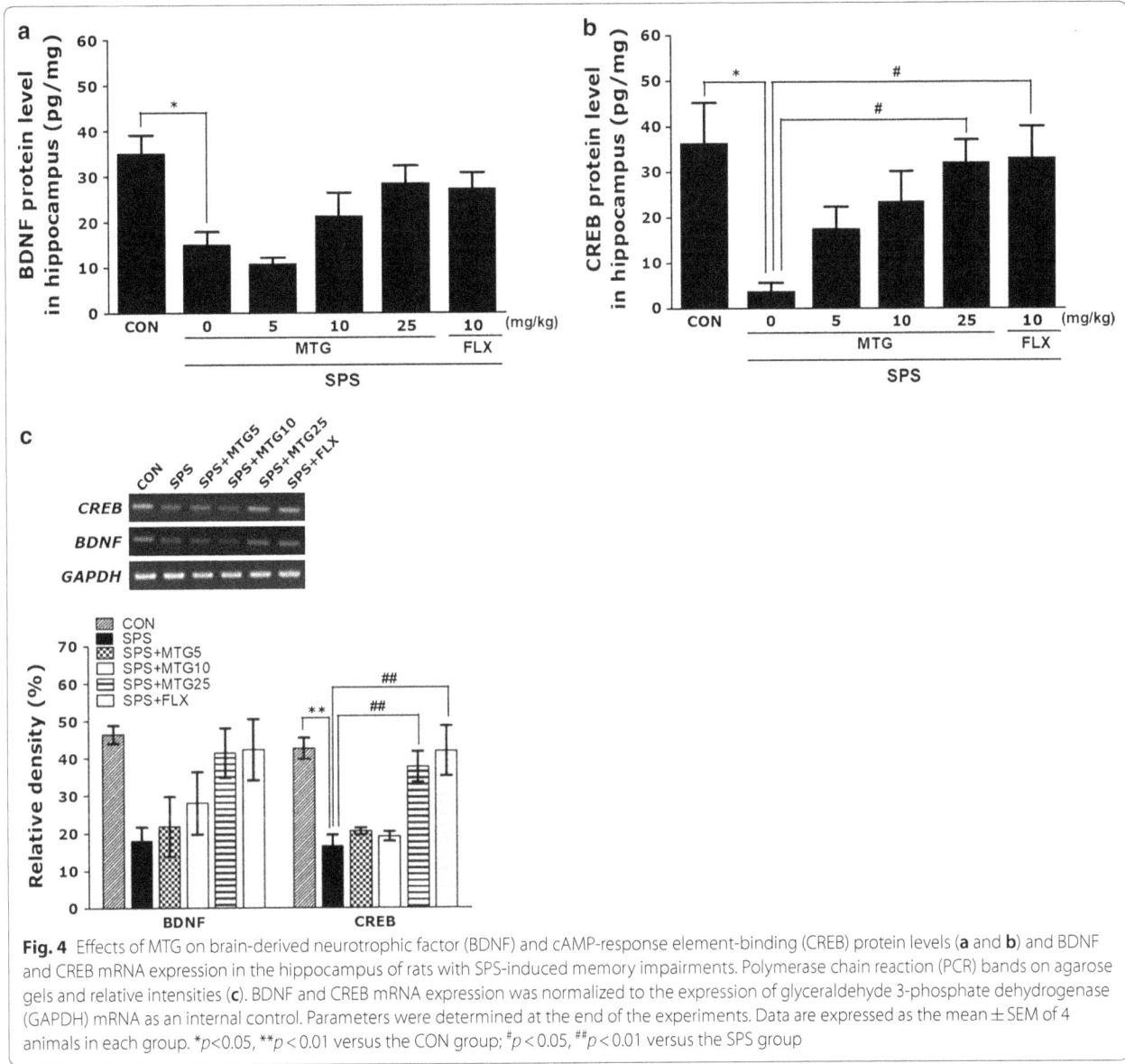

Fig. 4 Effects of MTG on brain-derived neurotrophic factor (BDNF) and cAMP-response element-binding (CREB) protein levels (**a** and **b**) and BDNF and CREB mRNA expression in the hippocampus of rats with SPS-induced memory impairments. Polymerase chain reaction (PCR) bands on agarose gels and relative intensities (**c**). BDNF and CREB mRNA expression was normalized to the expression of glyceraldehyde 3-phosphate dehydrogenase (GAPDH) mRNA as an internal control. Parameters were determined at the end of the experiments. Data are expressed as the mean ± SEM of 4 animals in each group. *$p < 0.05$, **$p < 0.01$ versus the CON group; #$p < 0.05$, ##$p < 0.01$ versus the SPS group

Effects of MTG on SPS-stimulated changes in neuroinflammatory cytokines in the hippocampus

Figure 5 indicates that the hippocampal concentrations of TNF-α and IL-6 were significantly different in comparisons among the groups. One-way ANOVA of the concentrations of TNF-α and IL-6 in the hippocampus disclosed a significant difference among the groups (($F_{(5,23)} = 4.678$, $p < 0.01$) and (($F_{(5,23)} = 4.189$, $p < 0.05$). The *post hoc* test results showed a significant increase in TNF-α and IL-6 levels in the hippocampus of the SPS groups compared to those in the CON group ($p < 0.05$ and $p < 0.01$; Fig. 5). Furthermore, MTG (5 and 10 mg/kg) treatment could not completely reverse the increased concentration of hippocampal TNF-α or

IL-6 observed in the SPS group. However, daily administration of 25 mg/kg MTG significantly reversed the SPS-stimulated increase in the TNF-α level in the hippocampus ($p < 0.05$), and daily treatment of 25 mg/kg MTG reversed the SPS-stimulated increase in IL-6 in the hippocampus, although this result was only marginally significant. Additionally, the TNF-α concentration in the hippocampus of rats treating 10 mg/kg FLX was similar to that of rats treating 25 mg/kg MTG.

To investigate the effects of MTG on the expression of neuroinflammatory cytokines in the hippocampus of rats exposed to SPS, the mRNA expression of TNF-α and IL-6 was analyzed by RT-PCR. The mRNA levels of TNF-α and IL-6 in the SPS group were significantly

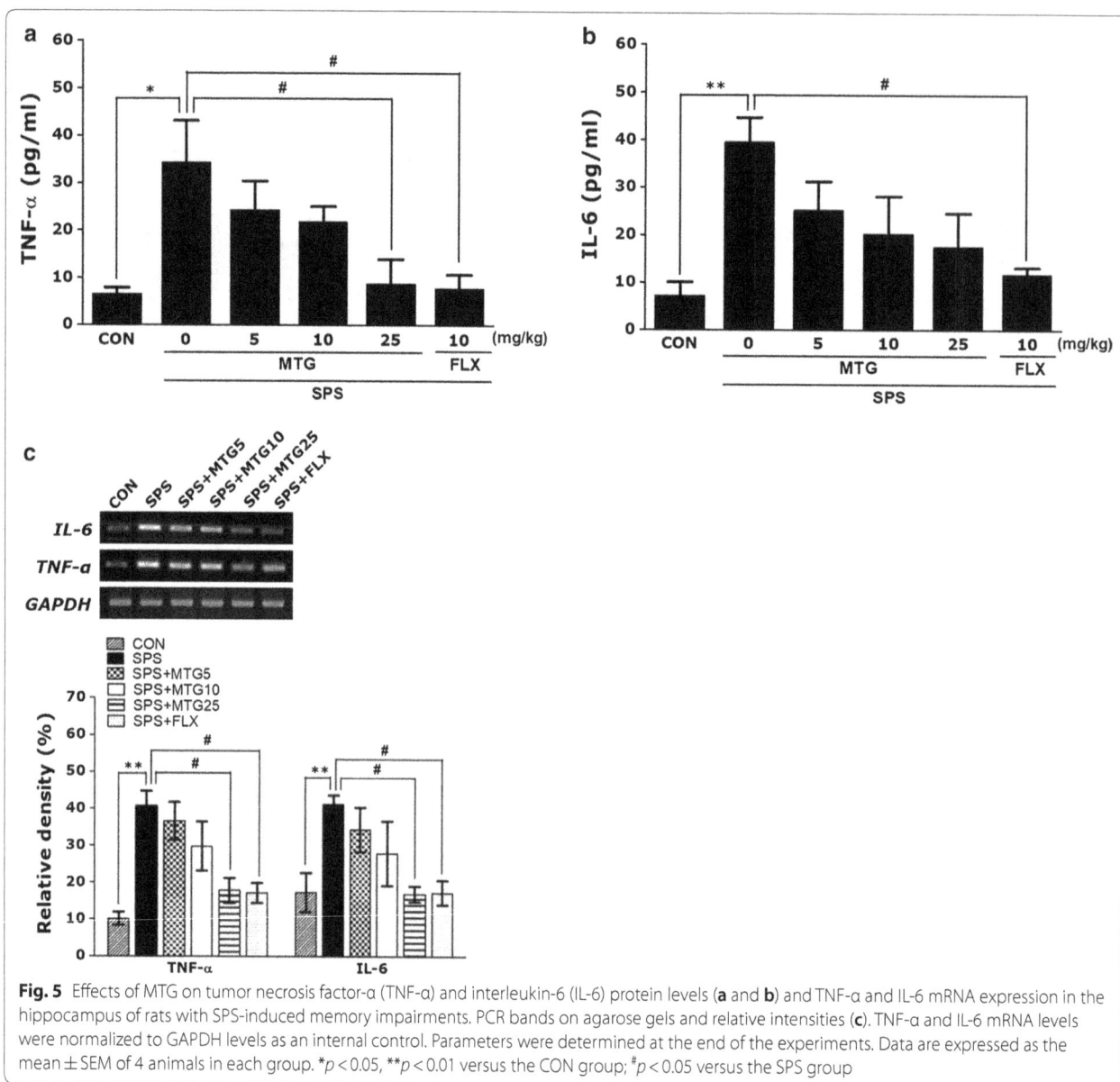

Fig. 5 Effects of MTG on tumor necrosis factor-α (TNF-α) and interleukin-6 (IL-6) protein levels (**a** and **b**) and TNF-α and IL-6 mRNA expression in the hippocampus of rats with SPS-induced memory impairments. PCR bands on agarose gels and relative intensities (**c**). TNF-α and IL-6 mRNA levels were normalized to GAPDH levels as an internal control. Parameters were determined at the end of the experiments. Data are expressed as the mean ± SEM of 4 animals in each group. *$p < 0.05$, **$p < 0.01$ versus the CON group; #$p < 0.05$ versus the SPS group

increased compared with that in the CON group ($p < 0.01$), but the increased TNF-α and IL-6 mRNA expression in the SPS group was significantly reinstated to levels similar to those in the CON group by 25 mg/kg MTG ($p < 0.05$). Finally, TNF-α and IL-6 mRNA expression in the hippocampus of rats treating 25 mg/kg MTG was similar to that of rats treating 10 mg/kg FLX.

Effect of MTG on SPS-stimulated changes in CREB in the hippocampus

Following the behavioral tests, brain tissue from the rats were analyzed using immunohistochemistry to examine the effect of MTG treatment on the neuronal loss related

to the SPS-stimulated memory deficits. The quantification of CREB immunoreactive cells in the hippocampus are shown in Fig. 6. In the SPS group, the number of CREB-immunoreactive neurons in the CA1 and CA3 of the hippocampus was decreased to 60.86 and 68.66% relative to those in the CON group, respectively. One-way ANOVA of the number of CREB immunoreactive cells disclosed a significant difference among the six groups (($5,95$) = 3.868, $p < 0.01$) and (($5,95$) = 3.735, $p < 0.01$). *Post hoc* comparisons showed that CREB reaction in the hippocampus of the SPS group was significantly lower than that of the CON group ($p < 0.01$ in the CA1 and $p < 0.05$ in the CA3). The number of CREB-immunoreactive

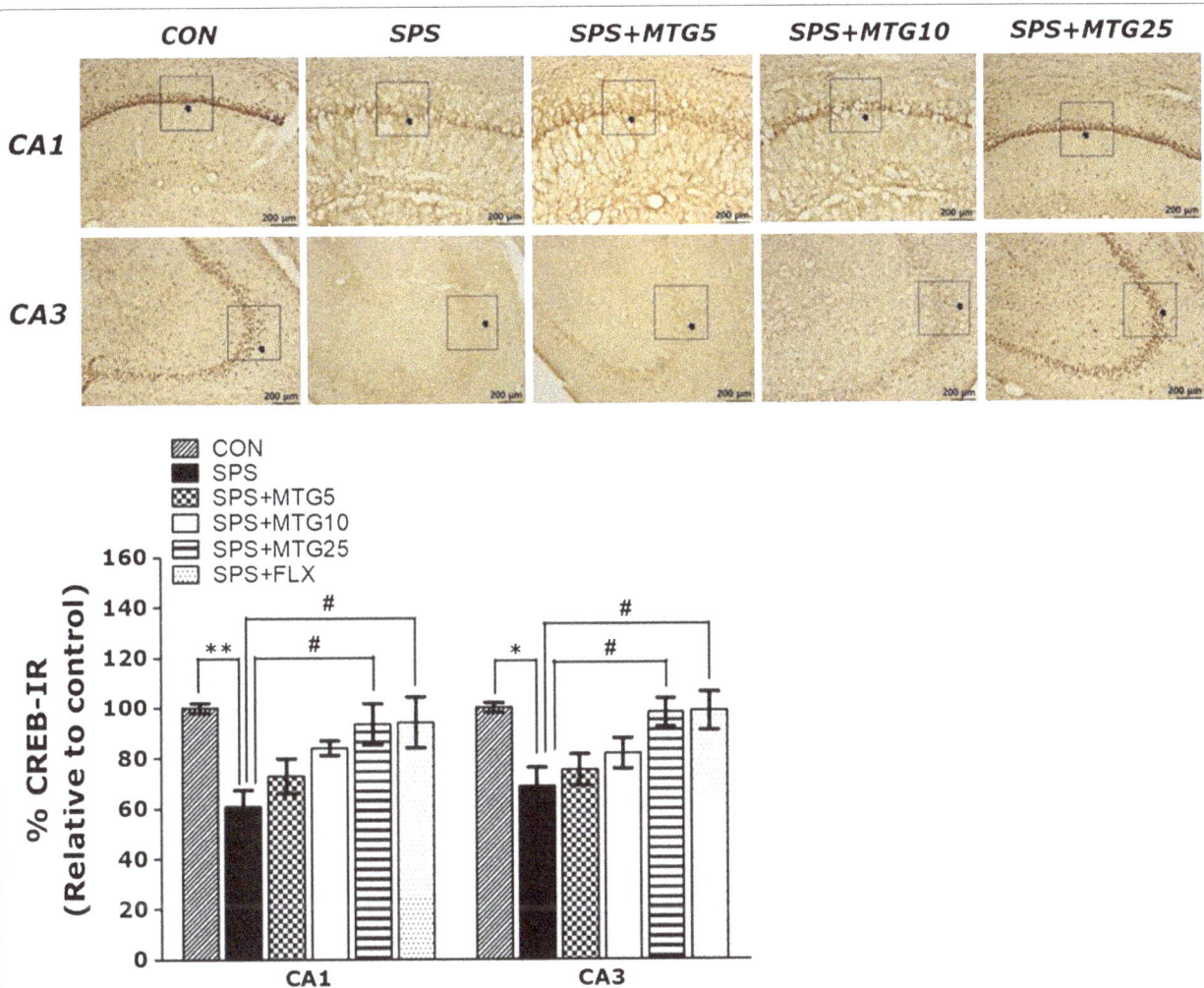

Fig. 6 Effects of MTG on the mean number of CREB-stained hippocampal areas after the MWM test. Representative photographs and relative percentages are shown in Fig. 6. The scale bar represents 100 μm. Representative images of immunoreactive neurons are shown above each graph. Their values were calculated as a percentage of the corresponding value of the control (CON) group. Data are expressed as the mean ± SEM of 3 animals in each group. *$p < 0.05$, **$p < 0.01$ versus the CON group; #$p < 0.05$ versus the SPS group

neurons in the SPS + MTG25 group was significantly higher in the CA1 and CA3 of the hippocampal region than in those of the SPS group ($p < 0.05$). This results also showed that the number of CREB-activity neuronal cells in the hippocampus in rats treating 25 mg/kg MTG was similar to that in rats treating 10 mg/kg FLX.

Discussion

The present results demonstrated that SPS-stimulated memory impairments were associated with serious impairment in performance on tests of learning and memory function as well as corresponding signs of neurodegeneration in the brain, including decreased BDNF and CREB expression and increased proinflammatory cytokine levels in the hippocampus. However,

treatment with MTG in a rat model of PTSD significantly advanced cognitive functions on the ORT and enhanced the number of platform crossings in the MWM test. Additionally, MTG treatment enhanced CREB activities in the hippocampus of male rats exposed to SPS-stimulated memory impairments and inhibited the increase in proinflammatory mediators in the hippocampus of rats with SPS-stimulated PTSD symptoms.

The SPS procedure is a well-validated animal model of PTSD with high face validity that addresses the core etiological factors of this disorder, including maladaptive cognitive processes, altered neuroplasticity, and enhanced negative feedback in the HPA axis [13]. SPS in rats transiently produces several impairment in learning acquisition and short-term memory that are associated with be similar to PTSD or chronic stress [12, 13]. Therefore, in the present study, rats were subjected to SPS to mimic the psychosocial and physiological stressors associated with PTSD and then treated with various doses of MTG.

In this model, the compulsory sustaining of high CORT levels affects cognition by decreasing memory ability, which may be associated with the progression or exacerbation of traumatic stress in humans [55]. The SPS procedure increased the plasma CORT level in the rats, which is in line with chronic stress models. In rat models, compulsory maintenance of high CORT levels can affect cognition by decreasing memory ability under experimental conditions and might be closely correlated with the progression or exacerbation of a chronically stressful condition in humans [55]. The HPA axis is an important component of the neuroendocrine system that controls immune function, energy expenditure, emotions and mood, and stress [59]. HPA axis dysfunction is a specific neuroendocrine role in experimental animals and humans with PTSD [59].

MTG is the primary secretory product of the pineal gland [60, 61]. The secretion of MTG with the circadian rhythm in the blood of mammals is functionally linked to the adjustment of 24-h cycles and to circannual rhythm control. The opposing circadian alternation in MTG and HPA-related hormones may suggest a connection between these two factors. MTG has been showed to be able to reverse HPA-axis activity caused by stress, which is similar to this results [61, 62]. In addition, MTG has also been showed to cause an inhibitory effect on both stimulated and spontaneous HPA axis activation [63]. Stress stimulates the HPA axis and influences several biological effects at both the peripheral and central level. In the present study, MTG treatment after application of the SPS procedure significantly reduced serum CORT levels and improved the behavioral alternations stimulated by SPS. Our results showed that the SPS procedure produced severe impairment in the performance of cognitive functioning tests and decreases in BDNF and CREB expression in the hippocampus, suggestive of neurodegeneration in the brain. MTG restored plasma CORT to near normal levels toward the end of the 2-week treatment period, which suggests that this treatment inhibited stress-related dysfunction in the HPA axis, alleviated associated behavioral diseases, and increased CREB expression and anti-inflammatory activity. Thus, the present findings indicate that MTG treatment prevented the dysfunction of the HPA axis. These findings may elucidate the mechanisms underlying the effects of MTG in the hippocampus as well as the biochemical and behavioral signals caused by low plasma levels of CORT.

The ORT and MWM test were used to investigate the effects of MTG on cognitive memory and spatial learning and memory, respectively, and the present findings showing that SPS impaired recognition memory are consistent with those of a previous study [16]. Cognitive impairments were significantly more pronounced after exposure to SPS, as indicated by a significant enhance in time spent exploring familiar objects, reduced exploration of novel objects, and a reduction in the discrimination index. These findings suggest that, following exposure to memory-impairing agents, there is a profound deterioration in the brain that contributes to a diminished episodic memory and recognition capacity [58]. Accordingly, the this study showed that SPS significantly reduced time spent sniffing novel objects and reduced the discrimination index, whereas treatment with MTG significantly enhanced time spent sniffing novel objects and improved recognition memory. The present study used the MWM test because it is more useful for assessing spatial learning and memory in rats than other conventional mazes, such as the radial-arm maze and T-maze [58]. The MWM is a hippocampus-associated memory test that is frequently used to investigate cognitive impairment and study constant spatial learning and memory abilities and reference memory in rats [64]. In the present study, the chronically stressed animals had a significantly longer escape latency to reach the platform than the non-stressed animals and exhibited spatial learning deficits in the MWM test. The chronically stressed animals that received MTG learned faster and had shorter escape latency than the untreated chronic stress group. Moreover, compared with the non-stressed rats, the chronically stressed rats that did not receive MTG treatment exhibited poorer performances on probe trials administered 24 h after task acquisition, which is indicative of damaged memory recall and retrieval. MTG reversed these behavioral abnormalities and reinstated spatial learning and memory in the chronically stressed rats. A similar effect was seen following chronic treatment with fluoxetine [65]. Thus, the this findings support and prove the hypothesis that MTG ameliorates spatial learning and memory impairment caused by traumatic stress.

An OFT was performed to rule out the potentially confounding effects of motor deficits, which could influence the outcomes of behavioral tests of anxiety and depression. However, no significant individual differences in locomotor activity were discovered between the groups, which suggests that MTG treatment did not affect sensorimotor performance. Thus, the improved performance in the MWM test was more likely due to improved learning and memory than to differences in limb flexibility, motor output, or sensorimotor function. Furthermore, no rats in either group appeared anxiety-like behaviors in the OFT after stress exposure in the MWM test, which indicates that MTG did not alter psychomotor function or active responses as measured by performance in the MWM test.

To identify additional MTG-related mechanisms underlying the improvements in memory, the effects of MTG on BDNF and CREB levels in the hippocampus were investigated. The change in the levels of BDNF and CREB proteins in the brain supplies a novel treatment strategy for the amelioration of memory impairment [66]. In addition to its roles in neuronal cell survival and the prevention of neurodegeneration, recent experimental evidence strongly supports the role of BDNF in the regulation of synaptic function and plasticity in the CNS for learning and memory processes [67]. However, in the present study, no significant individual differences in BDNF level were observed following treatment with MTG, which suggests that MTG did not affect the BDNF level. CREB is also believed to play a critical role in the formation of memories [66]. SPS-stimulated memory impairment are associated with significant reductions in CREB mRNA expression in the hippocampus as well as poor performance on hippocampus-dependent tests [5, 65]. In the present study, MTG treatment significantly reversed SPS-stimulated decreases in CREB mRNA expression, which suggests that the beneficial effects of MTG were mediated by increases in CREB expression that may be associated with enhanced neuronal function and performance in learning and memory tests. Furthermore, the present findings indicate that there is a correlation between protein and gene function and decreased CREB expression in the hippocampus.

Additionally, the current results also strongly suggest a close correlation between hippocampal CREB expression and number of CREB-immunoreactive neurons in the hippocampus. CREB dysfunction interrupts hippocampus-dependent memory formation, and CREB has been suggested to be required for memory solidity [68, 69]. Thus, BDNF transcriptional activity, up-regulated by CREB, may also play an important role in adaptive neuronal activations underlying memory function [70, 71]. The administration of MTG is proposed to significantly prevent the reduction in CREB in the hippocampus stimulated by SPS exposure, leading to memory deficits. Although MTG reversed the decrease in CREB expression in the hippocampus to some degree, the effect of MTG on other upstream or downstream pathways involving CREB was not determined [72]. The changes in CREB associated with memory impairment have been found to be accompanied by enhances in the phosphorylation of extracellular signal-related kinase [72]. Thus, further studies will be necessary to clarify more precisely

the effects of MTG on the CREB-mediated signaling pathway.

In the present study, SPS also significantly increased the expression of TNF-α and IL-6 in the hippocampus, which ultimately led to a chronic neuroinflammatory activation in the brain. Many studies have demonstrated that SPS-stimulated TNF-α and IL-1β expression are upregulated in PTSD and that these cytokines play a role in several events associated with the pathological cascade of PTSD [73]. Thus, inflammatory reactions may be associated with the pathogenesis of degenerative changes as well as cognitive impairments [74]. In this study, SPS induced an increase in the levels of the proinflammatory cytokines TNF-α and IL-6 and produced learning and memory impairment. However, MTG inhibited the increased expression of TNF-α and IL-6 in SPS-treated rats. MTG decreased the SPS-stimulated increase in the mRNA expression of TNF-α and IL-6, eventually resulting in the reversal of chronic inflammation and the amelioration of persistent brain dysfunction [65, 73]. According to the inflammation hypothesis, memory impairments in PTSD are due to selective and irreversible dysfunction and chronic inflammation in the brain [65, 73]. Thus, the anti-inflammatory effects of MTG are proposed here to significantly reverse the impaired memory retention and the increased expression of proinflammatory cytokines.

Conclusions

In summary, the present study demonstrated that SPS impaired neuronal function and produced associated memory and cognitive impairment in a rat model of progressive memory impairment in neurodegenerative disease. This was evidenced by performance on the ORT and MWM tests and by protein and gene expression analyses of CREB and BDNF. However, MTG treatment significantly attenuated the SPS-stimulated deficits as indicated by improved cognitive function on the behavioral tests, increased CREB expression, and normalization of the HPA axis. Moreover, MTG suppressed increases in the mRNA expressions of TNF-α and IL-6, which are proinflammatory mediators, in the hippocampus. Thus, MTG may be a useful agent for the prevention of neuronal impairments and the attenuation of anti-inflammatory effects such as those observed in patients with PTSD.

Abbreviations
PTSD: Post-traumatic stress disorder; MTG: Melatonin; SPS: Single prolonged stress; CREB: cAMP-response element-binding protein; HPA: Hypothalamic-pituitary-adrenal; BDNF: Brain-derived neurotrophic factor; SSRIs: Selective reuptake inhibitors; AD: Alzheimer disease; PD: Parkinson's disease; ORT: Object recognition task; MWM: Morris water maze; SD: Sprague-Dawley; FLX: Fluoxetine; CORT: Corticosterone; OFT: Open field test; TNF-α: Tumor necrosis factor-α; IL-6: Interleukin-6; ELISA: Enzyme-linked immunoassay; RT-PCR:

Reverse transcription-polymerase chain reaction; GAPDH: Glyceraldehyde-3-phosphate dehydrogenase; PBS: Phosphate-buffered saline; ABC: Avidin-biotin-peroxidase complex; DAB: 3,3'-Diaminobenzidine; ANOVA: Analysis of variance.

Authors' contributions

BL performed most experiments, data analysis and wrote the first draft of the paper. BL participated in animal experiments including behavioral tests. DHH directed the study, contributed to the discussion, edited and approved the manuscript. IS helped with concept development and data analysis. HL contributed to data analysis, wrote and revised the manuscript. All authors read and approved the final manuscript.

Author details

Acupuncture and Meridian Science Research Center, College of Korean Medicine, Kyung Hee University, 26, Kyungheedae-ro, Dongdaemun-gu, Seoul 02447, Republic of Korea. [2] Center for Converging Humanities, Kyung Hee University, Seoul 02447, Republic of Korea. [3] Department of Physiology, College of Medicine, Kyung Hee University, Seoul 02447, Republic of Korea.

Acknowledgements

This research was supported by a Grant from the National Research Foundation of Korea funded by the Korean government (2016R1D1A1A09917012).

Competing interests

The authors declared that they have no competing interests.

References

1. Lu CY, Liu X, Jiang H, Pan F, Ho CS, Ho RC. Effects of traumatic stress induced in the juvenile period on the expression of gamma-amin-obutyric acid receptor type A subunits in adult rat brain. Neural Plast. 2017;2017:5715816.
2. Anda RF, Felitti VJ, Bremner JD, Walker JD, Whitfield C, Perry BD, Dube SR, Giles WH. The enduring effects of abuse and related adverse experiences in childhood. A convergence of evidence from neurobiology and epidemiology. Eur Arch Psychiatry Clin Neurosci. 2006;256(3):174–86.
3. Brunello N, Davidson JR, Deahl M, Kessler RC, Mendlewicz J, Racagni G, Shalev AY, Zohar J. Posttraumatic stress disorder: diagnosis and epidemiology, comorbidity and social consequences, biology and treatment. Neuropsychobiology. 2001;43(3):150–62.
4. Nemeroff CB, Bremner JD, Foa EB, Mayberg HS, North CS, Stein MB. Posttraumatic stress disorder: a state-of-the-science review. J Psychiatr Res. 2006;40(1):1–21.
5. Shafia S, Vafaei AA, Samaei SA, Bandegi AR, Rafiei A, Valadan R, Hosseini-Khah Z, Mohammadkhani R, Rashidy-Pour A. Effects of moderate treadmill exercise and fluoxetine on behavioural and cognitive deficits, hypothalamic-pituitary-adrenal axis dysfunction and alternations in hippocampal BDNF and mRNA expression of apoptosis-related proteins in a rat model of post-traumatic stress disorder. Neurobiol Learn Mem. 2017;139(1):165–78.
6. Buckley TC, Blanchard EB, Neill WT. Information processing and PTSD: a review of the empirical literature. Clin Psychol Rev. 2000;20(8):1041–65.
7. Burke HM, Robinson CM, Wentz B, McKay J, Dexter KW, Pisansky JM, Talbot JN, Zoladz PR. Sex-specific impairment of spatial memory in rats following a reminder of predator stress. Stress. 2013;16(4):469–76.
8. Gilbertson MW, Gurvits TV, Lasko NB, Orr SP, Pitman RK. Multivariate assessment of explicit memory function in combat veterans with post-traumatic stress disorder. J Trauma Stress. 2001;14(1):413–32.
9. Brewin CR, Smart L. Working memory capacity and suppression of intrusive thoughts. J Behav Ther Exp Psychiatry. 2005;36(1):61–8.
10. McNally RJ. Debunking myths about trauma and memory. Can J Psychiatry. 2005;50(1):817–22.
11. Zoladz PR, Woodson JC, Haynes VF, Diamond DM. Activation of a remote (1-year old) emotional memory interferes with the retrieval of a newly formed hippocampus-dependent memory in rats. Stress. 2010;13(1):36–52.
12. Serova LI, Laukova M, Alaluf LG, Pucillo L, Sabban EL. Intranasal neuropeptide Y reverses anxiety and depressive-like behavior impaired by single prolonged stress PTSD model. Eur Neuropsychopharmacol. 2014;24(1):142–7.
13. Yamamoto S, Morinobu S, Takei S, Fuchikami M, Matsuki A, Yamawaki S, Liberzon I. Single prolonged stress: toward an animal model of posttraumatic stress disorder. Depress Anxiety. 2009;26(12):1110–7.
14. Serova LI, Laukova M, Alaluf LG, Sabban EL. Intranasal infusion of melanocortin receptor four (MC4R) antagonist to rats ameliorates development of depression and anxiety related symptoms induced by single prolonged stress. Behav Brain Res. 2013;250(1):139–47.
15. Lin CC, Tung CS, Lin PH, Huang CL, Liu YP. Traumatic stress causes distinctive effects on fear circuit catecholamines and the fear extinction profile in a rodent model of posttraumatic stress disorder. Eur Neuropsychopharmacol. 2016;26(9):1484–95.
16. Li XM, Han F, Liu DJ, Shi YX. Single-prolonged stress induced mitochondrial-dependent apoptosis in hippocampus in the rat model of posttraumatic stress disorder. J Chem Neuroanat. 2010;40(3):248–55.
17. Li X, Han F, Liu D, Shi Y. Changes of Bax, Bcl-2 and apoptosis in hippocampus in the rat model of post-traumatic stress disorder. Neurol Res. 2010;32(6):579–86.
18. Takei S, Morinobu S, Yamamoto S, Fuchikami M, Matsumoto T, Yamawaki S. Enhanced hippocampal BDNF/TrkB signaling in response to fear conditioning in an animal model of posttraumatic stress disorder. J Psychiatr Res. 2011;45(4):460–8.
19. Loganovsky KN, Zdanevich NA. Cerebral basis of posttraumatic stress disorder following the Chernobyl disaster. CNS Spectr. 2013;8(2):95–102.
20. Ragu Varman D, Rajan KE. Environmental enrichment reduces anxiety by differentially activating serotonergic and neuropeptide Y (NPY)-Ergic System in Indian field mouse (Mus booduga): an animal model of post-traumatic stress disorder. PLoS ONE. 2015;10(5):e0127945.
21. Ebenezer PJ, Wilson CB, Wilson LD, Nair AR, J F. The anti-inflammatory effects of blueberries in an animal model of post-traumatic stress disorder (PTSD). PLoS ONE. 2016;11(9):e0160923.
22. Han F, Xiao B, Wen L, Shi Y. Effects of fluoxetine on the amygdala and the hippocampus after administration of a single prolonged stress to male Wistar rates: in vivo proton magnetic resonance spectroscopy findings. Psychiatry Res. 2015;232(2):154–61.
23. Schoenfeld FB, Marmar CR, Neylan TC. Current concepts in pharmacotherapy for posttraumatic stress disorder. Psychiatr Serv. 2004;55(5):519–31.
24. Penn E, Tracy DK. The drugs don't work? Antidepressants and the current and future pharmacological management of depression. Ther Adv Psychopharmacol. 2012;2(5):179–88.
25. Liberzon I, López JF, Flagel SB, Vázquez DM, Young EA. Differential regulation of hippocampal glucocorticoid receptors mRNA and fast feedback: relevance to post-traumatic stress disorder. J Neuroendocrinol. 1999;11(1):11–7.
26. Fu W, Xie H, Laudon M, Zhou S, Tian S, You Y. Piromelatine ameliorates memory deficits associated with chronic mild stress-induced anhedonia in rats. Psychopharmacology. 2016;233(12):2229–39.

27. Sharif R, Aghsami M, Gharghabi M, Sanati M, Khorshidahmad T, Vakilzadeh G, Mehdizadeh H, Gholizadeh S, Taghizadeh G, Sharifzadeh M. Melatonin reverses H-89 induced spatial memory deficit: involvement of oxidative stress and mitochondrial function. Behav Brain Res. 2017;316(1):115–24.

28. Hardeland R, Cardinali DP, Brown GM, Pandi-Perumal SR. Melatonin and brain inflammaging. Prog Neurobiol. 2017;217–128(1):46–63.

29. Manchester LC, Coto-Montes A, Boga JA, Andersen LP, Zhou Z, Galano A, Vriend J, Tan DX, Reiter RJ. Melatonin: an ancient molecule that makes oxygen metabolically tolerable. J Pineal Res. 2015;59(4):403–19.

30. Moretti R, Zanin A, Pansiot J, Spiri D, Manganozzi L, Kratzer I, Favero G, Vasiljevic A, Rinaldi VE, Pic I, Massano D, D'Agostino I, Baburamani A, La Rocca MA, Rodella LF, Rezzani R, Ek J, Strazielle N, Ghersi-Egea JF, Gressens P, Titomanlio L. Melatonin reduces excitotoxic blood-brain barrier breakdown in neonatal rats. Neuroscience. 2015;311(1):382–97.

31. Rudnitskaya EA, Muraleva NA, Maksimova KY, Kiseleva E, Kolosova NG, Stefanova NA. Melatonin attenuates memory impairment, amyloid-β accumulation, and neurodegeneration in a rat model of sporadic alzheimer's disease. J Alzheimers Dis. 2015;47(1):103–16.

32. Zhang S, Wang P, Ren L, Hu C, Bi J. Protective effect of melatonin on soluble Aβ1-42-induced memory impairment, astrogliosis, and synaptic dysfunction via the Musashi1/Notch1/Hes1 signaling pathway in the rat hippocampus. Alzheimers Res Ther. 2016;8(1):40–5.

33. Huang F, Yang Z, Liu X, Li CQ. Melatonin facilitates extinction, but not acquisition or expression, of conditional cued fear in rats. BMC Neurosci. 2014;15(1):86–91.

34. Rawashdeh O, Maronde E. The hormonal Zeitgeber melatonin: role as a circadian modulator in memory processing. Front Mol Neurosci. 2012;5(1):27–31.

35. Morgan PJ, Barrett P, Howell HE, Helliwell R. Melatonin receptors: localization, molecular pharmacology and physiological significance. Neurochem Int. 1994;24(2):101–46.

36. Bertaina-Anglade V, Drieu-La-Rochelle C, Mocaër E, Seguin L. Memory facilitating effects of agomelatine in the novel object recognition memory paradigm in the rat. Pharmacol Biochem Behav. 2011;98(4):511–7.

37. He P, Ouyang X, Zhou S, Yin W, Tang C, Laudon M, Tian S. A novel melatonin agonist Neu-P11 facilitates memory performance and improves cognitive impairment in a rat model of Alzheimer' disease. Horm Behav. 2013;64(1):1–7.

38. Argyriou A, Prast H, Philippu A. Melatonin facilitates short-term memory. Eur J Pharmacol. 1998;349(2–3):159–62.

39. Barceló P, Nicolau C, Gamundí A, Fiol MA, Tresguerres JA, Akaârir M, Rial RV. Comparing the behavioural effects of exogenous growth hormone and melatonin in young and old Wistar rats. Oxid Med Cell Longev. 2016;2016:5863402.

40. Pandi-Perumal SR, BaHammam AS, Brown GM, Spence DW, Bharti VK, Kaur C, Hardeland R, Cardinali DP. Melatonin antioxidative defense: therapeutical implications for aging and neurodegenerative processes. Neurotox Res. 2013;23(3):267–300.

41. Furio AM, Brusco LI, Cardinali DP. Possible therapeutic value of melatonin in mild cognitive impairment: a retrospective study. J Pineal Res. 2007;43(4):404–9.

42. Esteban S, Nicolaus C, Garmundi A, Rial RV, Rodríguez AB, Ortega E, Ibars CB. Effect of orally administered L-tryptophan on serotonin, melatonin, and the innate immune response in the rat. Mol Cell Biochem. 2004;267(1–2):39–46.

43. Rosales-Corral SA, Acuña-Castroviejo D, Coto-Montes A, Boga JA, Manchester LC, Fuentes-Broto L, Korkmaz A, Ma S, Tan DX, Reiter RJ. Alzheimer's disease: pathological mechanisms and the beneficial role of melatonin. J Pineal Res. 2012;52(2):167–202.

44. Mukda S, Panmanee J, Boontem P, Govitrapong P. Melatonin administration reverses the alteration of amyloid precursor protein-cleaving secretases expression in aged mouse hippocampus. Neurosci Lett. 2016;621(1):39–46.

45. Rudnitskaya EA, Maksimova KY, Muraleva NA, Logvinov SV, Yanshole LV, Kolosova NG, Stefanova NA. Beneficial effects of melatonin in a rat model of sporadic Alzheimer's disease. Biogerontology. 2015;16(3):303–16.

46. Cardinali DP, Vigo DE, Olivar N, Vidal MF, Furio AM, Brusco LI. Therapeutic application of melatonin in mild cognitive impairment. Am J Neurodegener Dis. 2012;3:280–91.

47. Lee CH, Park JH, Ahn JH, Won MH. Effects of melatonin on cognitive impairment and hippocampal neuronal damage in a rat model of chronic cerebral hypoperfusion. Exp Ther Med. 2016;11(6):2240–6.

48. Lee CH, Yoo KY, Choi JH, Park OK, Hwang IK, Kwon YG, Kim YM, Won MH. Melatonin's protective action against ischemic neuronal damage is associated with up-regulation of the MT2 melatonin receptor. J Neurosci Res. 2010;88(12):2630–40.

49. Lee EJ, Lee MY, Chen HY, Hsu YS, Wu TS, Chen ST, Chang GL. Melatonin attenuates gray and white matter damage in a mouse model of transient focal cerebral ischemia. J Pineal Res. 2005;38(1):42–52.

50. Letechipía-Vallejo G, López-Loeza E, Espinoza-González V, González-Burgos I, Olvera-Cortés ME, Moralí G, Cervantes M. Long-term morphological and functional evaluation of the neuroprotective effects of post-ischemic treatment with melatonin in rats. J Pineal Res. 2007;42(2):138–46.

51. Lee MY, Kuan YH, Chen HY, Chen TY, Chen ST, Huang CC, Yang IP, Hsu YS, Wu TS, Lee EJ. Intravenous administration of melatonin reduces the intracerebral cellular inflammatory response following transient focal cerebral ischemia in rats. J Pineal Res. 2007;42(3):297–309.

52. Tyagi E, Agrawal R, Nath C, Shukla R. Effect of melatonin on neuroinflammation and acetylcholinesterase activity induced by LPS in rat brain. Eur J Pharmacol. 2010;640(1–3):206–10.

53. Keskin-Aktan A, Akbulut KG, Yazici-Mutlu Ç, Sonugur G, Ocal M, Akbulut H. The effects of melatonin and curcumin on the expression of SIRT2, Bcl-2 and Bax in the hippocampus of adult rats. Brain Res Bull. 2018;137:306–10.

54. Rebai R, Jasmin L, Boudah A. The antidepressant effect of melatonin and fluoxetine in diabetic rats is associated with a reduction of the oxidative stress in the prefrontal and hippocampal cortices. Brain Res Bull. 2017;134:142–50.

55. Lee B, Sur B, Cho SG, Yeom M, Shim I, Lee H, Hahm DH. Ginsenoside Rb1 rescues anxiety-like responses in a rat model of post-traumatic stress disorder. J Nat Med. 2016;70(2):133–44.

56. Patki G, Li L, Allam F, Solanki N, Dao AT, Alkadhi K, Salim S. Moderate treadmill exercise rescues anxiety and depression-like behavior as well as memory impairment in a rat model of posttraumatic stress disorder. Physiol Behav. 2014;130(1):47–53.

57. Okuda S, Roozendaal B, McGaugh JL. Glucocorticoid effects on object recognition memory require training-associated emotional arousal. Proc Natl Acad Sci USA. 2004;101(3):853–8.

58. Lee B, Sur B, Cho SG, Yeom M, Shim I, Lee H, Hahm DH. Wogonin attenuates hippocampal neuronal loss and cognitive dysfunction in trimethyltin-intoxicated rats. Biomol Ther. 2016;24(3):328–37.

59. Kim BK, Seo JH. Treadmill exercise alleviates post-traumatic stress disorder-induced impairment of spatial learning memory in rats. J Exerc Rehabil. 2013;9(4):413–9.

60. Tan DX, Manchester LC, Hardeland R, Lopez-Burillo S, Mayo JC, Sainz RM, Reiter RJ. Melatonin: a hormone, a tissue factor, an autocoid, a paracoid, and an antioxidant vitamin. J Pineal Res. 2003;34:75–8.

61. Zhang L, Guo HL, Zhang HQ, Xu TQ, He B, Wang ZH, Yang YP, Tang XD, Zhang P, Liu FE. Melatonin prevents sleep deprivation-associated anxiety-like behavior in rats: role of oxidative stress and balance between GABAergic and glutamatergic transmission. Am J Transl Res. 2017;9(5):2231–42.

62. Saito S, Tachibana T, Choi YH, Denbow DM, Furuse M. ICV melatonin reduces acute stress responses in neonatal chicks. Behav Brain Res. 2005;165:197–203.

63. Giordano R, Pellegrino M, Picu A, Bonelli L, Balbo M, Berardelli R, Lanfranco F, Ghigo E, Arvat E. Neuroregulation of the hypothalamus-pituitary-adrenal (HPA) axis in humans: effects of GABA-, mineralocorticoid-, and GH-Secretagogue-receptor modulation. Sci World J. 2006;6:1–11.

64. Janasson Z. Meta-analysis of sex differences in rodent models of learning and memory: a review of behavioral and biological data. Neurosci Biobehav Rev. 2005;28(8):811–25.

65. Lee B, Sur B, Yeom M, Shim I, Lee H, Hahm DH. Effects of systemic administration of ibuprofen on stress response in a rat model of post-traumatic stress disorder. Korean J Physiol Pharmacol. 2016;20(4):357–66.

66. Tyagi E, Agrawal R, Zhuang Y, Abad C, Waschek JA, Gomez-Pinilla F. Vulnerability imposed by diet and brain trauma for anxiety-like phenotype: implications for post-traumatic stress disorders. PLoS ONE. 2013;8(3):e57945.

67. Bollen E, Vanmierlo T, Akkerman S, Wouters C, Steinbusch HM, Prickaerts J. 7,8-Dihydroxyflavone improves memory consolidation processes in rats and mice. Behav Brain Res. 2013;257(1):8–12.

68. Saura CA, Valero J. The role of CREB signaling in Alzheimer's disease and other cognitive disorders. Rev Neurosci. 2011;22(2):153–69.

69. Pittenger C, Huang YY, Paletzki RF, Bourtchouladze R, Scanlin H, Vronskaya S, Kandel ER. Reversible inhibition of CREB/ATF transcription factors in region CA1 of the dorsal hippocampus disrupts hippocampus-dependent spatial memory. Neuron. 2002;34(3):447–62.

70. Vaynman S, Ying Z, Gomez-Pinilla F. Interplay between brain-derived neurotrophic factor and signal transduction modulators in the regulation of the effects of exercise on synaptic-plasticity. Neuroscience. 2003;122(3):647–57.

71. Tyler WJ, Alonso M, Bramham CR, Pozzo-miller LD. From acquisition to consolidation: on the role of brain-derived neurotrophic factor signaling in hippocampal-dependent learning. Learn Mem. 2002;9(5):224–37.

72. Rang OhS, Jin Kim S, Hyun Kim D, Hoon Ryu J, Ahn EM, Wook Jung J. *Angelica keiskei* ameliorates scopolamine-induced memory impairments in mice. Biol Pharm Bull. 2013;36(1):82–8.

73. Peng Z, Wang H, Zhang R, Chen Y, Xue F, Nie H, Chen Y, Wu D, Wang Y, Wang H, Tan Q. Gastrodin ameliorates anxiety-like behaviors and inhibits IL-1beta level and p38 MAPK phosphorylation of hippocampus in the rat model of posttraumatic stressdisorder. Physiol Res. 2013;62(5):537–45.

74. Wang Y, Cao X, Ma H, Tan W, Zhang L, Li Z, Gao Y. Prior stressor exposure delays the recovery of surgery-induced cognitive impairment and prolongs neuroinflammation in aged rats. Brain Res. 2016;1648(Pt A):380–6.

9

Involvement of Akt/CREB signaling pathways in the protective effect of EPA against interleukin-1β-induced cytotoxicity and BDNF down-regulation in cultured rat hippocampal neurons

YiLong Dong[1]*⬥, KangJing Pu[1], WenJing Duan[2], HuiCheng Chen[1], LiXing Chen[2] and YanMei Wang[2]*

Abstract

Background: Our published data have indicated that the omega-3 polyunsaturated fatty acid eicosapentaenoic acid (EPA) provides beneficial effects by attenuating neuronal damage induced by interleukin-1β (IL-1β), and up-regulation of the expression of brain-derived neurotrophic factor (BDNF) represents a crucial part in the neuroprotective effect of EPA. However, the mechanisms of how EPA regulates BDNF expression remains incompletely understood. The present study investigated the role of Akt/CREB signaling in the effect of EPA on BDNF expression and its neuroprotective effect.

Results: The present results showed that IL-1β reduced hippocampal neuronal viability and that EPA showed a concentration-dependent neuroprotective effect, but the neuroprotective effects of EPA were abolished by inhibition of Akt using KRX-0401, an inhibitor of Akt. Treatment of hippocampal neurons with EPA also ameliorated the decrease in Akt and CREB phosphorylation induced by IL-1β and BDNF down-regulation mediated by IL-1β. However, inhibition of Akt reversed the effect of EPA on levels of p-Akt, p-CREB, and BDNF.

Conclusions: Our data indicate that EPA elicited neuroprotection toward IL-1β-induced cell damage and BDNF decrease and that its effects potentially occurred via the Akt/CREB signaling pathway.

Keywords: Eicosapentaenoic acid, Brain-derived neurotrophic factor, Akt, Interleukin-1β

Background

Although the pathogenesis of neurodegenerative diseases, such as Alzheimer's disease (AD) and Parkinson's disease (PD), remains to be elucidated, neuroinflammation is considered one of the underlying factors of these disorders [1, 2]. Inflammation occurs in vulnerable brain regions of individuals with neurodegenerative disease, including the cortex, striatum and hippocampus, which is characterized by microglia activation and abnormally elevated levels of proinflammatory cytokines, such as interleukin-1β (IL-1β), IL-6 and tumor necrosis factor-alpha (TNF-α) [3]. The excessive proinflammatory factors may cause persistent neuronal damage through different signaling pathways, including suppression of brain-derived neurotrophic factor (BDNF) [4]. BDNF is a critical neurotrophin associated with neuronal survival, differentiation and synaptic plasticity [5]. Accumulating studies have demonstrated the link between low BDNF levels and increased neuronal injury during a neurodegenerative disorder [6, 7]. Therefore, BDNF-augmenting treatments shall be beneficial to rescue neurons from neurodegenerative disease.

*Correspondence: dongyilongmail@126.com; yaner6922@126.com
[1] School of Medicine, Yunnan University, 2 Cuihu Bei Road, Kunming 650091, Yunnan, People's Republic of China
[2] The First Affiliated Hospital of Kunming Medical University, 295 Xichang Road, Kunming 650031, Yunnan, People's Republic of China

Eicosapentaenoic acid (EPA) is an omega-3 polyunsaturated fatty acid that cannot be synthesized by the human body. Our main sources of EPA are cold-water fish. There is increasing scientific evidence from epidemiology and animal studies linking EPA intake with brain health, which demonstrated parallel alterations between diets high in EPA and reduced risk of neurodegenerative disease [8–12]. Previously, we have reported that EPA markedly attenuated the IL-1β-induced BDNF decrease in the hippocampus, which may provide beneficial effects against inflammation-associated neurodegenerative changes [13]. However, the mechanisms underlying how EPA modulates BDNF still remain unclear.

Previous studies have shown that cAMP-response element binding protein (CREB) acts as a transcription factor and is present in many types of neurons [14–16]. Importantly, CREB-binding sequences have been identified in the BDNF gene [17]. CREB may be located upstream of BDNF and may up-regulate the expression of BDNF [18]. Before it works, some protein kinases, such as protein kinase A (PKA), Akt (also known as protein kinase B) or mitogen-activated protein kinase 2, are required to phosphorylate CREB at serine-133 and convert CREB to its active form [19]. Recently, since research has suggested that EPA can modify the activity of several protein kinases, including Akt [20], we therefore hypothesized that EPA would protect neurons by rescuing low levels of BDNF from IL-1β toxicity by regulating the Akt/CREB signaling pathways. In the present study, using the IL-1β-induced neuronal degeneration model, we investigated the protective role of EPA against cellular toxicity and examined the potential involvement of the Akt/CREB pathway in EPA-mediated neuroprotection and BDNF regulation.

Methods

Materials

IL-1β was purchased from R&D Systems (Minneapolis, MN, USA). 3-(4,5-Dimethylthiazol-2-yl)-2,5-dimethyltetrazolium bromide (MTT), DNAase1 and 1-β-D-arabinofuranosylcytosine were obtained from Sigma-Aldrich (Saint Louis, MO, USA). Neurobasal medium, B27 supplement, trypsin and TRIzol were purchased from Invitrogen Corporation (Carlsbad, CA, USA). The protease inhibitor mixture, phosphatase inhibitor, BCA protein assay kit and enhanced chemiluminescence substrate kit were obtained from Pierce Biotechnology (Rockford, IL, USA). RIPA lysis buffer was purchased from Beyotime Biotechnology (Shanghai, China). Akt (catalog No. 9272), phospho-Akt (catalog No. 5012S, Ser473), CREB (catalog No. 4820) and phospho-CREB (catalog No. 9198, Ser133) antibody were purchased from Cell Signaling Technology (Danvers, MA,

USA). BDNF (catalog No. ab108319) and GAPDH (catalog No. ab37168) antibody were obtained from Abcam (Abcam, England). KRX-0401 (catalog No. S1037) was purchased from Selleck Chemicals LLC (Houston, TX, USA). An Ominiscript RT Kit and SYBR Green Kit were purchased from QIAGEN (Hilden, Germany). All other chemicals used were of the highest grade commercially available.

Cell culture

The primary hippocampal neurons were prepared as previously described with minor alterations [21]. Briefly, hippocampal tissues from Sprague–Dawley rats at embryonic day 18 were dissected in cold Ca^{2+} and Mg^{2+}-free Hank's balanced salt solution (HBSS), the tissues were mechanical dissociation using a Pasteur pipette after incubation with 0.25% trypsin and 50 µg/mL DNAase1 at 37 °C for 10 min. The cell suspensions were then transferred to a new tube, centrifuged at 1200 rpm for 3 min. The cell pellet was resuspended in serum-free neurobasal medium supplemented with 2% B27 supplement, 100 U/mL penicillin, and 100 µg/mL streptomycin, and then seeded on cell culture plates pre-coated with poly-L-lysine-coated. The cultures were grown in a humidified 5% CO_2 atmosphere at 37 °C. 1-β-D-arabinofuranosylcytosine was added to the neuronal cultures on day in vitro 3 (DIV 3) to a final concentration of 2 µM to reduce glial cells proliferate. All treatments were performed on DIV 7. The animals obtained from Weitong Lihua Experimental Animal Central (Beijing, China). Before to remove the fetuses, the pregnant rats were placed in a euthanasia chamber ($40 \times 18.5 \times 25$ cm, Rurui Science and Technology Instruments Co., Ltd, Guangzhou, China), and then filled with 100% CO_2 at a delivered rate of 0.2 L/s from a compressed gas cylinder for 3 min. Heart, breath, pupil and pain were detected to make sure the animal's death before dissection. All animal experimental procedures were approved by the Animal Care Committee of Yunnan University.

Experimental treatments

For the assessment of cell viability, cells were plated onto 96-well culture plates at 1×10^5 cells per well. For western blot and PCR assays, cells were plated onto 6-well culture plates at 1×10^6 cells per well. To investigate the toxicity effects of IL-1β, cells were treated at various times and with different concentrations of IL-1β, and cell viability was measured by MTT assay. To study the protective effects of EPA against IL-1β, the cells were pretreated with EPA for 40 min and then exposed to IL-1β for another 48 h. To determine whether or not the Akt/CREB signaling pathway was involved in the cell protection and BDNF regulation mediated by EPA, cells were pretreated with an Akt inhibitor (KRX-0401) for 30 min in conjunction with EPA and IL-1β. All experiments were performed using 3 separate cultures to confirm reproducibility.

MTT assay

Cell viability was assessed by the MTT assay at a designated time after the various treatments. MTT was added to the culture media at a final concentration of 0.5 mg/mL, after 4 h incubation at 37 °C, the supernatant was removed, and the MTT formazan crystals were dissolved with dimethyl sulfoxide (DMSO), the absorbance at 578 nm was read using a scanning multiwell plate reader (Tecan, Switzerland) after shaking the plates.

Western blot analysis

After the treatments, the cells were washed twice with cold phosphate-buffered saline (PBS) and harvested using cell scraper, and then lysed in RIPA buffer containing protease inhibitor mixture and phosphatase inhibitors on ice for 30 min. The protein concentrations were measured by BCA Protein Assay Kit. 30 μg of protein was separated by SDS polyacrylamide gel. Proteins were transferred to a PVDF membrane, incubated with fat-free milk for 2 h at room temperature for blocking nonspecific binding sites and further incubated overnight at 4 °C in fat-free milk containing the following primary antibodies: anti-Akt (1:1000), anti-phospho-Akt (1:1000), anti-CREB (1:2000), anti-phospho-CREB (1:1000), anti-BDNF (1:1000) and anti-GAPDH (1:5000). After washing, horseradish peroxidase (HRP)-conjugated secondary antibodies (1:5000) were applied to the membranes for 2 h at room temperature, immunostained bands were detected by enhanced chemiluminescence kit and quantified using Image-Pro Express 4.0 software (Media Cybernetics Inc. Rockville, MD, USA).

Real-time PCR

The total RNA will be extracted from cultured hippocampal neurons using TRIzol reagent, and the first stranded cDNA synthesized from 1 μg total RNA using the Ominiscript RT kit according to the manufacturer's instructions. Polymerase chain reactions was performed by the Corbett Life Science Rotor-Gene (Sydney, Australia) 6000 system,the PCR reaction solution contained 7.5 μL SYBR Green Mix, 0.5 μL each primer (10 μM), 1 μL cDNA and 5.5 μL RNase-free water. Cycling parameters were set at an initial 15 min step at 95 °C, followed by 45 cycles of 94 °C for 15 s, 59 °C for 30 s and 72 °C for 30 s. All reactions were performed in triplicate. Gene expression levels were normalized to the expression of reference gene (beta actin) with the ΔΔCt method [13]. The specific

primer pairs (Shanghai SangonBiotech, Shanghai, China) were as follows: BDNF: 5′-CAAAAGGCCAACTGAAGC -3′ (forward) and 5′-CGCCAGCCAATTCTCTTT-3′ (reverse); β-actin: 5′-GTCGTACCA CTGGCATTGTG-3′ (forward) and 5′-CTCTCAGCTGTGGTGGTGAA-3′ (reverse).

Statistical analysis

The data are presented as the mean ± SEM and statistical significance was evaluated by two-way analysis of variance (ANOVA) followed by the Bonferroni post hoc test using SPSS 18.0 software, with P values less than 0.05 considered to be statistically significant.

Results

Cell viability in IL-1β-incubated hippocampal neurons

To determine the toxicity induced by IL-1β, we exposed the cultured hippocampal neurons to IL-1β (0.1–30 ng/mL) for 48 h, and the cell viability was assessed by the MTT assay. At the low IL-1β level (0.1 and 0.3 ng/mL), cell viability increased slightly, but there was no statistical difference compared to control cells (Fig. 1a). From 1 to 30 ng/mL, IL-1β induced cell damage in a dose-dependent manner, but only high concentration (20 and 30 ng/mL) IL-1β induced significant cell damage (both $P < 0.01$ compared to control cells), and the 30 ng/mL IL-1β elicited worse cell damage, which shown cell viability decreased sharply close to 60% of the control level. We then examined the time-dependent effect of IL-1β on cell damage. Figure 1b shows that cell viability was significantly decreased after hippocampal neurons were exposed to IL-1β for 24 h. Although cell viability showed more decline while the cells were exposed to IL-1β for 72 h, there was no significant difference compared to the cells exposed to IL-1β for 48 h. Based on this result, 20 ng/mL IL-1β and 48 h exposure time were selected for the subsequent experiments.

EPA reversed IL-1β-induced cell damage, but the protective effect was blocked by inhibiting Akt

We then investigated the effects of EPA on IL-1β-induced cell damage. The MTT assay showed that pretreatment with EPA enhanced cell viability in a concentration-dependent manner (Fig. 2a). The pro-survival effect of EPA was observed at 10 μM ($P < 0.01$ compared to IL-1β treated cells). We next investigated if Akt signaling is involved in EPA's neuroprotective effect. Hippocampal neurons were pretreated with KRX-0401 (45 μM) to inhibit Akt [22] and then exposed to IL-1β in the presence or absence of EPA (10 μM). Figure 2b shows that IL-1β triggered a significant decrease in cell viability, whereas EPA significantly alleviated cytotoxicity

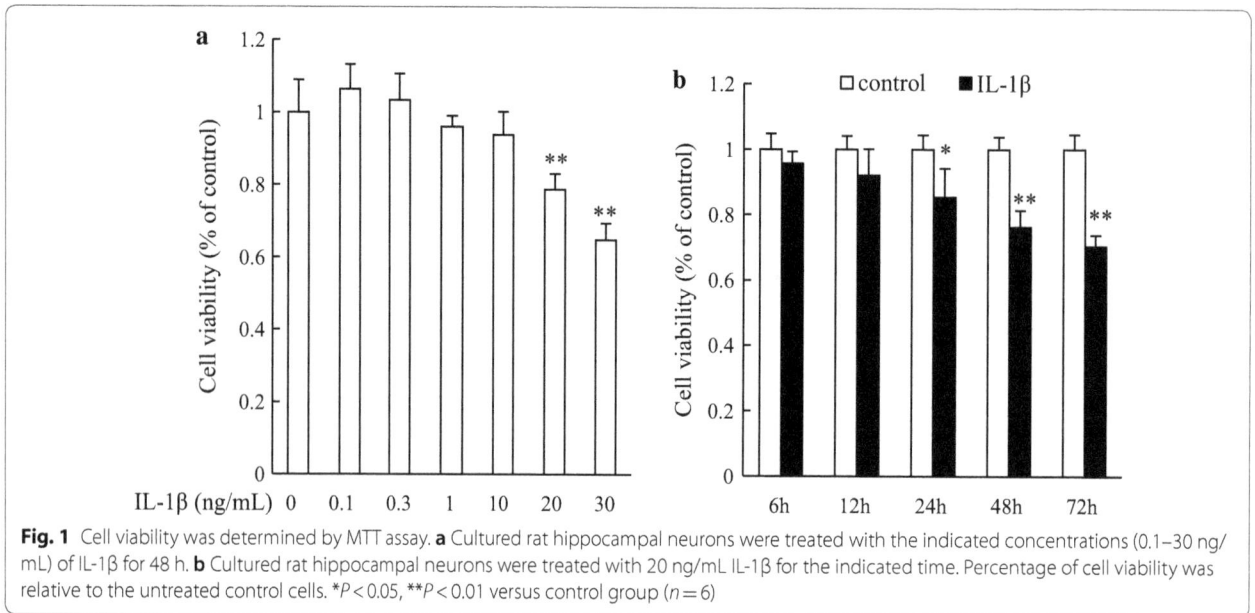

Fig. 1 Cell viability was determined by MTT assay. **a** Cultured rat hippocampal neurons were treated with the indicated concentrations (0.1–30 ng/mL) of IL-1β for 48 h. **b** Cultured rat hippocampal neurons were treated with 20 ng/mL IL-1β for the indicated time. Percentage of cell viability was relative to the untreated control cells. *$P < 0.05$, **$P < 0.01$ versus control group ($n = 6$)

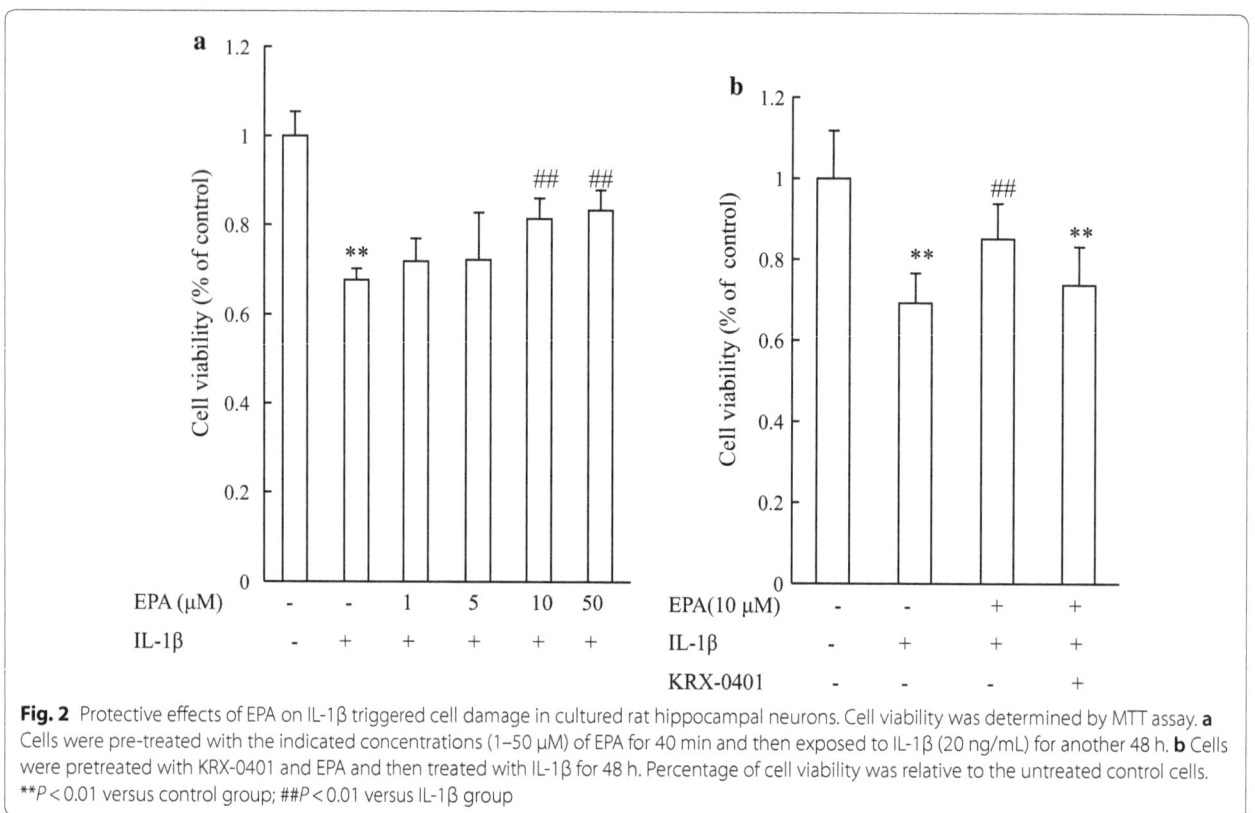

Fig. 2 Protective effects of EPA on IL-1β triggered cell damage in cultured rat hippocampal neurons. Cell viability was determined by MTT assay. **a** Cells were pre-treated with the indicated concentrations (1–50 μM) of EPA for 40 min and then exposed to IL-1β (20 ng/mL) for another 48 h. **b** Cells were pretreated with KRX-0401 and EPA and then treated with IL-1β for 48 h. Percentage of cell viability was relative to the untreated control cells. **$P < 0.01$ versus control group; ##$P < 0.01$ versus IL-1β group

mediated by IL-1β; however, the protective effect of EPA against IL-1β-induced cell damage was attenuated by KRX-0401, suggesting the involvement of the Akt pathways.

EPA rescued decline of Akt and CREB phosphorylation in IL-1β-treated hippocampal neurons, and this effect was blocked by Akt inhibitor

We assessed the role of the Akt/CREB pathway in the survival-promoting effect of EPA in hippocampal neurons.

As shown in Fig. 3, IL-1β inhibited the phosphorylation of Akt and CREB in hippocampal neurons, which was consistent with the finding that IL-1β decreased cell viability. While the cells were cultured with EPA, the inhibitory effect of IL-1β on protein phosphorylation was reversed, which was also consistent with the results that the effect of EPA against cell damage was induced by IL-1β. However, when the cells were pretreated with KRX-0401 and then treated with EPA and IL-1β, the improvement of EPA on Akt and CREB phosphorylation and cell viability was blocked, confirming that the neuroprotective effect is mediated by the Akt/CREB pathway.

EPA regulated BDNF levels via the Akt/CREB pathway

As shown in Fig. 4, IL-1β significantly down-regulated BDNF expression at both the mRNA and protein levels. The down-regulation of BDNF expression induced by IL-1β was also significantly attenuated by EPA. However, application of KRX-0401 inhibited the effects of EPA on BDNF expression, suggesting that EPA regulated BDNF expression in an Akt/CREB-dependent manner.

Discussion

The present results showed that IL-1β caused neurotoxicity in hippocampal neurons, and EPA attenuated cell damage and BDNF down-regulation in correlation with Akt/CREB pathway activation. This notion is supported by the following observations: (1) Treatment with IL-1β in cultured hippocampal neurons caused cell damage, while EPA significantly reversed the toxic effect of IL-1β; (2) Akt and CREB phosphorylation was inhibited by IL-1β, while EPA prevented this inhibition; (3) inhibition of Akt/CREB blocked the neuroprotective effect of EPA toward IL-1β-induced cell damage; (4) the beneficial effect of EPA on BDNF expression was blocked by inhibiting Akt/CREB signaling. The present study confirms that EPA acts as a neuroprotector in the hippocampus and that this is accompanied by improving phosphorylation of Akt and CREB to augment BDNF expression.

IL-1β is a pluripotent proinflammatory cytokine that may activate a host's defense system against infection and injury both in the peripheral immune system and in the central nervous system (CNS). Similar to Araujo and colleagues' study, which reported that IL-1β is neurotoxic only at high concentrations and after relatively long exposure [23], in the present study, we found that low IL-1β (0.1 and 0.3 ng/mL) promoted cell growth slightly instead of exacerbating neuron damage. The beneficial effect of IL-1β on cell viability maybe due to IL-1β functioning as a paracrine growth factor to promote cell proliferation [24]. Indeed, our previous data reported that acute IL-1β administration can up-regulate nerve growth

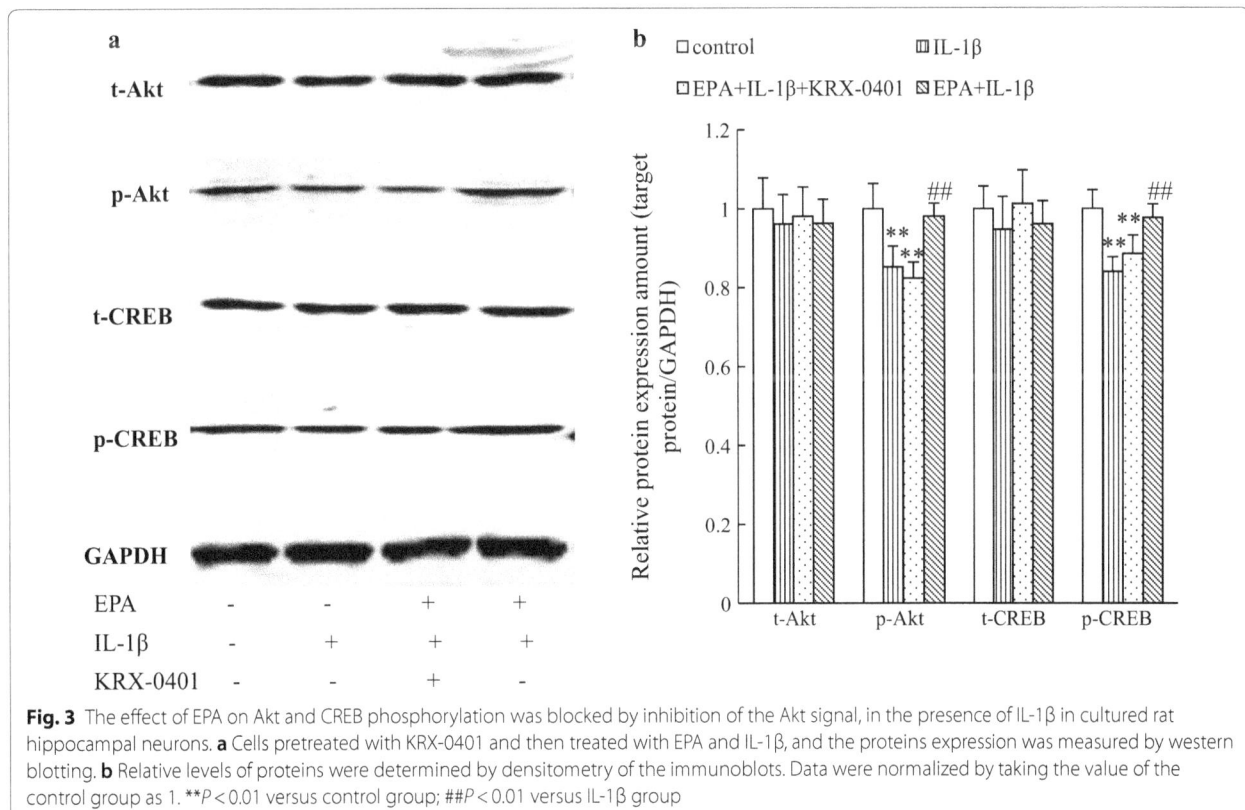

Fig. 3 The effect of EPA on Akt and CREB phosphorylation was blocked by inhibition of the Akt signal, in the presence of IL-1β in cultured rat hippocampal neurons. **a** Cells pretreated with KRX-0401 and then treated with EPA and IL-1β, and the proteins expression was measured by western blotting. **b** Relative levels of proteins were determined by densitometry of the immunoblots. Data were normalized by taking the value of the control group as 1. **P < 0.01 versus control group; ##P < 0.01 versus IL-1β group

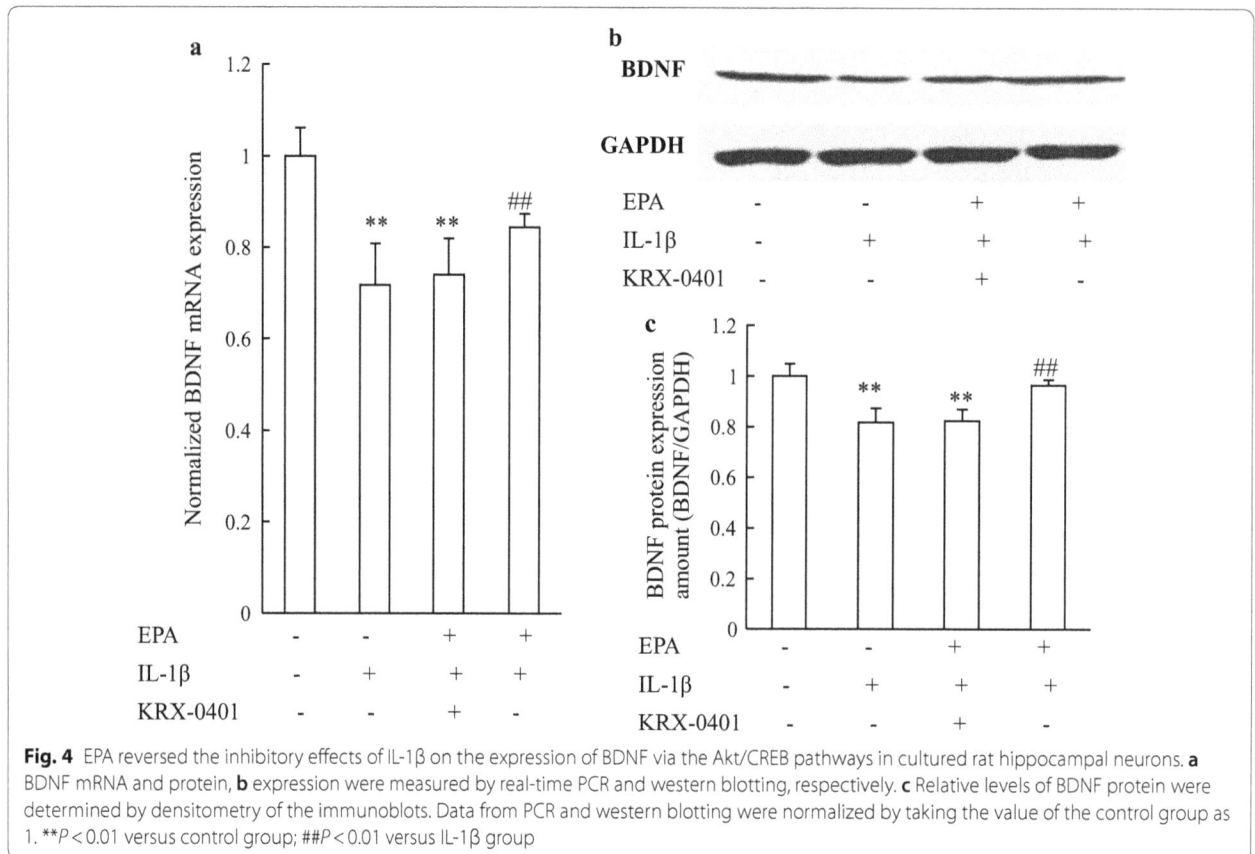

Fig. 4 EPA reversed the inhibitory effects of IL-1β on the expression of BDNF via the Akt/CREB pathways in cultured rat hippocampal neurons. **a** BDNF mRNA and protein, **b** expression were measured by real-time PCR and western blotting, respectively. **c** Relative levels of BDNF protein were determined by densitometry of the immunoblots. Data from PCR and western blotting were normalized by taking the value of the control group as 1. **$P < 0.01$ versus control group; ##$P < 0.01$ versus IL-1β group

factor (NGF) expression, the increase in NGF levels could contribute to improving neuronal vitality [25]. Taking our findings together, we speculated that physiologically, even a slight increase in IL-1β levels benefit neuron health and regulate the expression of neurotrophic factors that play a role in this effect. In particular, the interrelations between low IL-1β and neurotrophic factor should also be investigated in the future.

Under abnormal conditions, such as in neurodegenerative disease, microglia can be over-activated in the CNS, and the over-activation of microglia can produce excessive proinflammatory cytokines, especially IL-1β [26]. Elevated IL-1β could cause a state of chronic inflammation and evoke multiple signaling, such as NF-κB and MAPK pathways, leading to cell damage [27–29]. Thus, we are not surprised to find that cell viability decreased significantly in the neurons that received high IL-1β in this study. More importantly, when the cells were preincubated with EPA, the cell viability was improved. This finding supports that EPA is highly neuroprotective against IL-1β. It should be pointed out that IL-1β can affect signal transduction associated with BDNF. For instance, it is has been reported that IL-1β suppressed Akt activation, the upstream signaling pathway involved

in BDNF expression [30], it also demonstrated that IL-1β compromised phosphorylation of CREB, a transcription factor regulating BDNF expression [31], suggesting IL-1β places neurons at risk by interfering with BDNF signaling involving a Akt/CREB-associated mechanism. Our past work found EPA treatment restored BDNF decline induced by IL-1β administration rats provides a plausible explanation for the EPA's neuroprotective effects maybe BDNF dependent [13]. Furthermore, the present findings showed that the protective effect of EPA against IL-1β-induced cell damage was attenuated by KRX-0401, it should be surmised that Akt/CREB may be a candidate to contribute the BDNF regulation mediated by EPA.

Akt is a member of the AGC (cAMP-dependent, cGMP-dependent and protein kinase C) kinase family. Activation of Akt via phosphorylation involved in multiple physiological and pathological effects response by phosphorylate a variety downstream molecules including of CREB [32–35]. Reportedly, the decrease in Akt and CREB phosphorylation was associated with neuron loss in neurodegenerative disease animal models, whereas enhanced Akt/CREB activity in the brain produced a beneficial effect on inhibiting neuroinflammation and improving neuronal function [36]. Under our experimental conditions, IL-1β decreased the phosphorylation of Akt and CREB. This is consistent with the finding of Soiampornkul et al. [37], who observed that the phosphorylation of Akt and CREB has been inhibited in cortical neurons that received IL-1β. Additionally, in our study, EPA antagonized the decline in Akt and CREB phosphorylation induced by IL-1β. However, in the presence of an Akt inhibitor, the EPA-mediated increase in Akt and CREB phosphorylation was partially blocked, as well as the EPA-dependent protective effect on neurons. Collectively, our data indicated that EPA may neutralize neurotoxicity mediated by IL-1β via Akt/CREB phosphorylation.

As stated above, BDNF is a direct target of CREB, and phosphorylated CREB binds to the cAMP response element (CRE) sequence 5′-TGACGTCA-3′ in the BDNF promoter region, this binding may promote the transcription activity of BDNF and increase its expression [38]. Consistent with the changes in CREB, we found that IL-1β suppresses CREB phosphorylation accompanied by a low BDNF expression, while EPA acted against these alterations. The deficiency of BDNF is believed to be a cause of neurodegeneration, and the up-regulation of BDNF may reduce neuroinflammation and hippocampal damage [39, 40]. Therefore, with the elevation of BDNF, the present results indicated EPA exposure restored cell viability that was inhibited by IL-1β; however, the application of an Akt inhibitor is sufficient to attenuate the positive effect of EPA on BDNF expression. Thus, it can be suggested that the regulation of BDNF by EPA under neuroinflammatory conditions is mediated by the Akt/CREB signaling pathway.

Conclusions

Our findings extend previous data on the role of EPA in neuronal protection and show that EPA promoted the expression of BDNF, probably via activation of the Akt/CREB pathway. These results confirmed that EPA might constitute a promising alternative for the prevention of neuroinflammation-associated neurodegenerative diseases.

Abbreviations

AD: Alzheimer's disease Parkinson's disease (PD); AGC: cAMP-dependent, cGMP-dependent and protein kinase C; BDNF: brain-derived neurotrophic factor; CNS: central nervous system; CRE: cAMP response element; CREB: cAMP-response element binding protein; DMSO: dimethyl sulfoxide; EPA: eicosapentaenoic acid; IL-1β: interleukin-1β; MTT: methyl thiazolyl tetrazolium; NGF: nerve growth factor; PBS: phosphate-buffered saline; PD: Parkinson's disease; PKA: protein kinase A; NF-α: tumor necrosis factor-alpha.

Authors' contributions

This study is based on an original idea of YLD and YMW. YLD and YMW performed statistical analysis, drafted the manuscript, which was discussed and critically edited by all coauthors. KJP, WJD and HCC did the experiments including cell culture, MTT and western blot. KJP and LXC performed PCR assay. All authors read and approved the final manuscript.

Acknowledgements
Thanks are expressed to all co-investigators and laboratory technicians' assistants.

Competing interests
The authors declare that they have no competing interests.

Funding
This work was supported by grants from the National Nature Science Foundation of China (Nos. 81360179; 81560197) and the Science and Technology project of Yunnan Provincial Science and Technology Department (2016FB132; 2015FB118). The funders do not participate in the experimental research, or preparation the manuscript.

References

1. Alam Q, Alam MZ, Mushtaq G, Damanhouri GA, Rasool M, Kamal MA, Haque A. Inflammatory process in Alzheimer's and Parkinson's diseases: central role of cytokines. Curr Pharm Des. 2016;22(5):541–8.
2. Bolós M, Perea JR, Avila J. Alzheimer's disease as inflammatory disease. Biomol Concepts. 2017;8(1):37–43.
3. Kempuraj D, Thangavel R, Natteru PA, Selvakumar GP, Saeed D, Zahoor H, Zaheer S, Iyer SS, Zaheer A. Neuroinflammation induces neurodegeneration. J Neurol Neurosurg Spine. 2016;1(1):1003.
4. Carlos AJ, Tong L, Prieto GA, Cotman CW. IL-1β impairs retrograde flow of BDNF signaling by attenuating endosome trafficking. J Neuroinflammation. 2017;14(1):29.
5. Benarroch EE. Brain-derived neurotrophic factor: regulation, effects, and potential clinical relevance. Neurology. 2015;84(16):1693–704.
6. Braun DJ, Kalinin S, Feinstein DL. Conditional depletion of hippocampal brain-derived neurotrophic factor exacerbates neuropathology in a mouse model of Alzheimer's disease. ASN Neuro. 2017;9(2):1759091417696161.
7. Hernandez-Chan NG, Bannon MJ, Orozco-Barrios CE, Escobedo L, Zamudio S, De la Cruz F, et al. Neurotensin-polyplex-mediated brain-derived neurotrophic factor gene delivery into nigral dopamine neurons prevents nigrostriatal degeneration in a rat model of early Parkinson's disease. J Biomed Sci. 2015;22:59.
8. Hjorth E, Zhu M, Toro VC, Vedin I, Palmblad J, Cederholm T, et al. Omega-3 fatty acids enhance phagocytosis of Alzheimer's disease-related amyloid-β42 by human microglia and decrease inflammatory markers. J Alzheimers Dis. 2013;35(4):697–713.
9. Luchtman DW, Meng Q, Song C. Ethyl-eicosapentaenoate (E-EPA) attenuates motor impairments and inflammation in the MPTP-probenecid mouse model of Parkinson's disease. Behav Brain Res. 2012;226(2):386–96.
10. Robertsa RO, Cerhana JR, Geda YE, Knopman DS, Cha RH, Christianson TJ, et al. Polyunsaturated fatty acids and reduced odds of MCI: the mayo clinic study of aging. J Alzheimers Dis. 2010;21(3):853–65.
11. Solfrizzi V, D'Introno A, Colacicco AM, Capurso C, Del Parigi A, Capurso S, et al. Dietary fatty acids intake: possible role in cognitive decline and dementia. Exp Gerontol. 2005;40(4):257–70.
12. Solfrizzi V, Frisardi V, Capurso C, D'Introno A, Colacicco AM, Vendemiale G, et al. Dietary fatty acids in dementia and predementia syndromes: epidemiological evidence and possible underlying mechanisms. Ageing Res Rev. 2010;9(2):184–99.
13. Dong Y, Xu M, Kalueff AV, Song C. Dietary eicosapentaenoic acid normalizes hippocampal omega-3 and 6 polyunsaturated fatty acid profile, attenuates glial activation and regulates BDNF function in a rodent model of neuroinflammation induced by central interleukin-1β administration. Eur J Nutr. 2017;57:1751–91. https://doi.org/10.1007/s0039 4-017-1462-7.
14. Landeira BS, Santana TT, Araújo JA, Tabet EI, Tannous BA, Schroeder T, et al. Activity-independent effects of CREB on neuronal survival and differentiation during mouse cerebral cortex development. Cereb Cortex. 2018;28(2):538–48.

15. Gao HL, Xu H, Xin N, Zheng W, Chi ZH, Wang ZY. Disruption of the CaMKII/ CREB signaling is associated with zinc deficiency-induced learning and memory impairments. Neurotox Res. 2011;19(4):584–91.

16. Stern CM, Luoma JI, Meitzen J, Mermelstein PG. Corticotropin releasing factor-induced CREB activation in striatal neurons occurs via a novel Gβγ signaling pathway. PLoS ONE. 2011;6(3):e18114.

17. Yossifoff M, Kisliouk T, Meiri N. Dynamic changes in DNA methylation during thermal control establishment affect CREB binding to the brain-derived neurotrophic factor promoter. Eur J Neurosci. 2008;28(11):2267–77.

18. Palomer E, Carretero J, Benvegnù S, Dotti CG, Martin MG. Neuronal activity controls Bdnf expression via Polycomb de-repression and CREB/CBP/ JMJD3 activation in mature neurons. Nat Commun. 2016;7:11081.

19. Rosa E, Fahnestock M. CREB expression mediates amyloid β-induced basal BDNF downregulation. Neurobiol Aging. 2015;36(8):2406–13.

20. Marzuca-Nassr GN, Vitzel KF, De Sousa LG, Murata GM, Crisma AR, Junior CFR, et al. Effects of high EPA and high DHA fish oils on changes in signaling associated with protein metabolism induced by hindlimb suspension in rats. Physiol Rep. 2016;4(18):e12958.

21. Dong YL, Zuo PP, Li Q, Liu FH, Dai SL, Ge QS. Protective effects of phytoestrogen α-zearalanol on beta amyloid 25–35 induced oxidative damage in cultured rat hippocampal neurons. Endocrine. 2007;32(2):206–11.

22. Zeng B, Li Y, Niu B, Wang X, Cheng Y, Zhou Z, et al. Involvement of PI3 K/ Akt/FoxO3a and PKA/CREB signaling pathways in the protective effect of fluoxetine against corticosterone-induced cytotoxicity in PC12 cells. J Mol Neurosci. 2016;59(4):567–78.

23. Araujo DM, Cotman CW. Differential effects of interleukin-1β and interleukin-2 on glia and hippocampal neurons in culture. Int J Dev Neurosci. 1995;13(3–4):201–12.

24. Lonnemann G, Shapiro L, Engler-Blum G, Muller GA, KochK M, Dinarello CA. Cytokines in human renal interstitial fibrosis. I. Interleukin-1 is a paracrine growth factor for cultured fibrosis-derived kidney fibroblasts. Kidney Int. 1995;47(3):837–44.

25. Song C, Zhang Y, Dong Y. Acute and subacute IL-1β administrations differentially modulate neuroimmune and neurotrophic systems: possible implications for neuroprotection and neurodegeneration. J Neuroinflammation. 2013;10:59.

26. Ramirez AI, de Hoz R, Salobrar-Garcia E, Salazar JJ, Rojas B, Ajoy D, et al. The role of microglia in retinal neurodegeneration: Alzheimer's disease, Parkinson, and glaucoma. Front Aging Neurosci. 2017;9:214.

27. Swaroop S, Sengupta N, Suryawanshi AR, Adlakha YK, Basu A. HSP60 plays a regulatory role in IL-1β-induced microglial inflammation via TLR4-p38 MAPK axis. J Neuroinflammation. 2016;13:27.

28. Rossi S, Motta C, Studer V, Macchiarulo G, Volpe E, Barbieri F, et al. Interleukin-1β causes excitotoxic neurodegeneration and multiple sclerosis disease progression by activating the apoptotic protein p53. Mol Neurodegener. 2014;9:56.

29. Ji B, Guo W, Ma H, Xu B, Ma W, Zhang Z, et al. Isoliquiritigenin suppresses IL-1β induced apoptosis and inflammation in chondrocyte-like ATDC5 cells by inhibiting NF-κB and exerts chondroprotective effects on a mouse model of anterior cruciate ligament transection. Int J Mol Med. 2017;40(6):1709–18.

30. Tong L, Balazs R, Soiampornkul R, Thangnipon W, Cotman CW. Interleukin-1β impairs brain derived neurotrophic factor-induced signal transduction. Neurobiol Aging. 2008;29(9):1380–93.

31. Tong L, Prieto GA, Kramar EA, Smith ED, Cribbs DH, Lynch G, et al. Brain-derived neurotrophic factor-dependent synaptic plasticity is suppressed by interleukin-1β via p38 mitogen-activated protein kinase. J Neurosci. 2012;32(49):17714–24.

32. Hu M, Liu Z, Lv P, Wang H, Zhu Y, Qi Q, et al. Autophagy and Akt/ CREB signalling play an important role in the neuroprotective effect of nimodipine in a rat model of vascular dementia. Behav Brain Res. 2017;325(3):79–86.

33. Zhang L, Zhao H, Zhang X, Chen L, Zhao X, Bai X, et al. Nobiletin protects against cerebral ischemia via activating the p-Akt, p-CREB, BDNF and Bcl-2 pathway and ameliorating BBB permeability in rat. Brain Res Bull. 2013;96:45–53.

34. Simão F, Matté A, Pagnussat AS, Netto CA, Salbego CG. Resveratrol prevents CA1 neurons against ischemic injury by parallel modulation of both GSK-3β and CREB through PI3-K/Akt pathways. Eur J Neurosci. 2012;36(7):2899–905.

35. Brazil DP, Hemmings BA. Ten years of protein kinase B signaling: a hard Akt to follow. Trends Biochem Sci. 2001;26(11):657–64.

36. Braidy N, Essa MM, Poljak A, Selvaraju S, Al-Adawi S, Manivasagm T, et al. Consumption of pomegranates improves synaptic function in a transgenic mice model of Alzheimer's disease. Oncotarget. 2016;7(40):64589–604.

37. Soiampornkul R, Tong L, Thangnipon W, Balazs R, Cotman CW. Interleukin-1β interferes with signal transduction induced by neurotrophin-3 in corticalneurons. Brain Res. 2008;1188:189–97.

38. Suzuki A, Fukushima H, Mukawa T, Toyoda H, Wu LJ, Zhao MG, et al. Upregulation of CREB-mediated transcription enhances both short- and long-term memory. J Neurosci. 2011;31(24):8786–802.

39. Khallaf WAI, Messiha BAS, Abo-Youssef AMH, El-Sayed NS. Protective effects of telmisartan and tempol on lipopolysaccharide-induced cognitive impairment, neuroinflammation, and amyloidogenesis: possible role of brain-derived neurotrophic factor. Can J Physiol Pharmacol. 2017;95(7):850–60.

40. Xu D, Lian D, Wu J, Liu Y, Zhu M, Sun J, et al. Brain-derived neurotrophic factor reduces inflammation and hippocampal apoptosis in experimental Streptococcus pneumoniae meningitis. J Neuroinflammation. 2017;14(1):156.

10

Altered functional connectivity of the default mode network by glucose loading in young, healthy participants

Kenji Ishibashi[1]* , Keita Sakurai[2], Keigo Shimoji[2], Aya M. Tokumaru[2] and Kenji Ishii[1]

Abstract

Background: The functional connectivity of the default mode network (DMN) decreases in patients with Alzheimer's disease (AD) as well as in patients with type 2 diabetes mellitus (T2DM). Altered functional connectivity of the DMN is associated with cognitive impairment. T2DM is a known cause of cognitive dysfunction and dementia in the elderly, and studies have established that T2DM is a risk factor for AD. In addition, recent studies with positron emission tomography demonstrated that increased plasma glucose levels decrease neuronal activity, especially in the precuneus/posterior cingulate cortex (PC/PCC), which is the functional core of the DMN. These findings prompt the question of how increased plasma glucose levels decrease neuronal activity in the PC/PCC. Given the association among DMN, AD, and T2DM, we hypothesized that increased plasma glucose levels decrease the DMN functional connectivity, thus possibly reducing PC/PCC neuronal activity. We conducted this study to test this hypothesis.

Results: Twelve young, healthy participants without T2DM and insulin resistance were enrolled in this study. Each participant underwent resting-state functional magnetic resonance imaging in both fasting and glucose loading conditions to evaluate the DMN functional connectivity. The results showed that the DMN functional connectivity in the PC/PCC was significantly lower in the glucose loading condition than in the fasting condition ($P=0.014$).

Conclusions: Together with previous findings, the present results suggest that decreased functional connectivity of the DMN is possibly responsible for reduced PC/PCC neuronal activity in healthy individuals with increased plasma glucose levels.

Keywords: Resting-state functional MRI, Default mode network, Glucose, Precuneus, Posterior cingulate

Background

The default mode network (DMN), one of the resting-state brain networks, is characterized by hyperactivity when the brain is not engaged in specific behavioral tasks and low activity when the brain is focused on the external environment [1]. While performing various active tasks including novel, non-self-referential, and goal-directed tasks, the functional connectivity of the DMN consistently decreases [2, 3]. Although the mechanisms are not completely known, the DMN plays an important role in regulating complex cognition and behavior [4–6].

Its functional connectivity is impaired in patients with Alzheimer's disease (AD) [7], and impairment worsens with disease progression [8]. Furthermore, altered functional connectivity of the DMN is associated with cognitive decline [9, 10]. Interestingly, the DMN functional connectivity can also decrease in patients with type 2 diabetes mellitus (T2DM) [11–13]. Although T2DM, characterized by insulin resistance and increased plasma glucose levels, is intuitively far from AD pathophysiology, T2DM is reportedly associated with cognitive decline and is a risk factor for AD [14]. Although it is unclear why T2DM is a risk factor for AD, the shared vulnerability of the DMN in the two diseases may reveal a functional association between them.

*Correspondence: ishibashi@pet.tmig.or.jp
[1] Research Team for Neuroimaging, Tokyo Metropolitan Institute of Gerontology, 35-2 Sakae-cho, Itabashi-ku, Tokyo 173-0015, Japan
Full list of author information is available at the end of the article

The functional connectivity in resting-state brain networks is measured by detecting spontaneous fluctuations in the blood-oxygen-level-dependent (BOLD) signals with functional magnetic resonance imaging (fMRI) [15]. Positive BOLD signals are presumably caused by altered cerebral blood flow, an index of neuronal activity [16]. Therefore, the functional connectivity in resting-state brain networks may be associated with neuronal activity [17]. As one of the most fundamental resting-state brain networks, the DMN comprises a set of interconnected brain regions, such as the precuneus/posterior cingulate cortex (PC/PCC), medial prefrontal cortex (MPFC), and lateral parietotemporal cortex (LPTC), with the PC/PCC being the functional core of the DMN [4, 5]. In AD patients, functional connectivity of the DMN is impaired [7, 8]; glucose metabolism, another index of neuronal activity, is compromised primarily in the PC/PCC [18, 19]. Therefore, in AD patients, decreased functional connectivity of the DMN is possibly associated with reduced neuronal activity in the PC/PCC.

Resting-state glucose metabolism, measured by fluorine-18-labeled fluorodeoxyglucose (^{18}F-FDG) PET, is physiologically associated with neuronal activity [20]. Interestingly, recent studies using ^{18}F-FDG PET showed that neuronal activity in the PC/PCC significantly decreases with increased plasma glucose levels in young, healthy individuals [21] as well as in cognitively normal elderly individuals [22–24]. The reduction in PC/PCC neuronal activity has been shown to occur in cognitively normal individuals with plasma glucose levels between 100 and 110 mg/dL [25] as well as in individuals developing insulin resistance [26]. Reversibly increasing and decreasing plasma glucose levels decease and increase PC/PCC neuronal activity, respectively, in cognitively normal individuals with T2DM [27]. Cerebral blood flow can also decrease in the PC/PCC as plasma glucose levels increase [21]. More recently, we measured net glucose metabolism using ^{18}F-FDG PET with arterial blood sampling in young, healthy individuals under fasting and glucose loading conditions, and confirmed that glucose loading can reduce glucose metabolism (i.e., neuronal activity), especially in the PC/PCC [28]. These findings prompt the question of how increased plasma glucose levels decrease neuronal activity, especially in the PC/PCC.

Given the association among the DMN, AD, and T2DM, decreased functional connectivity of the DMN may be responsible for reduced neuronal activity in the PC/PCC. Therefore, we hypothesized that increased plasma glucose levels decrease the functional connectivity of the DMN even in healthy individuals without T2DM and insulin resistance, possibly thus reducing PC/PCC neuronal activity. To test this hypothesis, we used resting-state fMRI to compare the functional connectivity of the DMN in young, healthy participants under fasting and glucose loading conditions.

Methods

Research participants

The study was conducted in accordance with the tenets of the Declaration of Helsinki, and was approved by the Ethics Committee of the Tokyo Metropolitan Institute of Gerontology. After a detailed explanation of the study, each participant provided written informed consent. The study was composed of 12 young, healthy participants [six males and six females, age: 30.3 ± 4.6 years (mean ± SD), range: 24–36 years]. None of the participants had a history of T2DM, and all were certified to be healthy based on the results of physical and neurological examinations, medical interviews with a neurologist, and MRI findings.

Study protocol

Each participant visited the Tokyo Metropolitan Institute of Gerontology twice to undergo a resting-state fMRI under each of two different conditions: fasting and glucose loading. The order in which the participants presented for imaging under the two conditions was randomized. Half of the male and half of the female participants underwent the first and second resting-state fMRI sessions under fasting and glucose loading conditions, respectively. The other participants underwent the two resting-state fMRI sessions in the reverse order. The time interval between the two visits was less than 30 days. In the fasting condition, each participant visited the institute to undergo a resting-state fMRI after fasting overnight for at least 8 h. In the glucose loading condition, each participant visited the institute without having been under any dietary restriction, and was administered 75 g of glucose orally (TRELAN-G75; AY Pharma, Tokyo, Japan) approximately 30 min prior to the resting-state fMRI.

The plasma glucose levels, plasma insulin levels, and HbA1c values were measured after each resting-state fMRI, using ultraviolet absorption spectrophotometry, chemiluminescent enzyme immunoassay, and latex agglutination, respectively (SRL, Tokyo, Japan). The homeostasis model assessment of insulin resistance (HOMA-IR) was calculated as an index of insulin resistance using the following formula: HOMA-IR = (fasting glucose (mmol/L) × fasting insulin (μU/mL))/22.5.

Magnetic resonance data acquisition

Imaging data were acquired on a Discovery MR 750w 3.0-T scanner (GE Healthcare, Milwaukee, WI) at the Tokyo Metropolitan Institute of Gerontology.

High-resolution anatomical data were collected using an SPGR sequence (repetition time = 7.648 ms, echo time = 3.092 ms, flip angle = 11°, matrix size = 196 × 256 × 256, voxel size = 1.2 mm × 1.0547 mm × 1.0547 mm). Whole-brain resting-state fMRI data were collected using an echo planar imaging (EPI) sequence (repetition time = 2500 ms, echo time = 30 ms, flip angle = 73°, slice thickness = 4 mm, matrix size = 64 × 64 × 41, FOV = 192 mm × 192 mm). The participants were instructed to rest quietly with their eyes open and to avoid specific thoughts during the resting-state fMRI sessions. Subsequently, the procedure was manually reviewed to verify that all participants followed the instructions correctly.

Resting-state fMRI data processing and independent component analysis (ICA)

The resting-state fMRI data were processed using the FMRIB Software Library version 5.0.9 (FSL; Oxford, UK) [29–31]. The first 10 volumes (images) were discarded to avoid transient signal changes before magnetization reached a steady state and to allow the participants to become accustomed to the fMRI scanning noise [32]. Then, the following 120 volumes, equivalent to 5 min of resting-state fMRI, were realigned to compensate for motion. Each motion-corrected EPI image was registered to the corresponding high-resolution SPGR image, and transformed into the Montreal Neurological Institute space using a 12-parameter affine transformation and a nonlinear transformation. The data were skull-stripped and spatially smoothed using a 5-mm full width at a half maximum Gaussian kernel, and a high-pass temporal filter of 100 s was applied.

Probabilistic independent component analysis (ICA) was then performed to identify the functional anatomy of the DMN, and to create a DMN mask for the subsequent seed-based analysis. A multi-session temporal concatenation approach was applied to all echo planar imaging sequence images. This approach allowed for a single 2D ICA run on the concatenated data matrix to be obtained by stacking the 2D data matrices of every data set on top of each other (https://fsl.fmrib.ox.ac.uk/fsl/fslwiki/MELODIC). FSL Melodic was used to carry out inference on the estimated maps using a mixture model and an alternative hypothesis testing approach. A threshold level of 0.5 was applied to each mixture model probability map. This threshold level implies that a voxel "survives" thresholding as soon as the probability of being in the "active" class exceeds that of being in the "background noise" class, and assumes that the probability of false-negative and false-positive findings is equal [33, 34]. Of the 25 IC maps created by FSL Melodic, we identified one IC map representing the default mode network (Fig. 1).

Seed-based analysis and statistical analysis

The thresholded IC map, shown in Fig. 1, included the representative components of the DMN: the PC/PCC, the MPFC, and the LPTC. These components were

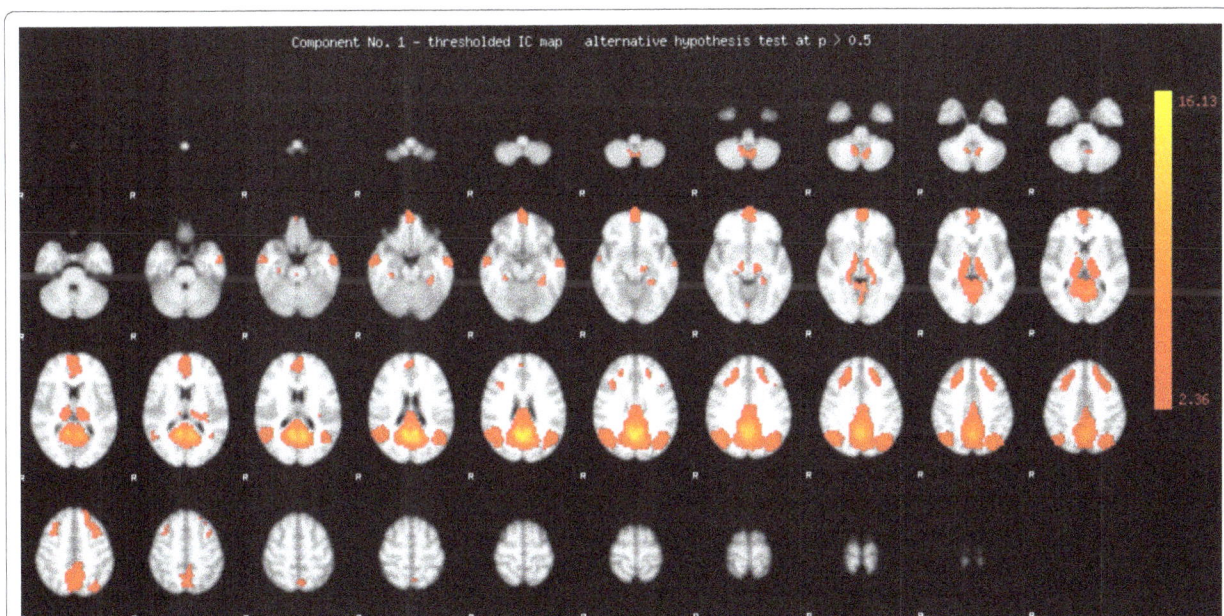

Fig. 1 Independent component map representing the default mode network. Independent component analysis was performed on all echo planar imaging sequence images using a multi-session temporal concatenation approach implemented in FSL Melodic. The mixture model probability map was transformed into a Z map. The red-yellow scale represents the magnitude of Z values ranging from 2.36 to 16.13

extracted from the IC map and used as a mask for the DMN (Fig. 2a). Using the mask for the DMN as a seed, the mean time series across all voxels within the seed was extracted from each EPI image. A first-level analysis was performed for each 4D EPI image. The extracted mean time series was set as a covariate. We added the following variables as nuisance regressors: mean signals of cerebrospinal fluid and white matter, and metrics of motion-related artifact created by FSL Mcflirt and Motion Outliers [35, 36]. A one-sample t test was then performed as a higher-level analysis for each of the two conditions to assess the within-group functional connectivity of the DMN, using FSL Feat (https://fsl.fmrib.ox.ac.uk/fsl/fslwiki/FEAT). Z statistic images were thresholded using clusters determined by $Z > 2.3$ and a corrected cluster significance of $P < 0.05$.

A between-group analysis was then performed to test the hypothesis that increased plasma glucose levels decrease the functional connectivity of the DMN. The central area of the PC/PCC was extracted from the IC map as shown in Fig. 1 and used as a mask for the PC/PCC (Fig. 2b). The mask was moved on each Z map that was created in the first-level analysis, as described above. The individual mean Z value within the mask was calculated, and used as the index of the magnitude of the functional connectivity of the DMN in the PC/PCC. To assess the effects of glucose loading on the functional connectivity of the DMN in the PC/PCC, Z values were compared between the fasting and glucose loading conditions using a one-tailed Wilcoxon signed-rank test. The null hypothesis was that the functional connectivity of the DMN in the glucose loading condition was not lower than in the fasting condition. Additionally, in order to assess whether any factors affected the changes in the functional connectivity of the DMN after glucose loading, a multiple regression analysis was

employed using the difference in Z values between the two conditions as a dependent factor and the order of conditions, gender, HOMA-IR, fasting plasma glucose and insulin levels, and HbA1c values as independent factors. Statistical significance was set at $P < 0.05$. All statistical analyses were conducted using SPSS Statistics version 22 (IBM, Armonk, NY).

Results

The demographic characteristics are presented in Table 1. After glucose loading, plasma glucose and insulin levels significantly increased (glucose: $Z = 2.158$, $P = 0.031$, insulin: $Z = 3.061$, $P = 0.002$, two-tailed Wilcoxon signed-rank test). All participants were confirmed to be free of T2DM and insulin resistance on the basis of HOMA-IR, fasting plasma glucose levels, and HbA1c values [37].

The results of the one-sample t tests ($Z > 2.3$, cluster-corrected $P < 0.05$) are shown in Fig. 3. The representative components of the DMN (PC/PCC, MPFC, and LPTC) were detected in the two conditions. The results of the between-group analysis of the magnitude of the DMN functional connectivity in the PC/PCC are shown in Fig. 4. The functional connectivity of the DMN in the PC/PCC was significantly lower in the glucose loading condition than in the fasting condition ($Z = 2.197$, $P = 0.014$, one-tailed Wilcoxon signed-rank test).

Multiple regression analyses revealed no significant factors that may have affected the changes in functional connectivity between the two conditions [$R^2 = 0.176$, $F(6, 5) = 0.178$, $P = 0.971$, order of conditions: $t = 0.380$, $P = 0.719$, gender: $t = 0.362$, $P = 0.732$, HOMA-IR: $t = 0.041$, $P = 0.969$, fasting plasma glucose: $t = 0.310$, $P = 0.769$, fasting plasma insulin: $t = 0.038$, $P = 0.971$, HbA1c: $t = 0.721$, $P = 0.503$].

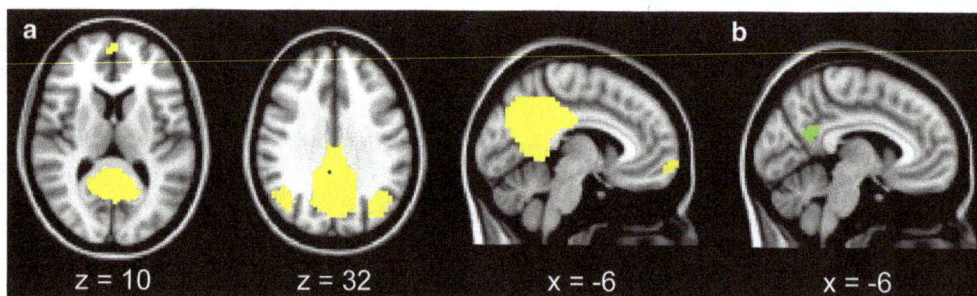

Fig. 2 Masks for the representative components of the DMN (**a**) and PC/PCC (**b**) in the Montreal Neurological Institute space. The representative components of the DMN were extracted from the IC map shown in Fig. 1, and used as a mask for the DMN (**a** yellow). The voxels with the highest statistical values were extracted from the IC map shown in Fig. 1, and used as a mask for the PC/PCC (**b** green). The mask volume for the PC/PCC was 2360 mm³. *DMN* default mode network, *IC* independent component, *PC/PCC* precuneus/posterior cingulate cortex

Table 1 Demographic and clinical characteristics

Subject	Age	Sex	HbA1c (%)	Fasting			Glucose loading	
				Glucose (mg/dL)	Insulin (μU/mL)	HOMA-IR	Glucose (mg/dL)	Insulin (μU/mL)
1	34	M	5.2	94	2.7	0.62	126	37.8
2	34	M	5.8	80	6.5	1.28	164	32.2
3	27	M	5.5	84	0.8	0.16	85	4.8
4	32	F	4.7	90	4.4	0.98	96	18.1
5	30	F	5.1	82	3.4	0.69	100	27.8
6	36	F	5.2	87	2.7	0.58	117	33.4
7	23	M	5.4	91	2.4	0.53	115	18.7
8	26	F	4.9	94	4.2	0.98	84	8.0
9	37	F	5.1	87	1.8	0.40	186	87.4
10	32	M	5.1	90	3.4	0.75	123	29.1
11	24	M	4.9	89	1.9	0.42	83	29.0
12	29	F	5.3	82	4.3	0.88	75	26.5
Mean			5.2	87.5	3.2	0.69	112.8	29.4

HOMA-IR homeostasis model assessment of insulin resistance

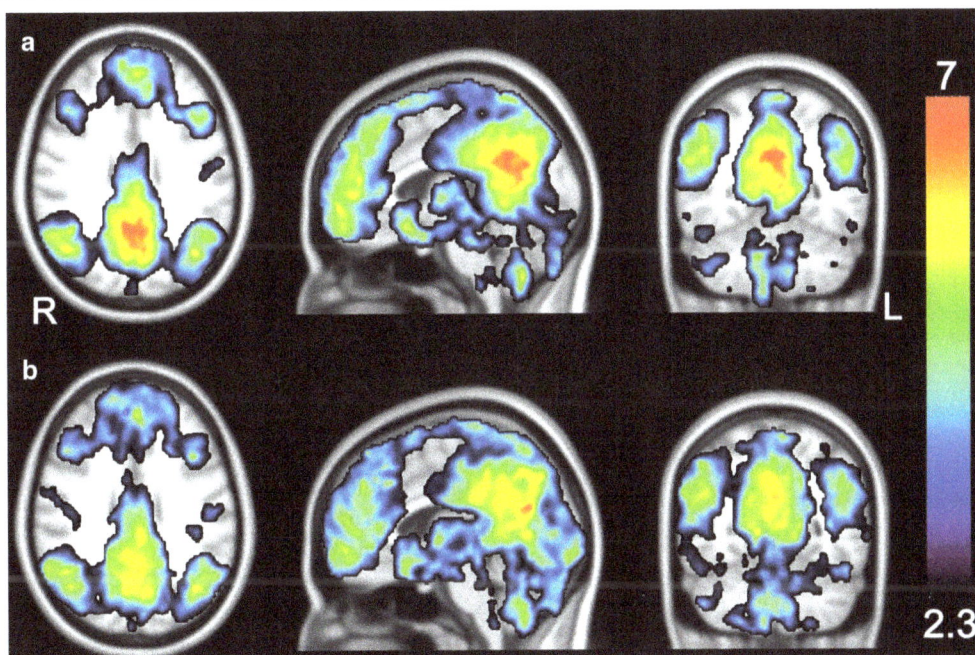

Fig. 3 Within-group functional connectivity of the DMN using a one-sample *t* test. A seed was placed on the representative components of the DMN as shown in Fig. 2a. The magnitude of the DMN functional connectivity is displayed in the fasting condition (**a**) and glucose loading condition (**b**). The threshold was set at $Z > 2.3$ and cluster-corrected $P < 0.05$. The rainbow scale represents the magnitude of the Z values. *R* right, *L* left, *DMN* default mode network

Discussion

The primary objective of this study was to investigate the effects of glucose loading on the functional connectivity of the DMN in young, healthy subjects free of T2DM and insulin resistance, using resting-state fMRI. The functional connectivity of the DMN is known to decrease in patients with T2DM, characterized by insulin resistance and increased plasma glucose levels [11–13]. To the best of our knowledge, this is the first study showing that after glucose loading, the functional connectivity of

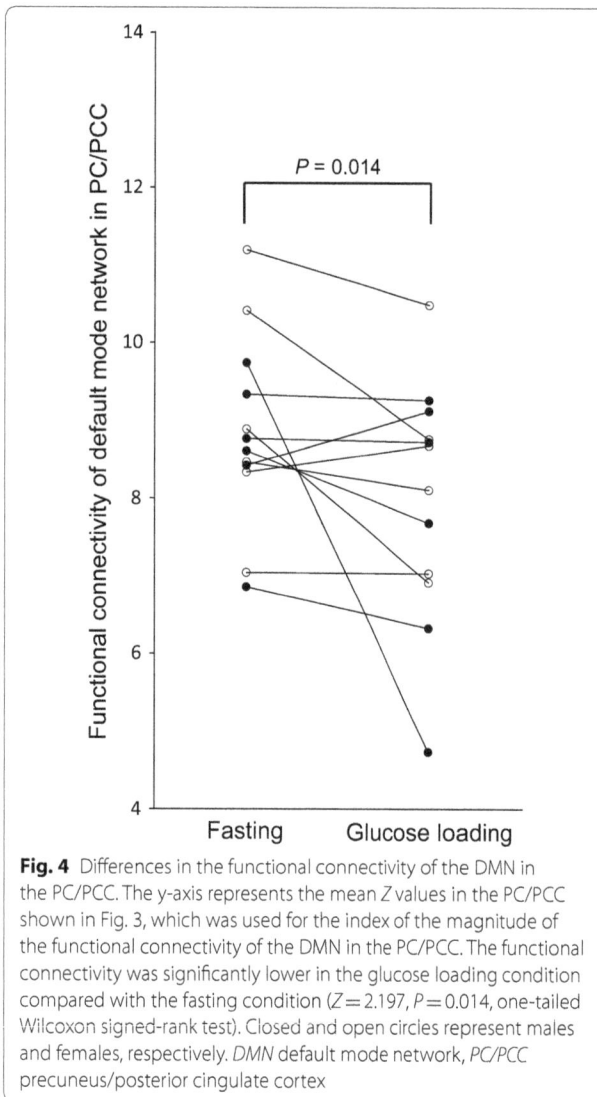

Fig. 4 Differences in the functional connectivity of the DMN in the PC/PCC. The y-axis represents the mean Z values in the PC/PCC shown in Fig. 3, which was used for the index of the magnitude of the functional connectivity of the DMN in the PC/PCC. The functional connectivity was significantly lower in the glucose loading condition compared with the fasting condition ($Z = 2.197$, $P = 0.014$, one-tailed Wilcoxon signed-rank test). Closed and open circles represent males and females, respectively. *DMN* default mode network, *PC/PCC* precuneus/posterior cingulate cortex

the DMN is decreased even in healthy individuals without T2DM and insulin resistance. Zhang and colleagues recently evaluated the acute effects of insulin administration on the resting-state brain network in patients with T2DM, and showed that insulin administration increased the functional connectivity between the hippocampus and the DMN [38]. Because insulin administration induces a reduction in plasma glucose levels, their findings could be restated as showing that a decrease in plasma glucose levels increases the functional connectivity of the DMN. Thus, their findings from patients with T2DM are consistent with our results. However, because the number of participants was relatively small in the present study, our results require further validation in a future study with a large number of participants.

One of the concerns of this study is a lack of understanding as to what the reduction in the functional

connectivity of the DMN by glucose loading physiologically reflects. There are several studies using ^{18}F-FDG PET, reporting that increased plasma glucose levels decrease glucose metabolism (i.e., neuronal activity), especially in the PC/PCC [24, 28]. In a dynamic ^{18}F-FDG PET study with arterial blood sampling, which directly measured net glucose metabolism, glucose loading decreased glucose metabolism in DMN-related regions, especially in the PC/PCC, in young, healthy individuals free of T2DM and insulin resistance [28]. Considering these findings, reduced functional connectivity of the DMN by glucose loading is possibly responsible for reduced neuronal activity in DMN-related regions, especially in the PC/PCC.

Interestingly, plasma glucose levels in the prediabetes range of 100–126 mg/dL [39] are associated with cognitive decline, as measured using a battery of neuropsychological tests [40–42]. There is an inverse association between plasma glucose levels and Mini Mental State Examination scores in individuals at high risk for cardiovascular disease [43]. In a sample of non-T2DM elderly subjects, individuals with higher plasma glucose levels tended to have lower Mini Mental State Examination scores [40]. A longitudinal study with a median follow-up of 6.8 years showed that higher glucose levels might be related to an increased risk for dementia, even among individuals without T2DM [44]. Although it remains unclear as to why mildly increased plasma glucose levels induce cognitive decline, the phenomenon may be speculated as follows: increased plasma glucose levels reduce the functional connectivity of the DMN as well as neuronal activity in its components, particularly the PC/PCC, which is a central core for regulating complex cognition and behavior [45, 46]. As a result, subclinical cognitive decline may occur even in individuals without T2DM. This speculation may be important to explain the functional link between T2DM and AD, although future studies are needed to elucidate this hypothesis.

In summary, glucose loading can reduce the DMN functional connectivity and PC/PCC neuronal activity in healthy participants. Although the mechanism underlying this phenomenon is unclear, cholinergic and glutamatergic neurotransmitter systems may play an important role in modulating the functional connectivity of the DMN and neuronal activity in the PC/PCC. This is because both the DMN and PC/PCC are anatomically crucial in regulating complex cognition and behavior [4–6, 45, 46], and cholinergic and glutamatergic systems are associated with cognitive function [47]. Moreover, cholinergic enhancement is reported to increase neuronal activity in the PC/PCC [48]. Hence, glucose loading may modulate these neurotransmitter systems, possibly reducing the functional connectivity of the DMN and neuronal activity in the PC/PCC. However, further investigation is needed to elucidate this speculation.

Conclusions

The present study showed that glucose loading reduces the functional connectivity of the DMN in the PC/PCC in young, healthy participants free of T2DM and insulin resistance. Taken together with the previous knowledge that glucose loading decreases neuronal activity in the PC/PCC, the present results suggest that decreased functional connectivity of the DMN is possibly responsible for reduced PC/PCC neuronal activity in healthy individuals with increased plasma glucose levels.

Abbreviations

DMN: default mode network; AD: Alzheimer's disease; T2DM: type 2 diabetes mellitus; PC/PCC: precuneus/posterior cingulate cortex; MPFC: medial prefrontal cortex; LPTC: lateral parietotemporal cortex; ^{18}F-FDG: fluorine-18-labeled fluorodeoxyglucose; PET: positron emission tomography; fMRI: functional magnetic resonance imaging; HOMA-IR: homeostasis model assessment of insulin resistance.

Author's contributions

KI and KI designed the study. KI, KS, KS, AMT, and KI obtained the data. KI carried out the data processing. KI, KS, KS, AMT, and KI interpreted the data. All authors were involved in drafting and revising the manuscript. All authors agreed to be accountable for all aspects of the work in ensuring that questions related to the accuracy or integrity of any part of the work are appropriately investigated and resolved. All authors read and approved the final manuscript.

Author details

[1] Research Team for Neuroimaging, Tokyo Metropolitan Institute of Gerontology, 35-2 Sakae-cho, Itabashi-ku, Tokyo 173-0015, Japan. [2] Department of Diagnostic Radiology, Tokyo Metropolitan Geriatric Hospital, 35-2 Sakae-cho, Itabashi-ku, Tokyo 173-0015, Japan.

Acknowledgements

The authors thank Dr. Dara Ghahremani at the Laboratory of Molecular Neuroimaging, UCLA for the advice and support on analyzing the resting-state fMRI data, and the people of Research Team for Neuroimaging at the Tokyo Metropolitan Institute of Gerontology and Department of Diagnostic Radiology at the Tokyo Metropolitan Geriatric Hospital for the technical assistance.

Competing interests

The authors declare that they have no competing interests.

Funding

This work was supported by Translational Research Grants 2016 of Tokyo Metropolitan Institute of Gerontology (to Kenji Ishibashi).

References

1. Anticevic A, Cole MW, Murray JD, Corlett PR, Wang XJ, Krystal JH. The role of default network deactivation in cognition and disease. Trends Cogn Sci. 2012;16(12):584–92.
2. Shulman GL, Corbetta M, Fiez JA, Buckner RL, Miezin FM, Raichle ME, Petersen SE. Searching for activations that generalize over tasks. Hum Brain Mapp. 1997;5(4):317–22.
3. Raichle ME. The brain's default mode network. Annu Rev Neurosci. 2015;38:433–47.
4. Fransson P, Marrelec G. The precuneus/posterior cingulate cortex plays a pivotal role in the default mode network: evidence from a partial correlation network analysis. NeuroImage. 2008;42(3):1178–84.
5. Utevsky AV, Smith DV, Huettel SA. Precuneus is a functional core of the default-mode network. J Neurosci. 2014;34(3):932–40.
6. Raichle ME, MacLeod AM, Snyder AZ, Powers WJ, Gusnard DA, Shulman GL. A default mode of brain function. Proc Natl Acad Sci USA. 2001;98(2):676–82.
7. Sperling RA, Laviolette PS, O'Keefe K, O'Brien J, Rentz DM, Pihlajamaki M, Marshall G, Hyman BT, Selkoe DJ, Hedden T, et al. Amyloid deposition is associated with impaired default network function in older persons without dementia. Neuron. 2009;63(2):178–88.
8. Zhu DC, Majumdar S, Korolev IO, Berger KL, Bozoki AC. Alzheimer's disease and amnestic mild cognitive impairment weaken connections within the default-mode network: a multi-modal imaging study. J Alzheimer's Dis. 2013;34(4):969–84.
9. Wang L, Brier MR, Snyder AZ, Thomas JB, Fagan AM, Xiong C, Benzinger TL, Holtzman DM, Morris JC, Ances BM. Cerebrospinal fluid Abeta42, phosphorylated Tau181, and resting-state functional connectivity. JAMA Neurol. 2013;70(10):1242–8.
10. Sheline YI, Raichle ME. Resting state functional connectivity in preclinical Alzheimer's disease. Biol Psychiatry. 2013;74(5):340–7.
11. Musen G, Jacobson AM, Bolo NR, Simonson DC, Shenton ME, McCartney RL, Flores VL, Hoogenboom WS. Resting-state brain functional connectivity is altered in type 2 diabetes. Diabetes. 2012;61(9):2375–9.
12. Zhou H, Lu W, Shi Y, Bai F, Chang J, Yuan Y, Teng G, Zhang Z. Impairments in cognition and resting-state connectivity of the hippocampus in elderly subjects with type 2 diabetes. Neurosci Lett. 2010;473(1):5–10.
13. Chen YC, Jiao Y, Cui Y, Shang SA, Ding J, Feng Y, Song W, Ju SH, Teng GJ. Aberrant brain functional connectivity related to insulin resistance in type 2 diabetes: a resting-state fMRI study. Diabetes Care. 2014;37(6):1689–96.
14. Ohara T, Doi Y, Ninomiya T, Hirakawa Y, Hata J, Iwaki T, Kanba S, Kiyohara Y. Glucose tolerance status and risk of dementia in the community: the Hisayama study. Neurology. 2011;77(12):1126–34.
15. Rosazza C, Minati L. Resting-state brain networks: literature review and clinical applications. Neurol Sci. 2011;32(5):773–85.
16. Heeger DJ, Ress D. What does fMRI tell us about neuronal activity? Nat Rev Neurosci. 2002;3(2):142–51.
17. Aiello M, Salvatore E, Cachia A, Pappata S, Cavaliere C, Prinster A, Nicolai E, Salvatore M, Baron JC, Quarantelli M. Relationship between simultaneously acquired resting-state regional cerebral glucose metabolism and functional MRI: a PET/MR hybrid scanner study. NeuroImage. 2015;113:111–21.
18. Friedland RP, Budinger TF, Ganz E, Yano Y, Mathis CA, Koss B, Ober BA, Huesman RH, Derenzo SE. Regional cerebral metabolic alterations in dementia of the Alzheimer type: positron emission tomography with [18F]fluorodeoxyglucose. J Comput Assist Tomogr. 1983;7(4):590–8.
19. Langbaum JB, Chen K, Lee W, Reschke C, Bandy D, Fleisher AS, Alexander GE, Foster NL, Weiner MW, Koeppe RA, et al. Categorical and correlational analyses of baseline fluorodeoxyglucose positron emission tomography images from the Alzheimer's Disease Neuroimaging Initiative (ADNI). NeuroImage. 2009;45(4):1107–16.
20. Phelps ME, Huang SC, Hoffman EJ, Selin C, Sokoloff L, Kuhl DE. Tomographic measurement of local cerebral glucose metabolic rate in humans with (F-18)2-fluoro-2-deoxy-D-glucose: validation of method. Ann Neurol. 1979;6(5):371–88.
21. Ishibashi K, Kawasaki K, Ishiwata K, Ishii K. Reduced uptake of ^{18}F-FDG and ^{15}O-H$_2$O in Alzheimer's disease-related regions after glucose loading. J Cereb Blood Flow Metab. 2015;35(8):1380–5.
22. Kawasaki K, Ishii K, Saito Y, Oda K, Kimura Y, Ishiwata K. Influence of mild hyperglycemia on cerebral FDG distribution patterns calculated by statistical parametric mapping. Ann Nucl Med. 2008;22(3):191–200.

23. Burns CM, Chen K, Kaszniak AW, Lee W, Alexander GE, Bandy D, Fleisher AS, Caselli RJ, Reiman EM. Higher serum glucose levels are associated with cerebral hypometabolism in Alzheimer regions. Neurology. 2013;80(17):1557–64.

24. Ishibashi K, Onishi A, Fujiwara Y, Ishiwata K, Ishii K. Effects of glucose, insulin, and insulin resistance on cerebral ^{18}F-FDG distribution in cognitively normal older subjects. PLoS ONE. 2017;12(7):e0181400.

25. Ishibashi K, Onishi A, Fujiwara Y, Ishiwata K, Ishii K. Relationship between Alzheimer disease-like pattern of ^{18}F-FDG and fasting plasma glucose levels in cognitively normal volunteers. J Nucl Med. 2015;56(2):229–33.

26. Baker LD, Cross DJ, Minoshima S, Belongia D, Watson GS, Craft S. Insulin resistance and Alzheimer-like reductions in regional cerebral glucose metabolism for cognitively normal adults with prediabetes or early type 2 diabetes. Arch Neurol. 2011;68(1):51–7.

27. Ishibashi K, Onishi A, Fujiwara Y, Ishiwata K, Ishii K. Plasma glucose levels affect cerebral ^{18}F-FDG distribution in cognitively normal subjects with diabetes. Clin Nucl Med. 2016;41(6):e274–80.

28. Ishibashi K, Wagatsuma K, Ishiwata K, Ishii K. Alteration of the regional cerebral glucose metabolism in healthy subjects by glucose loading. Hum Brain Mapp. 2016;37(8):2823–32.

29. Jenkinson M, Beckmann CF, Behrens TE, Woolrich MW, Smith SM. FSL. NeuroImage. 2012;62(2):782–90.

30. Smith SM, Jenkinson M, Woolrich MW, Beckmann CF, Behrens TE, Johansen-Berg H, Bannister PR, De Luca M, Drobnjak I, Flitney DE, et al. Advances in functional and structural MR image analysis and implementation as FSL. NeuroImage. 2004;23(Suppl 1):S208–19.

31. Woolrich MW, Jbabdi S, Patenaude B, Chappell M, Makni S, Behrens T, Beckmann C, Jenkinson M, Smith SM. Bayesian analysis of neuroimaging data in FSL. NeuroImage. 2009;45(1 Suppl):S173–86.

32. Lv XF, Qiu YW, Tian JZ, Xie CM, Han LJ, Su HH, Liu ZY, Peng JP, Lin CL, Wu MS, et al. Abnormal regional homogeneity of resting-state brain activity in patients with HBV-related cirrhosis without overt hepatic encephalopathy. Liver Int. 2013;33(3):375–83.

33. Beckmann CF, DeLuca M, Devlin JT, Smith SM. Investigations into resting-state connectivity using independent component analysis. Philos Trans R Soc Lond B Biol Sci. 2005;360(1457):1001–13.

34. Tuovinen T, Rytty R, Moilanen V, Abou Elseoud A, Veijola J, Remes AM, Kiviniemi VJ. The effect of gray matter ICA and coefficient of variation mapping of BOLD data on the detection of functional connectivity changes in Alzheimer's disease and bvFTD. Front Hum Neurosci. 2016;10:680.

35. Power JD, Barnes KA, Snyder AZ, Schlaggar BL, Petersen SE. Spurious but systematic correlations in functional connectivity MRI networks arise from subject motion. NeuroImage. 2012;59(3):2142–54.

36. Kohno M, Okita K, Morales AM, Robertson CL, Dean AC, Ghahremani DG, Sabb FW, Rawson RA, Mandelkern MA, Bilder RM, et al. Midbrain functional connectivity and ventral striatal dopamine D2-type receptors: link to impulsivity in methamphetamine users. Mol Psychiatry. 2016;21(11):1554–60.

37. Keskin M, Kurtoglu S, Kendirci M, Atabek ME, Yazici C. Homeostasis model assessment is more reliable than the fasting glucose/insulin ratio and quantitative insulin sensitivity check index for assessing insulin resistance among obese children and adolescents. Pediatrics. 2005;115(4):e500–3.

38. Zhang H, Hao Y, Manor B, Novak P, Milberg W, Zhang J, Fang J, Novak V. Intranasal insulin enhanced resting-state functional connectivity of hippocampal regions in type 2 diabetes. Diabetes. 2015;64(3):1025–34.

39. American Diabetes A. 2. Classification and diagnosis of diabetes. Diabetes Care. 2017;40(Suppl 1):S11–24.

40. Di Bonito P, Di Fraia L, Di Gennaro L, Vitale A, Lapenta M, Scala A, Iardino MR, Cusati B, Attino L, Capaldo B. Impact of impaired fasting glucose and other metabolic factors on cognitive function in elderly people. Nutr Metab Cardiovasc Dis. 2007;17(3):203–8.

41. Yaffe K, Blackwell T, Kanaya AM, Davidowitz N, Barrett-Connor E, Krueger K. Diabetes, impaired fasting glucose, and development of cognitive impairment in older women. Neurology. 2004;63(4):658–63.

42. Cukierman-Yaffe T, Gerstein HC, Anderson C, Zhao F, Sleight P, Hilbrich L, Jackson SH, Yusuf S, Teo K, Investigators OT. Glucose intolerance and diabetes as risk factors for cognitive impairment in people at high cardiovascular risk: results from the ONTARGET/TRANSCEND research programme. Diabetes Res Clin Pract. 2009;83(3):387–93.

43. Cukierman-Yaffe T. Diabetes, dysglycemia and cognitive dysfunction. Diabetes Metab Res Rev. 2014;30(5):341–5.

44. Crane PK, Walker R, Hubbard RA, Li G, Nathan DM, Zheng H, Haneuse S, Craft S, Montine TJ, Kahn SE, et al. Glucose levels and risk of dementia. N Engl J Med. 2013;369(6):540–8.

45. Cavanna AE, Trimble MR. The precuneus: a review of its functional anatomy and behavioural correlates. Brain. 2006;129(Pt 3):564–83.

46. Leech R, Sharp DJ. The role of the posterior cingulate cortex in cognition and disease. Brain. 2014;137(Pt 1):12–32.

47. Francis PT, Parsons CG, Jones RW. Rationale for combining glutamatergic and cholinergic approaches in the symptomatic treatment of Alzheimer's disease. Expert Rev Neurother. 2012;12(11):1351–65.

48. Iizuka T, Kameyama M. Cholinergic enhancement increases regional cerebral blood flow to the posterior cingulate cortex in mild Alzheimer's disease. Geriatr Gerontol Int. 2017;17(6):951–8.

11

Impact of brain arousal and time-on-task on autonomic nervous system activity in the wake-sleep transition

Jue Huang[1][*][†] [iD], Christine Ulke[1,2][†], Christian Sander[1,2], Philippe Jawinski[1,2], Janek Spada[1,2], Ulrich Hegerl[1,2] and Tilman Hensch[1]

Abstract

Background: Autonomic nervous system (ANS) activity has been shown to vary with the state of brain arousal. In a previous study, this association of ANS activity with distinct states of brain arousal was demonstrated using 15-min EEG data, but without directly controlling for possible time-on-task effects. In the current study we examine ANS-activity in fine-graded EEG-vigilance stages (indicating states of brain arousal) during two conditions of a 2-h oddball task while controlling for time-on-task. In addition, we analyze the effect of time-on-task on ANS-activity while holding the level of brain arousal constant.

Methods: Heart rate and skin conductance level of healthy participants were recorded during a 2-h EEG with eyes closed under simultaneous presentation of stimuli in an ignored (N = 39) and attended (N = 39) oddball condition. EEG-vigilance stages were classified using the Vigilance Algorithm Leipzig (VIGALL 2.1). The time-on-task effect was tested by dividing the EEG into four 30-min consecutive time blocks. ANS-activity was compared between EEG-vigilance stages across the entire 2 h and within each time block.

Results: We found a coherent decline of ANS-activity with declining brain arousal states, over the 2-h recording and in most cases within each 30-min block in both conditions. Furthermore, we found a significant time-on-task effect on heart rate, even when arousal was kept constant. It was most pronounced between the first and all subsequent blocks and could have been a consequence of postural change at the beginning of the experiment.

Conclusion: Our findings contribute to the validation of VIGALL 2.1 using ANS parameters in 2-h EEG recording under oddball conditions.

Keywords: VIGALL 2.1, Brain arousal, EEG-vigilance stages, Time-on-task effect, Heart rate, Skin conductance level

Background

Brain arousal fundamentally affects all dimensions of human behavior [1]. It can best be assessed using electroencephalography (EEG). According to the scoring systems by Rechtschaffen and Kales [2] and the American Academy of Sleep Medicine [3], different sleep stages can be differentiated, but only one uniform wake state has

been described. However, it has been demonstrated that different states of arousal can be discerned during the waking state [4–7]. For example, the wake-sleep transition is a period which is characterized by small arousal fluctuations [8] before stable sleep begins. To date, only a few studies have examined states of arousal in the period before sleep onset, which could be due to a lack of reliable research methods.

To fill this gap, the Vigilance Algorithm Leipzig (VIGALL), an EEG- and electrooculogram (EOG)-based algorithm, was introduced by Hegerl and colleagues [9–13]. VIGALL allows the automatic classification of brain arousal (assessed as EEG-vigilance stages) in the

*Correspondence: Jue.Huang@medizin.uni-leipzig.de
[†]Jue Huang and Christine Ulke contributed equally to this work and are co-first authors
[1] Department of Psychiatry and Psychotherapy, University of Leipzig, Semmelweisstrasse 10, 04103 Leipzig, Germany
Full list of author information is available at the end of the article

wake-sleep transition (see Table 1). Markers of autonomic nervous system (ANS) arousal (heart rate: HR; skin conductance levels: SCL; and temperature) can simultaneously be assessed.

Although situational factors substantially contribute to arousal states, the trait aspect of arousal is well-known and, in fact, a genetic component has been suggested [1, 14]. Moreover, arousal and regulatory systems have been posited as a fundamental domain for classifying mental disorders by the Research Domain Criteria Project (RDoC) of the National Institute of Mental Health (NIMH) [15]. In line with this, the Arousal Regulation Model posits a pathophysiological role of brain arousal in affective disorders and attention-deficit/hyperactivity disorder (ADHD) [9, 12, 16, 17]. VIGALL has been utilized in several clinical studies to identify distinct patterns of brain arousal regulation across these psychiatric disorders. For example, an unstable regulation of brain arousal was found in patients with bipolar disorder during manic episodes [18] and in patients with ADHD [19]. In contrast, a hyperstable pattern of arousal regulation was observed in patients with depression [20, 21] and bipolar patients during depressive episodes [18, 22].

Earlier versions of VIGALL have been validated using EEG-fMRI data [10], in a PET study [23], against evoked potentials [24] and relating ANS parameters to different EEG-vigilance stages [11].

Olbrich et al. [11] compared HR and SCL of healthy individuals in different EEG-vigilance stages using an earlier version of VIGALL to 15-min resting EEG data. High EEG-vigilance stages showed significantly higher HR and SCL activity in comparison to lower EEG-vigilance stages in regression analyses, but this was not the case for the comparisons between stage 0 and A1 (possibly due to the misclassification of stage 0, according to the authors). Concerning SCL, however, the effect of time explained more variance than did EEG-vigilance stages. Additionally, a direct effect of time on both central [25] and ANS arousal [26, 27] is well established elsewhere. However, no study to date has directly assessed this possible effect on ANS activity independent of the co-occurring arousal decline.

To gain more insight into the direct effect of time (i.e. time-on-task) on ANS activity, we analyzed a previously published dataset [24] of 2-h EEG data recorded in two conditions of an oddball experiment while controlling for arousal. We divided the 2-h EEG recording into four consecutive 30-min blocks, which enabled us to examine the time-on-task effect. The analyses were restricted to particular EEG-vigilance stages in order to control for the additional influence of brain arousal on ANS activity. The extended recording period also ensured a reliable comparison of ANS activity between different EEG-vigilance stages, since enough data from each arousal state could be obtained. Specifically, we analyzed whether the findings by Olbrich, (i.e. the decrease in ANS activity with the decline of EEG-vigilance stages) can be replicated in each of the four time blocks.

We hypothesize that there will be a decrease in ANS activity with the decline of EEG-vigilance stages over 2 h as well as within each time block (Hypothesis 1). We further hypothesize that there is a significant time-on-task effect on ANS activity across the four 30-min blocks when restricting the analysis to individual EEG-vigilance stages (Hypothesis 2). We are particularly interested in differences in ANS activity between EEG-vigilance stages 0 and A1 on account of the recently released VIGALL 2.1 which has greater classification accuracy. To this end, we set out to reexamine the shifts in ANS activity between fine-graded EEG-vigilance stages, for the first time in two different conditions (ignored and attended) of an oddball task.

Methods

Subjects

Healthy volunteers were recruited via local and online advertisements. None of the subjects reported a history of sleep disorder, psychiatric or neurological diseases, or current intake of psychotropic medication. All subjects were required to participate in two EEG

Table 1 Assessment of brain arousal states by applying VIGALL 2.1

EEG-vigilance stage	Corresponding behavioral state	EEG-characteristics
0	Cognitively active wakefulness	Low amplitude, desynchronized non-alpha EEG without horizontal SEM
A1	Relaxed wakefulness	Occipital dominant alpha activity
A2		Shifts of alpha to central and frontal cortical areas
A3		Continued frontalization of alpha
B1	Drowsiness	Low amplitude, desynchronized non-alpha EEG with SEM
B2/3		Dominant delta- and theta-power
C	Sleep onset	Occurrence of K-complexes and sleep spindles

VIGALL Vigilance Algorithm Leipzig, *EEG* electroencephalogram, *SEM* slow eye movements recordings (one ignored and one attended oddball condition, see below) with an interval of 7 days between the recordings. These two recordings were performed in a pseudorandom order. Not all subjects participated in the second session due to lack of compliance or availability, leaving 45 subjects in the ignored and 49 subjects in the attended condition. Within these participants, those who exhibited insufficient arousal variability during the 2-h recording (i.e. too much EEG-vigilance stage A1; n = 6 in the ignored and n = 10 in the attended condition) were further excluded. As result, the final sample consisted of 39 subjects in the ignored (22 females, age = 23.90 ± 3.93) and 39 in the attended condition (24 females, age = 24.46 ± 4.44), respectively. The study was approved by the local ethics committee of the University of Leipzig (075-13-11032013). Each subject gave written informed consent prior to the first recording. All subjects received 20€ or course credits (psychology students) for their participation.

Procedure

The 2-h EEG recordings began between 1 and 4 p.m. in a light-dimmed and sound attenuated room. The temperature in the booth was maintained around 25 °C at the beginning of each recording. For each individual, the time of assessment was the same in both sessions. During the EEG recording, subjects lay comfortably on a lounge chair while standard (500 Hz) and deviant (1000 Hz) tone were presented in an oddball sequence with stimuli probabilities of 80 and 20% respectively. In the ignored condition, subjects were instructed to ignore the tones, while in the attended condition they performed a simple cognitive task such as pressing a button to target stimuli. At the beginning of each recording, the body position was changed from upright to laid-back. During the recording, subjects were instructed to close their eyes, relax and not fight against an urge to sleep. When subjects did fall asleep, they were woken up after 5 min and asked to answer a common question (e.g. today's date) before they were allowed to continue the task. This process was repeated until the end of the experiment in order to acquire enough data from each arousal state.

EEG-recording and EEG-vigilance staging

The EEG was recorded at 1000 Hz with Ag/AgCl electrodes and DC amplifiers (QuickAmp; Brain Products GmbH, Gilching, Germany) from 31 sites (Fp1, Fp2, F3, F4, F7, F8, Fz, FC1, FC2, FC5, FC6, C3, C4, T7, T8, Cz, FT9, FT10, CP5, CP6, TP9, TP10, P3, P4, P7, P8, Pz, O1, O2, PO9, PO10) according to the extended international 10–20 system using EasyCap (EASYCAP Brain Products GmbH, Gilching, Germany), and referenced against

common average. Impedance of each electrode was kept below 10 kΩ. Bipolar electrodes were placed laterally to the left and right eyes to monitor horizontal eye movements and above and below the right eye to monitor vertical eye movements.

EEG data were analyzed using BrainVision Analyzer 2.1 software (Brain Products GmbH, Gilching, Germany). First, the EEG raw data were pre-processed according to standard operating procedures (see VIGALL manual [7] or refer to Additional file 1). After that, all 1-s EEG-segments were classified into seven different EEG-vigilance stages using VIGALL 2.1 (available at http://research.uni-leipzig.de/vigall/).

ANS parameters

To assess the R–R intervals of HR (in ms), an electrocardiogram (ECG) was recorded at a 1000 Hz sampling rate using a bipolar channel of the QuickAmp amplifier. Electrodes were placed on both forearms. R-peaks were marked using the CB correction module of BrainVision Analyzer (Brain Products GmbH, Gilching, Germany). The results were visually checked and corrected if necessary.

To assess SCL (in μSiemens), a bipolar channel of the QuickAmp amplifier was used with a constant voltage of 0.5 V (GSR module, Brain Products GmbH, Gilching, Germany). Two Ag/AgCl electrodes (with an overall diameter of 13 mm) were placed at the thenar and hypothenar of the non-dominant hand. A low pass filter of 1 Hz was applied to exclude phasic components of the electrodermal activity due to stimuli presentation (in both conditions) and response (only in the attended condition).

Segments identified as artifacts in the EEG were also marked as artifacts in the ECG and SCL channels. Only artifact-free segments were used in further analyses. VIGALL also provides calculations for R–R intervals and SCL values: R–R interval was computed as the mean of the R–R intervals across three consecutive artifact-free 1-s segments. The HR was calculated for each segment (indexed by 60,000/R–R intervals in ms). SCL value was computed as mean of all data points in each 1-s segment.

In order to account for the considerable degree of variability in SCL raw values between subjects, for each subject SCL values were z-transformed against the mean and standard deviation over 2 h when assessing overall SCL differences between EEG-vigilance stages. SCL values were also z-transformed against the mean and standard deviation in each corresponding time block for each subject when differences within each time block were examined.

Statistical analysis

A minimum criterion of 10 epochs for each EEG-vigilance stage was set in order to obtain reliable HR and SCL values. Subjects with an insufficient number of epochs were excluded from the comparisons of respective stages. This step resulted in different sample sizes for each EEG-vigilance stage. Some stages, such as A1 and B1, which were frequent, contained more subjects, whereas others, especially A3 and C, which rarely occurred, had fewer subjects (see Additional file 2).

To analyze differences in ANS activity between EEG-vigilance stages across the entire 2 h and within each time block, paired sample (within subject) t tests were used. The different sample sizes in the EEG-vigilance stages precluded adequate stage comparisons (due to list-wise deletion) by repeated measures analyses of variance (rmANOVAs). Hence, comparisons were only made for pairs with a sufficient sample size (n > 10). All statistical analyses were conducted using IBM SPSS Statistics version 20 (IBM, Armonk, NY, USA).

The time-on-task effect on HR and SCL was analyzed with rmANOVAs. In these analyses, the arousal stage was kept constant by restricting the analyses to a respective EEG-vigilance stage across the four consecutive time blocks (min 1–30, min 31–60, min 61–90, min 91–120). However, these analyses could only be performed in the EEG-vigilance stages A1, A2, B1 and B2/3 in the ignored condition and in stages A1, B1 and B2/3 in the attended condition because the sample sizes (n ≤ 10) across all four blocks were insufficient in the remaining stages. When significant main effects were present, post hoc tests for multiple comparisons were conducted with adjustments for significance level using the Bonferroni method ($p < 0.0125$). When analyzing the time-on-task effect on SCL we did not z-transform the data for two reasons. First, the time course and percentage of low EEG-vigilance stages in each time block may have increased with time (see Additional file 2), possibly resulting in a smaller z-score in low stages in earlier versus later time blocks. This could have led to an artificial time effect. Second, because we used rmANOVAs to examine within-subject effects over time, the inter-individual variations likely had little influence on the results.

Results

HR and SCL between EEG-vigilance stages during the total 2-h EEG recording

In the ignored condition, the analyses of HR across EEG-vigilance stages revealed a continuous decline from high (A1) to low (C) EEG-vigilance stages, with 14 out of 15 pair-wise comparisons (except pair B2/3 vs. C, $p = .103$) reaching the significance level (1.49E−13 ≤ p ≤ .023). HR in stage 0 was significantly higher than in the other far lower stages, i.e. B1, B2/3 and C (8.91E−8 ≤ p ≤ 8.05E−7), whereas no significant differences were found in comparisons with neighboring lower stages, i.e. A1, A2 and A3 (.063 ≤ p ≤ .260). Additionally, the HR value in stage 0 was even lower than in A1 and A2. For SCL, we also observed a continuous decrease from stage A1 to C (1.91E−13 ≤ p ≤ .019) with the exception of comparisons between some neighboring stages, i.e. A1 versus A2 ($p = .134$), A3 versus B1 ($p = .156$). SCL in stage 0 was higher than in other stages (except stage A1), wherein the comparisons with stage B1, B2/3 and C reached significance level (1.62E−6 ≤ p ≤ .005). SCL increased significantly from stage 0 to A1 ($p = 3.12E−5$). A visual illustration of ANS activity in the ignored condition is shown in Fig. 1. The detailed results of paired t tests are summarized in Table S2 in Additional file 3.

In the attended condition, a significant continuous decrease in HR from stage A1 to C was obtained from all pair-wise comparisons (6.80E−11 ≤ p ≤ .021). A significantly higher HR in stage 0 relative to stages ranging from A2 to C was observed (3.64E−8 ≤ p ≤ 1.25E−6), except for the comparison of 0 versus A2 ($p = .564$). A slightly higher but non-significant HR in stage A1 than in stage 0 was seen ($p = .301$). Similar results regarding SCL were demonstrated in 12 out of 15 pair-wise comparisons of stages ranging between A1 and C (2.86E−7 ≤ p ≤ .035). Exceptions included some comparisons between neighboring stages, i.e. A2 versus B1 ($p = .068$), A3 versus B1 ($p = .607$), A3 versus B2/3 ($p = .165$). A significant higher SCL in stage 0 was obtained as compared to stages from A2 to C (4.82E−5 ≤ p ≤ .002), with exception of stage A2 ($p = .106$). A non-significant increasing trend in SCL from stage 0 to A1 was observed ($p = .288$). A graphical representation is shown in Fig. 1. The detailed results of paired t tests are provided in Table S3 in Additional file 3.

The time-on-task effect on HR and SCL: restricting analyses to certain EEG-vigilance stages

Results of rmANOVAs for assessing the *time-on-task* effect are summarized in Table 2. HR and SCL in four time blocks in corresponding EEG-vigilance stages are presented in Fig. 2. Note that, subjects within one stage in the four time blocks were the same.

In the ignored condition, rmANOVAs revealed a significant main effect of *time-on-task* in stages A1 ($p = .002$) and B1 ($p = .021$) for HR, explaining about 20% and 10% of variance in stage A1 and B1, respectively (see Table 2). No significant *time-on-task* effect was found for SCL in any of the stages (.082 ≤ p ≤ .530).

For stage A1, HR was significantly higher in min 1–30 relative to min 61–90 (mean difference = 1.658, $p = .022$). For stage B1, HR in min 1–30 was significantly higher than in min 31–60 (mean difference = 1.532, $p = .037$).

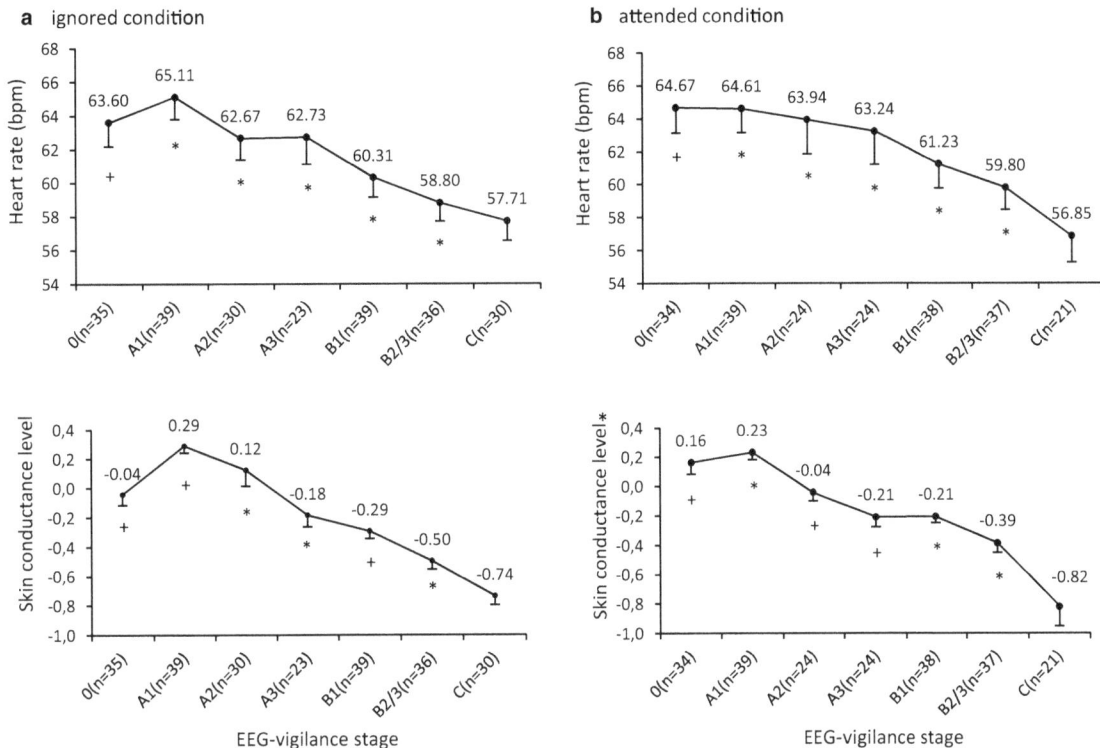

a ignored condition   **b** attended condition

Fig. 1 Averaged HR and SCL over 2-h in EEG-vigilance stage. The line diagrams show the mean of heart rate (HR) and skin conductance level (SCL, z transformed) in corresponding EEG-vigilance stages in ignored (**a**) and attended (**b**) condition. To note, the values were calculated based on different subjects. The numbers of subjects in each stage are shown in parentheses. Error bars reflect standard error of the means. The asterisk and plus sign represent results of pared sample *t* tests, which asterisk means significant different between this stage and all other lower stages, while plus sign means some of the comparisons between this stage and other lower stages reached significance level. Each pared sample *t* test was only made for pairs with a sufficient sample size (n > 10), therefore the degree of freedoms were different for each pair. For more details please refer to the Table S2 (ignored condition) and Table S3 (attended condition) in Additional file 3

In the attended condition, a significant main effect of *time-on-task* was obtained in stages B1 ($p = .006$) and B2/3 ($p = .036$) for HR, whereas no significant *time-on-task* effect was found for SCL ($.274 \leq p \leq .726$). 10% of the variance in HR in stages B1 and B2/3 was explained by the determined effect, whereas it explained only 2% of the variance in stage A1 (see Table 2).

For stage B1, HR in min 1–30 was significantly higher relative to min 31–60 (mean difference $= 1.296$, $p = .002$) and min 61–90 (mean difference $= 1.802$, $p = .023$). For stage B2/3, HR in min 1–30 was significantly higher when compared to min 61–90 (mean difference $= 1.735$, $p = .042$).

HR and SCL between EEG-vigilance stages during each time block

The detailed results from the analyses of HR and SCL across EEG-vigilance stages within each time block in the ignored and attended condition, as well as their summaries are provided in Additional file 4.

Comparisons in the ignored condition

The ANS differences in stage A1 versus A2/A3 were weakly pronounced in the first block, but present in most cases in the last three blocks. The differences between stages A2 and A3 in all blocks could not be confirmed, due to either non-significant results or insufficient sample sizes. The ANS values in stages B1 and B2/3 respectively differed significantly from other higher vigilance stages in most available cases in all blocks; and in most cases B1 and B2/3 also differed significantly from each other. Few comparisons with stage C could be conducted due to the rare occurrence of stage C. However, the ANS in stage C showed stable differences against all other stages in block min 31–60 and also differed from A1 in all other blocks. The differences between stages 0 versus A1 were only evidenced by SCL in all blocks except for min 61–90.

Comparisons in the attended condition

The differences in HR in stage A1 versus A2/A3 were most pronounced in the last two blocks, while SCL differences

Table 2 Results of repeated measures ANOVAs for assessing time-on-task effect on ANS parameters

	Heart rate					Skin conductance level				
	Time block (min)				Effect (η_p^2)	Time block (min)				Effect (η_p^2)
	1–30	31–60	61–90	91–120		1–30	31–60	61–90	91–120	
Ignored condition[a]										
A1	65.63 (7.38)	64.04 (7.60)	63.97 (7.59)	64.52 (7.78)	$F_{3,63} = 5.370^{**}$ (0.204)	3.75 (4.40)	3.81 (4.82)	4.02 (4.73)	4.37 (5.97)	$F_{1.183,24.852} = 0.472$ (0.022)
A2	62.30 (6.96)	60.74 (7.73)	60.90 (7.31)	61.91 (8.20)	$F_{3,42} = 1.574$ (0.101)	3.78 (4.80)	3.57 (5.39)	3.84 (5.12)	4.65 (7.13)	$F_{1.124,15.742} = 0.493$ (0.034)
B1	61.79 (6.85)	60.26 (6.96)	60.18 (7.76)	60.97 (8.01)	$F_{3,105} = 3.381^{*}$ (0.088)	2.77 (3.26)	2.68 (3.21)	2.94 (3.53)	3.55 (5.22)	$F_{1.153,40.351} = 2.263$ (0.061)
B2/3	61.42 (6.61)	59.87 (6.52)	59.52 (6.75)	60.89 (8.36)	$F_{1.981,45.573} = 2.314$ (0.091)	2.31 (3.27)	2.33 (3.56)	2.59 (3.60)	2.78 (3.68)	$F_{1.725,39.682} = 2.764$ (0.107)
Attended condition[b]										
A1	65.76 (9.49)	65.65 (9.55)	65.37 (9.18)	65.21 (9.10)	$F_{2.395,74.258} = 0.493$ (0.016)	2.66 (1.72)	2.54 (2.35)	2.76 (3.15)	2.66 (2.29)	$F_{1.366,42.343} = 0.208$ (0.007)
B1	63.45 (9.50)	62.16 (9.01)	61.65 (9.37)	61.81 (8.78)	$F_{2.023,66.757} = 5.509^{**}$ (0.143)	2.51 (1.48)	2.41 (1.95)	2.70 (3.04)	2.81 (2.68)	$F_{1.280,42.247} = 0.746$ (0.022)
B2/3	60.00 (8.08)	58.71 (7.31)	58.27 (7.67)	59.21 (8.45)	$F_{3,54} = 3.059^{*}$ (0.145)	2.03 (1.20)	1.86 (1.06)	1.78 (0.92)	1.85 (0.96)	$F_{1.378,24.810} = 1.323$ (0.068)

Standard deviations are presented in parentheses

$^{*}p < .05$; $^{**}p < .01$; $^{***}p < .001$

[a] The sample sizes in examination of time-on-task effect in the ignored condition during certain stage were different: n = 22 in stage A1, n = 15 in stage A2, n = 36 in stage B1, n = 24 in stage B2/3

[b] The sample sizes in examination time-on-task effect in the attended condition during certain stage were different: n = 32 in stage A1, n = 34 in stage B1, n = 19 in stage B2/3

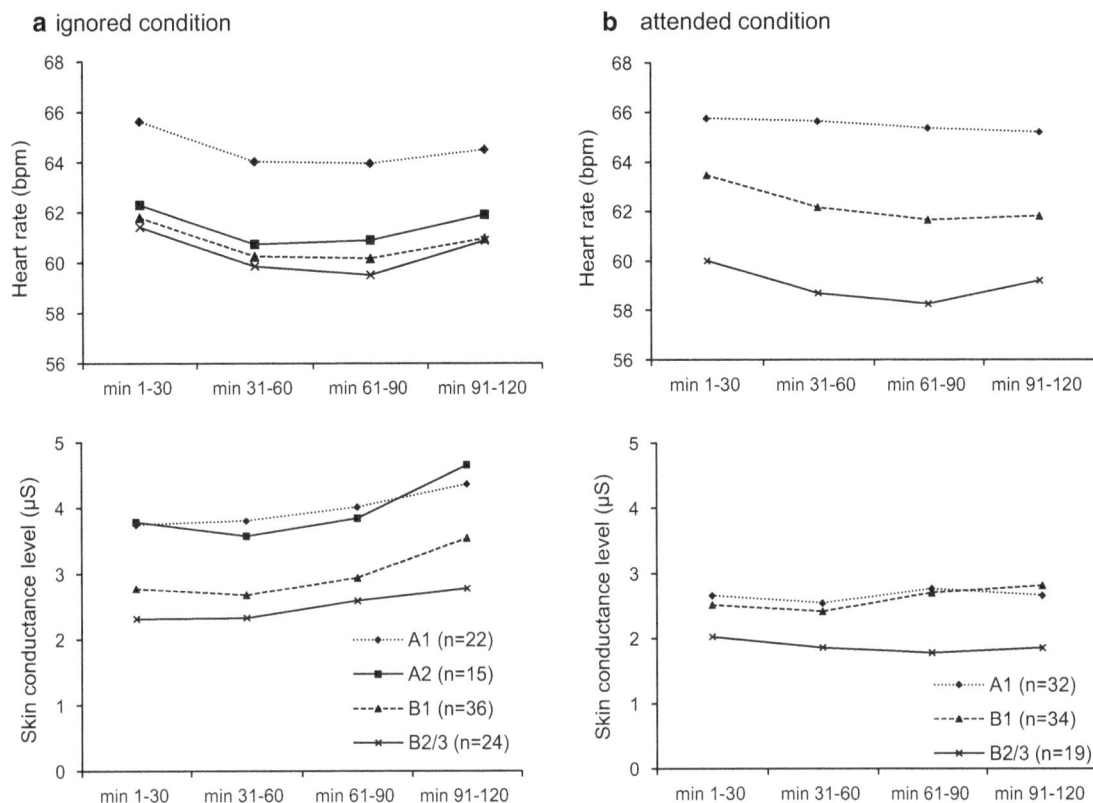

Fig. 2 Averaged HR and SCL within 30-min time block in EEG-vigilance stage. Heart rate (HR) and skin conductance level (SCL) values were calculated over available subjects in each time block (min 1–30, min 31–60, min 61–90, min 91–120) during corresponding EEG-vigilance stages in ignored (**a**) and attended (**b**) condition. The numbers of available subjects are presented in parentheses. To note, the tests in other stages could not be conducted due to insufficient sample size (n ≤ 10)

were obtained in most cases in all four blocks. ANS differences between stages A2 and A3 could not be confirmed in any block. The ANS values in stages B1 and B2/3 consistently differed from stages 0 and A1 in most cases in all blocks, but did not differ from other higher stages. Significant differences between stages B1 and B2/3 were consistently present in most cases. Comparisons concerning stage C were limited in most cases, except in block min 31–60 and min 61–90, wherein ANS differed significantly from stages A1 and B1. The differences between stages 0 versus A1 were only evidenced by SCL in the first two blocks.

Discussion

In the present study we examined ANS activity in different states of brain arousal (indexed by EEG-vigilance stages) in ignored and attended conditions of an auditory oddball task of a 2-h EEG. We examined the association of brain arousal and ANS activity within four subsequent 30-min time blocks to control for time-on-task (Hypothesis 1). We additionally examined the time-on-task effect on ANS activity, restricting analyses to individual EEG-vigilance stages (Hypothesis 2).

In line with Hypothesis 1, we found a clear decrease of HR and SCL from EEG-vigilance stage A1 to C over the entire 2-h EEG recording. This finding is in line with the study findings from Olbrich et al. [11] and more recently by Jawinski et al. [28], who demonstrated a gradual change of ANS activity in different states of brain arousal in 15-min resting EEG data. Most importantly, these gradual ANS changes were present in most cases within each 30-min time block. These findings demonstrate that changes in ANS activity correspond to declines in EEG-vigilance stages from A1 to C, even when controlling for time-on-task. The present study demonstrates this association for the first time under oddball conditions and therefore provides further validation of VIGALL 2.1.

In contrast, an unexpectedly lower HR and SCL in stage 0 (associated with cognitively active wakefulness) as compared to stage A1 (associated with relaxed wakefulness) was obtained over the 2-h recording time in both the ignored and attended conditions. This was also the case for SCL in all 30-min time blocks and in the most cases for HR, except for the second time block in the attended condition. In the Olbrich et al. [11] study, in which similar results were found using an earlier VIGALL version, the authors attributed this finding to the discriminative validity of EEG-vigilance stages 0 versus B1. Although 0/B1 separation has been improved upon in more recent VIGALL versions, this distinction remains a challenge, as both stages are characterized by desynchronized non alpha EEG via VIGALL (see Table 1). We also cannot rule out a possible 0/B1 misclassification in the present study. However, the difference obtained between stages 0 and A1 could be attributed to the wake-up reactions introduced by the experimenter. To acquire sufficient variability in EEG-vigilance, study participants were woken up 5-min after sleep-onset. To obtain a detailed assessment of individual temporal alterations in brain arousal and ANS activity, we plotted HR and SCL values with a resolution of 1 s for each subject in the ignored and the attended conditions, indicating different EEG-vigilance stages with colored points (see Fig. 3a, b). The wake-up reaction was characterized by a short episode of elevated HR and SCL values and during this episode stage A1 occurred almost exclusively. The HR and SCL during this episode were much higher than the HR and SCL in stage 0 and therefore led to an overall higher ANS value in stage A1 than in stage 0.

The simultaneous increase in cortical and ANS arousal during the wake-up reaction may reflect a protective mechanism to potential threatening stimuli [29]. Following this reaction, a subsequent steep decline in ANS activity in the absence of simultaneous cortical decline was observed in our healthy subjects. This is understood as a normal physiological return to baseline level (pattern: rapid decline of ANS but delayed decline of cortical arousal) as the experiment instructions necessitated. It would be interesting to examine whether there are similar patterns in clinical populations, for example in patients with depression or ADHD.

Hypothesis 2 was confirmed for HR. A strength of the current study is the extended recording period of 2 h compared to 15 min in prior work [11]. This allowed us to assess the direct time-on-task effect in the same subjects and to restrict the analyses to particular EEG-vigilance stages. Post hoc tests showed that the time-on-task effect was most evident between the first and all subsequent blocks. Regarding the direction of the change between the first and subsequent blocks, a decrease in HR in both the ignored and attended conditions was seen, although brain arousal was constant. One reason for this finding could be inherent in VIGALL's Standard Operating Procedure. At the beginning of the recording, the subject's body position was changed from an upright to a semi-supine position and individuals were asked to close their eyes [7]. This postural change may have induced an increase in cutaneous blood flow due to a deactivation of sympathetic vasoconstriction reflexes, resulting in reduced sympathetic outflow and decrease in HR [30]. In addition, the semi-supine position is associated with a considerable increase in venous return from the extremities to the heart, minimizing the effort against gravity which then consequently results in down-regulated HR [31]. The effect of postural change on brain arousal [32–34] and ANS activity [33, 35] has been evidenced in several studies, which may indicate the possible confounding effect of postural change in examinations requiring change body positions such as in fMRI studies.

Interestingly, concerning the time-on-task effect on HR in stage A1, we observed a clear difference—about 18% in explained variance—between the ignored and attended conditions. This finding illustrates the influence of a cognitive task on HR within a waking state, where most stimuli are perceived and a behavioral response must be maintained [24]. However, the influence of the cognitive task on HR became smaller upon occurrence of the drowsy state.

Our results underscore that the waking state is, at the physiological level, not a uniform state. Study participants displayed broad variability in EEG-vigilance stages during both conditions of the oddball task. Thus, in study designs where attention and cognitive processing are crucial, controlling for EEG-vigilance stages seems important, because arousal states influence performance, for example, reaction times [24]. This could also have implications for creating apps or devices for real-world situations such as commercial driving.

As a limitation of this study, we did not control for changes in temperature in the booth during the recording period, which might have resulted in increased temperature and humidity and therefore contributed to SCL [36]. The lack of time-on-task effect on SCL may be due to this environmental factor. Our finding of a numeric increase in SCL values across time blocks (Fig. 2) may therefore be attributed to the increased temperature in the booth $(4–5 \text{ m}^2)$ over 2 h recording.

A second limitation is the individual difference in arousal variability across the EEG recording and a minimum criterion of 10 epochs for every subject in EEG-vigilance stages. Because sufficient sample sizes were not obtained for each time block, some comparisons could not be made (e.g. stage A3 vs. C). This was especially pronounced in the attended condition. Because subjects were performing a task, they fell asleep less frequently and more often stayed awake, which resulted in more frequent higher EEG-vigilance stages in the attended condition. Further, we acknowledge that the relatively small and selected sample limits the generalizability of our findings.

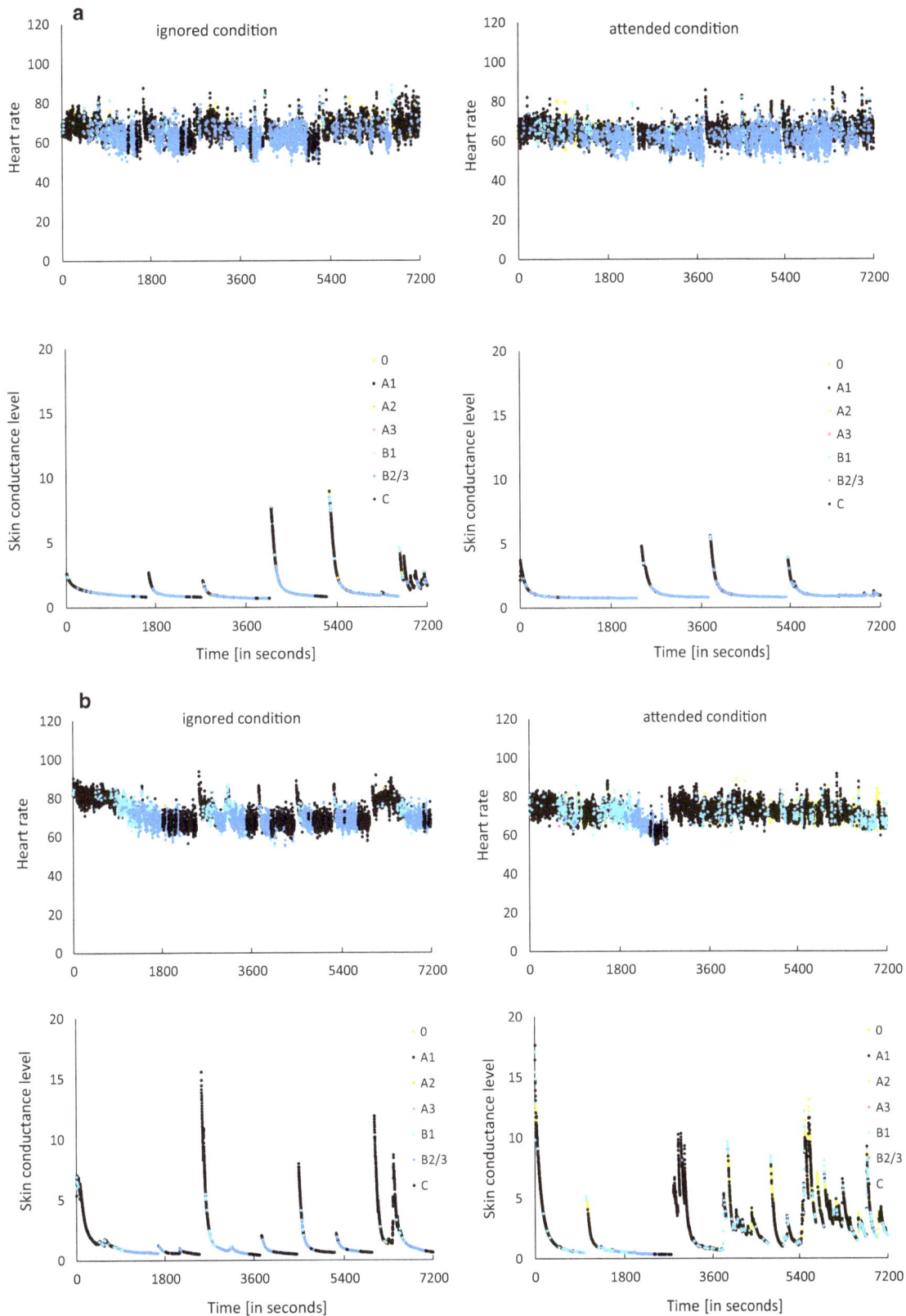

Fig. 3 HR and SCL for two individuals (**a**, **b**) over 2-h EEG. Each dot represents the corresponding ANS value in 1 s. The visible gaps between dots indicate possible wake-up reaction. After each wake-up, however, EEG-vigilance stage A1 (red dots) rather than stage 0 (yellow dots) occurred almost exclusively. Subsequently a steep decrease occurred in about 100 s but without change in level of brain arousal

Conclusion

In conclusion, this is the first study to directly determine a time-on-task effect on HR when restricting analyses to particular states of brain arousal. Concurrent changes in ANS activity and EEG-vigilance were found over the 2-h recording period and in most cases within each 30-min time block, contributing to the validation of VIGALL 2.1.

Abbreviations

EEG: electroencephalography; VIGALL: Vigilance Algorithm Leipzig; EOG: electrooculogram; ANS: autonomic nervous system; HR: heart rate; SCL: skin conductance level; RDoC: Research Domain Criteria Project; ADHD: attention-deficit/hyperactivity disorder; ECG: electrocardiogram; rmANOVA: repeated measures analyses of variance.

Authors' contributions

JH, CU, TH and UH conceptualized and designed the study. JH and CU contributed to the data analyses. JH, CU and TH interpreted the data. JH and CU drafted the manuscript. All authors read and approved the final manuscript.

Author details

[1] Department of Psychiatry and Psychotherapy, University of Leipzig, Semmelweisstrasse 10, 04103 Leipzig, Germany. [2] Depression Research Centre, German Depression Foundation, Leipzig, Germany.

Acknowledgements

We acknowledge support from University of Leipzig within the program of Open Access Publishing. This publication was written in the framework of the cooperation between the German Depression Foundation and the Deutsche Bahn Stiftung gGmbH. We thank Dr. Elise Paul of the German Depression Foundation for her English editing.

Competing interests

The authors declare that the research was conducted in the absence of any commercial or financial relationship which could be construed as a potential conflict of interest.

Funding

This study was supported by the Department of Psychiatry, University of Leipzig, which provided the expense allowances for subjects' participation. This funding body had no role in study design, data collection, evaluation and interpretation.

References

1. Pfaff D, Ribeiro A, Matthews J, Kow L. Concepts and mechanisms of generalized central nervous system arousal. Ann N Y Acad Sci. 2008;1129:11–25.
2. Rechtschaffen A, Kales A. A manual of standardized terminology, techniques and scoring system for sleep stages of human subjects. Washington, DC: Washington Public Health Service, US Government Printing Office; 1968.
3. Iber C, Ancoli-Isreal S, Chesson A, Quan SF. Das AASM-Manual zum Scoring von Schlaf und assoziierten Ereignissen: Regeln, Technologie und techinische Spezifikationen. 1st ed. Germany: Steinfopff; 2008.
4. Loomis AL, Harvey EN, Hobart GA. Cerebral states during sleep, as studied by human brain potentials. J Exp Psychol. 1937;21:127–44.
5. Bente D. Vigilanz, dissoziative Vigilanzverschiebung und Insuffizienz des Vigilanztonus. In: Kranz H, Heinrich K, editors. Begleitwirkungen und Misserfolge der psychiatrischen Pharmakotherapie. Stuttgart: Thieme; 1964.
6. Roth B. The clinical and theoretical importance of EEG rhythms corresponding to states of lowered vigilance. Electroencephalogr Clin Neurophysiol. 1961;13:395–9.
7. Hegerl U, Sander C, Ulke C, Böttger D, Hensch T, Huang J, Mauche N, Olbrich S. Vigilance Algorithm Leipzig (VIGALL) Version 2.1—Manual, 2017. http://research.uni-leipzig.de/vigall/.
8. Ulke C, Huang J, Schwabedal Justus T C, Surova G, Mergl R, Hensch T. Coupling and dynamics of cortical and autonomic signals are linked to central inhibition during the wake-sleep transition. Sci Rep. 2017;7:11804.
9. Hegerl U, Hensch T. The vigilance regulation model of affective disorders and ADHD. Neurosci Biobehav Rev. 2014;44:45–57.
10. Olbrich S, Mulert C, Karch S, et al. EEG-vigilance and BOLD effect during simultaneous EEG/fMRI measurement. Neuroimage. 2009;45:319–32.
11. Olbrich S, Sander C, Matschinger H, et al. Brain and body: associations between EEG-vigilance and the autonomous nervous system activity during rest. J Psychophysiol. 2011;25:190–200.
12. Sander C, Hensch T, Wittekind DA, Bottger D, Hegerl U. Assessment of wakefulness and brain arousal regulation in psychiatric research. Neuropsychobiology. 2015;72:195–205.
13. Huang J, Sander C, Jawinski P, et al. Test–retest reliability of brain arousal regulation as assessed with VIGALL 2.0. Neuropsychiatr Electrophysiol. 2015;1:13.
14. Jawinski P, Kirsten H, Sander C, et al. Human brain arousal in the resting state: a genome-wide association study. Mol Psychiatry. 2018 (**in press**)
15. Cuthbert BN, Insel TR. Toward the future of psychiatric diagnosis: the seven pillars of RDoC. BMC Med. 2013;11:126.
16. Geissler J, Romanos M, Hegerl U, Hensch T. Hyperactivity and sensation seeking as autoregulatory attempts to stabilize brain arousal in ADHD and mania? Atten Defic Hyperact Disord. 2014;6:159–73.
17. Hegerl U, Sander C, Hensch T. Arousal regulation in affective disorders. In: Frodl, Thomas (Hg.) Systems neuroscience in depression. 2016. p. 341–70.
18. Wittekind DA, Spada J, Gross A, et al. Early report on brain arousal regulation in manic vs depressive episodes in bipolar disorder. Bipolar Disord. 2016;18:502–10.
19. Strauss M, Ulke C, Paucke M, et al. Brain arousal regulation in adults with attention-deficit/hyperactivity disorder (ADHD). Psychiatry Res. 2018;261:102–8.
20. Ulke C, Sander C, Jawinski P, et al. Sleep disturbances and upregulation of brain arousal during daytime in depressed versus non-depressed elderly subjects. World J Biol Psychiatry. 2017;18:633–40.
21. Hegerl U, Wilk K, Olbrich S, Schoenknecht P, Sander C. Hyperstable regulation of vigilance in patients with major depressive disorder. World J Biol Psychiatry. 2012;13:436–46.
22. Ulke C, Mauche N, Makiol C, et al. Successful treatment in a case of ultra-rapid cycling bipolar disorder is reflected in brain arousal regulation. Bipolar Disord. 2018;20:77–80.
23. Guenther T, Schonknecht P, Becker G, et al. Impact of EEG-vigilance on brain glucose uptake measured with (18)FFDG and PET in patients with depressive episode or mild cognitive impairment. Neuroimage. 2011;56:93–101.
24. Huang J, Hensch T, Ulke C, et al. Evoked potentials and behavioral performance during different states of brain arousal. BMC Neurosci. 2017;18:21.
25. Lal SK, Craig A. A critical review of the psychophysiology of driver fatigue. Biol Psychol. 2001;55:173–94.
26. Lim CL, Barry RJ, Gordon E, Sawant A, Rennie C, Yiannikas C. The relationship between quantified EEG and skin conductance level. Int J Psychophysiol. 1996;21:151–62.
27. Nicoletti C, Muller C, Hayashi C, Nakaseko M, Tobita I, Laubli T. Circadian rhythm of heart rate and physical activity in nurses during day and night shifts. Eur J Appl Physiol. 2015;115:1313–20.
28. Jawinski P, Kittel J, Sander C, et al. Recorded and reported sleepiness: the association between brain arousal in resting state and subjective daytime sleepiness. Sleep. 2017;40:zsx099.
29. Horner RL, Sanford LD, Pack AI, Morrison AR. Activation of a distinct arousal state immediately after spontaneous awakening from sleep. Brain Res. 1997;778:127–34.

30. Sindrup JH, Kastrup J, Jorgensen B, Bulow J, Lassen NA. Nocturnal variations in subcutaneous blood flow rate in lower leg of normal human subjects. Am J Physiol. 1991;260:H480–5.

31. Pump B, Gabrielsen A, Christensen NJ, Bie P, Bestle M, Norsk P. Mechanisms of inhibition of vasopressin release during moderate antiorthostatic posture change in humans. Am J Physiol. 1999;277:R229–35.

32. Barra J, Auclair L, Charvillat A, Vidal M, Perennou D. Postural control system influences intrinsic alerting state. Neuropsychology. 2015;29:226–34.

33. Muehlhan M, Marxen M, Landsiedel J, Malberg H, Zaunseder S. The effect of body posture on cognitive performance: a question of sleep quality. Front Hum Neurosci. 2014;8:171.

34. Caldwell JA, Prazinko B, Caldwell JL. Body posture affects electroencephalographic activity and psychomotor vigilance task performance in sleep-deprived subjects. Clin Neurophysiol. 2003;114:23–31.

35. Krauchi K, Cajochen C, Wirz-Justice A. A relationship between heat loss and sleepiness: effects of postural change and melatonin administration. J Appl Physiol. 1985;1997(83):134–9.

36. Amano T, Gerrett N, Inoue Y, Nishiyasu T, Havenith G, Kondo N. Determination of the maximum rate of eccrine sweat glands' ion reabsorption using the galvanic skin conductance to local sweat rate relationship. Eur J Appl Physiol. 2016;116:281–90.

12

Expression of alternatively spliced variants of the Dclk1 gene is regulated by psychotropic drugs

Magdalena Zygmunt[1], Dżesika Hoinkis[1], Jacek Hajto[1], Marcin Piechota[1], Bożena Skupień-Rabian[2], Urszula Jankowska[2], Sylwia Kędracka-Krok[3], Jan Rodriguez Parkitna[1] and Michał Korostyński[1]*

Abstract

Background: The long-term effects of psychotropic drugs are associated with the reversal of disease-related alterations through the reorganization and normalization of neuronal connections. Molecular factors that trigger drug-induced brain plasticity remain only partly understood. Doublecortin-like kinase 1 (*Dclk1*) possesses microtubule-polymerizing activity during synaptic plasticity and neurogenesis. However, the *Dclk1* gene shows a complex profile of transcriptional regulation, with two alternative promoters and exon splicing patterns that suggest the expression of multiple isoforms with different kinase activities.

Results: Here, we applied next-generation sequencing to analyze changes in the expression of *Dclk1* gene isoforms in the brain in response to several psychoactive drugs with diverse pharmacological mechanisms of action. We used bioinformatics tools to define the range and levels of *Dclk1* transcriptional regulation in the mouse nucleus accumbens and prefrontal cortex. We also sought to investigate the presence of DCLK1-derived peptides using mass spectrometry. We detected 15 transcripts expressed from the *Dclk1* locus (FPKM > 1), including 2 drug-regulated variants (fold change > 2). Drugs that act on serotonin receptors (5-HT2A/C) regulate a subset of *Dclk1* isoforms in a brain-region-specific manner. The strongest influence was observed for the mianserin-induced expression of an isoform with intron retention. The drug-activated expression of novel alternative *Dclk1* isoforms was validated using qPCR. The drug-regulated isoform contains genetic variants of DCLK1 that have been previously associated with schizophrenia and hyperactivity disorder in humans. We identified a short peptide that might originate from the novel DCLK1 protein product. Moreover, protein domains encoded by the regulated variant indicate their potential involvement in the negative regulation of the canonical DCLK1 protein.

Conclusions: In summary, we identified novel isoforms of the neuroplasticity-related gene *Dclk1* that are expressed in the brain in response to psychotropic drug treatments.

Keywords: Dclk1, Alternative transcription, Psychotropic drugs, Nucleus accumbens, Prefrontal cortex

*Correspondence: michkor@if-pan.krakow.pl
[1] Department of Molecular Neuropharmacology, Institute
of Pharmacology of the Polish Academy of Sciences, Smetna 12,
31-343 Krakow, Poland
Full list of author information is available at the end of the article

Background

Psychiatric disorders are associated with complex patterns of abnormal neuronal activity and maladaptive plasticity [1]. Treatment with psychotropic drugs aims to restore the normal function of the affected circuits; long-term therapeutic benefits may depend on the ability of drugs to restore normal plasticity. Consistent with this notion, commonly used psychotropic drugs robustly induce molecular effects on the brain associated with neuroplastic alterations [2, 3].

The dynamic process of cytoskeletal reorganization is one of the key components of brain plasticity [4]. Based on findings from rodent studies, the canonical *Dclk1* transcript encodes a protein that mediates microtubule polymerization and is involved in neurogenesis and neuronal plasticity by regulating dendritic outgrowth and synapse formation [5]. This gene is widely expressed in the nervous system and has been reported to show persistent expression in adult neurons [6]. Moreover, genetic variants of *DCLK1* are associated with psychiatric disorders in humans [7, 8]. These observations suggest a potential role for *Dclk1* in the formation of drug-inducible changes in the brain.

The *Dclk1* gene consists of 20 exons that undergo alternative splicing, resulting in several known variants [6, 9, 10]. Previously identified *Dclk1* transcripts include both mRNAs coding for distinct proteins and noncoding, regulatory RNAs. The multiple isoforms of this gene are differentially expressed and have different kinase activities [6, 11]. The isoforms are classified into four groups expressed from the following two distinct promoters: the full-length variant (containing both DCX and kinase domains), a kinase-lacking isoform (DCL), a double-cortin-lacking isoform (CPG16) and the CaMK-related peptide (CARP/Ania-4) lacking both DCX and kinase domains. The mechanism involved in transcriptional regulation of the diverse alternatively spliced variants of *Dclk1* remains elusive. The importance of the expression of alternatively spliced gene products from a single gene locus in brain physiology and disease progression has been reported [10, 12]. Therefore, acquiring gene expression profiles from all gene variants is a necessary first step in understanding the specific functions of proteins and identification of disease-relevant isoforms.

Here, we investigate drug-induced alternative transcription from the *Dclk1* locus. We used next-generation sequencing to map all transcripts of the *Dclk1* gene, both currently annotated in the mouse genome as well as putative novel RNAs. We found that the gene expression patterns are both drug- and brain-region-specific. Moreover, we identified a new *Dclk1* variant that is specifically regulated by psychotropic drugs acting on the serotonin system.

Materials and methods

Animals

Adult male (8–10 weeks old) C57BL/6N mice (Charles River Laboratories, Wilmington, Massachusetts, USA) were housed in Plexiglas cages (Type II L, 2–5 animals per cage) containing Aspen Laboratory bedding (MIDI LTE E-002, Abedd) in a conventional facility on a 12 h light/dark cycle with ad libitum access to water and chow (RM1 A (P), Special Diets Services) and an ambient temperature of 22 ± 2 °C. All the experiments were conducted in accordance with the European Union guidelines for the care and use of laboratory animals (2010/63/EU). Experimental protocols were reviewed and approved by the 2nd Local Institutional Animal Care and Use Committee (IACUC), Institute of Pharmacology Polish Academy of Sciences in Kraków (permit number: 1156/2015).

Drug treatment

Mice received a single intraperitoneal injection (vol. 10 ml/kg) of haloperidol (1 mg/kg), risperidone (0.5 mg/kg), methamphetamine (2 mg/kg), venlafaxine (16 mg/kg), mianserin (20 mg/kg) or ketamine (20 mg/kg) dissolved in saline, or saline with a drop of 0.1 M HCl in the case of haloperidol and risperidone. Regarding peptide analyses, mice were injected with mianserin (20 mg/kg) daily over 5 days. All animals were decapitated 2 h after treatment, and brains were then extracted and dissected with needles under a binocular. Drug doses that produce robust and comparable gene expression alterations were selected based on our previous experience [2, 3, 13]. Doses were selected to provide a reasonable comparison of the effects of each drug on the molecular level. All of the drugs were shown to cross the blood–brain barrier [14] and accumulate in the brain within minutes of administration [15–18].

Tissue collection and RNA isolation

Tissue extraction was performed as described previously [3, 13]. Briefly, whole brains were incubated in RNAlater reagent (Ambion) overnight and then coronally sectioned into 125 μm slices using a Vibratome (Leica). The prefrontal cortex (PFCx) and nucleus accumbens (NAc) were dissected with needles under a binocular microscope with a Paxinos atlas as a Ref. [19]. The cingulate, prelimbic, infralimbic and part of the dorsal peduncular cortex were collected from the area approximately $+1.90$ to $+1.15$ mm from the bregma. The shapes of the corpus callosum and anterior commissure were used to assess the distance from the bregma. Tissue samples were placed in RNAlater reagent and preserved at -70 °C. The samples were homogenized in 1 ml of TRIzol reagent (Invitrogen, Carlsbad, CA, USA). RNA was isolated according to the manufacturer's protocol and was further purified using the RNeasy Mini Kit (Qiagen Inc.). The RNA quality was determined using an Agilent 2100 Bioanalyzer (Agilent, Palo Alto, CA, USA).

Microarray data analysis

In this study, we reanalyzed our previously published microarray data for striatal gene expression profiles produced by 18 major psychoactive drugs at 1, 2, 4 and 8 h after acute administration (Please see: [2] for details). Briefly, the analysis and quality control of 324 microarrays were performed using the BeadArray R package v1.10.0. After background subtraction, data were normalized using quantile normalization and then $\log_2$-transformed. The results were standardized to reduce the effects of hybridization batches using z-score transformation. Genes2mind was used to visualize the results (http://genes2mind.org) [20].

Whole-transcriptome sequencing

The procedure was performed as described previously [3, 13]. Total RNA (1 µg) was ribo-depleted using the RiboMinus Eukaryote Kit v2 (Ambion). rRNA-depleted RNA was used to prepare the RNA-seq library generated using the Ion Total RNA-seq Kit v2. Templates were prepared using emulsion PCR (ePCR) with the Ion One-Touch™ 2 Instrument and the Ion PI™ Template OT2 200 Kit v3. Sequencing was performed using an Ion PI™ Sequencing 200 Kit v3 and the Ion PI™ Chip v2 (Life Technologies). The template-positive ion sphere particles (ISPs) were loaded onto an Ion PITM Chip v2 and sequenced (single end reads > 100 bp).

NGS data analysis

The quality of the NGS data was assessed using FastQC. The RNA-seq reads were aligned using TopHat 2.0.1 followed by Tmap 3.0.2. The transcript FPKM (Fragments Per Kilobase of transcript per Million fragments mapped) levels were quantified using Cufflinks v2.2.1 and GTF from the Ensembl gene database. Statistical significance was tested using ANOVA on $\log_2(1+x)$ values [3]. The false discovery rate (FDR) was estimated using the Benjamini–Hochberg method. All statistical analyses were performed using R software v3.3.1. Transcript annotation and classification were performed using the BioMart interface to the Ensembl database. Identification of transcription factor binding sites in the promoter regions corresponding to the identified transcripts was performed using the seqinspector (seqinspector.cremag.org) [20]. The data stored in seqinspector included ENCODE ChIP-seq tracks and data deposited in the Gene Expression Omnibus (GEO).

Variant identification

Initial analysis of transcripts from the *Dclk1* locus was based on GRCm38.p5/mm10, which lists 15 variants. A new variant was identified in the mouse NAc after mianserin treatment using Cufflinks. The new transcript was selected based on the abundance level (FPKM) calculated by Cufflinks; selection criteria were F (min-isoform-fraction) = 0.005 and j (pre-mRNA-fraction) = 0.15. The depth parameter for each nucleotide of the *Dclk1* transcript was computed using Samtools depth v0.1.19. The abundance levels for intron regions were calculated as the median read coverage of the intron.

Quantitative PCR

Reverse transcription was performed with the Omniscript Reverse Transcriptase (Qiagen Inc.). qPCR was performed using TaqMan Gene Expression Assays ("probe 1": Mm00444950_m1—exons 4–5 of *Dclk1*; "probe 2": Mm01545304_m1—exons 6–7 of *Dcl*; "probe 5": Mm01512375_m1—exons 13–14 of *Cpg16*; "probe 3": custom designed for 5′ intron 6 of *Dclk1* using Custom TaqMan Assay Design Tool, assay ID: AJ20T2J, "probe 4": custom designed for 3′ intron 6 of *Dclk1*, assay ID: AI0IY5 V). The reactions were run on the CFX96 Real-Time system (Bio-Rad). Each template was generated from an individual animal. Expression of the hypoxanthine–guanine phosphoribosyltransferase 1 (*Hprt1*) transcript was used to control for variations in cDNA concentrations. The abundance of each RNA was calculated as $2^{-(\text{threshold cycle})}$. The data were analyzed using one-way analysis of variance (ANOVA) followed by Tukey's HSD.

Protein isolation

For the proteomics assessment, NAc samples were collected after 5 days of mianserin treatment. Immediately after removal, the tissue was homogenized in 1% SDS using the Rotor Stator Homogenizer (IKA®-Werke, Staufen, Germany) and cleared by centrifugation (16,000*g* for 3 min). The protein concentration in the supernatant was determined using the BCA Protein Assay Kit (Sigma-Aldrich). Samples containing 50 µg of protein were heated in Laemmli 6 × loading buffer for 5 min at 95 °C and resolved by sodium dodecyl sulphate–polyacrylamide gel electrophoresis (SDS-PAGE; 18% Criterion™ TGX™ Precast Gels, Bio-Rad). After electrophoresis, the gel was transferred to 40% methanol/20% acetic acid and stained with Coomassie brilliant blue R250 overnight. Bands corresponding to the < 10 kD fraction of peptides according to the Polypeptide 1.4–26.6 kD SDS-PAGE Standard (Bio-Rad, #1610326) were excised from the gel.

LC–MS/MS analysis

The procedure is based on a previously reported protocol [21]. First, we injected the heavy-labeled peptide for shotgun LC–MS/MS analysis at 1 pmol. Peptide retention time was determined and a spectral library was constructed in Skyline software version 3.7. Then, the peptide was measured using the scheduled parallel reaction monitoring (PRM) mode. At 10 fmol per injection no contamination with light counterparts was observed.

The gel band was alternately washed with 25% acetonitrile (ACN)/25 mM $(NH_4)HCO_3$ (ABC) and 50% ACN/25 mM ABC, dehydrated with 100% ACN and then air dried. Then, the band was re-swelled in 25 mM ABC containing endoproteinase LysC (Promega) and digested overnight at 37 °C. The reaction was stopped by addition of CF_3COOH (TFA), and peptides were collected, vacuum dried and resuspended in the solution containing heavy-labeled peptide.

The samples were analyzed using a Q-Exactive mass spectrometer (Thermo Scientific) coupled with nano-HPLC (UltiMate 3000 RSLCnano System, Thermo Scientific). Peptides were loaded onto a trap column (AcclaimPepMap100 C18, Thermo Scientific; ID 75 μm, length 20 mm, particle size 3 μm, pore size 100 Å) in 2% ACN/0.05% TFA at a flow rate of 5 μl/min and then separated on an analytical column (AcclaimPepMapRLSC C18, Thermo Scientific; ID 75 μm, length 500 mm, particle size 2 μm, pore size 100 Å) using a 30 min gradient of ACN from 2 to 40% in the presence of 0.05% formic acid at a flow rate of 300 nl/min. A digital PicoView 550 ion source (New Objective) was used for ionization. Labeled peptide and its light counterpart were isolated in scheduled PRM with a 2 m/z window and fragmented with a normalized collision energy of 25. Resulting ions were collected with a maximum injection time of 500 ms and an automatic gain control (AGC) target value of 2.0×10^4. Measurements were collected at a resolution of 140,000. Data were analyzed using Skyline software (version 3.7). The signal corresponding to the SPSPSPTSPGSLRK peptide

was verified by confirming its coelution with the heavy-labeled counterpart and by comparing the fragment ion area ratios in peptide pairs.

Results

Changes in Dclk1 expression in response to psychotropic drugs

First, we reexamined the expression of alternatively spliced transcripts from the Dclk1 locus based on the previously reported dataset describing the effects of various psychotropic drugs on the mouse striatum [2]. The results of the analysis are shown in Fig. 1. Panel A shows a schematic representation of the main transcripts of the mouse Dclk1 gene based on the NCBI37/mm9 mouse genome release. Regions corresponding to probes from the MouseWG-6 v2 BeadChip are marked with blue or red symbols. Probes correspond to nonoverlapping transcripts and neither detected the full-length canonical Dclk1 transcript. As shown in the reanalysis of the array data presented in panel B, levels of transcripts detected by the probes were differentially affected by treatments with psychotropic drugs.

The mRNA levels measured using the first microarray probe (ILMN_1259689, presented as a red star in Fig. 1; drug P value $= 4.14 \times 10^{-16}$, time P-value $= 9.9 \times 10^{-15}$, interaction P-value $= 4.2 \times 10^{-5}$) indicated increased expression after the administration of mianserin (1, 2 and 4 h after the injection), risperidone (1 and 2 h) and, to a lesser extent, haloperidol (2 h) treatments (Fig. 1b). The second probe (ILMN_2434274, blue star; drug P-value $= 4.68 \times 10^{-16}$, time P-value $= 1.2 \times 10^{-4}$, interaction P-value $= 2.5 \times 10^{-7}$) revealed a different pattern of regulation, with an increase in mRNA abundance levels 8 h after the tranylcypromine treatment. Analysis of the array profiling results showed isoform-specific regulation of Dclk1 expression by psychotropic drugs. However, the interpretation was also confounded by ambiguous detection of the Dclk1 transcripts.

(See figure on next page.)
Fig. 1 Schematic representation of the Dclk1 gene and psychotropic drug treatment-mediated regulation of its expression. **a** Main transcripts of the Dclk1 locus: two Cpg16 variants (ENSMUST00000198437, ENSMUST00000070418), Carp (ENSMUST00000199585), intron-retained isoform (RI, ENSMUST00000198757), Dcl (ENSMUST00000167204) and Dclk1 (ENSMUST00000054237). The positions of the microarray probes are indicated by the stars. The schematic was generated based on information in the Ensembl database and available literature [6, 26]. The functional protein domains are boxed (SP is the serine/proline-rich domain). **b** Results from the microarray gene expression analysis are presented as time courses (1, 2, 4 and 8 h) of fold changes in expression compared to levels observed in saline-treated controls (as described in the legend). The measurements from two microarray probes are presented. The left side of the figure shows Dclk1 levels based on the ILMN_1259689 probe, whereas the right side corresponds to ILMN_2434274. The list of analyzed drugs include mianserin (MIA), imipramine (IMI), fluoxetine (FLU), bupropion (BUP), tianeptine (TIA), tranylcypromine (TRA), methamphetamine (MET), cocaine (COC), nicotine (NIC), heroin (HER), morphine (MOR), ethanol (ETO), diazepam (DIA), buspirone (BUS), hydroxyzine (HYD), clozapine (CLO), risperidone (RIS), haloperidol (HAL), saline (SAL), and naive (NAI) control. *P < 0.01, **P < 0.001, ***P < 0.0001, one-way ANOVA of the drug factor

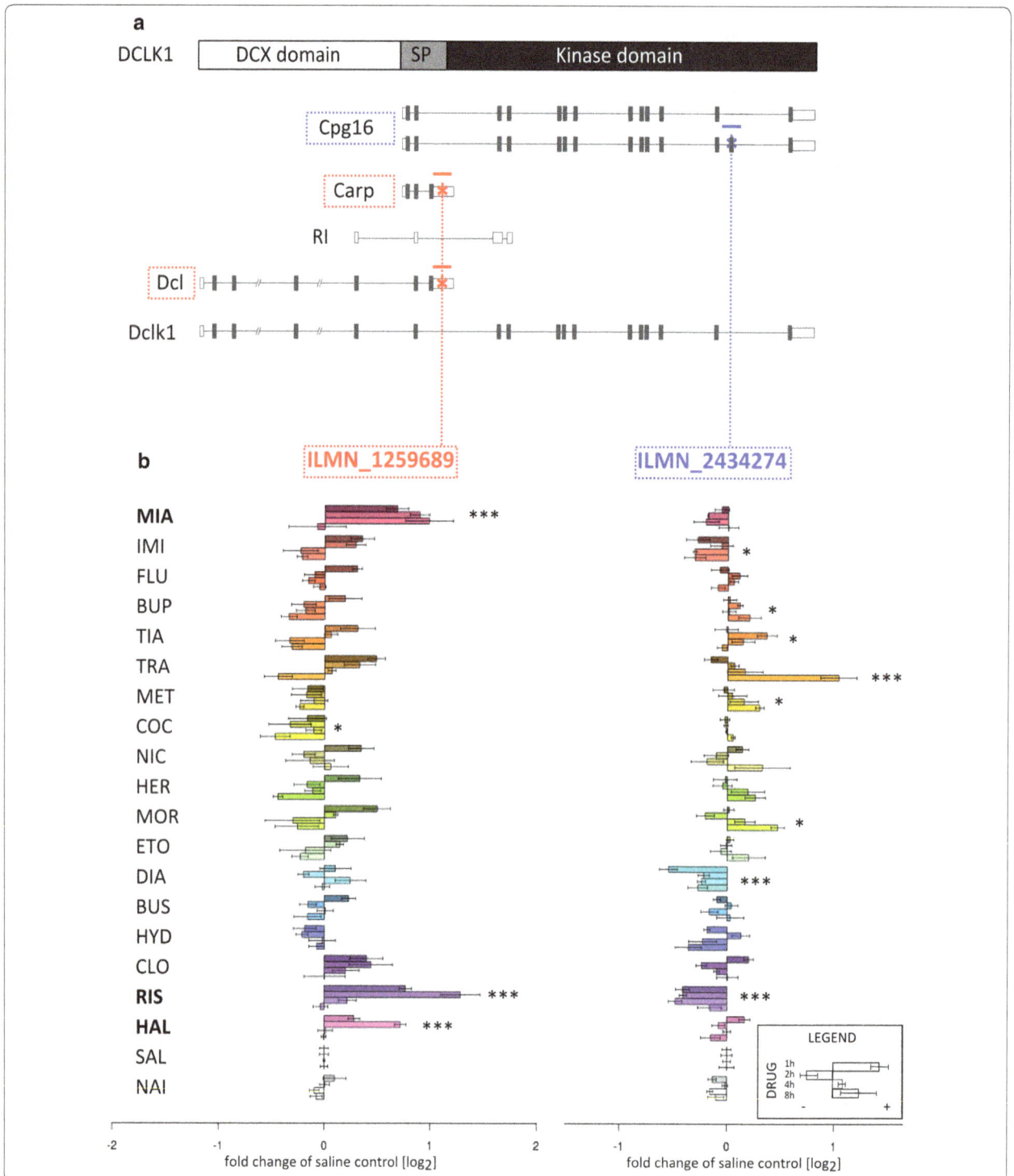

Transcriptome profiling of the effects of psychotropic drugs using RNA sequencing

We used next-generation sequencing to comprehensively examine drug-induced *Dclk1* gene expression at the level of specific transcriptional units. Sequencing was performed on ribo-depleted RNA samples derived from the mouse nucleus accumbens septi (NAc) and prefrontal cortex (PFCx) 2 h after treatment with antidepressants (venlafaxine and mianserin), antipsychotics (haloperidol and risperidone), a psychostimulant (methamphetamine) or a psychotomimetic (ketamine).

We measured normalized transcript abundance levels (FPKM) for all transcripts annotated in the GRCm38.p5 genome release using the Cufflinks package. A total of 110,327 different transcripts corresponding to 45,935 annotated genes were detected in the PFCx or NAc at the threshold of a mean FPKM ≥ 0.1.

The overall differences in drug-induced gene expression between the NAc and PFCx were assessed using a one-way ANOVA for drug factor performed separately in each tissue. We found 90 transcripts regulated by the treatment only in the NAc and 246 transcripts altered in the PFC (at FDR < 0.0001). The examples of regulated genes are *Map6* and *Cdkn1a* in the NAc, and *Bhlhe40* and *Fkbp5* in the PFC. We also identified 26 transcripts regulated in both the analyzed tissues above the threshold, including *Homer1*, *Sgk1* and *Fosb* (Additional file 1: Figure S1).

Drug-regulated changes in transcript levels were classified by biotypes and alternatively spliced events. Notably, 78% of regulated transcripts in the NAc and 65% of the transcripts in the PFCx encoded proteins, compared with 56% of the transcripts expressed in the NAc or PFCx under basal conditions (Additional file 2: Figure S2). Among the drug-induced alterations, an enrichment of protein-coding variants was observed, although the majority of noncoding, regulated transcripts were classified as intron-retained transcripts.

We used a two-way ANOVA with the drug and tissue as factors to identify drug-regulated changes in transcript levels (arbitrary cutoff at treatment effect FDR < 0.001; Additional file 3: Figure S3). Figure 2 shows the hierarchical clustering of the top 113 transcripts, grouped into four clusters. Transcripts from the four main branches were examined for overrepresented putative transcription factor binding sites in their promoter regions using seqinspector [20].

Transcripts from the first pattern were upregulated by mianserin in both brain regions. Their expression also increased in the NAc in response to risperidone and haloperidol treatments. Examples of transcripts clustered in this group included *Sgk1*, *Nfkbia* and the long noncoding RNA *Neat1*. Promoters of these transcripts exhibit a significant overrepresentation of the ChIP-seq signal for several transcriptional factors, including GR (P $= 9.7 \times 10^{-6}$, *t*-test with Bonferroni's correction, track GEO accession: GSM686976), E2F1 (P $= 1.1 \times 10^{-6}$, GSM881056) and NFKB1 (P $= 1 \times 10^{-5}$, GSM88115). Haloperidol, methamphetamine and, to a lesser extent, risperidone induced the expression of the greatest number of transcripts (pattern 2) in the NAc. The strongest induction in the PFCx was observed after methamphetamine treatment. Pattern

2 included several genes involved in the molecular control of neuronal plasticity, such as *Fosb*, *Arc*, *Junb* or *Homer1*. The promoters of these transcripts contained a different set of putative transcriptional regulator binding sites, including SRF (P $= 1.2 \times 10^{-22}$, GSM530190) and EGR2 (P $= 4.7 \times 10^{-12}$, GSM881094). The expression of the third group of transcripts (pattern 3, e.g., *Celf2* and *Dclk1*) was induced by mianserin, with stronger effects observed in the NAc. We only identified one overrepresented potential transcriptional regulator of these genes, TBP (P $= 3.5 \times 10^{-7}$). The TBP binding motif was present in 18 of the 28 total genes. The *Dclk1* transcript was clustered into pattern 3. Notably, at the statistical threshold used to analyze the whole transcriptome, we observed significant changes in the levels of the transcript for only one *Dclk1* isoform, a noncoding variant with a retained intron (ENSMUST00000198757). Finally, the expression of transcripts from pattern 4, including *Clk1* and *Hes5*, decreased after mianserin treatment in both brain regions. Significantly overrepresented TFB sites were not present in the upstream promoter regions of transcripts from this cluster.

The profile of the drug-specific transcripts corresponding to the *Dclk1* locus was obtained by comparing the results of two high-throughput gene profiling methods-microarray (Fig. 1) and RNA-sequencing (Fig. 2).

Isoform-specific regulation of *Dclk1* expression

Next, we performed a detailed analysis of the sequencing results mapped to the *Dclk1* locus. Based on the assignments from Cufflinks using the GRCm38.p5 mouse genome release, sequencing reads corresponded to 12 transcripts expressed from the *Dclk1* locus (at FPKM > 1), with 8 highly abundant isoforms (FPKM > 5). Three isoforms were not detected in the NAc or PFCx (ENSMUST00000198821, ENSMUST00000197870, and ENSMUST00000196745). The majority of the sequencing reads corresponded to Carp (ENSMUST00000199585), Dcl (ENSMUST00000167204) and Cpg16 (ENSMUST00000198437). Two of the transcripts assembled by Cufflinks contained retained introns and had not previously been described (Additional file 4: Figure S4). Relative changes in the abundance of the transcripts are shown in Fig. 3.

The expression of the Carp transcript in the NAc was induced in response to mianserin (log$_2$FC $= 1.78$, P $= 0.0002$), risperidone (log$_2$FC $= 1.07$, P $= 0.007$) and venlafaxine (log$_2$FC $= 1.01$, P $= 0.009$). Carp expression in the PFCx was only regulated only mianserin (log$_2$FC $= 1.57$, P $= 0.0027$). The level of the Cpg16 transcript was not significantly altered in any of the analyzed brain regions upon drug treatment. The venlafaxine treatment downregulated the expression of the Dcl isoform in

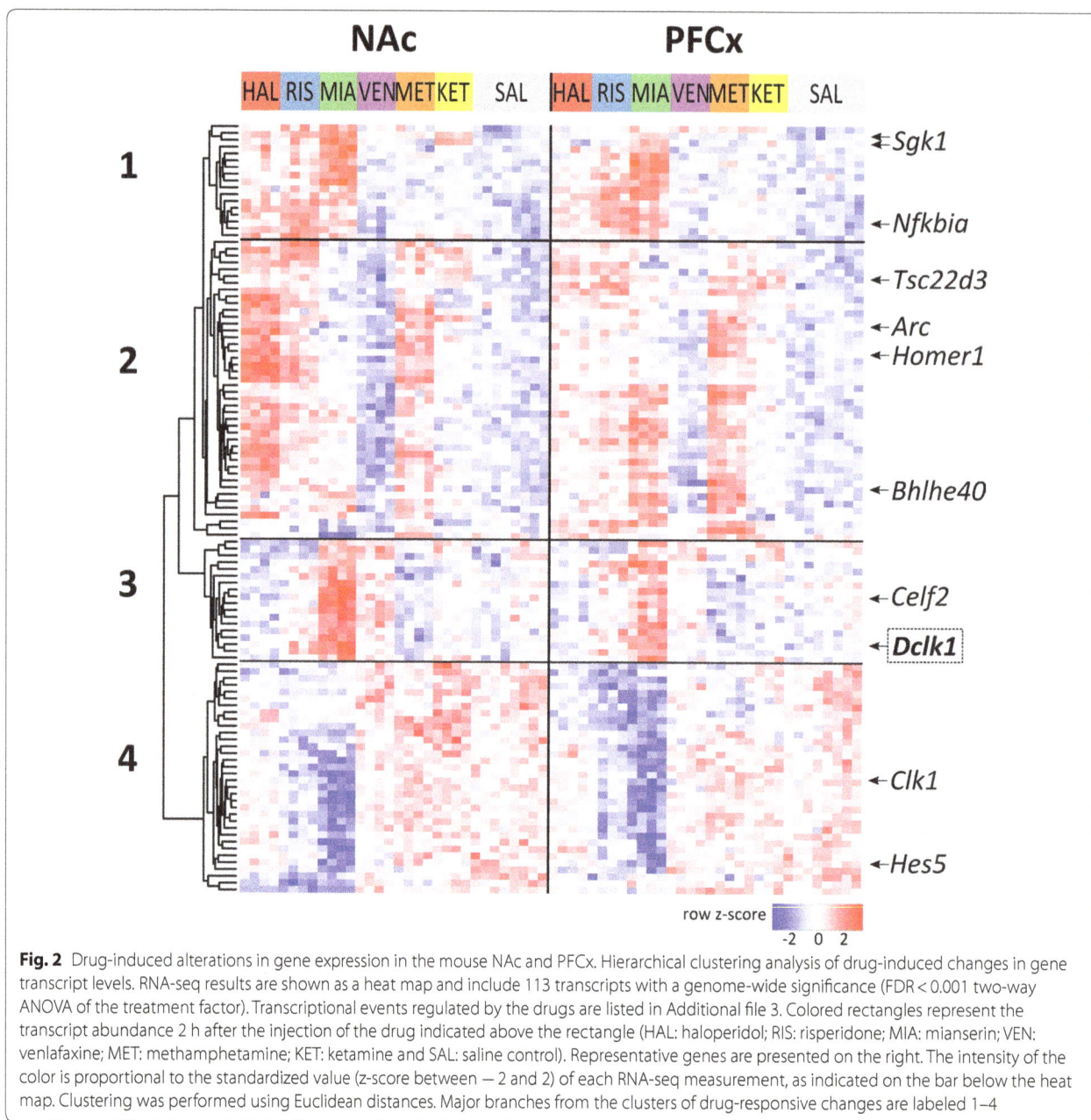

Fig. 2 Drug-induced alterations in gene expression in the mouse NAc and PFCx. Hierarchical clustering analysis of drug-induced changes in gene transcript levels. RNA-seq results are shown as a heat map and include 113 transcripts with a genome-wide significance (FDR < 0.001 two-way ANOVA of the treatment factor). Transcriptional events regulated by the drugs are listed in Additional file 3. Colored rectangles represent the transcript abundance 2 h after the injection of the drug indicated above the rectangle (HAL: haloperidol; RIS: risperidone; MIA: mianserin; VEN: venlafaxine; MET: methamphetamine; KET: ketamine and SAL: saline control). Representative genes are presented on the right. The intensity of the color is proportional to the standardized value (z-score between − 2 and 2) of each RNA-seq measurement, as indicated on the bar below the heat map. Clustering was performed using Euclidean distances. Major branches from the clusters of drug-responsive changes are labeled 1–4

the NAc ($\log_2$FC $= -0.74$, P $= 0.078$). However, the level of the Dcl transcript in the PFCx increased in response to the mianserin treatment ($\log_2$FC $= 0.46$, P $= 0.0009$). The expression of the full-length *Dclk1* transcript (ENS-MUST00000054237) was below the level of detection in the NAc, and no significant changes were observed in the PFCx. The expression of the intron-retained isoform (RI) was substantially upregulated by mianserin ($\log_2$FC $= 0.9$, P $= 2.8 \times 10^{-6}$) and risperidone ($\log_2$FC $= 0.49$, P $= 0.002$) in the NAc and by mianserin ($\log_2$FC $= 0.69$, P $= 0.0003$) in the PFCx.

Furthermore, when we mapped individual reads to the *Dclk1* locus, a considerable number of fragments did not match known transcripts and corresponded to a fragment annotated as an intronic region (Fig. 4b, red arrow). Exon-level analysis of the data suggested the presence of a novel transcript, referred to as Dclk1-m, with an alternative transcription start site (first exon), termination codon (last exon) and a sequence corresponding to the sixth intron of the canonical *Dclk1* transcript (ENS-MUST00000054237). The detected retention of intron 6 is unlikely to correspond to an unspliced pre-mRNA.

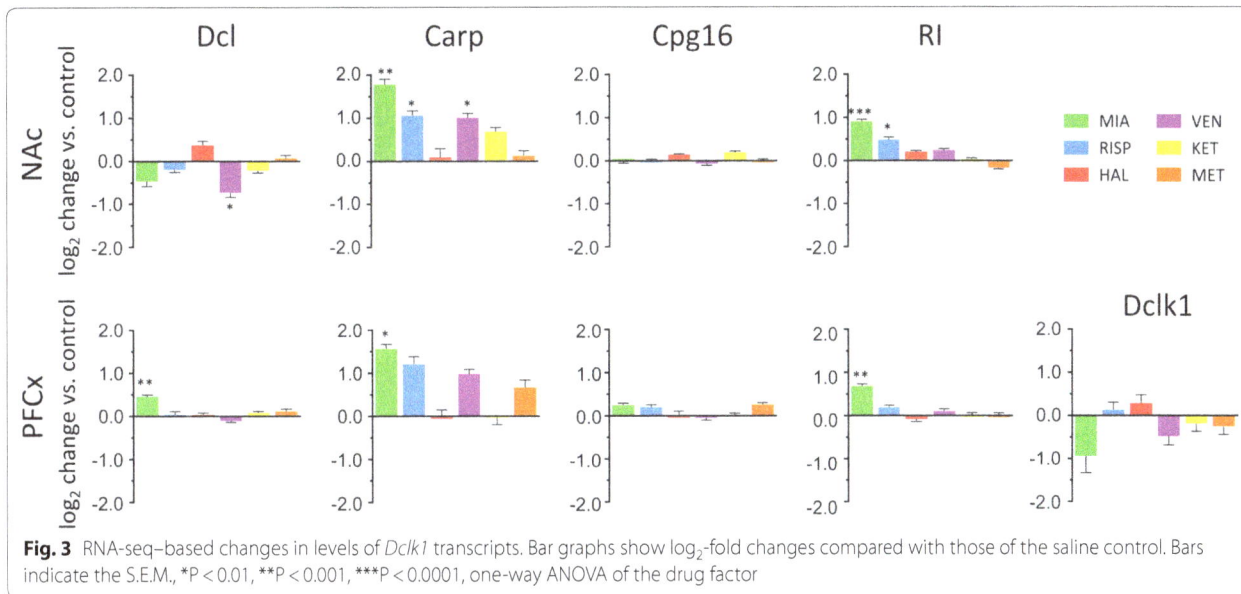

Fig. 3 RNA-seq–based changes in levels of *Dclk1* transcripts. Bar graphs show log$_2$-fold changes compared with those of the saline control. Bars indicate the S.E.M., *P < 0.01, **P < 0.001, ***P < 0.0001, one-way ANOVA of the drug factor

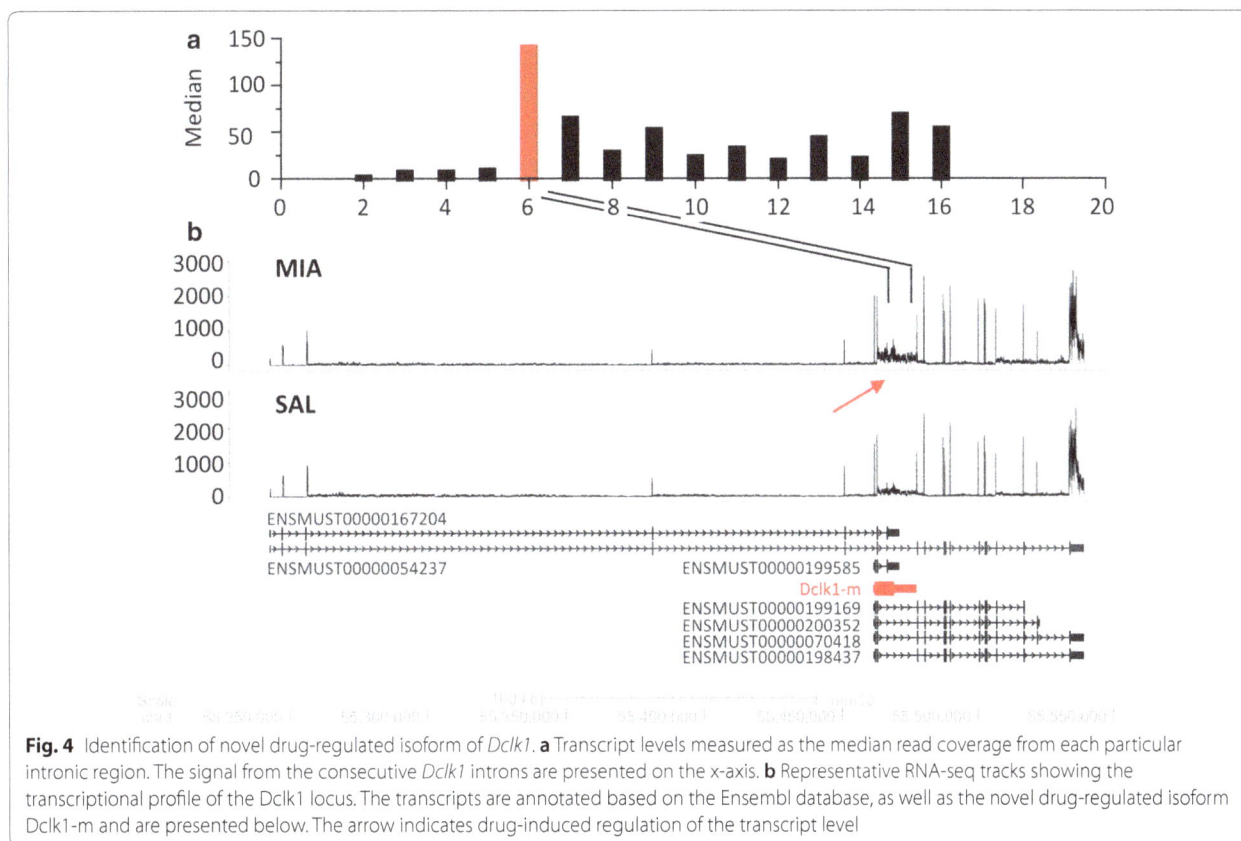

Fig. 4 Identification of novel drug-regulated isoform of *Dclk1*. **a** Transcript levels measured as the median read coverage from each particular intronic region. The signal from the consecutive *Dclk1* introns are presented on the x-axis. **b** Representative RNA-seq tracks showing the transcriptional profile of the Dclk1 locus. The transcripts are annotated based on the Ensembl database, as well as the novel drug-regulated isoform Dclk1-m and are presented below. The arrow indicates drug-induced regulation of the transcript level

The level of intron coverage calculated as the median read coverage for each position at each intron was significantly higher (P = 0.002) for this intron compared with that of other introns (Fig. 4a).

Based on the frequency of the sequence reads corresponding to the Dclk1-m variant, the expression of this isoform was upregulated in the PFCx by the mianserin treatment (log$_2$FC = 0.679, P = 0.0000253) and in

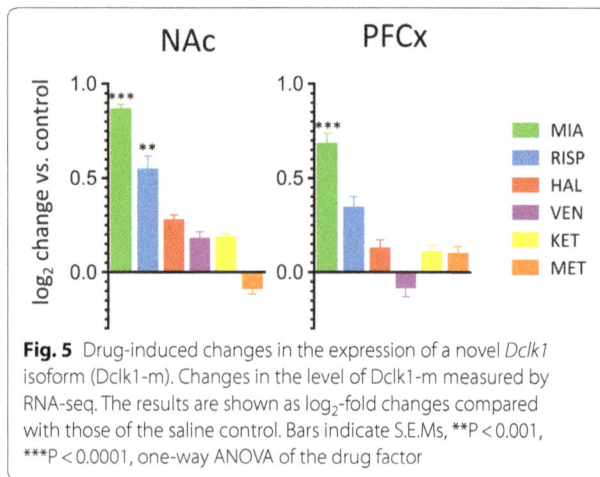

Fig. 5 Drug-induced changes in the expression of a novel *Dclk1* isoform (Dclk1-m). Changes in the level of Dclk1-m measured by RNA-seq. The results are shown as $\log_2$-fold changes compared with those of the saline control. Bars indicate S.E.Ms, $**P < 0.001$, $***P < 0.0001$, one-way ANOVA of the drug factor

the NAc by mianserin and risperidone ($\log_2 FC = 0.862$, $P = 3.8 \times 10^{-8}$; $\log_2 FC = 0.542$, $P = 0.00079$, respectively; Fig. 5 and Additional file 5: Figure S5). Notably, the ILMN_1259689 probe shown in Fig. 1 hybridized with Dclk1-m. In conclusion, next-generation sequencing analysis confirmed the drug-specific induction of transcription from the Dclk1 locus and showed that psychotropic drugs affected the transcription of a short region close to the sequence encoding the serine-proline rich domain. Most importantly, changes in transcription might actually represent a novel transcript, Dclk1-m.

Validation of drug-induced expression of *Dclk1* isoforms

We designed a series of isoform-specific probes for qPCR to confirm which of the transcripts exhibited increased expression in response to drug treatments. The analysis was performed on a new set of samples obtained from mice euthanized 2 h after the i.p. injection of mianserin (20 mg/kg), risperidone (0.5 mg/kg), haloperidol (1 mg/kg) or saline (n = 8). Five fluorescent probe assays were used to analyze changes in the expression of *Dclk1* transcripts; two of the assays were specifically designed to detect the isoform containing the retained intron (Fig. 6, 5′ region of intron 6 and 3′ region of intron 6).

The mianserin treatment increased the levels of transcripts containing intron 6 in the NAc (approximately 1.5-fold). The level of Cpg16 was slightly decreased, whereas levels of Dcl/Carp were not different from those of the saline-treated control group. Risperidone significantly induced the expression of the Dclk1/Dcl isoform (approximately 1.2-fold), as well as transcripts containing intron 6 (approximately 1.6- to 2.1-fold). The haloperidol treatment had no effect on the expression of *Dclk1* isoforms in the NAc. In the PFCx, the mianserin treatment upregulated the expression of Dcl/Carp isoforms (1.5-fold), as well as transcripts containing intron 6 (more

than twofold). Risperidone did not regulate the expression of *Dclk1* isoforms in the PFCx. The haloperidol treatment slightly decreased the expression of a variant containing part of intron 6 in the PFCx (Fig. 6 and Additional file 6: Figure S6).

We also performed two additional experiments and measured the transcript levels 4 h after a single treatment and 2 h after 5 days of treatment. The mianserin treatment significantly increased levels of Dclk1-m in the NAc. The effect of mianserin on *Dclk1* expression was not detected 5 days after repeated drug treatment (Additional file 7: Figure S7). Together, these data confirm that Dclk1-m expression is acutely increased in response to the mianserin treatment. Levels of other *Dclk1* transcripts were not increased in response to the mianserin treatment, with the possible exception of Carp.

Functional features of the newly detected *Dclk1* variant

Finally, we used mass spectrometry to determine whether protein products of the Dclk1-m transcript were detected. Dclk1-m and Carp sequences overlap on the 5′ side of the putative protein-coding sequences; only the C-termini differ. Both sequences include the proline- and serine-rich (SP-rich) region that interacts with other proteins. Mass spectrometry analysis of the SDS-PAGE-purified protein fraction with a molecular weight less than 10 kDa confirmed the presence of the SP-rich fragment (Fig. 7). Shotgun LC–MS/MS analysis, performed in addition to PRM, did not show a presence of other fragments derived from either CARP or DCLK1-M. Thus, we were only able to conclude that either or both the DCLK1-M and CARP proteins are translated.

Discussion

Our results reveal the existence of a novel *Dclk1* isoform (Dclk1-m), the expression of which is induced in the nucleus accumbens and prefrontal cortex of the brain after treatment with psychotropic drugs that affect 5HT2A/C receptor signaling (i.e., mianserin and risperidone). It should be noted here that these drug-related effects are relatively unspecific in pharmacological action, and transcription might be triggered by the activity of more than one type of neuronal receptors. Notably, Dclk1-m is the main, if not exclusive *Dclk1* transcript whose expression appears to be regulated by drugs. At present, we were not able to unequivocally establish whether Dclk1-m is translated; we were only able to confirm that protein products of Dclk1-m or Carp were present.

The identification of Dclk1-m revises and extends observations from our previous reports, where we detected an increase in *Dclk1* expression after treatment with mianserin and risperidone [2, 3, 13]. However, due

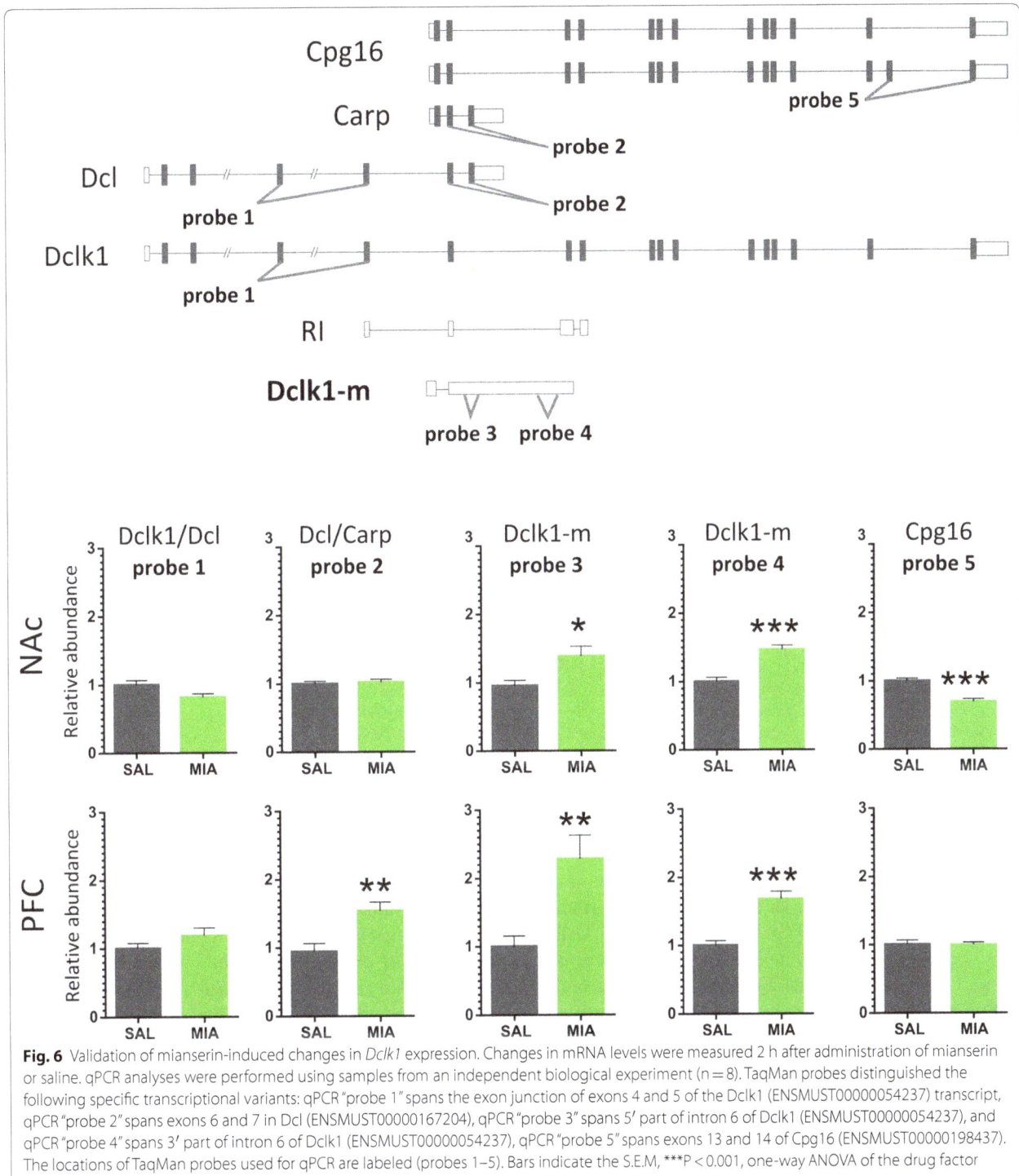

Fig. 6 Validation of mianserin-induced changes in *Dclk1* expression. Changes in mRNA levels were measured 2 h after administration of mianserin or saline. qPCR analyses were performed using samples from an independent biological experiment (n = 8). TaqMan probes distinguished the following specific transcriptional variants: qPCR "probe 1" spans the exon junction of exons 4 and 5 of the Dclk1 (ENSMUST00000054237) transcript, qPCR "probe 2" spans exons 6 and 7 in Dcl (ENSMUST00000167204), qPCR "probe 3" spans 5′ part of intron 6 of Dclk1 (ENSMUST00000054237), and qPCR "probe 4" spans 3′ part of intron 6 of Dclk1 (ENSMUST00000054237), qPCR "probe 5" spans exons 13 and 14 of Cpg16 (ENSMUST00000198437). The locations of TaqMan probes used for qPCR are labeled (probes 1–5). Bars indicate the S.E.M, ***P < 0.001, one-way ANOVA of the drug factor

to limitations regarding the array methodology used in our previous study, we were not able to discern exactly which transcripts were induced by drug actions in many cases. The array probes used in gene expression arrays may actually be detecting Dclk1-m, Carp and Dcl. Furthermore, we postulate that other previous reports may

have been reporting changes in Dclk1-m expression, as well. We concluded that drug treatment regulated the expression of brain-specific isoforms of *Dclk1* with an alternatively spliced last exon—either Dcl or Carp. In-depth analysis of RNA-seq data revealed that psychotropic drug treatments induced the expression of a

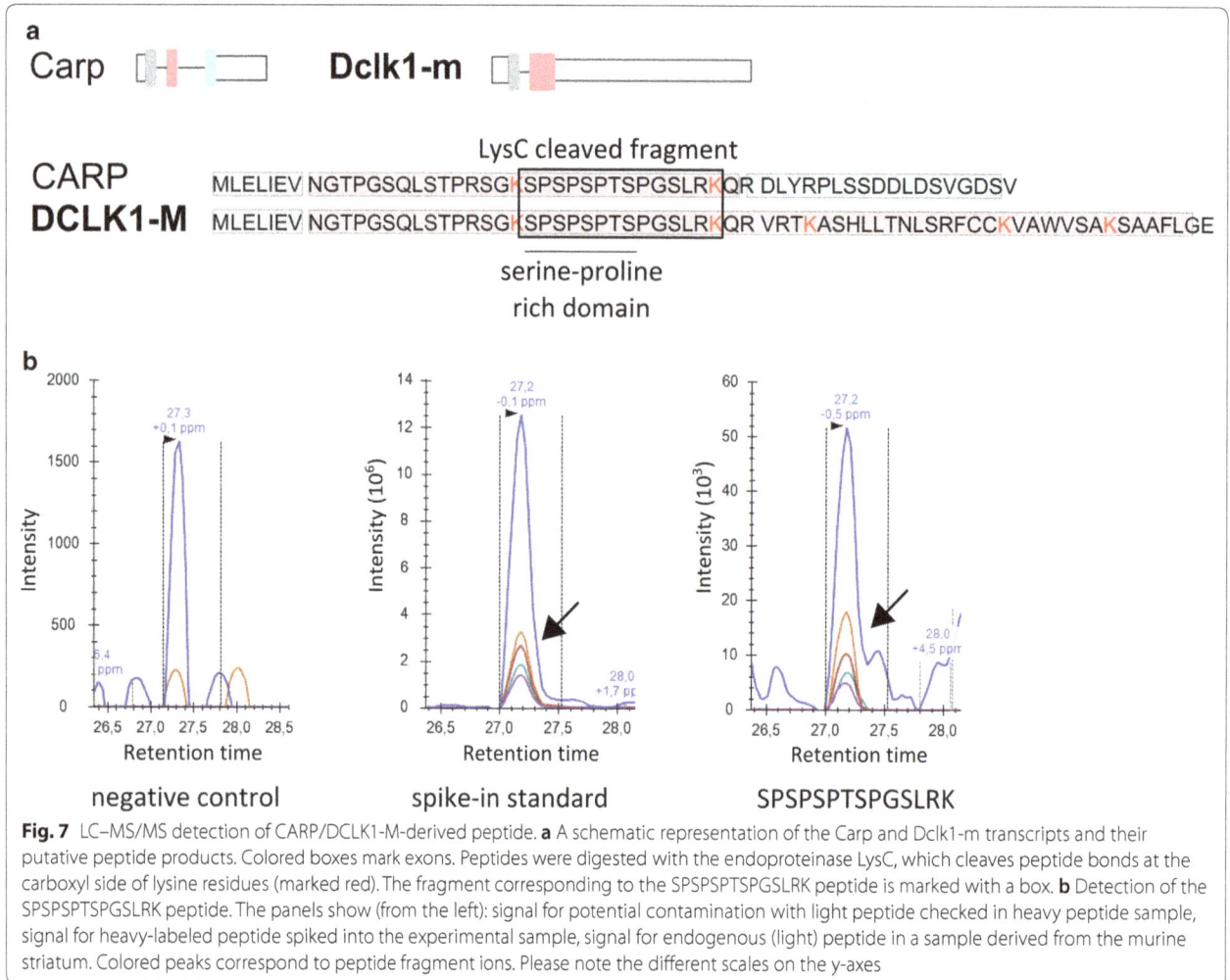

Fig. 7 LC–MS/MS detection of CARP/DCLK1-M-derived peptide. **a** A schematic representation of the Carp and Dclk1-m transcripts and their putative peptide products. Colored boxes mark exons. Peptides were digested with the endoproteinase LysC, which cleaves peptide bonds at the carboxyl side of lysine residues (marked red). The fragment corresponding to the SPSPSPTSPGSLRK peptide is marked with a box. **b** Detection of the SPSPSPTSPGSLRK peptide. The panels show (from the left): signal for potential contamination with light peptide checked in heavy peptide sample, signal for heavy-labeled peptide spiked into the experimental sample, signal for endogenous (light) peptide in a sample derived from the murine striatum. Colored peaks correspond to peptide fragment ions. Please note the different scales on the y-axes

previously unannotated transcript. The expression of this transcript was upregulated in the NAc by mianserin and risperidone and in the PFCx by mianserin. The Dclk1-m isoform contains a retained intron covering the middle part of the *Dclk1* locus. Thus, this intron is a region of the gene important for the mechanisms of action of those drugs. Both mianserin and risperidone are potent antagonists of 5-HT2a receptors, which might mediate the effect on Dclk1-m transcription. Moreover, the addition of mianserin to typical antipsychotics improves their therapeutic efficacy in patients with schizophrenia [22]. Polymorphisms in the *Dclk1* gene are associated with the development of schizophrenia. Thus, the altered function of the *Dclk1* gene may be involved in both the etiology and treatment of this psychopathology. From our results, we can't ascertain whether the increase in Dclk1 isoform is sufficient to produce the therapeutic effects of the drugs. It is likely a more complex phenomenon and no single gene or transcript is solely responsible for the therapeutic effect.

The *Dclk1* gene has a complex structure and comprises at least 15 known transcriptional variants. Although *Dclk1* was first described as a brain-specific gene, the roles of *Dclk1* outside the nervous system have recently been the main area of study. *Dclk1* is expressed in a variety of cancer cells [23], with a functional role in tumor growth and progression. However, its general role in carcinogenesis and clinical significance as a potential diagnostic marker remain unclear [24]. The present analysis reveals the brain-region-specific regulation of the expression of *Dclk1* isoforms in response to treatments with various classes of psychotropic drugs. A comparative meta-analysis of drug-induced *Dclk1* expression profiles is difficult to perform due to the use of different experimental designs (organism, time and tissue selection) and methodologies. To our knowledge, this study is the first to show that *Dclk1* expression is regulated at the single-exon level. In general, our results are consistent with previous findings and complement them in many ways. The short, the *Dclk1* transcript Carp (also known as Ania-4) is considered an immediate early gene (IEG). The expression of this variant increases in striatal neurons within minutes of dopamine receptor D1 (D1) stimulation [25]. In the hippocampus, the Carp mRNA was upregulated following kainate-elicited seizures [9], adrenalectomy [26], brain-derived neurotrophic factor-induced long-term potentiation [27] and repeated exposures to glutamate in hippocampal slice cultures [28]. We only identified one study showing the regulation of *Dclk1* expression by psychotropic drugs; this study reported that chronic haloperidol, but not clozapine or olanzapine treatments [29], affect *Dclk1* transcription. However, based on the reported results, we were not able to distinguish between Dcl, Carp and Dclk1-m. Based on our results, the upregulation of Dclk1-m expression is transient, likely lasting only hours, and was not detected after repeated treatment with mianserin.

Interestingly, Dclk1-m potentially encodes a protein that includes the serine- and protein-rich peptide. Using mass spectrometry, we confirmed the presence of small proteins containing the SP-rich domain that were potentially derived from CARP or DCLK1-M. Therefore, the newly identified variant might be translated into a protein. The SP-rich domain shared by the CARP and DLCK1-M peptides is postulated to be responsible for interactions with other proteins. To our knowledge, the endogenous CARP peptide has never been identified in vivo. This domain is predicted to interact with proteins containing the Src homology (SH3) domain [30]. Indeed, CARP interacts with the adapter protein growth factor receptor-bound 2 (Grb2) that contains the SH3 domain in vitro [26]. Grb2 plays a role in the formation of dendritic spines, which is critical for synaptic development [31] and is implicated in regulating actin cytoskeleton dynamics [32] and in Ras-ERK kinase activation [33]. Thus, the observed effects on Dclk1-m expression may correspond to alterations at the protein level. We were not able to unequivocally establish whether Dclk1-m is translated, although we did confirm that protein products translated from Dclk1-m or Carp were indeed present.

Recent results suggest the involvement of DCLK1 in dendrite development, as the depletion of endogenous DCLK1 affects the complexity of dendritic branching and total dendritic length in neurons in vitro [34]. DCLK1 plays a critical role in cargo transport into dendrites; in particular, DCX domains are required for dense-core vesicle (DCV) trafficking that causes dendritic growth through the release of peptide neuromodulators [35]. Notably, DCLK1 kinase activity is not required for its ability to bind and bundle microtubules. One of the C-terminal variants (Cpg16) has also been suggested to be a candidate neural plasticity gene with a potential role in synaptic remodeling. In vitro,

CPG16 autophosphorylates and phosphorylates myelin basic protein, but the in vivo target of CPG16 remains unknown. CPG16 may be activated by a PKA-induced pathway. CARP was proposed to both modulate kinase activity [9] and enhance DCL-induced tubulin polymerization [36] in vitro. The proposed roles in synaptic plasticity were based in large part on in silico structural analysis. Taken together, the effects of the drug-induced expression of Dclk1-m on controlling synaptic dynamics might be mediated at multiple molecular levels.

Another interesting observation from our study is the expression levels of specific *Dclk1* isoforms. Generally, isoforms driven by the upstream promoter are expressed at high levels in mice during early stages of life (P0–P5), whereas downstream promoter-derived transcripts are adult-specific [37]. In our study, the most abundant isoform in both the NAc and PFCx is Cpg16, which is consistent with the literature [6]. Carp was reported to be exclusively expressed in adulthood, although some reports show that its expression in the mouse brain is undetectable under basal conditions but dramatically increases upon stimulation [25]. One of the unexpected findings from our study is that the full-length *Dclk1* isoform was detected in PFCx, although it was reported to only be expressed during brain development [6, 36]. Dcl expression has been reported in specific neuronal cell populations and implicated in adult neurogenesis [38, 39]. We concluded that the expression level of *Dclk1* isoforms might exhibit brain region-specific patterns. The number and different proportions of *Dclk1* isoforms make it very difficult to study in vitro. We aim to evaluate the expression of *Dclk1* isoforms in primary cultures of neurons and astrocytes [3]. We observed significant differences in the levels of *Dclk1* isoforms between primary cultures and brain tissues. Notably, the *Cpg16* isoform was expressed at high levels in vivo but was virtually undetectable in cell cultures. The full-length *Dclk1* transcript was expressed at higher levels in cultured neurons than in brain tissues. This finding is not surprising because primary neuronal cultures are derived from mouse embryos. Moreover, stimulation of neurons with kainic acid (activity-regulated gene expression) and astrocytes with dexamethasone (GR-dependent gene expression) did not change the expression of any *Dclk1* isoforms. Thus, studies of the mechanisms regulating the expression of *Dclk1* isoforms in the brain should not be conducted in vitro.

Conclusions

In conclusion, we identified a previously unknown *Dclk1* transcript, which is expressed in response to treatment with psychotropic drugs. This study enhances our understanding of brain plasticity by revealing that the expression of alternative *Dclk1* transcripts is an important component of the pharmacological treatment of neuropsychiatric disorders. Although further studies will allow researchers to determine the precise role of the newly discovered Dclk1-m variant, our findings reveal a previously unknown molecular mechanism of mianserin action. Moreover, our research also emphasizes the need to carefully analyze the raw data obtained from high-throughput gene expression profiling experiments, as analyses that are restricted to previously annotated transcripts might provide us with false-positive results, as in the case of *Dclk1* transcripts. The data reported here may also serve as a set of drug-specific transcriptional signatures in the PFCx and NAc.

Additional files

Additional file 1. The lists of transcripts and corresponding gene names that are altered by drug treatment after one-way ANOVA in each tissue (FDR < 0.0001).

Additional file 2. The charts presenting the distribution of transcripts biotypes among the drug-regulated transcripts in comparison to the entire transcriptome of the mouse nucleus accumbens and prefrontal cortex.

Additional file 3. Results from two-way ANOVA for 113 drug-responsive transcripts (FDR for drug factor < 0.001) are included. For each transcript, a fold change over control, p-value and FDR for drug and tissue factors and all the interactions are presented. Table also includes biotypes annotation and classification using the BioMart interface to the Ensembl gene database.

Additional file 4. RNA-seq results from two-way ANOVA for all Dclk1 isoforms reported in Ensembl gene database (GRCm38.p5/mm10). For each transcript, a fold change over control, p-value and FDR for drug and tissue factors and all the interactions are presented.

Additional file 5. Table summarizing the RNA-seq re-analysis for Dclk1 locus with Dclk1-m variant added. The first sheet presents the results from one-way ANOVA for NAc, the second sheet for PFCx. For each transcript, a fold change over control, p-value and FDR for drug is presented.

Additional file 6. Changes in mRNA levels were measured 2 h after administration of risperidone, haloperidol or saline control. qPCR analyses were performed using samples from an independent biological experiment (n = 8). TaqMan probes distinguished the following specific transcriptional variants: qPCR "probe 1" spans the exon junction of exons 4 and 5 of the Dclk1 (ENSMUST00000054237) transcript, qPCR "probe 2" spans exons 6 and 7 in Dcl (ENSMUST00000167204), qPCR "probe 3" spans 5′ part of intron 6 of Dclk1 (ENSMUST00000054237), qPCR "probe 4" spans 3′ part of intron 6 of Dclk1 (ENSMUST00000054237), qPCR "probe 5" spans exons 13 and 14 of Cpg16 (ENSMUST00000198437). The locations of TaqMan probes used for qPCR are labeled in Figure 6. Bars indicate the S.E.M., *P < 0.01, one-way ANOVA of the drug factor.

Additional file 7. Changes in mRNA levels were measured (A) 4 h after administration of mianserin or saline control (B) 2 h after 5 days of treatment with mianserin or saline. qPCR analyses were performed using samples from an independent biological experiment (n = 4). The locations of TaqMan probes used for qPCR are labeled in Figure 6. Bars indicate the S.E.M., **P < 0.001, one-way ANOVA of the drug factor.

Abbreviations

Dclk1: doublecortin-like kinase 1; FDR: false discovery rate; FPKM: fragments per kilobase of transcript per million fragments mapped; MS: mass spectrometry; NAc: nucleus accumbens; NGS: next-generation sequencing; PFCx: prefrontal cortex; PRM: parallel reaction monitoring.

Authors' contributions

DH, JH and MP performed statistical and bioinformatics analyses. MZ performed whole-transcriptome resequencing and qPCR validation. MZ, MK and JRP interpreted the results, designed the study and drafted the manuscript. BSR, UJ and SKK performed the LC–MS/MS analysis. All authors agreed to be accountable for all aspects of the work in ensuring that questions related to the accuracy or integrity of any part of the work are appropriately investigated and resolved. All authors read and approved the final manuscript.

Author details

[1] Department of Molecular Neuropharmacology, Institute of Pharmacology of the Polish Academy of Sciences, Smetna 12, 31-343 Krakow, Poland. [2] Laboratory of Proteomics and Mass Spectrometry, Malopolska Centre of Biotechnology, Jagiellonian University, Krakow, Poland. [3] Department of Physical Biochemistry, Faculty of Biochemistry, Biophysics and Biotechnology, Jagiellonian University, Krakow, Poland.

Acknowledgements

Not applicable.

Competing interests

The authors declare that they have no competing interests.

Funding

This work was supported by the National Science Centre Poland Grant [2011/03/D/NZ3/01686] and statutory funds of the Institute of Pharmacology PAS. MZ was supported by National Science Centre Poland Grant [2016/23/N/NZ3/00133].

References

1. Brennand KJ, Simone A, Tran N, Gage FH. Modeling psychiatric disorders at the cellular and network levels. Mol Psychiatry. 2012;17(12):1239–53.
2. Korostynski M, Piechota M, Dzbek J, Mlynarski W, Szklarczyk K, Ziolkowska B, Przewlocki R. Novel drug-regulated transcriptional networks in brain reveal pharmacological properties of psychotropic drugs. BMC Genom. 2013;14:606.
3. Piechota M, Golda S, Ficek J, Jantas D, Przewlocki R, Korostynski M. Regulation of alternative gene transcription in the striatum in response to antidepressant drugs. Neuropharmacology. 2015;99:328–36.
4. Gordon-Weeks PR, Fournier AE. Neuronal cytoskeleton in synaptic plasticity and regeneration. J Neurochem. 2014;129(2):206–12.
5. Shin E, Kashiwagi Y, Kuriu T, Iwasaki H, Tanaka T, Koizumi H, Gleeson JG, Okabe S. Doublecortin-like kinase enhances dendritic remodelling and negatively regulates synapse maturation. Nat Commun. 2013;4:1440.
6. Burgess HA, Reiner O. Alternative splice variants of doublecortin-like kinase are differentially expressed and have different kinase activities. J Biol Chem. 2002;277(20):17696–705.
7. Havik B, Degenhardt FA, Johansson S, Fernandes CP, Hinney A, Scherag A, Lybaek H, Djurovic S, Christoforou A, Ersland KM, et al. DCLK1 variants are associated across schizophrenia and attention deficit/hyperactivity disorder. PLoS ONE. 2012;7(4):e35424.
8. Wu JQ, Wang X, Beveridge NJ, Tooney PA, Scott RJ, Carr VJ, Cairns MJ. Transcriptome sequencing revealed significant alteration of cortical promoter usage and splicing in schizophrenia. PLoS ONE. 2012;7(4):e36351.
9. Vreugdenhil E, Datson N, Engels B, de Jong J, van Koningsbruggen S, Schaaf M, de Kloet ER. Kainate-elicited seizures induce mRNA encoding a CaMK-related peptide: a putative modulator of kinase activity in rat hippocampus. J Neurobiol. 1999;39(1):41–50.

10. Burgess HA, Martinez S, Reiner O. KIAA0369, doublecortin-like kinase, is expressed during brain development. J Neurosci Res. 1999;58(4):567–75.
11. Silverman MA, Benard O, Jaaro H, Rattner A, Citri Y, Seger R. CPG16, a novel protein serine/threonine kinase downstream of cAMP-dependent protein kinase. J Biol Chem. 1999;274(5):2631–6.
12. Engels BM, Schouten TG, van Dullemen J, Gosens I, Vreugdenhil E. Functional differences between two DCLK splice variants. Brain Res Mol Brain Res. 2004;120(2):103–14.
13. Ficek J, Zygmunt M, Piechota M, Hoinkis D, Rodriguez Parkitna J, Przewlocki R, Korostynski M. Molecular profile of dissociative drug ketamine in relation to its rapid antidepressant action. BMC Genom. 2016;17:362.
14. van de Waterbeemd H, Camenisch G, Folkers G, Chretien JR, Raevsky OA. Estimation of blood–brain barrier crossing of drugs using molecular size and shape, and H-bonding descriptors. J Drug Target. 1998;6(2):151–65.
15. Altamura AC, De Novellis F, Mauri MC, Gomeni R. Plasma and brain pharmacokinetics of mianserin after single and multiple dosing in mice. Prog Neuropsychopharmacol Biol Psychiatry. 1987;11(1):23–33.
16. Zetler G, Baumann GH. Pharmacokinetics and effects of haloperidol in the isolated mouse. Pharmacology. 1985;31(6):318–27.
17. Higashino K, Ago Y, Umehara M, Kita Y, Fujita K, Takuma K, Matsuda T. Effects of acute and chronic administration of venlafaxine and desipramine on extracellular monoamine levels in the mouse prefrontal cortex and striatum. Eur J Pharmacol. 2014;729:86–93.
18. Riviere GJ, Gentry WB, Owens SM. Disposition of methamphetamine and its metabolite amphetamine in brain and other tissues in rats after intravenous administration. J Pharmacol Exp Ther. 2000;292(3):1042–7.
19. Paxinos G, Franklin KBJ. The mouse brain in stereotaxic coordinates. 2nd ed. Cambridge: Academic Press; 2001.
20. Piechota M, Korostynski M, Ficek J, Tomski A, Przewlocki R. Seqinspector: position-based navigation through the ChIP-seq data landscape to identify gene expression regulators. BMC Bioinform. 2016;17:85.
21. Gabruk M, Nowakowska Z, Skupien-Rabian B, Kedracka-Krok S, Mysliwa-Kurdziel B, Kruk J. Insight into the oligomeric structure of PORA from A. thaliana. Biochem Biophys Acta. 2016;1864(12):1757–64.
22. Shiloh R, Zemishlany Z, Aizenberg D, Valevski A, Bodinger L, Munitz H, Weizman A. Mianserin or placebo as adjuncts to typical antipsychotics in resistant schizophrenia. Int Clin Psychopharmacol. 2002;17(2):59–64.
23. Shi W, Li F, Li S, Wang J, Wang Q, Yan X, Zhang Q, Chai L, Li M. Increased DCLK1 correlates with the malignant status and poor outcome in malignant tumors: a meta-analysis. Oncotarget. 2017;8(59):100545–57.
24. Westphalen CB, Quante M, Wang TC. Functional implication of Dclk1 and Dclk1-expressing cells in cancer. Small GTPases. 2017;8(3):164–71.
25. Berke JD, Paletzki RF, Aronson GJ, Hyman SE, Gerfen CR. A complex program of striatal gene expression induced by dopaminergic stimulation. J Neurosci Off J Soc Neurosci. 1998;18(14):5301–10.
26. Schenk GJ, Engels B, Zhang YP, Fitzsimons CP, Schouten T, Kruidering M, de Kloet ER, Vreugdenhil E. A potential role for calcium/calmodulin-dependent protein kinase-related peptide in neuronal apoptosis: in vivo and in vitro evidence. Eur J Neurosci. 2007;26(12):3411–20.
27. Wibrand K, Messaoudi E, Havik B, Steenslid V, Lovlie R, Steen VM, Bramham CR. Identification of genes co-upregulated with Arc during BDNF-induced long-term potentiation in adult rat dentate gyrus in vivo. Eur J Neurosci. 2006;23(6):1501–11.

28. Kawaai K, Tominaga-Yoshino K, Urakubo T, Taniguchi N, Kondoh Y, Tashiro H, Ogura A, Tashiro T. Analysis of gene expression changes associated with long-lasting synaptic enhancement in hippocampal slice cultures after repetitive exposures to glutamate. J Neurosci Res. 2010;88(13):2911–22.
29. Duncan CE, Chetcuti AF, Schofield PR. Coregulation of genes in the mouse brain following treatment with clozapine, haloperidol, or olanzapine implicates altered potassium channel subunit expression in the mechanism of antipsychotic drug action. Psychiatr Genet. 2008;18(5):226–39.
30. Zarrinpar A, Bhattacharyya RP, Lim WA. The structure and function of proline recognition domains. Sci STKE Signal Transduct Knowl Environ. 2003;2003(179):RE8.
31. Moeller ML, Shi Y, Reichardt LF, Ethell IM. EphB receptors regulate dendritic spine morphogenesis through the recruitment/phosphorylation of focal adhesion kinase and RhoA activation. J Biol Chem. 2006;281(3):1587–98.
32. Buday L, Wunderlich L, Tamas P. The Nck family of adapter proteins: regulators of actin cytoskeleton. Cell Signal. 2002;14(9):723–31.
33. Katz ME, McCormick F. Signal transduction from multiple Ras effectors. Curr Opin Genet Dev. 1997;7(1):75–9.
34. Lipka J, Kapitein LC, Jaworski J, Hoogenraad CC. Microtubule-binding protein doublecortin-like kinase 1 (DCLK1) guides kinesin-3-mediated cargo transport to dendrites. EMBO J. 2016;35(3):302–18.
35. Lazo OM, Gonzalez A, Ascano M, Kuruvilla R, Couve A, Bronfman FC. BDNF regulates Rab11-mediated recycling endosome dynamics to induce dendritic branching. J Neurosci Off J Soc Neurosci. 2013;33(14):6112–22.
36. Vreugdenhil E, Kolk SM, Boekhoorn K, Fitzsimons CP, Schaaf M, Schouten T, Sarabdjitsingh A, Sibug R, Lucassen PJ. Doublecortin-like, a microtubule-associated protein expressed in radial glia, is crucial for neuronal precursor division and radial process stability. Eur J Neurosci. 2007;25(3):635–48.
37. Pal S, Gupta R, Kim H, Wickramasinghe P, Baubet V, Showe LC, Dahmane N, Davuluri RV. Alternative transcription exceeds alternative splicing in generating the transcriptome diversity of cerebellar development. Genome Res. 2011;21(8):1260–72.
38. Saaltink DJ, Havik B, Verissimo CS, Lucassen PJ, Vreugdenhil E. Doublecortin and doublecortin-like are expressed in overlapping and non-overlapping neuronal cell population: implications for neurogenesis. J Comp Neurol. 2012;520(13):2805–23.
39. Kunze A, Achilles A, Keiner S, Witte OW, Redecker C. Two distinct populations of doublecortin-positive cells in the perilesional zone of cortical infarcts. BMC Neurosci. 2015;16:20.

13

Modulation of long-term potentiation-like cortical plasticity in the healthy brain with low frequency-pulsed electromagnetic fields

Enrico Premi[1,2]* ⓘ, Alberto Benussi[2], Antonio La Gatta[3], Stefano Visconti[4], Angelo Costa[1], Nicola Gilberti[1], Valentina Cantoni[2], Alessandro Padovani[2], Barbara Borroni[2] and Mauro Magoni[1]

Abstract

Background: Non-depolarizing magnetic fields, like low frequency-pulsed electromagnetic fields (LF-PEMFs) have shown the ability to modulate living structures, principally by influencing synaptic activity and ion channels on cellular membranes. Recently, the CTU Mega 20 device was presented as a molecular accelerator, using energy up to 200 J and providing high-power (2 Tesla) pulsating fields with a water-repulsive (diamagnetic) action and tissue biostimulation. We tested the hypothesis that LF-PEMFs could modulate long-term corticospinal excitability in healthy brains by applying CTU Mega 20®. Ten healthy subjects without known neurological and/or psychiatric diseases entered the study. A randomized double-blind sham-controlled crossover design was employed, recording TMS parameters (amplitude variation of the motor evoked potential as index of cortical excitability perturbations of the motor system) before (pre) and after (post $+0$, $+15$, $+30$ min) a single CTU Mega 20 session on the corresponding primary right-hand motor area, using a real (magnetic field $= 2$ Tesla; intensity $= 90$ J; impulse frequency $= 7$ Hz; duration $= 15$ min) or sham device. A two-way repeated measures ANOVA with TIME (pre, post $+0$, $+15$, $+30$ min) and TREATMENT (real vs. sham stimulation) as within-subjects factor was applied.

Results: A significant TIME × TREATMENT interaction was found ($p < 0.001$). Post hoc comparisons showed a significant effect of TIME, with significant differences at $+0$, $+15$ and $+30$ min compared to baseline after real stimulation (all $p < 0.05$) but not after sham stimulation (all $p < 0.05$) and significant effects of TREATMENT, with significant differences at $+0$, $+15$ and $+30$ min for real stimulation compared to sham stimulation (all $p < 0.005$). No significant depolarizing effects were detected throughout the (real) stimulation.

Conclusions: Our proof-of-concept study in healthy subjects supports the idea that non-ionizing LF-PEMFs induced by the CTU Mega 20 diamagnetic acceleration system could represent a new approach for brain neuromodulation. Further studies to optimize protocol parameters for different neurological and psychiatric conditions are warranted.

Trial Registration The present work has been retrospectively registered as clinical trial on ClinicalTrials.gov NCT03537469 and publicly released on May 24, 2018

Keywords: Long-term potentiation-like cortical plasticity, Low frequency-pulsed electromagnetic fields, Diamagnetism, Neuroplasticity

*Correspondence: zedtower@gmail.com
[1] Stroke Unit, Azienda Socio Sanitaria Territoriale "Spedali Civili", "Spedali Civili" Hospital, Piazza Spedali Civili 1, 25123 Brescia, Italy
Full list of author information is available at the end of the article

Modulation of long-term potentiation-like cortical plasticity in the healthy brain with low frequency-pulsed...

149

Background

Several studies have investigated the effects of different stimulation methods in modulating human brain plasticity [1–3]. Among these, the paired associative stimulation (PAS) paradigms were shown to modulate the excitability of corticospinal fibers related to the primary motor cortex, as a form of long-term modulation, including long-term potentiation (LTP) or depression (LTD) linked to synaptic plasticity [4, 5]. All these approaches induce electric currents to obtain a depolarization in the stimulated brain regions [6, 7]. However, even non-depolarizing magnetic fields, as in static magnets [8–10] or Low Frequency-Pulsed Electromagnetic Fields (LF-PEMFs) [11, 12], have shown the potential to modulate living structures [8, 13]. In particular, these non-depolarizing approaches seem to influence synaptic activity and ion channels on cellular membranes [8]. Indeed, it has been suggested that LF-PEMF can influence numerous types of changes in cells including migration, cell differentiation, stress response, potentially affecting morphology, migration of embryonic cells, and cell reprogramming [13–17]. Furthermore, it has been reported that LF-PEMF promotes osteogenic and neurogenic differentiation, which has been clinically used to repair bone fractures, promote wound healing [18, 19], and has been shown to have a neuroprotective effect after ischemic stroke in mice during the recovery process [11]. Several trials have also assessed the effects of LF-PEMF on major depressive disorder and unipolar or bipolar depression [20–22]. Moreover, LF-PEMF has been reported to influence brain glucose metabolism, thus affecting local brain activity [23]. Collectively, these studies indicate that LF-PEMF may be involved in neuroprotection.

LF-PEMFs (< 50 Hz) can be considered as a class of non-ionizing radiation with an associate energy < 12 electronvolt (eV), not enough to induce ionization phenomena [24], but with potential effects on biological components [25]. Recently, the CTU Mega 20® device (see Fig. 1) was presented as a molecular accelerator, using an energy up to 200 J and providing high-power (2 Tesla) pulsating fields with a water-repulsive (diamagnetic) action with a consequent tissue biostimulation [25, 26]. In this research we tested the hypothesis that LF-PEMFs could modulate long-term corticospinal excitability in the healthy brain by applying transcranial pulsed magnetic fields with CTU Mega 20® (http://www.periso.ch/). Therefore, we employed single-pulse transcranial magnetic stimulation (TMS), which allows an in vivo registration of the amplitude variation of the motor evoked potentials as a tool to explore cortical excitability perturbations of the motor system after CTU Mega 20 application.

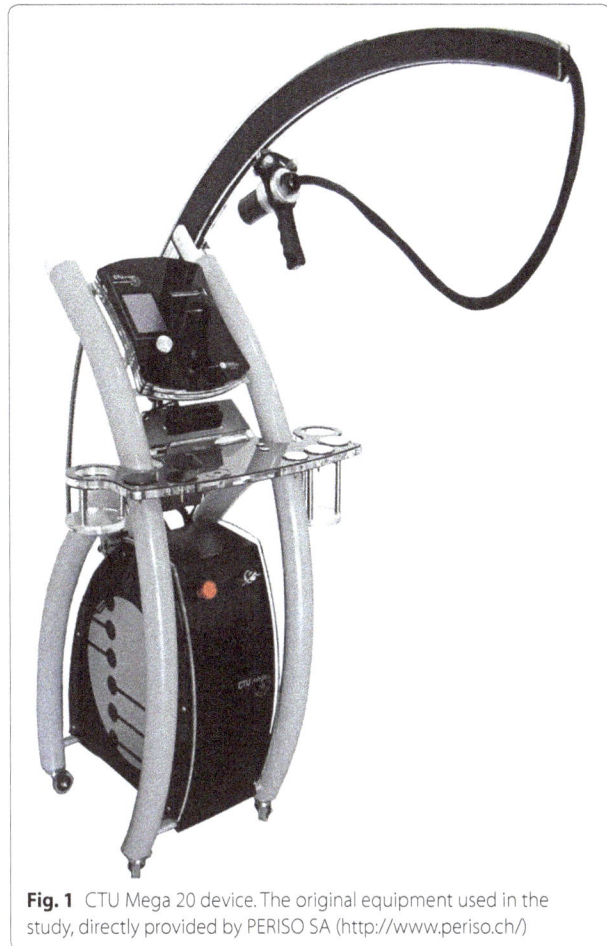

Fig. 1 CTU Mega 20 device. The original equipment used in the study, directly provided by PERISO SA (http://www.periso.ch/)

Methods

Subjects

Ten healthy subjects without known neurological or psychiatric diseases were recruited for this study (mean age ± standard deviation: 25.5 ± 3.8 years) (see Table 1).

The subjects and operators who performed TMS were blinded to the type of stimulation applied.

Written informed consent was obtained from all subjects according to the Declaration of Helsinki. The study protocol was approved by the local ethics committee. This study adheres to CONSORT guidelines (http://www.consort-statement.org/) (see Additional file 1 for CONSORT checklist).

CTU Mega 20 stimulation

The CTU Mega 20 diamagnetic acceleration system discharges high-field magnetic impulses (with a duration of 5 ms and a period of 1000 ms), generating a magnetic field up to 2 Tesla, with a frequency of 7500 Hz in a volume of approximately 27 cm^3 [12]. See Additional file 2

Table 1 Demographic characteristics and neurophysiological parameters

Variable	Real (n = 10)	Sham (n = 10)	p
Age (mean ± SD)	25.5 ± 3.8	25.5 ± 3.8	–
Gender % (no female)	50 (5)	50 (5)	–
Educational level, years	21.5 ± 1.9	21.5 ± 1.9	–
Handedness % (no right)	100 (10)	100 (10)	–
Correct hypothesis on treatment %	50	50	–
rMT (% of MSO)	46.4 ± 6.5	46.2 ± 6.5	n.s.
Corticospinal excitability baseline (mV)	1.01 ± 0.12	1.05 ± 0.05	n.s.
Corticospinal excitability post + 0 (mV)	1.60 ± 0.19	1.10 ± 0.14	p = 0.001
Corticospinal excitability post + 15 (mV)	1.69 ± 0.18	1.12 ± 0.21	p < 0.001
Corticospinal excitability, post + 30 (mV)	1.57 ± 0.34	1.07 ± 0.20	p = 0.002

MSO max stimulator output, *SD* standard deviation, *mV* millivolt

for a detailed technical description of CTU Mega 20 physics principles and function.

To assess the effect of LF-PEMFs provided by CTU Mega 20 we employed a randomized double-blind sham-controlled crossover design, recording TMS parameters before (pre) and after (post +0, +15, +30 min) a single-session of CTU Mega 20 on the corresponding primary right-hand motor area, using a real (magnetic field = 2 Tesla; intensity = 90 J; frequency of impulses = 7 Hz; duration = 15 min) or the sham device. Subjects were randomly assessed for real or sham protocol stimulation, in a 1:1 ratio, with a mean interval of 16.9 ± 2.1 days between sessions.

To detect differences in the perception of the stimulation, we asked the patients whether they thought they were receiving real or sham stimulation at the end of each treatment.

Transcranial magnetic stimulation

TMS was performed with a figure-eight coil (loop diameter 70 mm) connected to a Magstim 200^2 stimulator (Magstim Company, Oxford, UK). The magnetic stimuli had a monophasic current waveform (rise time of 100 µs, decaying back to zero over 800 µs). The motor evoked potentials (MEPs) were registered from the right first dorsal interosseous muscle (FDI) through surface Ag/AgCl electrodes placed in a belly-tendon montage and acquired using a Biopac MP-150 electromyograph (BIOPAC Systems Inc., Santa Barbara, CA, USA), as previously reported [27].

The TMS coil was held tangentially over the scalp zone related to the primary hand motor area contralateral to the target muscle, with the coil handle pointed 45° posteriorly and laterally to the sagittal plane. The motor region was considered as the location where TMS consistently produced the largest MEP size at 120% of the resting motor threshold (rMT) in the target muscle. The region was marked with a felt tip pen on the scalp to guarantee

constant placement of the coil during the whole experiment. The stimulator intensity was set to evoke a MEP approximately 1 mV peak-to-peak in the relaxed FDI at baseline, and was kept constant during the whole session. MEP amplitude measurements (average of 25 responses) were performed at baseline and at 0, 15, and 30 min after sham or real stimulation. The inter trial interval was set at 5 s (± 10%).

Throughout the experiment, complete muscle relaxation was guaranteed by audio-visual feedback where appropriate. Trials were discarded if EMG activity exceeded 100 µV in the 250 ms prior to TMS stimulus delivery. All participants were able to understand instructions, obtaining a full muscle relaxation.

Statistical analysis

Neurophysiological parameters were compared by means of two-way repeated measures ANOVA with TIME (pre, post +0, +15, +30 min) and TREATMENT (real vs. sham stimulation) as within-subjects factor. When a significant main effect was reached, post hoc tests with Bonferroni correction for multiple comparisons were conducted to analyze group-differences at respective interstimulus intervals s or time points. Mauchly's test was used to test for assumption of sphericity, while the Greenhouse–Geisser epsilon determination was used to correct in case of sphericity violation.

Spearman's rank-order correlation was used to assess the association between the percentage of increase in MEP amplitude and baseline rMT.

Statistical significance was assumed at $p < 0.05$. Data analyses were carried out using SPSS 21.0 software.

Results

Regarding the differences in the subjects' perception of the stimulation, there was no statistically significant association between the type of stimulation and its perception, as assessed by Fisher's exact test, $p = 1.00$, suggesting that real stimulation could not be distinguished from sham stimulation.

Two-way repeated measures ANOVA performed on corticospinal excitability revealed a significant TIME × TREATMENT interaction, $F(3, 27) = 0.453$, $p < 0.001$, partial $\eta^2 = 0.645$. A significant main effect of TIME was observed, with significant differences in post hoc tests at $+0$, $+15$ and $+30$ min compared to baseline after real stimulation (all $p < 0.05$) but not after sham stimulation (all $p > 0.05$). There was also a significant main effect of TREATMENT, with significant differences at $+0$, $+15$ and $+30$ min versus baseline, for real stimulation but not for sham stimulation (all $p < 0.005$) (see Table 1, Fig. 2).

There was no significant association between the percentage of increase in average MEP amplitude and baseline rMT in both groups (real stimulation: $r_s = 0.10$, $p = 0.776$; sham stimulation: $r_s = -0.46$, $p = 0.177$).

During the treatment phase (application of real or sham CTU Mega 20 protocol), EMG activity at high-gain amplification was monitored to highlight possible depolarizing effects, which were however absent throughout the stimulation.

Discussion

In this study, we employed a randomized double-blind sham-controlled crossover design (to control for known and unknown factors that could potentially influenced brain activity and TMS registration) to demonstrate that Low Frequency-Pulsed Electromagnetic Fields (LF-PEMFs) induced by CTU Mega 20 were able to modulate cortical excitability in human brains, even after a single-shot application. As described above, these findings were not influenced by subject treatment expectation (real stimulation versus sham), considering its potential effect on brain activity and consequently on TMS parameters [28]. In line with transcranial static magnetic field stimulation [10, 23, 29], cortical excitability enhancement was not directly related to induced electric currents, as is the case for other neuromodulation TMS-based techniques.

In our experiment, by providing 15-min pulsed-magnetic stimulus on the primary motor area, we obtained a persistent increase of more than 60% in corticospinal excitability (as an index of Long-Term Potentiation-Like Cortical Plasticity), recording the MEP from the contralateral first dorsal interosseous muscle. This perturbation lasted for at least for 30 min after the stimulation protocol, potentially maintaining a significant difference

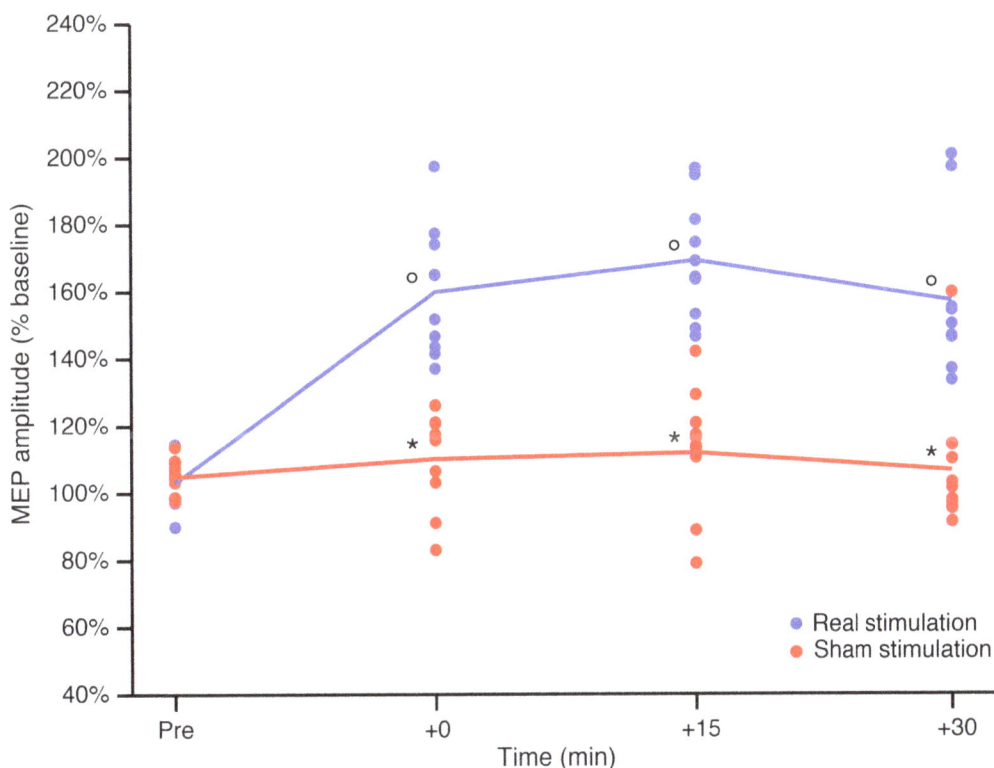

Fig. 2 Corticospinal excitability after real and sham stimulation. Real and sham stimulation effects on corticospinal excitability, as measured by change in 1 mV MEP amplitude at various time points, in the real (blue line) and sham (red line) stimulation groups. Error bars represent standard errors. *$p < 0.05$ versus real stimulation. °$p < 0.05$ versus baseline (T0). *MEP* motor evoked potential, *mV* millivolt, *min* minutes

(at least 30%), for even a longer time. As reported above, tissue biostimulation provided by CTU Meg 20 was based on non-ionizing LF-PEMFs, which could act primarily at synapse level, altering membrane ion channel function. In particular, it was shown that Ca^{2+} and Na^+ channel activity can be perturbed by magnetic fields, considering the diamagnetic anisotropic characteristics of membrane phospholipids [8, 30, 31]. Interestingly, CTU Mega 20 is defined as a diamagnetic acceleration system, allowing high-field magnetic impulses potentially capable of inducing magnetic reorientation of membrane phospholipids and consequently inducing a biological effect on nervous system function. From this point of view, there are three points in our proof of concept study that support the idea that non-ionizing LF-PEMFs induced by the CTU Mega 20 could represent a new approach for brain neuromodulation. They are (1) CTU Mega 20 provided a larger stimulation volume (up to 27 cm^3 compared to 1–2 cm^3 for TMS) allowing the modulation of an extended portion of cortical surface, compared to TMS; (2) as acommercially available device, the CTU Mega 20 is ready to use, with predefined programs to perform stimulation of the nervous system, not requiring specialized staff and can be easily adapted to everyday clinical application; (3) as a completely programmable system, the CTU Mega 20 can be optimized for different types of stimulation and different neurological diseases. In conclusion, the CTU Mega 20 diamagnetic acceleration system may well be of interest in the field of neuromodulation. Further studies to optimize protocol parameters for different neurological and psychiatric conditions are warranted [32, 33].

Conclusions

This proof-of-concept study in healthy subjects supports the idea that non-ionizing LF-PEMFs induced by the CTU Mega 20 diamagnetic acceleration system could represent a new approach for brain neuromodulation. Further studies to optimize protocol parameters for different neurological and psychiatric conditions are warranted.

Abbreviations

PAS: Paired associative stimulation; LTP: Long-term potentiation; LTD: Long-term depression; LF-PEMFs: Low frequency-pulsed electromagnetic fields; Hz: Hertz; eV: Electronvolt; CTU Mega 20: Name of the device used in the present study; TMS: Transcranial magnetic stimulation; MEP: Motor evoked potential; ms: Millisecond; min: Minute; J: Joule; μs: Microsecond; FDI: First dorsal interosseous muscle; Ag/AgCl: Silver chloride; rMT: Resting motor threshold; EMG: Electromyography; μV: Microvolts; ANOVA: Analysis of variance.

Authors' contributions

All authors made substantial contributions to the study concept and design, and/or the acquisition of data, and/or the analysis and interpretation of the data. In detail, EP: first draft of the manuscript, patient cohort, interpretation of data, study conceptualization and design, AB: TMS data recording, TMS data analysis and interpretation of data, study conceptualization and design, critical revision of the manuscript for content, ALG: original developer of the (CTU) device used, technical description of the device, critical revision of the manuscript for content, SV, AC, NG: subject cohort, critical revision of the manuscript for content, VC: subject cohort, TMS data recording, AP: critical revision of the manuscript for content, BB, MM: study conceptualization and design, critical revision of the manuscript for content. All authors read and approved the final manuscript.

Author details

[1] Stroke Unit, Azienda Socio Sanitaria Territoriale "Spedali Civili", "Spedali Civili" Hospital, Piazza Spedali Civili 1, 25123 Brescia, Italy. [2] Neurology Unit, Department of Clinical and Experimental Sciences, University of Brescia, Brescia, Italy. [3] cNVR Consorzio Veneto di Ricerca, Padua, Italy. [4] Rehabilitation Unit, Casa di Cura "Villa Barbarano", Salò, Brescia, Italy.

Acknowledgements

We would like to thank all the partecipants (medical students, residents in Neurology, neuropsychologists) involved in the study.

Competing interests

This study was supported by PERISO SA (http://www.periso.ch/).

Funding

This study was supported by PERISO SA (http://www.periso.ch/), which provided the CTU devices (real and sham) and the written technical description of the CTU device (see Additional file 2).

References

1. Stefan K, Kunesch E, Cohen LG, Benecke R, Classen J. Induction of plasticity in the human motor cortex by paired associative stimulation. Brain. 2000;123(Pt 3):572–84.
2. Huang YZ, Edwards MJ, Rounis E, Bhatia KP, Rothwell JC. Theta burst stimulation of the human motor cortex. Neuron. 2005;45(2):201–6.
3. Nitsche MA, Paulus W. Excitability changes induced in the human motor cortex by weak transcranial direct current stimulation. J Physiol. 2000;527(Pt 3):633–9.
4. Rossini PM, Burke D, Chen R, Cohen LG, Daskalakis Z, Di Iorio R, Di Lazzaro V, Ferreri F, Fitzgerald PB, George MS, et al. Non-invasive electrical and magnetic stimulation of the brain, spinal cord, roots and peripheral nerves: basic principles and procedures for routine clinical and research application. An updated report from an I.F.C.N. Committee. Clin Neurophysiol. 2015;126(6):1071–107.
5. Benussi A, Cosseddu M, Filareto I, Dell'Era V, Archetti S, Sofia Cotelli M, Micheli A, Padovani A, Borroni B. Impaired long-term potentiation-like cortical plasticity in presymptomatic genetic frontotemporal dementia. Ann Neurol. 2016;80(3):472–6.
6. Di Lazzaro V, Oliviero A, Pilato F, Saturno E, Dileone M, Mazzone P, Insola A, Tonali PA, Rothwell JC. The physiological basis of transcranial motor cortex stimulation in conscious humans. Clin Neurophysiol. 2004;115(2):255–66.
7. Hallett M. Transcranial magnetic stimulation and the human brain. Nature. 2000;406(6792):147–50.
8. Rosen AD. Mechanism of action of moderate-intensity static magnetic fields on biological systems. Cell Biochem Biophys. 2003;39(2):163–73.
9. Coots A, Shi R, Rosen AD. Effect of a 0.5-T static magnetic field on conduction in guinea pig spinal cord. J Neurol Sci. 2004;222(1–2):55–7.
10. Oliviero A, Mordillo-Mateos L, Arias P, Panyavin I, Foffani G, Aguilar J. Transcranial static magnetic field stimulation of the human motor cortex. J Physiol. 2011;589(Pt 20):4949–58.
11. Urnukhsaikhan E, Mishig-Ochir T, Kim SC, Park JK, Seo YK. Neuroprotective effect of low frequency-pulsed electromagnetic fields in ischemic stroke. Appl Biochem Biotechnol. 2017;181(4):1360–71.

12. Izzo MNL, Coscia V, La Gatta A, Mariani F, Gasbarro V. The role of diamagnetic pump (CTU Mega 18) in the physical treatment of limbs lymphoedema. A clinical study. Eur J Lymphol. 2010;21(61):24–9.

13. Juutilainen J. Developmental effects of electromagnetic fields. Bioelectromagnetics. 2005;Suppl 7:S107–115.

14. Seo TB, Kim TW, Shin MS, Ji ES, Cho HS, Lee JM, Kim TW, Kim CJ. Aerobic exercise alleviates ischemia-induced memory impairment by enhancing cell proliferation and suppressing neuronal apoptosis in hippocampus. Int Neurourol J. 2014;18(4):187–97.

15. Ceccarelli G, Bloise N, Mantelli M, Gastaldi G, Fassina L, De Angelis MG, Ferrari D, Imbriani M, Visai L. A comparative analysis of the in vitro effects of pulsed electromagnetic field treatment on osteogenic differentiation of two different mesenchymal cell lineages. Int Neurourol J. 2013;2(4):283–94.

16. Maaroufi K, Save E, Poucet B, Sakly M, Abdelmelek H, Had-Aissouni L. Oxidative stress and prevention of the adaptive response to chronic iron overload in the brain of young adult rats exposed to a 150 kilohertz electromagnetic field. Neuroscience. 2011;186:39–47.

17. Levin M. Large-scale biophysics: ion flows and regeneration. Trends Cell Biol. 2007;17(6):261–70.

18. Pesce M, Patruno A, Speranza L, Reale M. Extremely low frequency electromagnetic field and wound healing: implication of cytokines as biological mediators. Eur Cytokine Netw. 2013;24(1):1–10.

19. Kang KS, Hong JM, Kang JA, Rhie JW, Jeong YH, Cho DW. Regulation of osteogenic differentiation of human adipose-derived stem cells by controlling electromagnetic field conditions. Exp Mol Med. 2013;45:e6.

20. Martiny K, Lunde M, Bech P. Transcranial low voltage pulsed electromagnetic fields in patients with treatment-resistant depression. Biol Psychiatry. 2010;68(2):163–9.

21. Rohan ML, Yamamoto RT, Ravichandran CT, Cayetano KR, Morales OG, Olson DP, Vitaliano G, Paul SM, Cohen BM. Rapid mood-elevating effects of low field magnetic stimulation in depression. Biol Psychiatry. 2014;76(3):186–93.

22. Straaso B, Lauritzen L, Lunde M, Vinberg M, Lindberg L, Larsen ER, Dissing S, Bech P. Dose-remission of pulsating electromagnetic fields as augmentation in therapy-resistant depression: a randomized, double-blind controlled study. Acta Neuropsychiatr. 2014;26(5):272–9.

23. Volkow ND, Tomasi D, Wang GJ, Fowler JS, Telang F, Wang R, Alexoff D, Logan J, Wong C, Pradhan K, et al. Effects of low-field magnetic stimulation on brain glucose metabolism. Neuroimage. 2010;51(2):623–8.

24. Bassett CA. Fundamental and practical aspects of therapeutic uses of pulsed electromagnetic fields (PEMFs). Crit Rev Biomed Eng. 1989;17(5):451–529.

25. Luben RA. Effects of low-energy electromagnetic fields (pulsed and DC) on membrane signal transduction processes in biological systems. Health Phys. 1991;61(1):15–28.

26. Patino O, Grana D, Bolgiani A, Prezzavento G, Mino J, Merlo A, Benaim F. Pulsed electromagnetic fields in experimental cutaneous wound healing in rats. J Burn Care Rehabil. 1996;17(6 Pt 1):528–31.

27. Benussi A, Cotelli MS, Cosseddu M, Bertasi V, Turla M, Salsano E, Dardis A, Padovani A, Borroni B. Preliminary results on long-term potentiation-like cortical plasticity and cholinergic dysfunction after miglustat treatment in niemann-pick disease type C. In: JIMD Report 2017.

28. Fiorio M, Emadi Andani M, Marotta A, Classen J, Tinazzi M. Placebo-induced changes in excitatory and inhibitory corticospinal circuits during motor performance. J Neurosci. 2014;34(11):3993–4005.

29. Rivadulla C, Foffani G, Oliviero A. Magnetic field strength and reproducibility of neodymium magnets useful for transcranial static magnetic field stimulation of the human cortex. Neuromodulation. 2014;17(5):438–41 **(Discussion 441–432)**.

30. Lu XW, Du L, Kou L, Song N, Zhang YJ, Wu MK, Shen JF. Effects of moderate static magnetic fields on the voltage-gated sodium and calcium channel currents in trigeminal ganglion neurons. Electromagn Biol Med. 2015;34(4):285–92.

31. Ye SR, Yang JW, Chen CM. Effect of static magnetic fields on the amplitude of action potential in the lateral giant neuron of crayfish. Int J Radiat Biol. 2004;80(10):699–708.

32. Rohan M, Parow A, Stoll AL, Demopulos C, Friedman S, Dager S, Hennen J, Cohen BM, Renshaw PF. Low-field magnetic stimulation in bipolar depression using an MRI-based stimulator. Am J Psychiatry. 2004;161(1):93–8.

33. Capone F, Dileone M, Profice P, Pilato F, Musumeci G, Minicuci G, Ranieri F, Cadossi R, Setti S, Tonali PA, et al. Does exposure to extremely low frequency magnetic fields produce functional changes in human brain? J Neural Transm (Vienna). 2009;116(3):257–65.

14

Cochlear morphology in the developing inner ear of the porcine model of spontaneous deafness

Wei Chen[1], Qing-Qing Hao[1], Li–Li Ren[1], Wei Ren[1], Hui-sang Lin[2], Wei-Wei Guo[1*] and Shi-Ming Yang[1*]

Abstract

Background: Auditory function and cochlear morphology have previously been described in a porcine model with spontaneous WS2-like phenotype. In the present study, cochlear histopathology was further investigated in the inner ear of the developing spontaneous deafness pig.

Results: We found that the stria vascularis transformed into a complex tri-laminar tissue at embryonic 85 days (E85) in normal pigs, but not in the MITF$^{-/-}$ pigs. As the neural crest (NC) of cochlea was derived by melanocytes. MITF mutation caused failure of development of melanocytes which caused a subsequent collapse of cochlear duct and deficits of the epithelium after E100. Furthermore, the spiral ganglion neurons of cochlea in the MITF$^{-/-}$ pigs began to degenerate at postnatal 30 days (P30). Thus, our histopathological results indicated that the malformation of the stria vascularis was a primary defect in MITF$^{-/-}$ induced WT pigs which was resulted from the loss of NC-derived melanocytes. Subsequently, the cochleae underwent secondary degeneration of the vestibular organs. As the degeneration of spiral ganglion neurons happened after P30, it suggests that WS patients should be considered as candidates for cochlear implant.

Conclusions: Our porcine model of MITF-M mutation may provide a crucial animal model for cochlear implant, cell therapy in patients with congenital hereditary hearing loss.

Keywords: Stria vascularis, MITF-M mutation, Waardenburg syndrome, Porcine model

Background

Waardenburg syndrome (WS) is one of the most common types of syndromic sensorineural hearing loss, characterized abnormal pigmentation in heterochromia irides, depigmented patches of skin or early greying [1]. The incidence of WS is estimated about 1/42,000 and is responsible for approximately 1–5% of congenital deafness [1–3]. WS is classified into four types (WS1, WS2, WS3 and WS4) with clinical and genetic hetero-geneses caused by mutations of six candidate genes, i.e., PAX3 (OMIM #606597), MITF (OMIM #156845), EDN3 (OMIM #131242), EDNRB (OMIM #131244), SOX10 (OMIM #602229) and SNAI2 (OMIM #602150) [1, 3]. WS2 (OMIM #193510) is similar to WS1, but is absent of distopia canthorum. About 15–21% of WS2 cases are involved with mutation in MITF gene [1, 4, 5]. MITF (microphthalmia-associated transcription factor) protein, which contains a basic helix–loop–helix leucine zipper (bHLH-LZ) domain, is crucial for the development of pigmental cells [6–8]. The MITF gene contains multiple promoters consecutively followed by a different first exon and common downstream exons. It consequently encodes distinct isoforms with different N-termini and uniform C-termini where the bHLH-LZ structures are located [9, 10]. Accordingly, these MITF isoforms exhibit tissue-specific expression and functions, of which the melanocyte-specific isoforms (MITF-M) plays a critical

*Correspondence: gwent001@163.com; yangsm301@263.net
[1] Department of Otolaryngology, Head & Neck Surgery, Institute of Otolaryngology, Chinese PLA General Hospital, Beijing Key Laboratory of Hearing Impairment Prevention and Treatment, Key Laboratory of Hearing Impairment Science, Chinese PLA Medical School, Ministry of Education, Beijng, China
Full list of author information is available at the end of the article

role in development of neural crest-derived melanocytes in inner ear and optic cup-derived retinal pigment epitheliums [11–13]. It is indicated that the correct expression level of MITF-M is required for early development and migration of melanoblasts in the neural tube, as well as their differentiation into intermediate cells in the stria vascularis (SV) of the mammalian cochlea which secrete potassium ions and produce the endolymphatic potential (both are essential for hearing) [13–16].

In our previous studies, a porcine model with spontaneous WS2-like phenotype exhibits a spontaneous sensorineural deafness and depigmentation, and a de novo short insertion in the distal regulatory region of MITF-M isoform [17]. As the effects of MITF-M isoform defection on development of cochlea is still not clear, we studied the development of the cochlea, especially on the stria vascularis (SV), of this MITF-M specific mutation porcine model in order to have a better insight of the role of MITF-M in auditory system. Our results provide the first detailed record that degradation rule and schedule of SV, hair cells and SGNs in the MITF-M mutation porcine model.

Methods

Animals

Pigs used in this study were provided by the Animal Breeding Facility of Chongqing Academy of Animal Science (from embryonic 65 days to postnatal 1 month). The porcine model with *MITF-M* specific mutation was characterized by albino and heterochromia irides [16] and the wild type were used as the control group. This study was approved by the Institutional Animal Care and Use Committee of General Hospital of People's Liberation Army (PLA).

Specific methods of animal care-taking

All pregnant sows were housed separately. The piglets in the first month after birth were reared in the same column of the sows, and the weaned pigs were housed in separate barns. The pregnant sows were subjected to deep anesthesia, and then the embryos were obtained utilizing the cesarean section. Before the operation, these pigs were fasted for 12 h, and water was cut-off for 24 h. The animals were given an injection into the muscles of their neck with Sumianxin II at the dose of 0.1 ml/kg. Moreover, 10 min later, isofurane was introduced with a ventilator at 0.2 ml/min. At the end, the sows were over-anesthetized with increasing the most amount of inhaled anesthesia, 0.5 ml/min isofurane until breathing and the heartbeat stopped. There was no pain in the entire process.

After birth, animals were deeply anesthetized-excessively anesthetized as described above, after the termination of breathe and heartbeat, the specimens of the iliac crest were taken without pain. Animal carcasses were handed over to the management department for unified treatment approach.

Based on the National Institutes of Health Guidelines on Use of Laboratory Animals, all experiments were conducted and approved by the General Hospital of People's Liberation Army (PLA) Committee on Animal Care (Beijing, China).

Tissue preparations

Inner ear of pigs were collected after deep anesthetized at different developmental stages (E65, E75, E85, E100, P1, P30 and P60). Their cochleae were dissected out immediately, then perfused with 4% paraformaldehyde fixative (through a hole made in the apical turn). All the cochlear samples were immersed in 4% formalin (for light microscopy) or 2.5% glutaraldehyde (for scanning and transmission electron microscopy) overnight at 4 °C. The cochleae from older embryos or postnatal pigs were decalcified with 10% ethylene diamine tetraacetic acid (EDTA) until the bone was soft enough for sectioning. At least three pigs were used for each age group in morphological analysis.

Morphologic analysis

Stria vascularis semi-thin sections stained in 1% toluidine blue and cochlear celloidin embedding sections stained in hematoxylin-eosin (H&E) at different stages were observed under a light microscope (Olympus).

For the transmission electron microscopy (TEM), the cochleae were washed with 0.1 M PB, post-fixed in 1% osmium tetroxide, dehydrated in a graded series of ethanol and embedded in plastic Agar 100 resin. After polymerisation, the third cochlear turn was embedded on a blank block of Agar 100 for sectioning. Then, the sections stained with toluidine blue were examined under a transmission electron microscope (PHILIPS TECNAI10).

For the scanning electron microscopy (SEM), the cochlear samples, after being washed, post-fixed and dehydrated by the same methods as for TEM, were embedded on aluminum stubs, coated with gold particles, then examined under a scanning electron microscope (JEOL JSM35C).

Spiral ganglion cell (SGCs) counts

The number of SGCs was determined as described previously [16]. Briefly, neurons were counted in the basal turns on the same side of the modiolus. We counted ten fields of a light microscope at $400 \times$ magnification in each H&E taining collodion section. Six cochleae were examined at P1, P30 and P60, respectively with six normal (wild type) cochleae at the same stage used as the reference.

Statistical analysis

All data were recorded and analyzed using the statistical software SPSS19. The mean ± standard deviation (SD) of MITF$^{-/-}$ (MT) group was contrasted with MITF$^{+/+}$ (WT) group using the Student's t test. One-way ANOVA was used to contrast whether the number of SGCs at different stages had statistic difference. A P value of 0.05 was considered significant.

Results

Morphology change of stria vascularis (SV)

Semi-thin Sections of the SV: To investigate the development of SV in the MITF-M specific mutation porcine model, we examined the morphology of the SV at different embryonic and postnatal stages (E65, E75, E85, E100, P1 and P13) using light microscopy (LM) and transmission electron microscopy (TEM). The semi-thin sections of SV stained with xylidine blue were observed though LM to monitor the morphogenesis of SV. For the wild-type Rongchang Pig (MITF$^{+/+}$), a dense area could be observed at the lateral wall of the cochlear scala media, but no clear boundary with the adjacent spiral ligament at embryonic Day 65 (E65) was found (Fig. 1A1). The SV became thickened from E65 to E85 and then became increasingly compact from E85 to E100, and matured

after E100 (Fig. 1A1–6). For the mutant-type (MITF $^{-/-}$), the distinctions with the wild-type were showed at E85, when the SV became thinner and looser.

The SV under transmission electron microscopy revealed ultrastructural differences of the developing SV between the MITF$^{+/+}$ and MITF $^{-/-}$ genotypes (Fig. 2). The intermediate cells (IC) of SV could be identified in both genotypes at E65. For the wild-type, the SV developed three layers at E75, consisting of the marginal cell (MC) layer, the intermediate cell layer and the basal cell (BC) layer. At E85, the marginal cells exhibited numerous microvilli at the apical membrane and extended processes at the basal membrane with centrally located nuclei, while the spindle-shaped basal cells were paralleled to the SV. At E100, marginal cells showed decreased microvilli, flattened nuclei and elongated processes that interacted with the intermediate cells and capillaries. At P1 and P13, the marginal cells were lengthened and connected with each other through tight junctions to form a barrier of the SV after birth. In contrast, the SV of mutant-type appeared totally under developed since E75 when processes at the basal membrane of marginal cells were gradually aggregated and failed to interact with the intermediate cells and mesenchymal capillaries. The intermediate cells began to reduce at E85. After E100, the differences of the SV between two genotypes were more apparent. A discernable boundary was formed between the marginal cell layer and the basal cell layer with only a

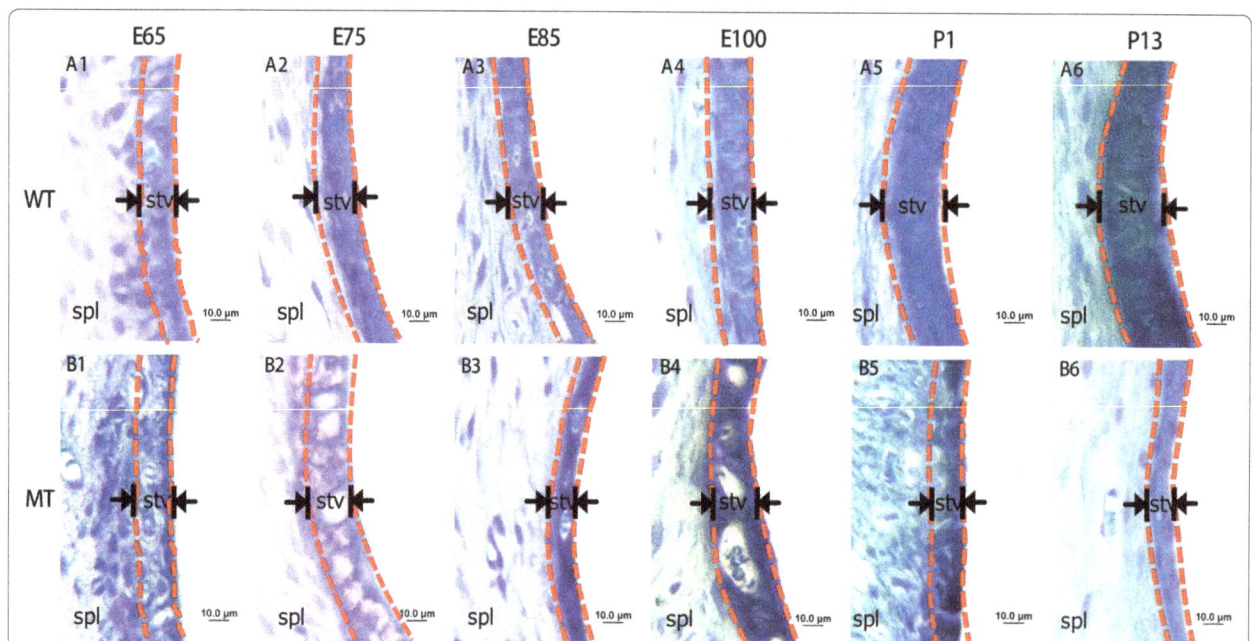

Fig. 1 Malformation of the stria vascularis (SV) in developing cochleae of pigs with MITF-M mutation. **A1–6** Illustrate the SV in the wild type cochleae from E65 to P13. **B1–6** Illustrate the SVs in mutant pigs from E65 to P13. Images show that the SV of MITF-M mutant pigs are remarkably thinner than the normal pigs after E85. All images were taken from the basal turn of cochleae (Wild type, WT; mutant type, MT; spiral ligament, Spl; stria vascularis, stv. Bar = 10 μm)

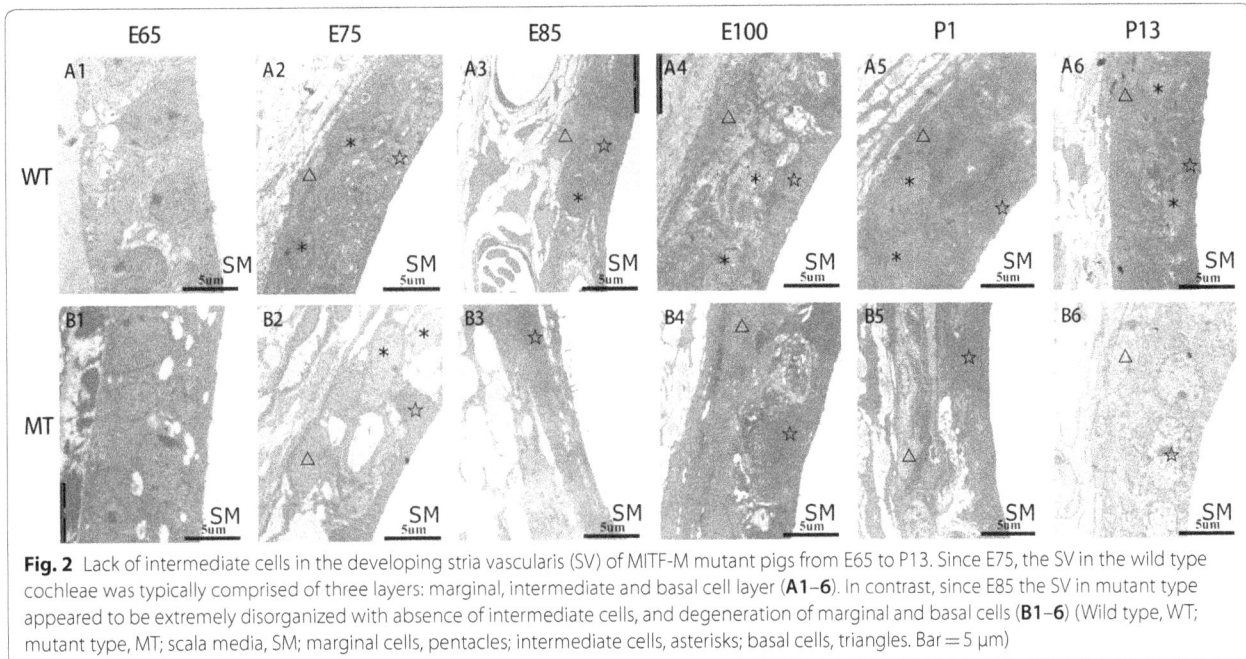

Fig. 2 Lack of intermediate cells in the developing stria vascularis (SV) of MITF-M mutant pigs from E65 to P13. Since E75, the SV in the wild type cochleae was typically comprised of three layers: marginal, intermediate and basal cell layer (**A1–6**). In contrast, since E85 the SV in mutant type appeared to be extremely disorganized with absence of intermediate cells, and degeneration of marginal and basal cells (**B1–6**) (Wild type, WT; mutant type, MT; scala media, SM; marginal cells, pentacles; intermediate cells, asterisks; basal cells, triangles. Bar = 5 μm)

few intermediate cells embedded in processes at the basal membrane of marginal cells. Subsequently, intermediate cells were rarely observed in the postnatal SV (P1 and P13), leading an extremely thin SV. In summary, the SV of the MITF$^{-/-}$ cochlea was initially under developed and degenerated progressively over time.

Defective hair cells

We further examined the morphology of the developed organ of Corti at high magnification of LM and the hair cells using scanning electron microscopy (SEM).

The organ of Corti in MITF$^{-/-}$ embryos was similar to that in MITF$^{+/+}$ embryos between E75 and E85. From E100, the organ of Corti degenerated with loss of sensory epithelia in the MITF $^{-/-}$ cochlea, when the Reissner's membrane began to collapse (Fig. 3).

To have a better understanding of the altered structures of hair cells, we observed the hair cells through SEM at E75, E85, E100, P1 and P13 (Fig. 3). It is showed that porcine cochleae were extremely similar with human, as four rows of hair cells arranged along the entire cochlear duct. There were only one row of inner hair cells (IHCs) located in the inner most row toward the central region of the cochlea and three rows of outer hair cells (OHCs) located toward the peripheral region of the cochlea. The hair bundles of OHCs are in a "V"—pattern in the basal

and middle turns, whereas in a "C"—pattern in the apical turn. The stereocilia of hair cells lengthened from the basal turn to the apical turn. Until E85, no significant difference was observed between two genotypes. The loss of hair cells and stereocilia bundles in the mutant-type cochleae were manifested and deteriorated since E100.

Collapsed cochlear duct

To investigate the time course of cochlear duct formation along with the under developed SV, we compared the mid-modiolar cross celloidin sections through the cochlea in both genotypes at E75, E85, E100, P1 and P13 (Fig. 4). At E75 and E85, the morphology and size of the cochlear duct appeared similar in two genotypes that the volume of the cochlear duct gradually increased with elongation of the SV. The inner spiral sulcus space was first spotted at E75. At E85, the tunnel of Corti and the space of Nuel were distinguishable, while the amorphous tectorial membrane developed to lay over the greater epithelial ridge. By E100, the cochlear gross morphology of wild-type Rongchang pig had matured, whereas the volume of cochlear duct had shrunk and the fine structure of the organ of Corti had deteriorated due to the collapse of Reissner's membrane in the mutant-type. These pathological changes occurred similarly at all cochlear turns of the mutant-type.

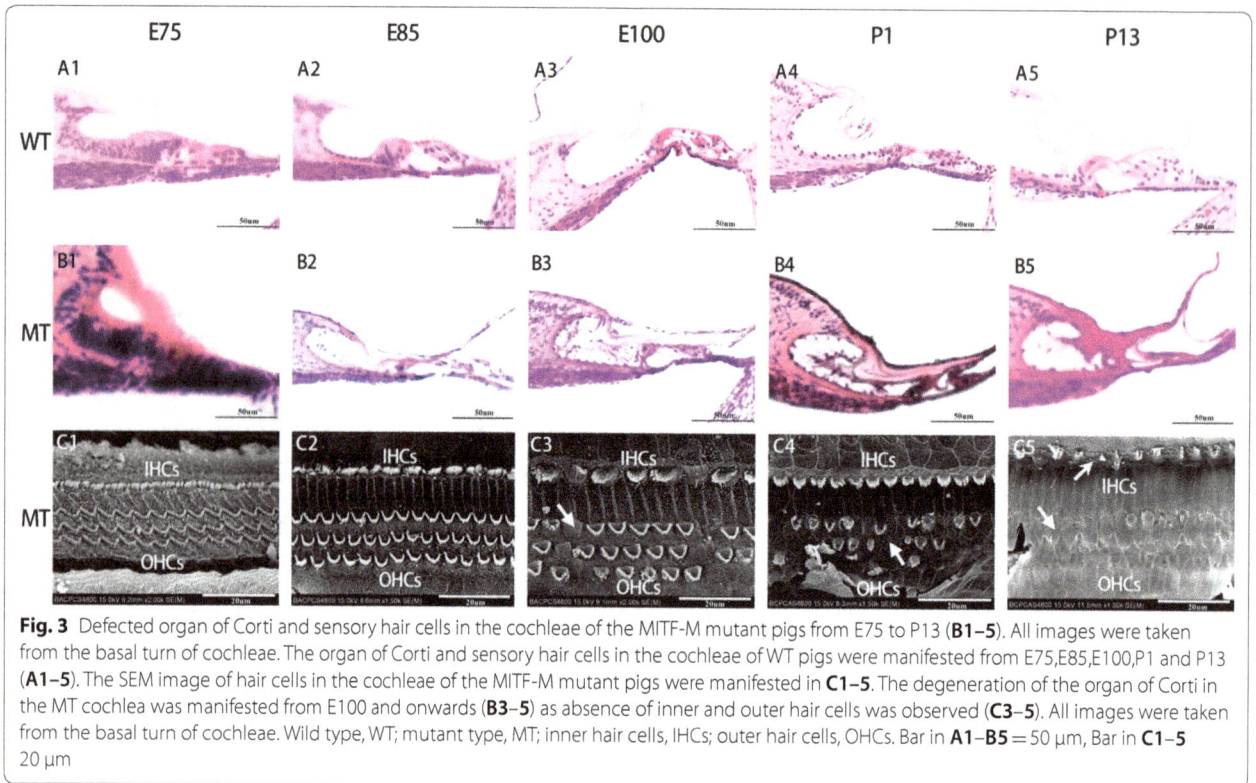

Fig. 3 Defected organ of Corti and sensory hair cells in the cochleae of the MITF-M mutant pigs from E75 to P13 (**B1–5**). All images were taken from the basal turn of cochleae. The organ of Corti and sensory hair cells in the cochleae of WT pigs were manifested from E75,E85,E100,P1 and P13 (**A1–5**). The SEM image of hair cells in the cochleae of the MITF-M mutant pigs were manifested in **C1–5**. The degeneration of the organ of Corti in the MT cochlea was manifested from E100 and onwards (**B3–5**) as absence of inner and outer hair cells was observed (**C3–5**). All images were taken from the basal turn of cochleae. Wild type, WT; mutant type, MT; inner hair cells, IHCs; outer hair cells, OHCs. Bar in **A1–B5** = 50 μm, Bar in **C1–5** 20 μm

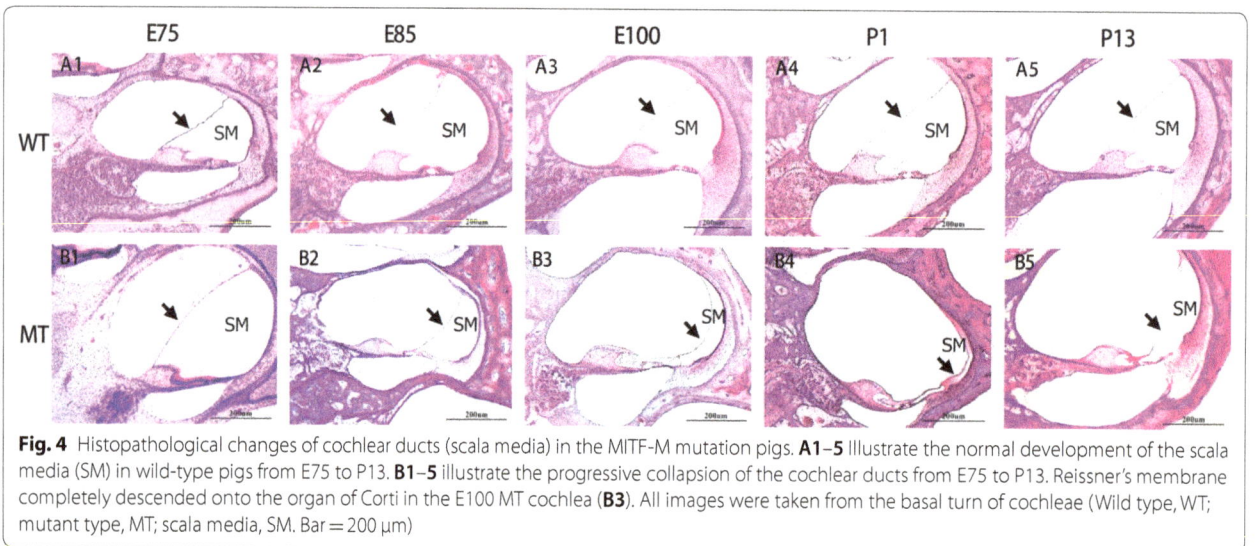

Fig. 4 Histopathological changes of cochlear ducts (scala media) in the MITF-M mutation pigs. **A1–5** Illustrate the normal development of the scala media (SM) in wild-type pigs from E75 to P13. **B1–5** illustrate the progressive collapse of the cochlear ducts from E75 to P13. Reissner's membrane completely descended onto the organ of Corti in the E100 MT cochlea (**B3**). All images were taken from the basal turn of cochleae (Wild type, WT; mutant type, MT; scala media, SM. Bar = 200 μm)

Figure 5 showed the different degree of degeneration of inner and outer hair cells in the cochleae of the postnatal MITF$^{-/-}$ mutation pigs. The loss of stereocilias of hair cells, both inner hair cells (IHCs) and outer hair cells (OHCs), were most severe in the basal turn.

SGC degeneration

In addition, we observed cochlear SGCs at high magnification of LM to study their pathologic changes at E65,

E100, P1, P30 and P60. The results (Fig. 6) showed no distinct difference of cochlear spiral ganglions between the mutant-type and the wild-type Rongchang pig from E65 to P1. However, the number of SGNs decreased significantly at P30 with other changes including swollen cells, shrunken nuclei and increased intercellular gaps.

The number of SGNs in the MITF$^{-/-}$ pigs was counted at different stages (P1, P30 and P60) after hair cell loss. The SGNs in the basal turns of each slice were counted

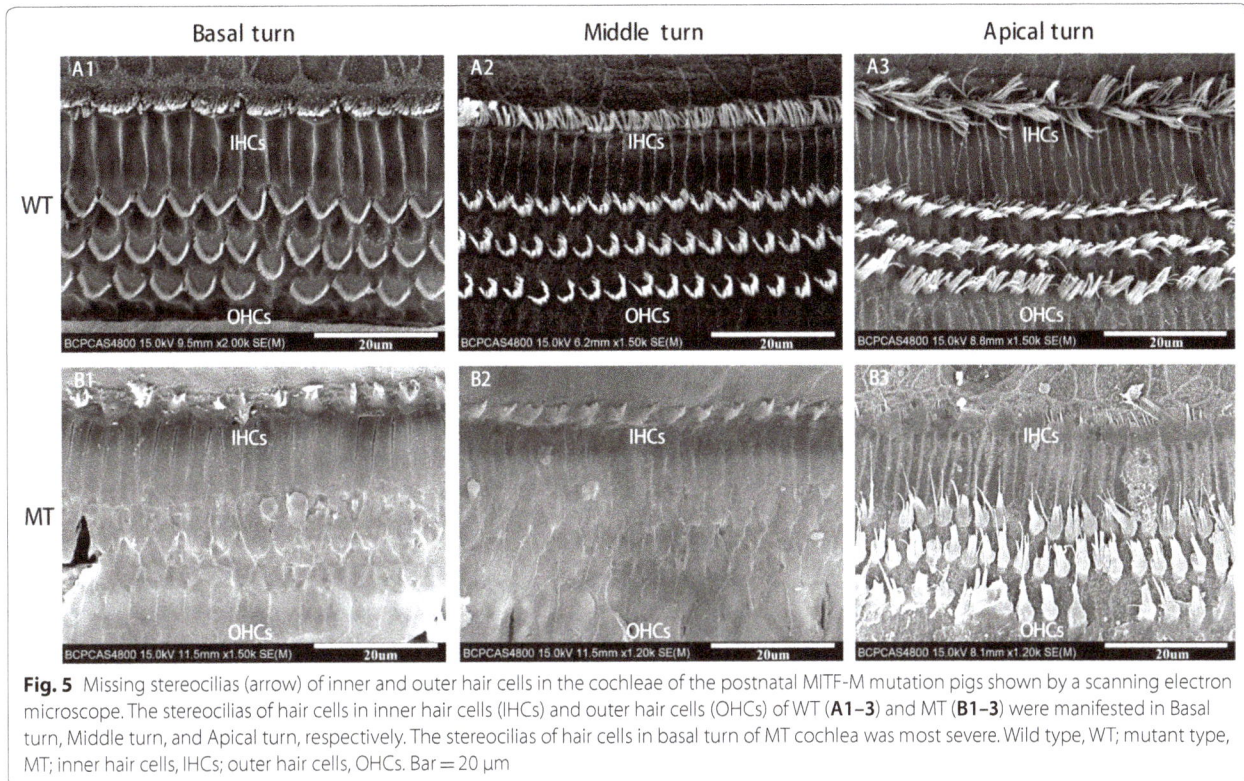

Fig. 5 Missing stereocilias (arrow) of inner and outer hair cells in the cochleae of the postnatal MITF-M mutation pigs shown by a scanning electron microscope. The stereocilias of hair cells in inner hair cells (IHCs) and outer hair cells (OHCs) of WT (**A1–3**) and MT (**B1–3**) were manifested in Basal turn, Middle turn, and Apical turn, respectively. The stereocilias of hair cells in basal turn of MT cochlea was most severe. Wild type, WT; mutant type, MT; inner hair cells, IHCs; outer hair cells, OHCs. Bar = 20 μm

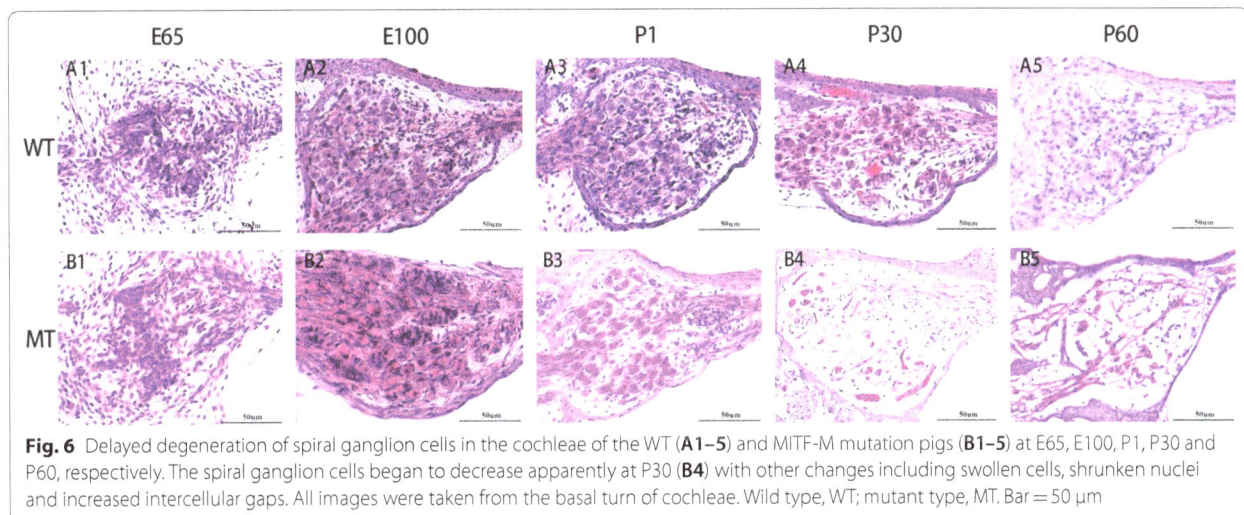

Fig. 6 Delayed degeneration of spiral ganglion cells in the cochleae of the WT (**A1–5**) and MITF-M mutation pigs (**B1–5**) at E65, E100, P1, P30 and P60, respectively. The spiral ganglion cells began to decrease apparently at P30 (**B4**) with other changes including swollen cells, shrunken nuclei and increased intercellular gaps. All images were taken from the basal turn of cochlea. Wild type, WT; mutant type, MT. Bar = 50 μm

at high magnification (400 ×). The results were presented as mean ± SD. As shown in Fig. 7, the number of SGNs of MITF$^{-/-}$ cochleae 732.0 ± 27.7 at P1, 17.0 ± 4.7 at P30 and 6.2 ± 3.0 at P60. There was a significant difference between P1 with P30 and P60 (One-way ANOVA, P < 0.01 in P1 vs. P30 and P1 vs. P60) and no significant difference after P30 (One-way ANOVA, P > 0.01). There was no significant difference of the SGNs at P1 between the mutant and wild types (Student's t test). However, the SGNs number in MITF$^{-/-}$ cochleae at P30 and P60 were both significantly less than that in MITF$^{+/+}$ cochleae (both P < 0.01).

Discussion

It is known that hearing loss in the WS is due to the abnormal proliferation, survival, migration, or differentiation of neural crest-derived melanocytes in inner ear which are situated in the middle layer of the SV called

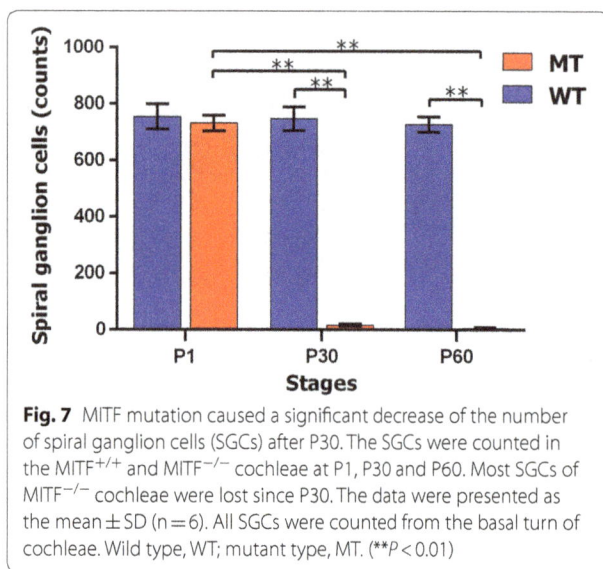

Fig. 7 MITF mutation caused a significant decrease of the number of spiral ganglion cells (SGCs) after P30. The SGCs were counted in the MITF$^{+/+}$ and MITF$^{-/-}$ cochleae at P1, P30 and P60. Most SGCs of MITF$^{-/-}$ cochleae were lost since P30. The data were presented as the mean ± SD (n = 6). All SGCs were counted from the basal turn of cochleae. Wild type, WT; mutant type, MT. (**$P < 0.01$)

intermediate cells. Histopathologic findings of WS both in patients and animal models indicate that the primary alteration is loss of the intermediate cells in the SV, whereas all the other alterations are secondary, including atrophy of the organ of Corti, collapse of the endolymphatic space and degeneration of the SGCs [18–20]. In our previous studies, we had described the morphological changes found in the postnatal cochlear of Rongchang pigs induced by MITF-M mutation [17]. In this study, we further examined the morphological changes in embryonic stages in this porcine model. Our results revealed that the hearing loss in the MITF-M mutant pigs are primarily caused by the malformation of the SVs and the progressive reduction of the cochlear duct and the degeneration of sensory epithelium of the developing inner ears. Our findings on this MITF-M mutant pig model is consistent with previous reports.

In the MITF$^{-/-}$ porcine cochleae, the reduction and absence of intermediate cells in the SV was observed since E85, which indicates that melanocytes in MITF-M mutation pigs are still able to migrate to the cochlea, but have a deficiency in survival during embryogenesis. Subsequently, the Reissner's membrane descended and cochlear duct finally collapsed with apoptosis of hair cells by E100. Unlike other altricial species that cochleosaccular degenerations were mainly observed at postnatal period, the pig models and humans showed a similar pattern that cochlear disorder happened embryonic stages [21–23]. Cochlear implant, which mainly depend on the survival of cochlear SGCs, is an effective treatment for deaf patients with WS. It is confirmed that outcomes of cochlear implant in WS children are similar to other non-syndromic SNHL children [24–26]. It is also suggested

that patients who received early intervention show a better hearing and language skills [27]. However few studies have identified the intervention time and the outcome of the cochlear implants. It is manifested in the current study that the SGNs in the MITF-M mutation pigs began to degenerate gradually one month after birth. However, the morphology of the survival SGNs seemed to be normal. The number of SGCs in MITF$^{-/-}$ cochleae significantly decreased since P30, which had no significant difference among MITF$^{+/+}$ cochleae at P1, P30 and P60. Delayed degeneration of the SGNs in the MITF$^{-/-}$ pigs indicates that cochlear implant is an effective option for auditory rehabilitation of patients with WS and it appears that the earlier of cochlear implant, the better outcomes. This porcine model may also be used to study whether the SGNs in WS patients would remain after the cochlear implant.

Conclusions

In summary, the malformation of the SV was the primary defect in the cochleae of the MITF-M mutation porcine model. The neural crest-derived melanocytes might migrate to the developing SV but fail to survive leading to malformation of the marginal and basal cells. Subsequently, the cochlear duct collapsed and hair cells degenerated are the secondary cochleosaccular degeneration caused by the MIFT mutation. However, no significant change was found in the SGNs of MITF$^{-/-}$ pigs until one month after birth. This result suggests that WS patients should be good candidates for cochlear implant. Earlier receiving cochlear implant, better outcomes after the surgery. This MITF-M mutation porcine model will provide a crucial animal model for further research on cochlear implant, cell therapy in patients with congenital hereditary deafness.

Abbreviations

WS: Waardenburg syndrome; E85: embryonic 85 days; NC: neural crest; P30: postnatal 30 days; MITF: microphthalmia-associated transcription factor; bHLH-LZ: basic helix–loop–helix leucine zipper; MITF-M: melanocyte-specific isoforms; SV: stria vascularis; SGNs: sprial ganglion cells; PLA: People's Liberation Army; EDTA: ethylene diamine tetraacetic acid; HE: hematoxylin–eosin; TEM: transmission electron microscopy; SEM: scanning electron microscopy; SD: standard deviation; MT: mutate type; WT: wild type; ANOVA: analysis of variance; LM: light microscopy; IC: intermediate cells; MC: marginal cell; BC: basal cell; IHCs: inner hair cells; OHCs: outer hair cells.

Authors' contributions

WWG and SMY led the experiments. HSL performed animal work and prepared biological samples. WC, QQH, WR and LLR performed the cochlear morphology experiments. WC wrote the paper. QQH revised the paper. Moreover, all authors were involved in drafting the manuscript or revising it critically for important intellectual content. All authors read and approved the final manuscript.

Author details

[1] Department of Otolaryngology, Head & Neck Surgery, Institute of Otolaryngology, Chinese PLA General Hospital, Beijing Key Laboratory of Hearing

Impairment Prevention and Treatment, Key Laboratory of Hearing Impairment Science, Chinese PLA Medical School,Ministry of Education, Beijng, China.
[2] Department of Biotechnology, Dalian Medical University, Dalian 116044, Liaoning, China.

Acknowledgements
None.

Competing interests
The authors declare that they have no competing interests.

Funding
The funding body and sponsors had no role in study design, data collection, data analysis, data interpretation, and in writing the manuscript. This work was supported by grants from the National Natural Science Foundation of China (Nos. 81670940, 81670941, 81570933, and 81400472), and Special Cultivating and Developing Program of Beijing Science and Technology Innovation Base (z151100001615050). Youth cultivation project of military medical science (16QNP133), the major project of Twelfth Five-Year Plan (BWS14J045).

References

1. Pingault V, Ente D, Dastot-Le MF, et al. Review and update of mutations causing Waardenburg syndrome. Hum Mutat. 2010;31(4):391–406.
2. Read AP, Newton VE. Waardenburg syndrome. J Med Genet. 1997;34(8):656–65.
3. Song J, Feng Y, Acke FR, et al. Hearing loss in Waardenburg syndrome: a systematic review. Clin Genet. 2016;89(4):416–25.
4. Tassabehji M, Newton VE, Read AP. Waardenburg syndrome type 2 caused by mutations in the human microphthalmia (MITF) gene. Nat Genet. 1994;8(3):251–5.
5. Yang S, Dai P, Liu X, et al. Genetic and phenotypic heterogeneity in Chinese patients with Waardenburg syndrome type II. PLoS ONE. 2013;8(10):e77149.
6. Grill C, Bergsteinsdottir K, Ogmundsdottir MH, et al. MITF mutations associated with pigment deficiency syndromes and melanoma have different effects on protein function. Hum Mol Genet. 2013;22(21):4357–67.
7. Vachtenheim J, Borovansky J. "Transcription physiology" of pigment formation in melanocytes: central role of MITF. Exp Dermatol. 2010;19(7):617–27.
8. Grill C, Bergsteinsdottir K, Ogmundsdottir MH, et al. MITF mutations associated with pigment deficiency syndromes and melanoma have different effects on protein function. Hum Mol Genet. 2013;22(21):4357–67.
9. Steingrimsson E, Copeland NG, Jenkins NA. Melanocytes and the microphthalmia transcription factor network. Annu Rev Genet. 2004;38:365–411.
10. Hozumi H, Takeda K, Yoshida-Amano Y, et al. Impaired development of melanoblasts in the black-eyed white Mitf(mi-bw) mouse, a model for auditory-pigmentary disorders. Genes Cells. 2012;17(6):494–508.
11. Fuse N, Yasumoto K, Suzuki H, et al. Identification of a melanocyte-type promoter of the microphthalmia-associated transcription factor gene. Biochem Biophys Res Commun. 1996;219(3):702–7.
12. Saito H, Yasumoto K, Takeda K, et al. Melanocyte-specific microphthalmia-associated transcription factor isoform activates its own gene promoter through physical interaction with lymphoid-enhancing factor 1. J Biol Chem. 2002;277(32):28787–94.
13. Hozumi H, Takeda K, Yoshida-Amano Y, et al. Impaired development of melanoblasts in the black-eyed white Mitf(mi-bw) mouse, a model for auditory-pigmentary disorders. Genes Cells. 2012;17(6):494–508.
14. Tachibana M. Sound needs sound melanocytes to be heard. Pigment Cell Res. 1999;12(6):344–54.
15. Toriello HV. Pigmentary anomalies and hearing loss. Adv Otorhinolaryngol. 2011;70:50–5.
16. Ma L, Yi HJ, Yuan FQ, et al. An efficient strategy for establishing a model of sensorineural deafness in rats. Neural Regen Res. 2015;10(10):1683–9.
17. Chen L, Guo W, Ren L, et al. A de novo silencer causes elimination of MITF-M expression and profound hearing loss in pigs. BMC Biol. 2016;14:52.
18. Nakashima S, Sando I, Takahashi H, et al. Temporal bone histopathologic findings of Waardenburg's syndrome: a case report. Laryngoscope. 1992;102(5):563–7.
19. Tachibana M, Kobayashi Y, Matsushima Y. Mouse models for four types of Waardenburg syndrome. Pigment Cell Res. 2003;16(5):448–54.
20. Ni C, Zhang D, Beyer LA, et al. Hearing dysfunction in heterozygous Mitf(Mi-wh)/+ mice, a model for Waardenburg syndrome type 2 and Tietz syndrome. Pigment Cell Melanoma Res. 2013;26(1):78–87.
21. Jin Z, Mannstrom P, Jarlebark L, et al. Malformation of stria vascularis in the developing inner ear of the German waltzing guinea pig. Cell Tissue Res. 2007;328(2):257–70.
22. Bibas A, Liang J, Michaels L, et al. The development of the stria vascularis in the human foetus. Clin Otolaryngol Allied Sci. 2000;25(2):126–9.
23. Guo W, Yi H, Ren L, et al. The morphology and electrophysiology of the cochlea of the miniature pig. Anat Rec (Hoboken). 2015;298(3):494–500.
24. Kontorinis G, Lenarz T, Giourgas A, et al. Outcomes and special considerations of cochlear implantation in waardenburg syndrome. Otol Neurotol. 2011;32(6):951–5.
25. De Sousa AS, Monteiro AR, Martins JH, et al. Cochlear implant rehabilitation outcomes in Waardenburg syndrome children. Int J Pediatr Otorhinolaryngol. 2012;76(9):1375–8.
26. Koyama H, Kashio A, Sakata A, et al. The Hearing Outcomes of Cochlear Implantation in Waardenburg Syndrome. Biomed Res Int. 2016;2016:2854736.
27. Magalhaes AT, Samuel PA, Goffi-Gomez MV, et al. Audiological outcomes of cochlear implantation in Waardenburg Syndrome. Int Arch Otorhinolaryngol. 2013;17(3):285–90.

15

Assessment of brain beta-amyloid deposition in transgenic mouse models of Alzheimer's disease with PET imaging agents ^{18}F-flutemetamol and ^{18}F-florbetaben

Hye Joo Son[1], Young Jin Jeong[1], Hyun Jin Yoon[1], Sang Yoon Lee[1], Go-Eun Choi[2], Ji-Ae Park[3], Min Hwan Kim[3], Kyo Chul Lee[3], Yong Jin Lee[3], Mun Ki Kim[4], Kook Cho[2] and Do-Young Kang[1,2]* [iD]

Abstract

Background: Although amyloid beta (Aβ) imaging is widely used for diagnosing and monitoring Alzheimer's disease in clinical fields, paralleling comparison between ^{18}F-flutemetamol and ^{18}F-florbetaben was rarely attempted in AD mouse model. We performed a comparison of Aβ PET images between ^{18}F-flutemetamol and ^{18}F-florbetaben in a recently developed APPswe mouse model, C57BL/6-Tg (NSE-hAPPsw) Korl.

Results: After an injection (0.23 mCi) of ^{18}F-flutemetamol and ^{18}F-florbetaben at a time interval of 2–3 days, we compared group difference of SUVR and kinetic parameters between the AD (n = 7) and control (n = 7) mice, as well as between ^{18}F-flutemetamol and ^{18}F-florbetaben image. In addition, bio-distribution and histopathology were conducted. With visual image and VOI-based SUVR analysis, the AD group presented more prominent uptake than did the control group in both the ^{18}F-florbetaben and ^{18}F-flutemetamol images. With kinetic analysis, the ^{18}F-florbetaben images showed differences in K1 and k4 between the AD and control groups, although ^{18}F-flutemetamol images did not show significant difference. ^{18}F-florbetaben images showed more prominent cortical uptake and matched well to the thioflavin S staining images than did the ^{18}F-flutemetamol image. In contrast, ^{18}F-flutemetamol images presented higher K1, k4, K1/k2 values than those of ^{18}F-florbetaben images. Also, ^{18}F-flutemetamol images presented prominent uptake in the bowel and bladder, consistent with higher bio-distribution in kidney, lung, blood and heart.

Conclusions: Compared with ^{18}F-flutemetamol images, ^{18}F-florbetaben images showed prominent visual uptake intensity, SUVR, and higher correlations with the pathology. In contrast, ^{18}F-flutemetamol was more actively metabolized than was ^{18}F-florbetaben (Son et al. in J Nucl Med 58(Suppl 1):S278, 2017].

Keywords: PET/CT imaging, Alzheimer's disease, transgenic mouse model, ^{18}F-flutemetamol, ^{18}F-florbetaben

*Correspondence: dykang@dau.ac.kr
[1] Department of Nuclear Medicine, Dong-A University Medical Center, Dong-A University College of Medicine, 26 Daesingongwon-ro, Seo-gu, Busan 602-812, Korea
Full list of author information is available at the end of the article

Background

Recently, Aβ imaging with ^{18}F labeled radiotracers has been widely used for patients with Alzheimer's disease (AD). ^{18}F-flutemetamol is ^{18}F labeled analogue of ^{11}C-PiB produced by GE Healthcare (Buckinghamshire, UK) [2]. It has been useful in differentiating between patients with AD and healthy subjects with high specificity (96%) and sensitivity (93%) in the detection of AD, as well as high test–retest reliability [3, 4]. ^{18}F-florbetaben is an ^{18}F labeled polyethylene glycol stilbene derivative showing high in vitro affinity and specificity for β-amyloid plaques [3].

[18]F-florbetaben and ^{18}F-flutemetamol are widely used for the diagnosis and monitoring of AD in a routine medical field. However, there are many unknown issues regarding the difference in tracer dynamics and biodistribution between ^{18}F-flutemetamol and ^{18}F-florbetaben. Because of the difficulty conducting the direct comparison between two tracers for humans due to the weighted exposure to radiation, a preclinical animal study is a good alternative option for a baseline study.

Recently, several imaging studies using newly developed ^{18}F labeled Aβ PET tracers were reported in AD mouse models. In a previous study, the in vivo ^{18}F-flutemetamol binding of Aβ deposits was tested in various AD mouse models [5]. In old APP23 mice, significant ^{18}F-flutemetamol retention was observed in the brain. But, ^{18}F-flutemetabmol did not show a outstanding advantage in APPswe-PS1dE9 and Tg2576 mice.

However, transgenic mice with various genetic backgrounds have been related with different pathologies, which make it difficult to interpret the overlapping study results [6]. Therefore, comparisons between β-amyloid imaging regarding AD mouse have to be accomplished with some caution as brain sizes and anatomic landmarks of target VOIs greatly affect accurate PET signal quantification. Until now, there has been no antecedent report comparing between ^{18}F-flutemetamol and

[18]F-florbetaben images in an AD mouse model, so comparative conclusions draw special interest.

Herein, we tested a recently developed APPsw mouse model (C57BL/6-Tg(NSE-hAPPsw)Korl) enhancing expressing Swedish double mutation form of human APP (K670 N, M671L) under regulation of the neuron specific enolase (NSE) promoter. For this mouse model, there has been no attempt regarding its application for the evaluation of new Aβ imaging ligands. Hence, we performed a small animal study conducting direct comparisons between two ^{18}F labeled Aβ PET tracers, ^{18}F-flutemetamol and ^{18}F-florbetaben in (C57BL/6-Tg(NSE-hAPPsw)Korl) mouse model in terms of following aspects: the ability to discriminate a transgenic from a control mouse, intensity of uptake and distribution pattern in visual images, difference of static ratio and kinetic parameters, bio-distribution and correlation with neuropathologic findings.

Methods

Animals

Experiments were conducted with 7 APPsw transgenic mice (genetic background C57BL/6-Tg(NSE-hAPPsw) Korl) augmenting human APP with the Swedish double mutation (K670N, M671L) under regulation of the NSE promoter. As controls, 7 littermates with the corresponding genetic background, C57BL/6J, were used. Age and sex were matched between the two groups (mean age and mean weight: 18 weeks and 24.84 ± 1.01 g for APPsw mice and 18 weeks and 29.20 ± 3.49 g for C57BL/6 J control mice). The mice used in the study were donated from the Division of Laboratory Animal Resources, Korea FDA (Food and Drug safety administration, National Institute of Toxicological Research, registration number: KNL-HYD-TG0615). Details on number of animals per study group, sex, mean age and mean body weight are summarized in Table 1. Two mice from each AD and control group were sacrificed for pathology at 18 weeks

Table 1 Basic characteristics of AD transgenic and control mouse model

ID	AD transgenic			Control		
	Age (weeks)	Sex	Weight (g)	Age (weeks)	Sex	Weight (g)
1	18	Male	23.41	18	Male	27.20
2	18	Male	26.34	18	Male	27.68
3	18	Male	25.12	18	Male	31.32
4	18	Male	24.16	18	Male	26.27
5	18	Male	24.12	18	Male	36.26
6	18	Male	25.68	18	Male	27.74
7	18	Male	25.11	18	Male	27.99
Mean ± SD	18	Male	24.84 ± 4.8	18	Male	29.20 ± 3.4

and correlated with imaging. The remaining mice were sacrificed for pathology at 48 weeks. Animal experiments were conducted with the approval of the institutional animal care committee (IRB number: LML 16-970, Dong-A university, Busan, Korea).

PET/CT imaging

Seven transgenic and 7 control mice underwent sequential PET imaging for direct comparison of the two tracers (total 28 scans). The time interval between ^{18}F-florbetaben and ^{18}F-flutemetamol PET imaging was 2–3 days. Inhalation anesthesia was maintained by 3.5 L/min oxygen and 0.6–2% isoflurane, 15 min prior to scanning. The body temperature was kept at 37 °C with a temperature-controlled heating pad, and the respiratory rate stayed at 80–100/min. Small animal PET data was acquired with a nanoscan PET scanner (Mediso Medical Imaging Systems, USA). After the induction of anesthesia, the animals were positioned with their heads in the center of the field of view and were fixed in the PET scanner in the prone head first position (HFP). At the beginning of the PET scanning procedure, computed tomography (CT) scans were acquired for attenuation correction and anatomical reference (50 kVp, 250 mA). Next, simultaneous with an i.v. injection of 8.51 MBq (0.23 mCi) of ^{18}F-flutemetamol or ^{18}F-florbetaben, a 90-min dynamic emission scan was started. Dynamic acquisition was performed in the 3D list mode for 90 min. The emission data were normalized and corrected for decay and dead time. The sinograms were reconstructed with FBP (filtered back-projection using a ramp filter with a cut-off at the Nyquist frequency). Static images and dynamic images with 20 imaging frames were generated.

Radiosynthesis

The radiosynthesis of ^{18}F-florbetaben (4-ethoxy)phenyl] vinyl}-N-methylaniline, commercial name: Neuraceq) was performed using an auto-synthesizer according to the protocol of Piramal Enterprises Ltd. The radiochemical purity was > 99%, as determined by analytical HPLC. The radiochemical yield averaged 45% (decay-corrected) at the end of synthesis (EOS) based on ^{18}F-fluorine. The specific activity averaged 774 GBq/umol at the EOS. The commercial products were purchased from the company (Duchem Bio, South Korea). The radiosynthesis of ^{18}F-flutemetamol (6-Benzothiazolol, 2-[3-(^{18}F) fluoro-4-(methylamino) phenyl], commercial name: Visamyl) was performed to using an auto-synthesizer according to the protocol of GE Healthcare. The radiochemical purity was > 96% as determined by analytical HPLC. The radiochemical yield averaged 27% (decay-corrected) at the end of synthesis (EOS) based on ^{18}F-fluorine. The specific activity averaged 1862 GBq/umol at the EOS. The

commercial products were purchased from the company (Carecamp Co., Ltd., South Korea).

Analysis of PET data

PET data was analyzed with the fusion toolbox embedded in PMOD version 3.7.0 software (PMOD Technologies, Zurich, Switzerland). The CT image was thresholded at 2/3 of the maximal value (approximately 1340 Hounsfield units), and the skull image was obtained. For the shape of an atlas to properly fit with the skull CT, the thresholded CT image was manually fused with the magnetic resonance brain template, called M.Mirrione. Then, the transformation information was saved in a MAT-file format. Using the Initialize/Match function of the fusion toolbox, the PET image was re-sliced to match M.Mirrione template [7]. Then, the transformation information between the thresholded CT and the mouse magnetic resonance template was loaded on re-sliced PET image. Then, the re-sliced PET image was co-registered manually using the shift, rotate and scale functions and normalized to the mouse MR brain template (M. Mirrione) [7, 8]. The final co-registered PET image was masked with the M. Mirrione brain mask. The corresponding template and mask files can be found in the resources/usertemplates directory embedded in PMOD version 3.7.0 software (Pmod Technologies, Zurich, Switzerland). The same step was applied to all frames of dynamic data.

Volumes of interest (VOIs) of embedded mouse brains are presented in Fig. 1. The areas of the VOIs are the cortex (Cor), right hippocampus (Rhip), left hippocampus (Lhip), thalamus (Thal), right striatum (Rstr), left striatum (Lstr) and the cerebellum (Crbl). To investigate the difference between ^{18}F-florbetaben and ^{18}F-flutemetamol images, different images using the image algebra option embedded in PMOD fusion tool (version 3.7.0; Pmod Technologies, Zurich, Switzerland) were created. For the analysis of static PET image, the standardized uptake value (SUV) and the standardized uptake value ratio (SUVR) between the cortex and cerebellum was calculated with a VOI based method.

To determine the optimal compartment model for amyloid specific tracers, the 2 tissue compartment model from previous studies was used [9–11]. For the 2 tissue compartment model analysis with the Image Derived Input Function (IDIF) method, 1 mm^3 volumes of interest (VOIs) were drawn on the center of the left ventricle on the initial time frame image.

Pathology

Sample preparation

The animals were deeply anesthetized with zoletil and xylazine and were sacrificed by intra-cardiac perfusion with 4% paraformaldehyde (pH 7.4). The brains were

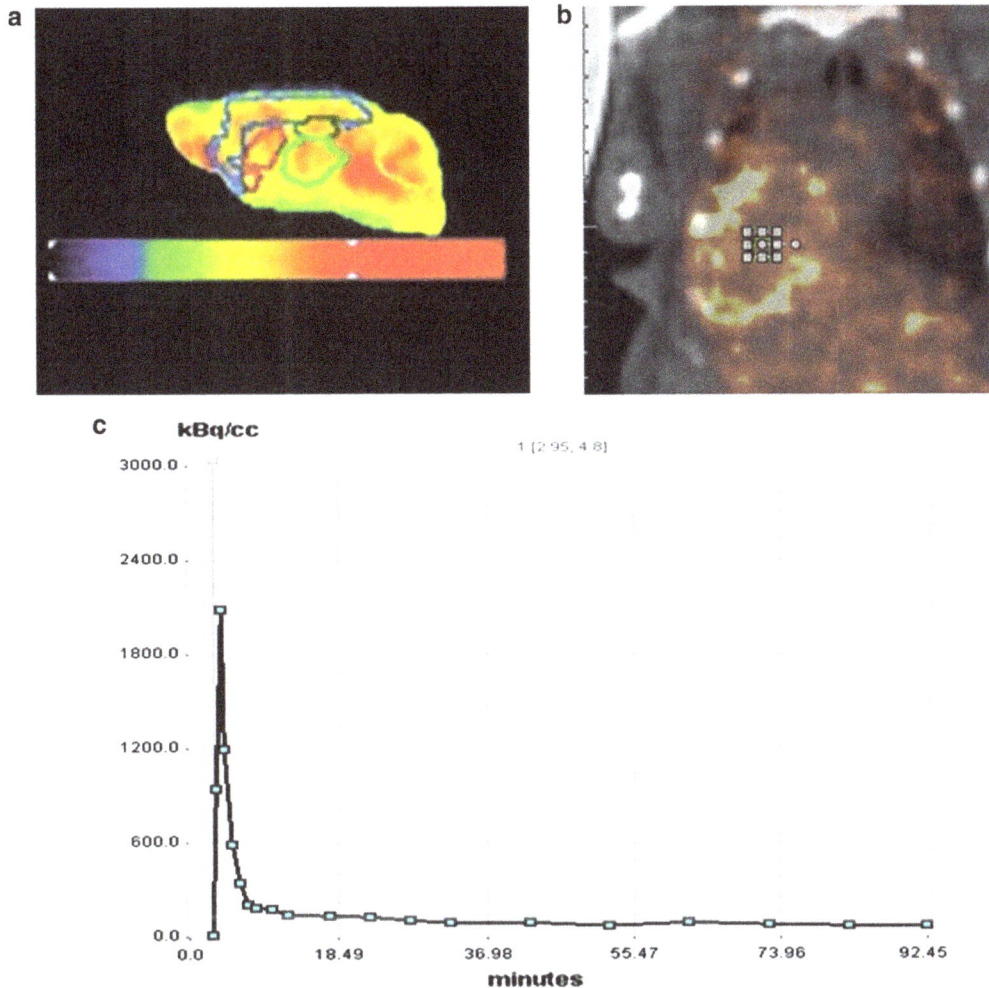

Fig. 1 a Volume of interest (VOI) of mouse brain. VOI was drawn under guidance of the PMOD embedded mouse brain atlas (Mouse (M. Mirrione)-T2 MRI atlas) to cover the cortex (Cor: blue), right hippocampus (Rhip: dark green), left hippocampus (Lhip: dark green), thalamus (Thal: light green), right striatum (Rstr: red), left striatum (Lstr: red) and the cerebellum (Crbl: yellow), **b** volume of interest in blood input area, **c** time activity curve of blood input area

embedded in paraffin wax for 48 h. The tissue samples were serially sectioned at a thickness of 10 μm on a rotary microtome for immuno-histochemical analysis.

Thioflavin S staining

The sections were deparaffinated and rehydrated before staining. The sections were incubated in a 1% (1 g per 100 ml water) thioflavin S (TfS, T1892, Sigma Aldrich, St. Louis, MI, USA) solution for 30 min. The sections were washed with water three times for 2 min, 80% ethanol for 6 min, washed again with water and cover slip mounted with VectaShield as the mounting medium. The slides were stored for 4 °C. The sections were washed with water three times for 2 min and with 80% ethanol for fluorescence microscopy using filter sets for

DAPI and GFP. The DAPI (contained in the mounting medium) fluorescence was used by the scanner to set the optical focus, and the GFP contained the specific signal of thioflavin S.

Immunohistochemistry for amyloid beta 40

Non-specific reactions were blocked with 3% fetal bovine serum in phosphate buffered saline (PBS) for 1 h. Slides were incubated with mouse monoclonal primary amyloid beta 40 antibody (diluted 1:150; Millipore, USA). The secondary antibody was Streptavidin Alexa fluor 594 conjugated anti-mouse IgG (1:400, Invitrogen, USA). The fluorescence was observed using Nikon-80i fluorescence microscopy using filter sets for

DAPI and RFP. The DAPI (contained in the mounting medium) fluorescence was used by the scanner to set the optical focus, and the RFP contained the specific signal of amyloid beta 40.

Bio-distribution

The ^{18}F-florbetaben and ^{18}F-flutemetamol binding to different brain regions and peripheral organs in AD transgenic (N=1) and control mice (N=1) using ex vivo gamma counting. Mice were anaesthetized with isoflurane and injected with 0.23 mCi of ^{18}F-florbetaben and ^{18}F-flutemetamol. The tracer was allowed to distribute for 90 min. Mice were sacrificed by cervical dislocation and the brain was rapidly removed. Then, the blood, heart, lung, liver, kidney, medulla, cerebellum, right cortex, left cortex, olfactory bulb were dissected. ^{18}F-radioactivity was measured with a gamma counter.

Statistics

For the analysis of static PET data, group comparison of SUVR and kinetic parameters were conducted with the Mann–Whitney U. A threshold of P less than 0.05 was considered significant. All statistical analyses were performed using IBM SPSS Statistics (version 20.0; SPSS) and Medcalc 16.8.4.

Results
Comparative overview of representative visual brain PET image

A comparative overview of the representative brain PET images is presented in Fig. 2. On the ^{18}F-florbetaben PET image, the AD transgenic mice showed significantly higher tracer retention in the cortical regions than did the control mice. On the ^{18}F-flutemetamol PET image, the transgenic mice showed mild, focal uptake in cortical brain regions; however, higher uptake was shown in the transgenic mice than in the control mice. Overall, regardless of the AD transgenic and control group, ^{18}F-florbetaben imaging showed much higher retention than did ^{18}F-flutemetamol imaging. Both the AD transgenic and control groups showed high tracer retention in the cerebellum and pons than did the cortical regions.

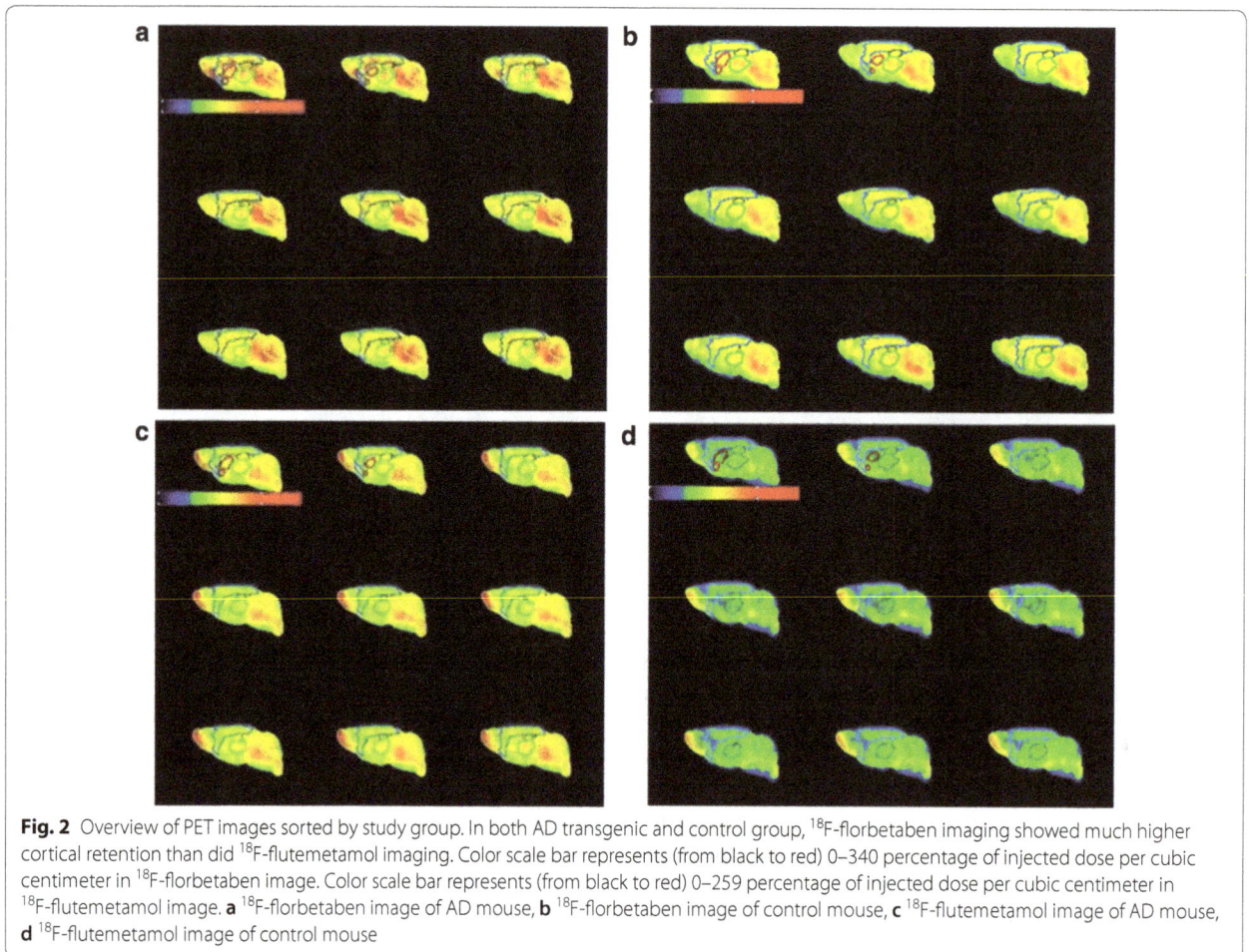

Fig. 2 Overview of PET images sorted by study group. In both AD transgenic and control group, ^{18}F-florbetaben imaging showed much higher cortical retention than did ^{18}F-flutemetamol imaging. Color scale bar represents (from black to red) 0–340 percentage of injected dose per cubic centimeter in ^{18}F-florbetaben image. Color scale bar represents (from black to red) 0–259 percentage of injected dose per cubic centimeter in ^{18}F-flutemetamol image. **a** ^{18}F-florbetaben image of AD mouse, **b** ^{18}F-florbetaben image of control mouse, **c** ^{18}F-flutemetamol image of AD mouse, **d** ^{18}F-flutemetamol image of control mouse

Difference image obtained from image algebra calculation: (^{18}F-florbetaben- ^{18}F-flutemetamol)

A visual representation of comparisons of the difference between ^{18}F-florbetaben and ^{18}F-flutemetamol is presented in Fig. 3. In the AD transgenic group, ^{18}F-florbetaben showed higher and more extensive cortical uptakes compared with ^{18}F-flutemetamol.

Comparative overview of representative visual whole body PET image

Figure 4 provides a comparative overview of the representative whole body PET images. The color bar of

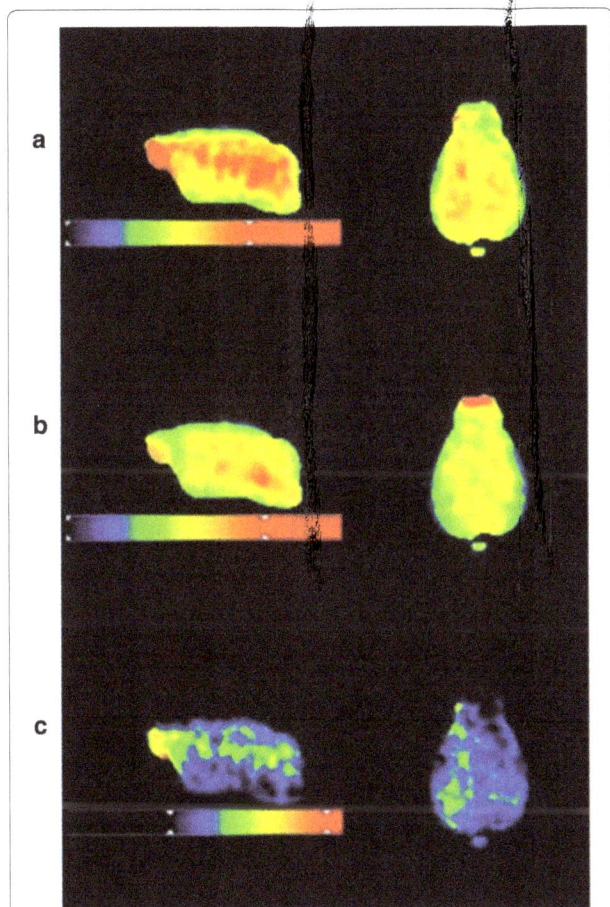

Fig. 3 Difference between ^{18}F-florbetaben and ^{18}F-flutemetamol in AD transgenic group. Each image represents PET image of **a** ^{18}F-florbetaben (upper column), **b** ^{18}F-flutemetamol (middle column) and **c** algebra calculation (^{18}F-florbetaben-^{18}F-flutemetamol, lower column). In the AD transgenic group, ^{18}F-florbetaben showed higher and more extensive cortical uptakes compared with ^{18}F-flutemetamol. Color scale bar represents 0–340 percentage of injected dose per cubic centimeter in ^{18}F-florbetaben image. Color scale bar represents 0–270 percentage of injected dose per cubic centimeter in ^{18}F-flutemetamol image. Color scale bar represents 0–280 percentage of injected dose per cubic centimeter in difference image

the PET image was adjusted to (0–30% ID/g) to optimize for visualization of the peripheral organ uptakes. ^{18}F-flutemetamol PET imaging showed much more intense uptake in the bowel and bladder than did ^{18}F-florbetaben.

Bio-distribution

Bio-distribution data of both ^{18}F-florbetaben and ^{18}F-flutemetamol are presented in Fig. 5. The highest radioactivity in the brain was measured in the cortex, followed by the medulla and cerebellum. ^{18}F-florbetaben (Rt. cortex: 1.39 ID/g (%), Lt. cortex: 1.209 ID/g (%)) showed higher absolute differences between AD transgenic mice and control mice than did ^{18}F-flutemetamol (Rt. cortex: 0.619 ID/g (%), Lt. cortex: 0.608 ID/g (%)). In AD transgenic mouse, ^{18}F-florbetaben showed higher uptake in the cortex than did ^{18}F-flutemetamol. In addition, for both ^{18}F-florbetaben and ^{18}F-flutemetamol, the right cortex in the AD mouse showed higher uptake, showing right side laterality. In terms of the visceral distribution of ^{18}F-florbetaben, the highest radioactivity was measured in the liver, followed by the kidney, lung, blood and heart in both transgenic and control mice. In terms of visceral distribution of ^{18}F-flutemetamol, the highest radioactivity was measured in the kidney, followed by the liver, lung, blood and heart in transgenic mice. In control mice, the highest radioactivity was measured in the kidney, followed by the lung, liver, blood and heart. Comparative analysis of ^{18}F-florbetaben and ^{18}F-flutemetamol biodistribution revealed that ^{18}F-florbetaben imaging showed higher radioactivity in the cortex than did ^{18}F-flutemetamol. In contrast, ^{18}F-flutemetamol showed higher radioactivity in the kidney, lung, blood and heart, although the liver showed higher radioactivity with ^{18}F-florbetaben. In contrast with the imaging findings, the bio-distribution data showed higher uptake in the cortex than in the cerebellum.

SUVmean and SUVR based analysis of static PET image

The SUVmean and SUVR values of PET images in both the AD transgenic and control groups are presented in Tables 2, 3. The mean SUVmean values of the ^{18}F-florbetaben images in the AD and control mice were 0.804 and 0.699, respectively. In contrast, the mean SUVmean values of the ^{18}F-flutemetamol images in the AD and control mice were 0.332 and 0.297, respectively. The mean SUVR values of the ^{18}F-florbetaben images in the AD and control mice were 0.926 and 0.829, respectively. In contrast, the mean SUVR values of the ^{18}F-flutemetamol images in the AD and control mice were 0.854 and 0.687, respectively. On both the ^{18}F-florbetaben and ^{18}F-flutemetamol scans, the mean SUVmean and SUVR values of the AD transgenic group showed higher values

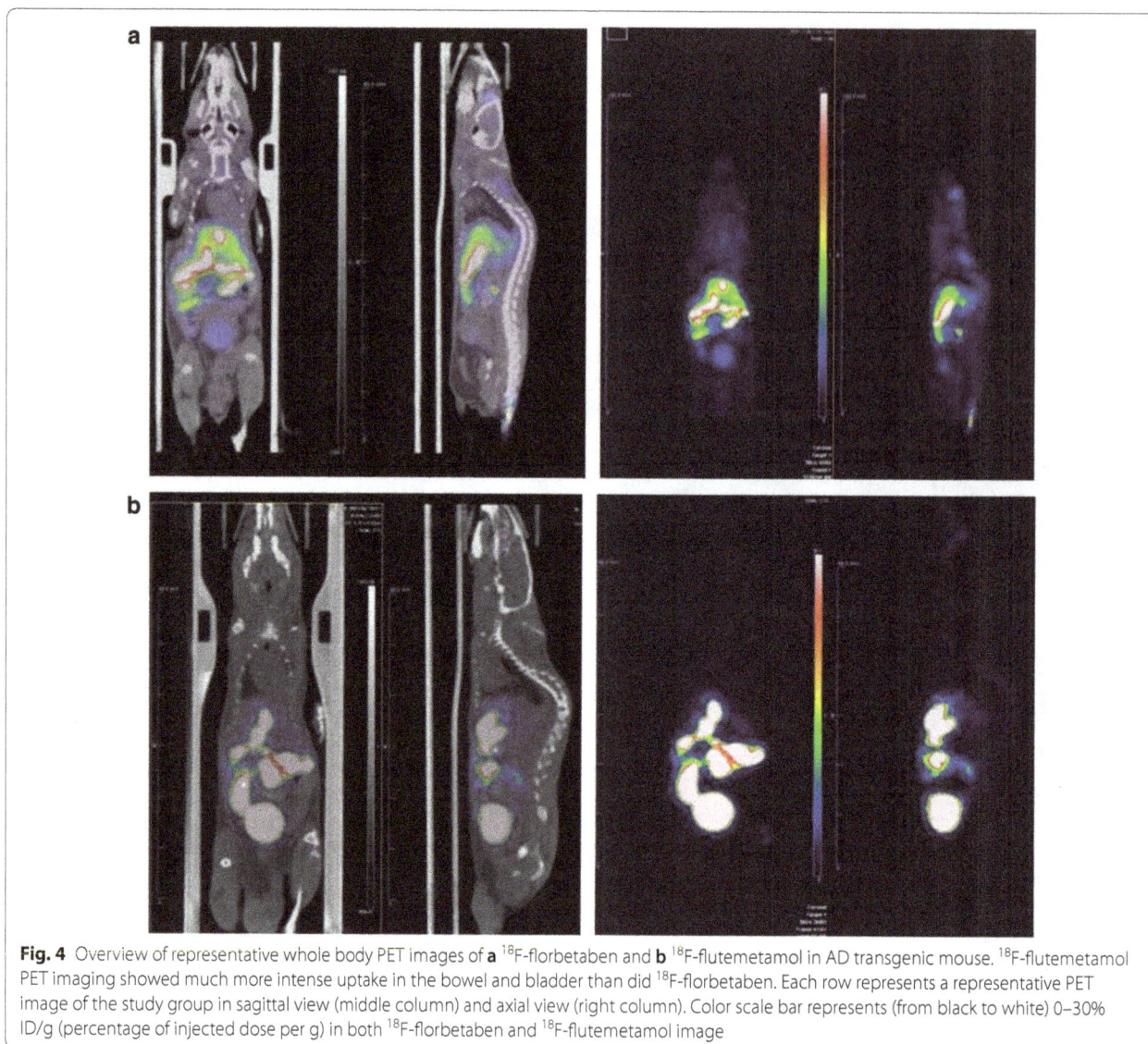

Fig. 4 Overview of representative whole body PET images of **a** ^{18}F-florbetaben and **b** ^{18}F-flutemetamol in AD transgenic mouse. ^{18}F-flutemetamol PET imaging showed much more intense uptake in the bowel and bladder than did ^{18}F-florbetaben. Each row represents a representative PET image of the study group in sagittal view (middle column) and axial view (right column). Color scale bar represents (from black to white) 0–30% ID/g (percentage of injected dose per g) in both ^{18}F-florbetaben and ^{18}F-flutemetamol image

than those of the control group. The mean SUVmean and SUVR of ^{18}F-florbetaben showed higher values than those of ^{18}F-flutemetamol in the AD transgenic and control groups, respectively. The mean of the differences in the SUVmean between the AD and control group was 0.106 for ^{18}F-florbetaben and 0.03 for ^{18}F-flutemetamol.

Statistical analysis of static PET data: AD vs. control

The quantitative parameters of the static PET images (SUVR) in the AD transgenic and control groups were tested. On the ^{18}F-florbetaben images, the AD transgenic group showed significantly higher SUVR values ($p = 0.011$) than did the control group. On the ^{18}F-flutemetamol images, the AD group showed significantly higher SUVR values ($p = 0.001$) than did

the control group. Moreover, on the ^{18}F-flutemetamol images, the AD group showed significantly higher SUVR values than did the control group in all brain areas. However, on the ^{18}F-florbetaben images, the AD group showed significantly higher SUVR values than did the control group only in the cortex.

Statistical analysis of static PET data: ^{18}F-florbetaben vs. ^{18}F-flutemetamol

The quantitative parameters of the static PET images (SUVR) between the ^{18}F-florbetaben and ^{18}F-flutemetamol groups are presented in Table 4. The significant differences of the SUVR (cortex/cerebellum) between the scans of the two tracers in each AD and control group were compared. ^{18}F-florbetaben presented a higher

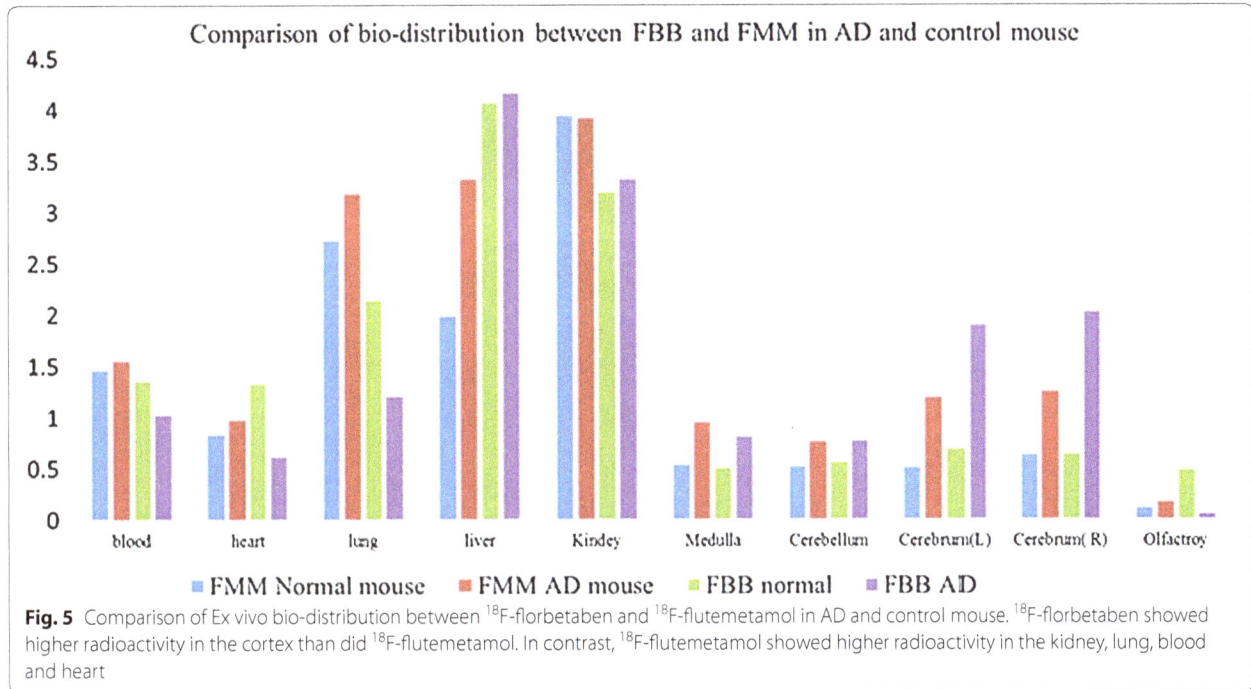

Fig. 5 Comparison of Ex vivo bio-distribution between ^{18}F-florbetaben and ^{18}F-flutemetamol in AD and control mouse. ^{18}F-florbetaben showed higher radioactivity in the cortex than did ^{18}F-flutemetamol. In contrast, ^{18}F-flutemetamol showed higher radioactivity in the kidney, lung, blood and heart

Table 2 SUVR values of ^{18}F-florbetaben image in both AD transgenic and control group

Group	ID	Cor	Rhip	Lhip	Thala	Rstr	Lstr
(a) SUVR values of ^{18}F-florbetaben image in AD transgenic group							
AD	1	0.879	0.912	0.941	1.017	0.917	0.979
	2	0.958	0.843	0.808	0.932	0.883	0.878
	3	0.929	0.988	1.004	1.083	1.015	1.014
	4	0.838	0.955	1.009	1.084	0.978	1.000
	5	0.966	0.996	0.966	1.030	0.870	0.856
	6	0.919	1.121	1.133	1.258	1.161	1.187
	7	0.994	1.074	1.133	1.216	1.071	1.144
Average		0.926	0.984	0.999	1.089	0.985	1.008
SD		0.054	0.094	0.113	0.114	0.106	0.123
(b) SUVR values of ^{18}F-florbetaben image in control group							
Control	1	0.663	0.901	0.966	1.023	0.948	0.956
	2	0.852	0.964	0.957	1.025	0.932	0.962
	3	0.872	0.944	1.006	1.098	1.016	1.035
	4	0.854	1.780	1.775	1.997	1.762	1.752
	5	0.876	0.894	1.003	1.054	0.960	0.988
	6	0.822	1.000	0.989	1.085	1.000	1.012
	7	0.862	0.918	0.972	1.084	0.966	1.007
Average		0.829	1.057	1.095	1.195	1.084	1.102
SD		0.070	0.297	0.278	0.329	0.278	0.267

Cor cortex, *Rhip* Rt. hippocampus, *Lhip* Lt. hippocampus, *Thala* Thalamus, *Rstr* Rt. striatum, *Lstr* Lt. striatum

Table 3 SUVR values of ^{18}F-flutemetamol image in both AD transgenic and control group

Group	ID	Cor	Rhip	Lhip	Thala	Rstr	Lstr
(a) *SUVR values of ^{18}F-flutemetamol image in AD transgenic group*							
AD	1	0.872	0.997	1.037	1.116	1.038	1.094
	2	0.849	0.913	0.882	1.086	0.978	0.974
	3	0.922	0.991	1.064	1.147	1.035	1.144
	4	0.782	0.922	0.939	1.016	0.897	0.889
	5	0.814	0.989	0.950	1.129	0.995	0.899
	6	0.946	0.989	1.003	1.134	1.035	1.123
	7	0.792	0.880	0.933	0.933	0.791	0.837
Average		0.854	0.954	0.973	1.080	0.967	0.994
SD		0.063	0.048	0.064	0.078	0.092	0.125
(b) *SUVR values of ^{18}F-flutemetamol image in control group*							
Control	1	0.589	0.623	0.633	0.720	0.650	0.638
	2	0.674	0.718	0.784	0.839	0.738	0.779
	3	0.765	0.839	0.862	0.940	0.814	0.829
	4	0.684	0.743	0.773	0.837	0.764	0.762
	5	0.706	0.904	0.912	1.015	0.923	0.950
	6	0.685	0.822	0.848	0.873	0.752	0.771
	7	0.703	0.736	0.864	0.928	0.818	0.850
Average		0.687	0.769	0.811	0.879	0.780	0.797
SD		0.053	0.093	0.092	0.094	0.084	0.095

Cor cortex, *Rhip* Rt. hippocampus, *Lhip* Lt. hippocampus, *Thala* Thalamus, *Rstr* Rt. striatum, *Lstr* Lt. striatum

Table 4 Comparison of SUVR values between ^{18}F-florbetaben and ^{18}F-flutemetamol in AD transgenic group

Group	Cor	Rhip	Lhip	Thala	Rstr	Lstr
^{18}F-flutemetamol	0.851 ± 0.063	0.950 ± 0.051	0.972 ± 0.064	1.081 ± 0.080	0.970 ± 0.092	0.9910 ± .092
^{18}F-florbetaben	0.931 ± 0.050	0.980 ± 0.090	1.000 ± 0.110	1.090 ± 0.113	0.991 ± 0.113	1.010 ± 0.124
p value	0.049**	0.805	0.456	0.805	1.000	0.805

Cor cortex, *Rhip* Rt. hippocampus, *Lhip* Lt. hippocampus, *Thala* Thalamus, *Rstr* Rt. striatum, *Lstr* Lt. striatum, ** $p < 0.05$ considered as significant

SUVR value in the cortex than did ^{18}F-flutemetamol in both the AD ($p = 0.049$) and control groups ($p = 0.017$).

Quantitative compartment model dynamic analysis of ^{18}F-florbetaben and ^{18}F-flutemetamol image
Statistical analysis of dynamic PET data: AD versus. control
In the ^{18}F-florbetaben group, there was a significant difference in the K1 ($p = 0.011$) and k4 ($p = 0.017$) parameters between the AD transgenic and control groups. However, in the ^{18}F-flutemetamol group, there was no significant difference in K1, k2, k3, k4, K1/k2, or k3/k4 between the AD transgenic and control groups.

Statistical analysis of dynamic PET data: ^{18}F-florbetaben and ^{18}F-flutemetamol
In the AD transgenic group, there were significant differences of K1 (Table 5), k4 (Table 6), and K1/k2 between ^{18}F-florbetaben and ^{18}F-flutemetamol. In the control

group, there were differences in k3 and k3/k4 between ^{18}F-florbetaben and ^{18}F-flutemetamol.

Difference in the time-activity curve between ^{18}F-florbetaben and ^{18}F-flutemetamol
Dynamic PET time activity curves of the cortex-VOI and cerebellum-VOI for the two tracer images in representative AD and control mice are illustrated in Fig. 6. Visual inspection of the time-activity curves revealed that ^{18}F-florbetaben showed higher initial uptake and later retention than did ^{18}F-flutemetamol. In contrast, ^{18}F-flutemetamol showed lower initial upstroke and faster washout than did ^{18}F-florbetaben.

Neuropathologic findings (at 18 weeks)
Hematoxylin and eosin (H & E) staining
In Fig. 7, the AD mice show a more immature pattern as a result of disarrangement of hippocampal cell migration

Table 5 Comparison of K1 values (2 compartment model) between ^{18}F-florbetaben and ^{18}F-flutemetamol in AD transgenic group

Group	Rstr	Lstr	Cor	Rhip	Lhip	Thal	Crbl
^{18}F-flutemetamol							
Mean + SD	7.380 ± 1.032	7.331 ± 1.103	6.861 ± 1.331	6.972 ± 1.303	7.3 ± 0.900	7.841 ± 0.240	7.400 ± 1.410
Median (IQR)	7.98 (6.95–8)	8 (6.84–8)	7.52 (5.85–7.95)	7.29 (6.38–8)	7.92 (6.31–8)	7.95 (7.61–8)	8 (7.66–8)
^{18}F-florbetaben							
Mean + SD	4.991 ± 3.091	4.581 ± 2.960	3.561 ± 2.160	4.182 ± 2.160	4.802 ± 2.160	4.891 ± 2.160	5.060 ± 2.160
Median (IQR)	4.9 (1–8)	4.51 (1–8)	3.92 (1–4.63)	3.84 (1–7.63)	4.78 (1–7.95)	4.88 (1.18–8)	5.84 (1.65–7.61)
p-value	0.128	0.053	0.011**	0.073	0.128	0.038**	0.073

Cor cortex, *Crbl* cerebellum, *Rhip* Rt. hippocampus, *Lhip* Lt. hippocampus, *Thala* Thalamus, *Rstr* Rt. striatum, *Lstr* Lt. striatum, ** $p < 0.05$ considered as significant

Table 6 Comparison of k4 values (2 compartment model) between ^{18}F-florbetabenand ^{18}F-flutemetamol in AD transgenic group

Group	Rstr	Lstr	Cor	Rhip	Lhip	Thal	Crbl
^{18}F-flutemetamol							
Mean + SD	2.281 ± 3.510	1.622 ± 2.793	2.950 ± 3.210	4.551 ± 3.982	2.432 ± 3.982	1.281 ± 3.982	2.403 ± 3.982
Median (IQR)	0.331 (0.18–6.77)	0.561 (0.35–1.06)	1.752 (0.37–7.23)	7.460 (0.32–7.87)	0.340 (0.13–7.71)	0.273 (0.11–0.44)	0.374 (0–7.28)
^{18}F-florbetaben							
Mean + SD	0.713 ± 1.010	1.327 ± 2.290	0.161 ± 0.150	0.321 ± 0.331	0.902 ± 1.880	2.190 ± 3.102	0.140 ± 0.141
Median (IQR)	0.312 (0.22–0.92)	0.283 (0.25–2.03)	0.240 (0–0.29)	0.282 (0–0.41)	0.281 (0–0.35)	0.383 (0.21–6.15)	0.110 (0–0.3)
p-value	0.902	0.383	0.017**	0.053	0.383	0.535	0.165

Cor cortex, *Crbl* cerebellum, *Rhip* Rt. hippocampus, *Lhip* Lt. hippocampus, *Thala* Thalamus, *Rstr* Rt. striatum, *Lstr* Lt. striatum, ** $p < 0.05$ considered as significant

(pathogenic sign of AD) along the dentate gyrus of the hippocampus compared with the wild type.

Thioflavin S staining image

On thioflavin S staining images, Aβ deposits were found broadly in various brain regions including the cortex, hippocampus and thalamus in AD mice. Thioflavin S positive plaque areas predominantly diffuse in a morphologic characteristic nature rather than in a compact nature (Fig. 8).

Immunohistochemistry for Aβ$_{40}$ staining

The results of immunohistochemistry for Aβ$_{40}$ staining in AD transgenic and wild type were represented in Figs. 9, 10. In wild type mouse, there was no Aβ $_{40}$ expression in the cortex and hippocampus. In contrast, the Aa$_{40}$ expression of AD transgenic mouse significantly increased, correlating our H & E staining findings.

Correlation with neuropathologic findings and visual PET image

Finally, as shown in Fig. 11, the ^{18}F-florbetaben PET images more closely correlated with the thioflavin S staining image in terms of spatial distribution pattern. However, the ^{18}F-flutemetamol images revealed less prominent signal intensity and poor correlation of spatial distribution with neuropathologic plaque distribution shown in thioflavin S staining images.

Follow-up neuropathologic findings (at 48 weeks)

The results of the follow-up immunohistochemistry for Ai$_{40}$ staining in AD mice at 48 weeks are shown in Figs. 12, 13. At 48 weeks, AD mice showed extensive At$_{40}$ expression in dentate gyrus of hippocampus (CA1, CA2, CA3) and cortex, compared with the images at 18 weeks.

Discussion

In this study, ^{18}F-florbetaben and ^{18}F-flutemetamol images could differentiate AD and control group on visual and SUVR analysis. The ^{18}F-florbetaben group presented differences in K1 and k4 kinetic parameters between AD and control groups, although ^{18}F-flutemetamol did not show difference. Several differences emerged between ^{18}F-florbetaben and ^{18}F-flutemetamol. ^{18}F-florbetaben images showed more prominent visual uptake intensity and higher SUVR than the ^{18}F-flutemetamol images did. Moreover, ^{18}F-florbetaben PET images more correlated well with the thioflavin S staining. However, according

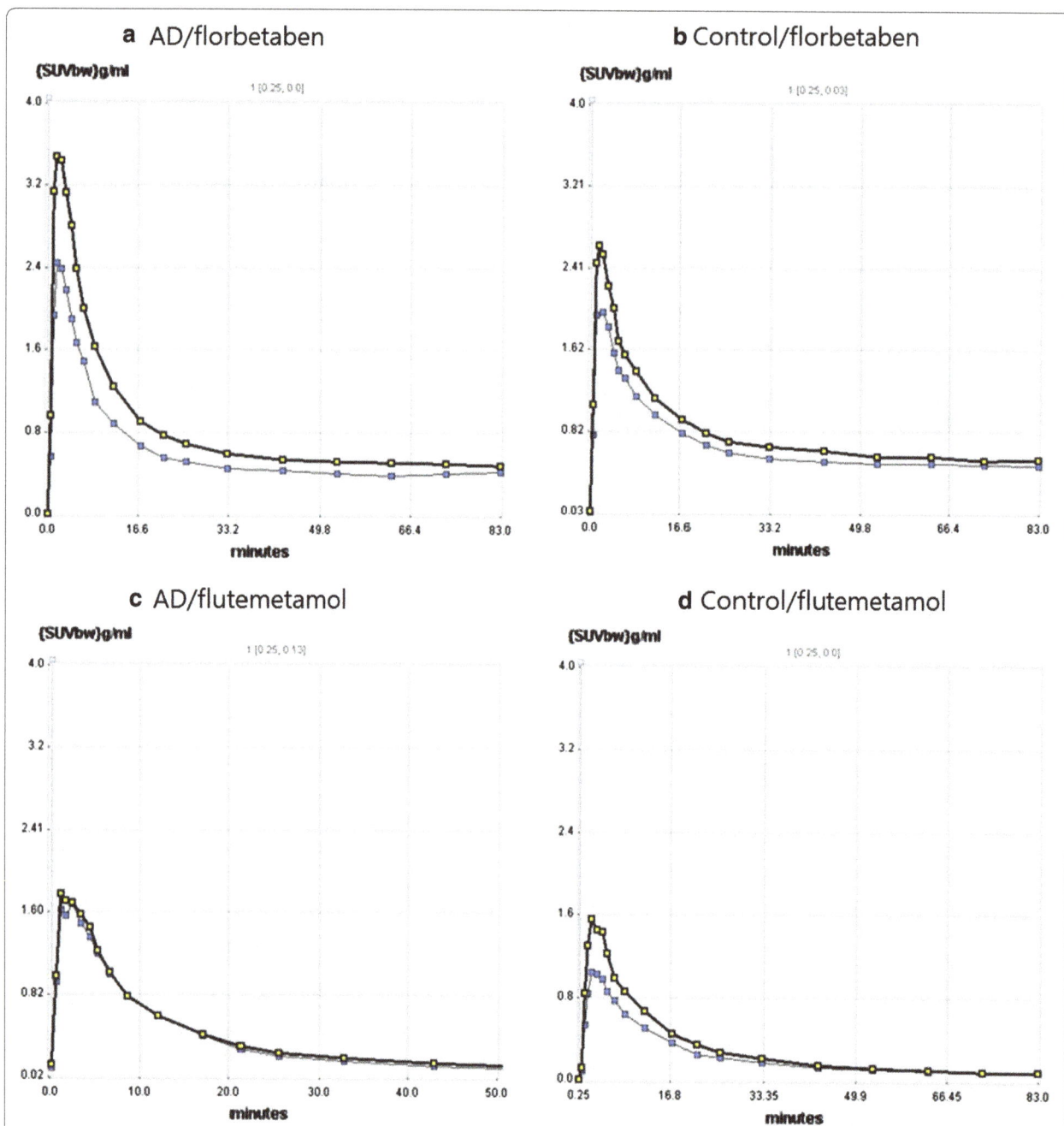

Fig. 6 Dynamic PET time activity curves of the cortex-VOI and the cerebellum-VOI. Time-activity curves of **a** ^{18}F-florbetaben in AD mouse, **b** ^{18}F-florbetaben in control mouse, **c** ^{18}F-flutemetamol in AD mouse, **d** ^{18}F-flutemetamol in control mouse, were illustrated. Values are SUVbw (g/ml) for a cortex VOI (blue line) and a cerebellum VOI (black line). ^{18}F-florbetaben showed higher initial uptake and later retention than did ^{18}F-flutemetamol. In contrast, ^{18}F-flutemetamol showed lower initial upstroke and faster washout than did ^{18}F-florbetaben

to bio-distribution and kinetic results, ^{18}F-flutemetamol is more actively metabolized than is ^{18}F-florbetaben, suggesting that ^{18}F-flutemetamol has faster transport from arterial plasma into the first tissue compartment and faster dissociation from the amyloid tracer complex.

In the static analysis data, the results were grossly consistent with a previous study [12]. In another ^{18}F-florbetaben PET study, the SUVR in APPswe/PS2 at 5 months was 0.95 ± 0.04, and the SUVR in APPswe/PS1G384A mice at 5 months was 0.93 [12]. The traditional SUVR method measures the radioactivity ratio of brain target

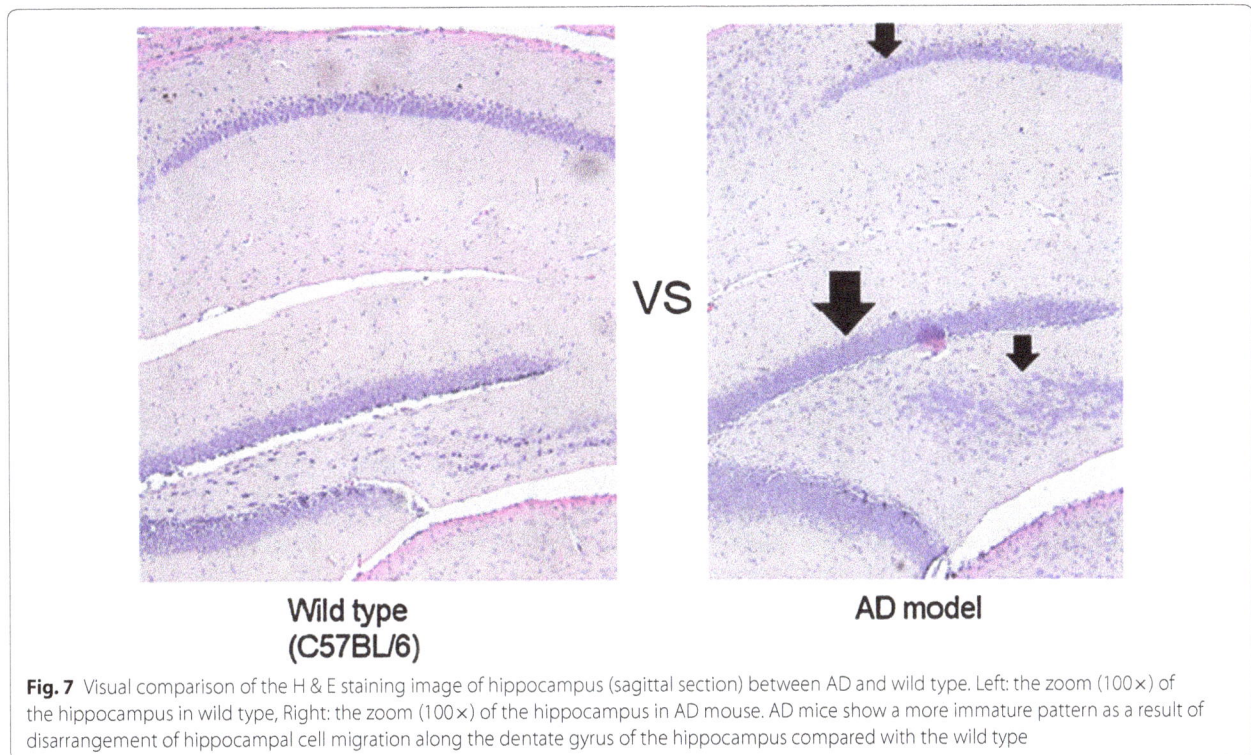

Fig. 7 Visual comparison of the H & E staining image of hippocampus (sagittal section) between AD and wild type. Left: the zoom (100×) of the hippocampus in wild type, Right: the zoom (100×) of the hippocampus in AD mouse. AD mice show a more immature pattern as a result of disarrangement of hippocampal cell migration along the dentate gyrus of the hippocampus compared with the wild type

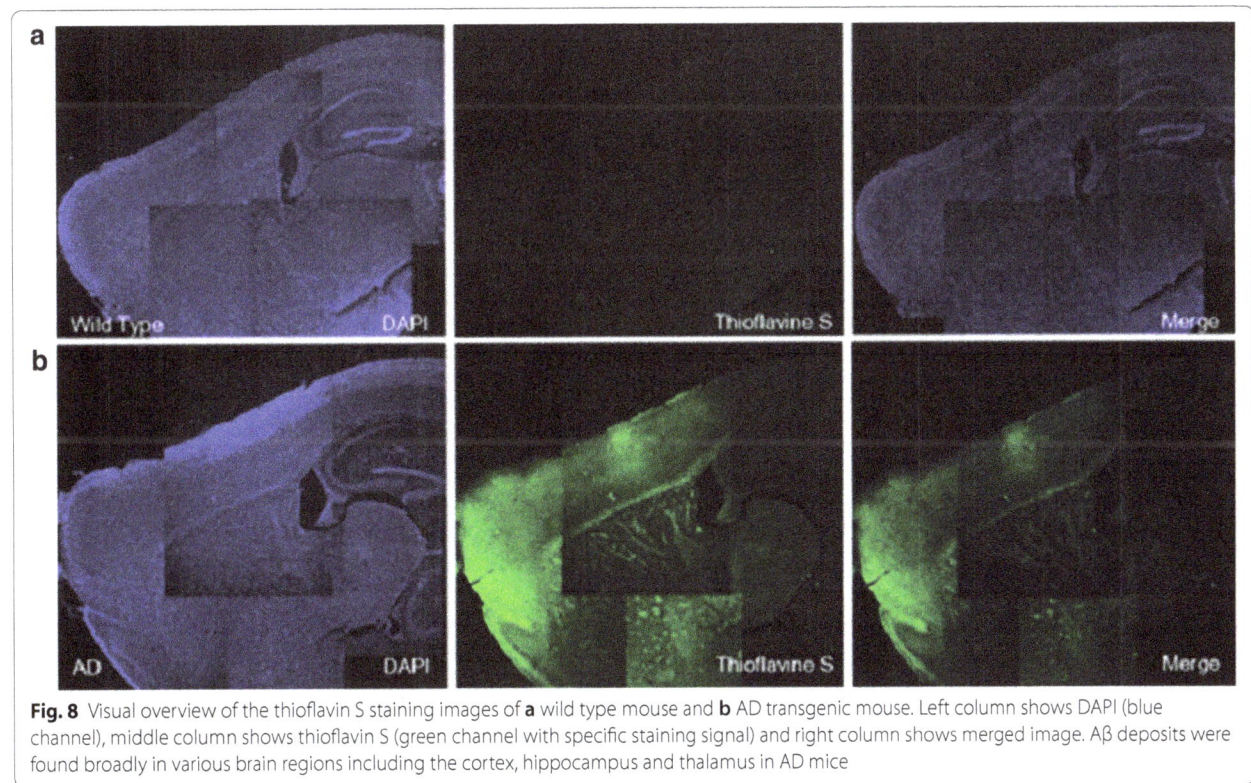

Fig. 8 Visual overview of the thioflavin S staining images of **a** wild type mouse and **b** AD transgenic mouse. Left column shows DAPI (blue channel), middle column shows thioflavin S (green channel with specific staining signal) and right column shows merged image. Aβ deposits were found broadly in various brain regions including the cortex, hippocampus and thalamus in AD mice

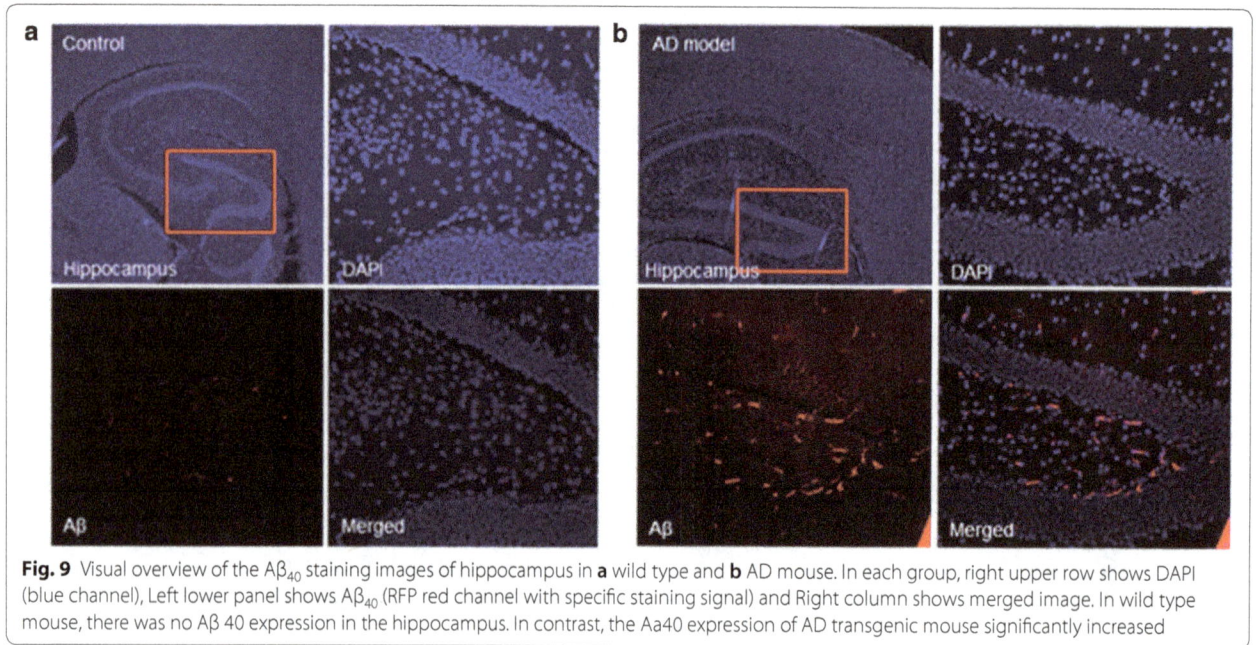

Fig. 9 Visual overview of the Aβ$_{40}$ staining images of hippocampus in **a** wild type and **b** AD mouse. In each group, right upper row shows DAPI (blue channel), Left lower panel shows Aβ$_{40}$ (RFP red channel with specific staining signal) and Right column shows merged image. In wild type mouse, there was no Aβ 40 expression in the hippocampus. In contrast, the Aa40 expression of AD transgenic mouse significantly increased

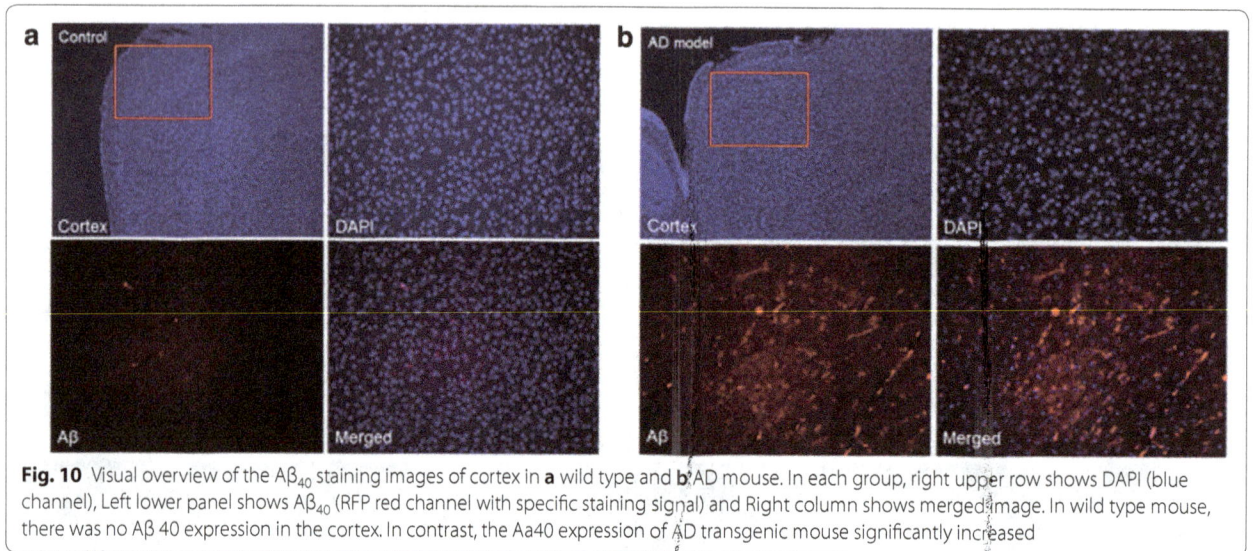

Fig. 10 Visual overview of the Aβ$_{40}$ staining images of cortex in **a** wild type and **b** AD mouse. In each group, right upper row shows DAPI (blue channel), Left lower panel shows Aβ$_{40}$ (RFP red channel with specific staining signal) and Right column shows merged image. In wild type mouse, there was no Aβ 40 expression in the cortex. In contrast, the Aa40 expression of AD transgenic mouse significantly increased

regions to reference tissue during a fixed time interval after injection of the tracer [11]. This relative quantitative approach for static PET data is practical for routine clinical setting. However, due to the kinetic compartment model for reversible binding radiotracers such as ^{18}F-florbetaben or ^{18}F-flutemetamol, the kinetic model reflects the available binding site density and also the perfusion signal and tracer clearance to and from brain tissue [11]. In this study, the 2 tissue compartment model with IDIF method was used, and the IDIF appears to be an attractive non-invasive alternative option obviating the need

for arterial cannulation, blood handling and analysis [13–15]. Furthermore, to avoid the effects of non-specific binding, we prolonged the uptake time, resulting in a longer wash-out of non-specifically bound tracer. A clinical protocol for ^{18}F-florbetaben involves a 90 min uptake periods [14]. A similar protocol was used in the previous APPPS1-21 mouse cohort study, allowing a 90-min uptake time [15].

The reasons for the disparity in imaging characteristics between ^{18}F-florbetaben and ^{18}F-flutemetamol are related to their chemico-physiological properties.

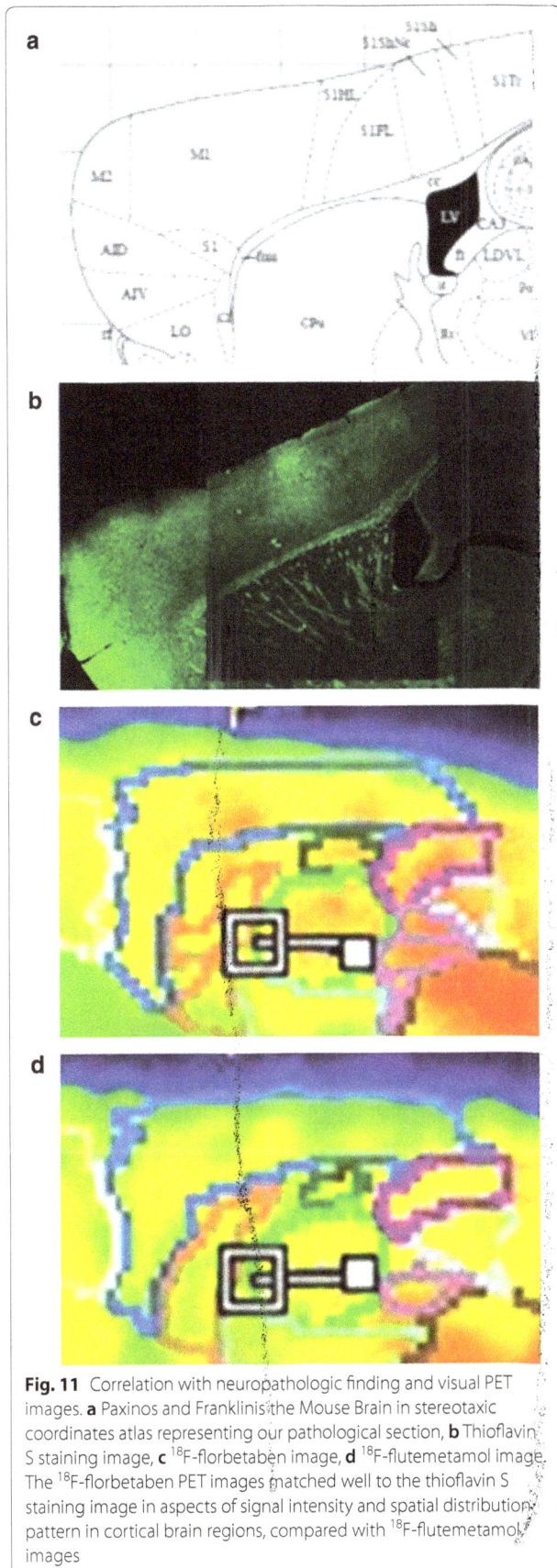

Fig. 11 Correlation with neuropathologic finding and visual PET images. **a** Paxinos and Franklinis the Mouse Brain in stereotaxic coordinates atlas representing our pathological section, **b** Thioflavin S staining image, **c** ^{18}F-florbetaben image, **d** ^{18}F-flutemetamol image. The ^{18}F-florbetaben PET images matched well to the thioflavin S staining image in aspects of signal intensity and spatial distribution pattern in cortical brain regions, compared with ^{18}F-flutemetamol images

[18]F-florbetaben and ^{18}F-flutemetamol belong to different families of imaging probes. ^{18}F-flutemetamol is a member of the thioflavin derivatives imaging probe family [16], and ^{18}F-florbetaben belongs to a different branch of imaging probe family, the trans-stilbene derivatives [16]. Because these two tracers belong to distinct chemical families, they showed differences in binding affinity. In the bio-distribution data, ^{18}F-flutemetamol showed lower brain and higher peripheral organ uptake responsible for metabolite excretion compared with ^{18}F-florbetaben. These findings and kinetic parameter results suggest that ^{18}F-flutemetamol is more actively metabolized than is ^{18}F-florbetaben. The tracer metabolites were more polar than were the parent molecules and therefore less able to enter the brain [17]. In a preclinical study comparing the pharmacokinetic characteristics of ^{18}F-flutemetamol with that of ^{11}C-PiB, the metabolism of ^{18}F-flutemetamol was faster than that of ^{11}C-PiB [18]. This finding can be explained by the higher lipophilicity of ^{18}F-flutemetamol ($logPC18 = 1.7$) than that of ^{11}C-PiB ($logPC18 = 1.2$) [19]. In another study, the lipophilicity of ^{18}F-florbetaben ($Log Doct/PBS = 1.58$) was higher than that of ^{11}C-PiB ($Log Doct/PBS = 1.50$) [20]. These results indirectly demonstrate that the rapid metabolism of ^{18}F-flutemetamol could be explained by the higher lipophilicity of ^{18}F-flutemetamol ($logPC18 = 1.7$) than of ^{18}F-florbetaben ($Log Doct/PBS = 1.58$).

Previous studies reported that various transgenic animal models showed differences in binding affinity with imaging tracers and this phenomenon was thought to be related with variations in plaques configurations. In this study, 18-week-old AD transgenic mice carrying NSE-controlled APPswe, C57BL/6-Tg (NSE-hAPPsw) Korl were selected due to their rapid and robust amyloid plaque development at that early age [21]. In contrast, Tg2576 mice showed late onset and slower accumulation [5]. In another previous report using APPPS1 mice co-expressing L166P mutated Presenilin 1 under the control of a neuron-specific Thy1 promoter and KM670/671NL mutated amyloid precursor protein, cortical amyloidosis was reported at the age of 6–8 weeks [22]. In APPPS1-21 mice, amyloid was known to accumulate in a 4-week and cortical microglia increased threefold from 1 to 8 months of age [22]. Hence, APPPS1 mice are good for investigating the mechanism of amyloidosis and treatment strategies because of their early onset of amyloid deposition and convenient cross-breeding with other genetically engineered mouse models.

In humans, the APPswe gene caused early presentation of familial AD [23]. In the NSE-controlled APPswe mouse model, the Swedish double mutation at the 670/671 codon in the human APP gene under the control of the NSE promoter caused increased cleavage by

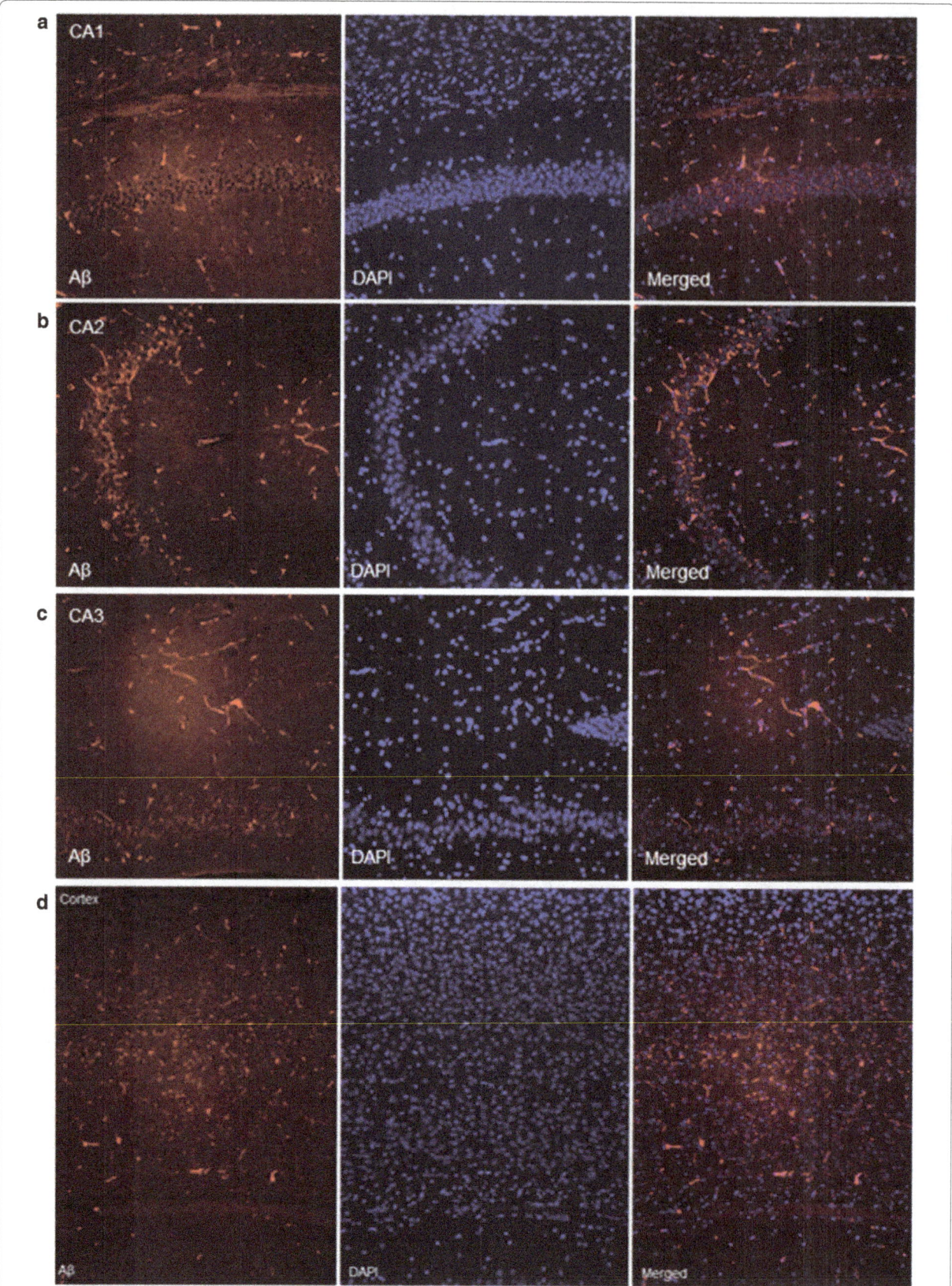

Fig. 12 Aβ$_{40}$ staining images of AD mouse at 48 weeks in **a** CA1, **b** CA2, **c** CA3 area of hippocampus and **d** cortex

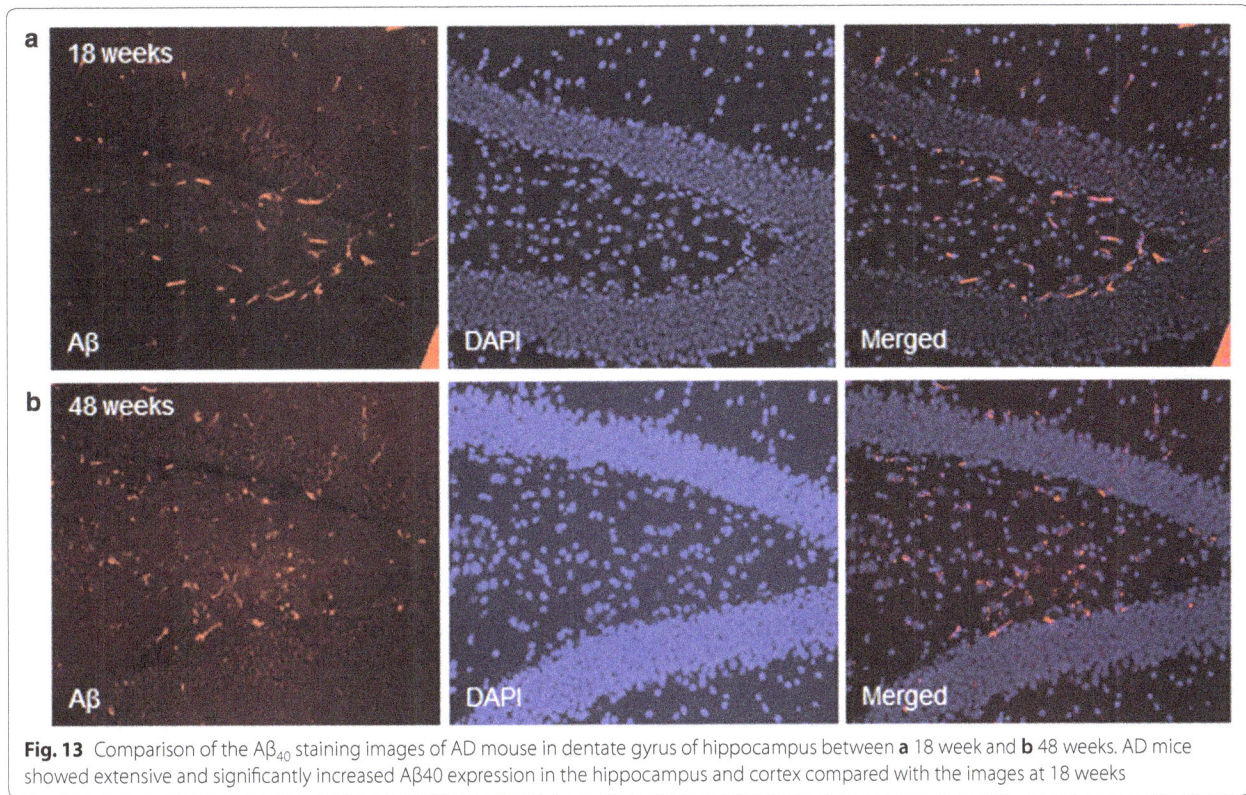

Fig. 13 Comparison of the $A\beta_{40}$ staining images of AD mouse in dentate gyrus of hippocampus between **a** 18 week and **b** 48 weeks. AD mice showed extensive and significantly increased Aβ40 expression in the hippocampus and cortex compared with the images at 18 weeks

the beta secretase and accelerated amyloid accumulation at young age [24]. Amyloid deposition in the NSE-controlled APPswe mouse induces subsequent neuronal apoptosis through the mechanisms of the mitogen-activated protein kinase (MAPK) and c-Jun N-terminal kinase (JNK) pathway or caspase-3 pathway [25, 26]. Although the mouse model in our study was relatively young, compelling evidence from previous studies regarding the dynamics of cerebral amyloidosis using a young APP mouse model indicates that NSE-augmented APPswe mice are suitable for the neuropathological phenotype of AD [27]. Moreover, we selected only male mice to control the effect of sex. Several studies reported the effect of sex on β-amyloid accumulation and AD phenotype. Latest studies have investigated the effects of sex on hippocampal atrophy in normal aging, MCI and AD [28]. Sex could regulate the relation of amyloid positivity and cognition [28]. Also, significant sex differences in pathology of 3xTg-AD mice suggested these differences may be due to organizational actions of sex hormones during development [29].

The results of this study are in contrary to those of antecedent ^{18}F-FDDNP study that presented affinity for both amyloid and neurofibrillary tangles [30]. There was no increase in cortical uptake even in 13–15-month-old Tg2576 mice, even if technical issues, such as low spatial

resolution, were regarded as the reasons for this negative PET finding [30]. However, in another ^{18}F-FDDNP study in triple-transgenic rats, previous partial volume effects were overcome and contrasting results were observed; prominent uptake was presented in the frontal cortex and hippocampus [31]. In an ^{11}C-PiB study, old Tg2576 mice showed prominent cortical binding than did control mice [9]. Those paradoxical results were explained by the confounding effects of cortical perfusion and the low distribution of ^{11}C-PiB binding sites per plaque [32]. However, following the ^{11}C-PiB study with high specific activity overcame such confounding effects, so significant cortical uptake and excellent correlation between PET uptake and a pathologic amyloid burden were observed in APP23 mice compared with age-matched healthy controls [33]. Additionally, in a recent ^{11}C-PiB PET study of APP/PS1 mice, an outstanding correlation can be found between imaging results and the plaque burden measure obtained ex vivo and in vitro in the same animals [34]. In a previous preclinical imaging study comparing ^{18}F-florbetaben and ^{11}C-PiB, which is of the same thioflavin T derivative family with ^{18}F-flutemetamol, two aged AD mouse models with contrasting levels of amyloid deposition to high (APPPS 1-21) and low (BRI 1-42) target state were investigated [15]. Compared with control mice, APPPS 1-21 mice (high target state) presented prominent fibrillary amyloid accumulation in both ^{11}C-PiB and ^{18}F-florbetaben, but the difference of uptake between AD and control mice was higher for ^{11}C-PiB than for ^{18}F-florbetaben [15]. However, BRI1-42 mice (low target state) did not show enhanced tracer uptake [15]. Taking into consideration the difference in the mouse ages, our results broadly resemble their findings. Another ^{18}F-florbetaben study using the same mouse cohort reported only a 14.5% difference between control and transgenic mice (5XFAD) found with ^{18}F-florbetapir in comparison to a 21% difference found with ^{11}C-PiB [35].

Before the interpretation of ^{18}F-florbetaben or ^{18}F-flutemetamol images in clinical settings, preclinical approaches can provide baseline information regarding differences in the kinetic and metabolic properties of two tracers. The visual image and SUVR of ^{18}F-florbetaben showed extensive cortical uptake in the same cohorts compared with ^{18}F-flutemetamol images in both the AD and control groups. On the ^{18}F-flutemetamol images, high lipophilicity and fast metabolism might complicate the analysis of PET data. In this study, the metabolism and kinetics of the tracer also have a great influence on the visual uptake of the amyloid tracers. Using these points, the human amyloid image should be read in consideration of the pharmacokinetic and metabolic properties of the tracer. Therefore, preclinical imaging might provide valuable information about the possibilities and limits of a given approach in humans by helping to better understand the in vivo binding characteristics of an imaging agent. The results of this study suggest that appropriate outcome measures are important in monitoring disease progression and response to therapeutic approaches in human settings. In this study, both tracers for VOI-based ratio analysis could discriminate the AD transgenic and control groups. However, on kinetic parameters from dynamic data, ^{18}F-flutemetamol images could not be used as an indicator to distinguish between AD transgenic and control groups. Moreover, the detection of amyloid PET signal in this early aged mouse model used in this study suggests the sensitivity of the PET imaging bio-marker, suggesting the possibility of early detection of amyloid pathology before the manifestation of behavioral abnormalities.

There are several limitations that should be mentioned. First, the distribution patterns between ^{18}F-florbetaben and ^{18}F-flutemetamol were compared at a single time point. Therefore, the current data are insufficient to judge the superiority between the two tracers based. In a follow-up study, the scope of the analysis should be extended to cover the comparison of serial and chronological accumulation pattern between ^{18}F-florbetaben and ^{18}F-flutemetamol.

Second, there are some issues regarding methodological perspectives. Herein, for the shape of the merged atlas to match well with the skull CT, the thresholded CT image was manually fused with the magnetic resonance template. However, limitations could exist regarding the method of manual registration. More accurate, automatic algorithm is required in the further study. Additionally, partial volume correction was not conducted when defining the VOI in the blood input area, because the VOI size of the blood input area was larger than the volumetric PET spatial resolution (0.343 mm^3). Therefore, the effect of the partial-volume correction should be investigated in a further study.

Moreover, in further studies, the different amyloid isoform structures and the range of fibrillarity influencing PET imaging results should be investigated. Amyloid plaques can be sub-classified according to the presence of dystrophic neuritis or reactive astrocytes and the morphological features as either diffuse, fibrillary or dense core types [36, 37]. In the thioflavin S image in our study, the thioflavin S positive plaque areas were predominantly diffuse rather than compact in terms of morphologic characteristic nature. Diffuse plaques are known to occur early in the disease course and to progress towards typical cored plaques [27, 38]. Dense-core plaques are often observed in AD mouse models, at an advanced age [39]. Morphological and biochemical compositional differences of plaques can influence the affinity binding sites for amyloid imaging tracers. Between ^{18}F-florbetaben and ^{18}F-flutemetamol, which tracer has higher binding affinity to diffuse type plaques? The answer to this question should be investigated in a further study including an in vitro binding assay. In addition, as plaques are amorphous three-dimensional configurations, further three-dimensional analysis of plaque structures with more precise detection stringency should be required.

Moreover, we have not performed Aβ 1-42 staining along with the Aβ 1-40 staining, in the follow-up of immunohistochemistry, because we simply wanted to demonstrate the establishment of AD mouse model and regarded Aβ 1-40 was better choice. Aβ 1-40 presents the most prominent Aβ isoform in the AD brain, while the Aβ 1-42 shows a substantial increase with specific forms of AD [40, 41]. Moreover, extraordinary expressions in AD mice carrying NSE-controlled APPsw presented that Aβ 1-40 was more prominent than Aβ 1-42 in the APPsw mice [42].

Conclusion

[18]F-florbetaben and ^{18}F-flutemetamol images could distinguish between the AD and control group by both visual and SUVR-based analysis. The ^{18}F-florbetaben

and ^{18}F-flutemetamol images showed disparate character in aspects of visual uptake intensity, quantitative parameters, bio-distribution and relations with neuropathological finding. ^{18}F-flutemetamol was more actively metabolized than was ^{18}F-florbetaben, although ^{18}F-florbetaben presented higher visual uptake intensity, SUVR and close correlation with the pathology.

Abbreviations
FBB: ^{18}F-florbetaben; FMM: ^{18}F-flutemetamol; AD: Alzheimer's disease; Aβ: amyloid plaque; APP: amyloid precursor protein; CSF: cerebrospinal fluid; FDG: fludeoxyglucose; MRI: magnetic resonance image; MCI: mild cognitive impairment; ND: neurodegenerative diseases; NFT: neurofibrillary tangles; PiB: Pittsburgh compound B; PET: positron emission tomography; RFP: red fluorescent protein; GFP: green fluorescent protein; APPswe: Swedish APP mutation; DAPI: diamidino-2-phenylindole.

Authors' contributions
HJS got the original idea, designed the study, analyzed and interpreted data, ran the statistics and wrote the draft. HJS, SYL, GEC, JAP, MHK, KCL, YJL, MKK, YJJ, HJY, KC, DYK performed the experiments and collected the data, revised and approved the final manuscript. Also, they agreed to be accountable for all aspect of the work in ensuring that questions related to the accuracy of the work are appropriately investigated. All authors read and approved the final manuscript.

Author details
[1] Department of Nuclear Medicine, Dong-A University Medical Center, Dong-A University College of Medicine, 26 Daesingongwon-ro, Seo-gu, Busan 602-812, Korea. [2] Institute of Convergence Bio-Health, Dong-A University, Busan, Korea. [3] Division of RI-Convergence Research, Korea Institute of Radiological and Medical Sciences, Seoul, Korea. [4] Pohang Center of Evolution of Biomaterials, Pohang Technopark, Pohang, Korea.

Acknowledgements
The authors are grateful to Ji-Ae Park, Min Hwan, Kyo Chul Lee, Yong Jin Lee (Division of RI-Convergence Research, Korea Institute of Radiological and Medical Sciences) for animal care and PET/CT imaging and to Mun Ki Kim (Pohang Center of Evolution of Biomaterials, Pohang Technopark) for pathology.

Competing interests
The authors declare that they have no competing interests.

Funding
This work was supported by the Busan Metropolitan City research fund. This research was partially supported by a grant of the Korea Institute of Radiological and Medical Science (KIRAMS) funded by the Ministry of Science and ICT (MSIT), Republic of Korea (No. 50461-2018).

References
1. Son HJ, Kang DY, Jeong YJ, Yoon HJ, Lee YJ, Kim MH, et al. Comparison analysis of brain beta-amyloid deposition in transgenic mouse models of Alzheimer's disease with PET imaging agents ^{18}F-flutemetamol and ^{18}F-florbetaben. J Nucl Med. 2017;58(Suppl 1):S278.
2. Henriksen G, Yousefi BH, Drzezga A, Wester HJ. Development and evaluation of compounds for imaging of beta-amyloid plaque by means of positron emission tomography. Eur J Nucl Med Mol Imaging. 2008;35(Suppl 1):S75–81.
3. Rinne JO, Wong DF, Wolk DA, Leinonen V, Arnold SE, Buckley C, et al. [(18)F]Flutemetamol PET imaging and cortical biopsy histopathology for fibrillar amyloid beta detection in living subjects with normal pressure hydrocephalus: pooled analysis of four studies. Acta Neuropathol. 2012;124:833–45.
4. Hatashita S, Yamasaki H, Suzuki Y, Tanaka K, Wakebe D, Hayakawa H. [18F]Flutemetamol amyloid-beta PET imaging compared with [11C]PIB across the spectrum of Alzheimer's disease. Eur J Nucl Med Mol Imaging. 2014;41:290–300.
5. Snellman A, Rokka J, Lopez-Picon FR, Eskola O, Salmona M, Forloni G, et al. In vivo PET imaging of beta-amyloid deposition in mouse models of Alzheimer's disease with a high specific activity PET imaging agent [(18)F] flutemetamol. EJNMMI Res. 2014;4:37.
6. Ashe KH, Zahs KR. Probing the biology of Alzheimer's disease in mice. Neuron. 2010;66:631–45.
7. Saigal N, Bajwa AK, Faheem SS, Coleman RA, Pandey SK, Constantinescu CC, et al. Evaluation of serotonin 5-HT(1A) receptors in rodent models using [(1)(8)F]mefway PET. Synapse. 2013;67:596–608.
8. PMOD Thechnologies. PMOD Image fusion (PFUS): II.PMOD. version 3.8. Switzerland: PMOD Technologies Ltd; 2016.
9. Su Y, Blazey TM, Snyder AZ, Raichle ME, Hornbeck RC, Aldea P, et al. Quantitative amyloid imaging using image-derived arterial input function. PLoS ONE. 2015;10:e0122920.
10. Price JC, Klunk WE, Lopresti BJ, Lu X, Hoge JA, Ziolko SK, et al. Kinetic modeling of amyloid binding in humans using PET imaging and Pittsburgh Compound-B. J Cereb Blood Flow Metab. 2005;25:1528–47.
11. Becker GA, Ichise M, Barthel H, Luthardt J, Patt M, Seese A, et al. PET quantification of 18F-florbetaben binding to beta-amyloid deposits in human brains. J Nucl Med. 2013;54:723–31.
12. Brendel M, Jaworska A, Griessinger E, Rotzer C, Burgold S, Gildehaus FJ, et al. Cross-sectional comparison of small animal [18F]-florbetaben amyloid-PET between transgenic AD mouse models. PLoS ONE. 2015;10:e0116678.
13. Zanotti-Fregonara P, Chen K, Liow JS, Fujita M, Innis RB. Image-derived input function for brain PET studies: many challenges and few opportunities. J Cereb Blood Flow Metab. 2011;31:1986–98.
14. Villemagne VL, Mulligan RS, Pejoska S, Ong K, Jones G, O'Keefe G, et al. Comparison of 11C-PiB and 18F-florbetaben for Abeta imaging in ageing and Alzheimer's disease. Eur J Nucl Med Mol Imaging. 2012;39:983–9.
15. Waldron AM, Verhaeghe J, Wyffels L, Schmidt M, Langlois X, Van Der Linden A, et al. Preclinical comparison of the amyloid-beta radioligands [(11)C]Pittsburgh compound B and [(18)F]florbetaben in Aged APPPS1-21 and BRI1-42 mouse models of cerebral amyloidosis. Mol Imaging Biol. 2015;17:688–96.
16. Rinne JO, Brooks DJ, Rossor MN, Fox NC, Bullock R, Klunk WE, et al. 11C-PiB PET assessment of change in fibrillar amyloid-beta load in patients with Alzheimer's disease treated with bapineuzumab: a phase 2, double-blind, placebo-controlled, ascending-dose study. Lancet Neurol. 2010;9:363–72.
17. Snellman A, Rokka J, Lopez-Picon FR, Eskola O, Wilson I, Farrar G, et al. Pharmacokinetics of [(1)(8)F]flutemetamol in wild-type rodents and its binding to beta amyloid deposits in a mouse model of Alzheimer's disease. Eur J Nucl Med Mol Imaging. 2012;39:1784–95.
18. Koivunen J, Verkkoniemi A, Aalto S, Paetau A, Ahonen JP, Viitanen M, et al. PET amyloid ligand [11C]PIB uptake shows predominantly striatal increase in variant Alzheimer's disease. Brain. 2008;131:1845–53.
19. Mathis C, Lopresti B, Mason N, Price J, Flatt N, Bi W, et al. Comparison of the amyloid imaging agents [F-18]3'-F-PIB and [C-11]PIB in Alzheimer's disease and control subjects. J Nucl Med. 2007;48:56.
20. Yousefi BH, von Reutern B, Scherubl D, Manook A, Schwaiger M, Grimmer T, et al. FIBT versus florbetaben and PiB: a preclinical comparison study with amyloid-PET in transgenic mice. EJNMMI Res. 2015;5:20.
21. Darvesh S, Cash MK, Reid GA, Martin E, Mitnitski A, Geula C. Butyrylcholinesterase is associated with beta-amyloid plaques in the transgenic APPSWE/PSEN1dE9 mouse model of Alzheimer disease. J Neuropathol Exp Neurol. 2012;71:2–14.
22. Radde R, Bolmont T, Kaeser SA, Coomaraswamy J, Lindau D, Stoltze L, et al. Abeta42-driven cerebral amyloidosis in transgenic mice reveals early and robust pathology. EMBO Rep. 2006;7:940–6.
23. Mullan M, Crawford F, Axelman K, Houlden H, Lilius L, Winblad B, et al. A pathogenic mutation for probable Alzheimer's disease in the APP gene at the N terminus of beta amyloid. Nat Genet. 1992;1:345–7.

24. Irizarry MC, McNamara M, Fedorchak K, Hsiao K, Hyman BT. APPSw transgenic mice develop age-related A beta deposits and neuropil abnormalities, but no neuronal loss in CA1. J Neuropathol Exp Neurol. 1997;56:965–73.

25. Troy CM, Rabacchi SA, Xu Z, Maroney AC, Connors TJ, Shelanski ML, et al. beta-Amyloid-induced neuronal apoptosis requires c-Jun N-terminal kinase activation. J Neurochem. 2001;77:157–64.

26. Gamblin TC, Chen F, Zambrano A, Abraha A, Lagalwar S, Guillozet AL, et al. Caspase cleavage of tau: linking amyloid and neurofibrillary tangles in Alzheimer's disease. Proc Natl Acad Sci USA. 2003;100:10032–7.

27. Hefendehl JK, Wegenast-Braun BM, Liebig C, Eicke D, Milford D, Calhoun ME, et al. Long-term in vivo imaging of beta-amyloid plaque appearance and growth in a mouse model of cerebral beta-amyloidosis. J Neurosci. 2011;31:624–9.

28. Caldwell JZK, Berg JL, Cummings JL, Banks SJ. Moderating effects of sex on the impact of diagnosis and amyloid positivity on verbal memory and hippocampal volume. Alzheimers Res Ther. 2017;9(1):72.

29. Carroll JC, Rosario ER, Kreimer S, Villamagna A, Gentzschein E, Stanczyk FZ, et al. Sex differences in beta-amyloid accumulation in 3xTg-AD mice: role of neonatal sex steroid hormone exposure. Brain Res. 2010;1366:233–45.

30. Kuntner C, Kesner AL, Bauer M, Kremslehner R, Wanek T, Mandler M, et al. Limitations of small animal PET imaging with [18F]FDDNP and FDG for quantitative studies in a transgenic mouse model of Alzheimer's disease. Mol Imaging Biol. 2009;11:236–40.

31. Teng E, Kepe V, Frautschy SA, Liu J, Satyamurthy N, Yang F, et al. [F-18] FDDNP microPET imaging correlates with brain Abeta burden in a transgenic rat model of Alzheimer disease: effects of aging, in vivo blockade, and anti-Abeta antibody treatment. Neurobiol Dis. 2011;43:565–75.

32. Saido TC, Iwatsubo T, Mann DM, Shimada H, Ihara Y, Kawashima S. Dominant and differential deposition of distinct beta-amyloid peptide species, A beta N3(pE), in senile plaques. Neuron. 1995;14:457–66.

33. Maeda J, Ji B, Irie T, Tomiyama T, Maruyama M, Okauchi T, et al. Longitudinal, quantitative assessment of amyloid, neuroinflammation, and anti-amyloid treatment in a living mouse model of Alzheimer's disease enabled by positron emission tomography. J Neurosci. 2007;27:10957–68.

34. Manook A, Yousefi BH, Willuweit A, Platzer S, Reder S, Voss A, et al. Small-animal PET imaging of amyloid-beta plaques with [11C]PiB and its multi-modal validation in an APP/PS1 mouse model of Alzheimer's disease. PLoS ONE. 2012;7:e31310.

35. Rojas S, Herance JR, Gispert JD, Abad S, Torrent E, Jimenez X, et al. In vivo evaluation of amyloid deposition and brain glucose metabolism of 5XFAD mice using positron emission tomography. Neurobiol Aging. 2013;34:1790–8.

36. Thal DR, Capetillo-Zarate E, Del Tredici K, Braak H. The development of amyloid beta protein deposits in the aged brain. Sci Aging Knowledge Environ. 2006;2006:re1.

37. Dickson TC, Vickers JC. The morphological phenotype of beta-amyloid plaques and associated neuritic changes in Alzheimer's disease. Neuroscience. 2001;105:99–107.

38. Iwatsubo T, Odaka A, Suzuki N, Mizusawa H, Nukina N, Ihara Y. Visualization of A beta 42(43) and A beta 40 in senile plaques with end-specific A beta monoclonals: evidence that an initially deposited species is A beta 42(43). Neuron. 1994;13:45–53.

39. Guntert A, Dobeli H, Bohrmann B. High sensitivity analysis of amyloid-beta peptide composition in amyloid deposits from human and PS2APP mouse brain. Neuroscience. 2006;143:461–75.

40. Mori H, Takio K, Ogawara M, Selkoe DJ. Mass spectrometry of purified amyloid beta protein in Alzheimer's disease. J Biol Chem. 1992;267(24):17082–6.

41. Naslund J, Schierhorn A, Hellman U, Lannfelt L, Roses AD, Tjernberg LO, et al. Relative abundance of Alzheimer A beta amyloid peptide variants in Alzheimer disease and normal aging. Proc Natl Acad Sci USA. 1994;91(18):8378–82.

42. Hwang DY, Cho JS, Lee SH, Chae KR, Lim HJ, Min SH, et al. Aberrant e xpressions of pathogenic phenotype in Alzheimer's diseased transgenic mice carrying NSE-controlled APPsw. Exp Neurol. 2004;186(1):20–32.

16

Limited effects of dysfunctional macroautophagy on the accumulation of extracellularly derived α-synuclein in oligodendroglia: implications for MSA pathogenesis

Lisa Fellner[1]* [ID], Edith Buchinger[1], Dominik Brueck[1], Regina Irschick[2], Gregor K. Wenning[1] and Nadia Stefanova[1]

Abstract

Background: The progressive neurodegenerative disorder multiple system atrophy (MSA) is characterized by α-synuclein-positive (oligodendro-) glial cytoplasmic inclusions (GCIs). A connection between the abnormal accumulation of α-synuclein in GCIs and disease initiation and progression has been postulated. Mechanisms involved in the formation of GCIs are unclear. Abnormal uptake of α-synuclein from extracellular space, oligodendroglial overexpression of α-synuclein, and/or dysfunctional protein degradation including macroautophagy have all been discussed. In the current study, we investigated whether dysfunctional macroautophagy aggravates accumulation of extracellular α-synuclein in the oligodendroglia.

Results: We show that oligodendroglia uptake monomeric and fibrillar extracellular α-synuclein. Blocking macroautophagy through bafilomycin A1 treatment or genetic knockdown of LC3B does not consistently change the level of incorporated α-synuclein in oligodendroglia exposed to extracellular soluble/monomeric or fibrillar α-synuclein, however leads to higher oxidative stress in combination with fibrillar α-synuclein treatment. Finally, we detected no evidence for GCI-like formation resulting from dysfunctional macroautophagy in oligodendroglia using confocal microscopy.

Conclusion: In summary, isolated dysfunctional macroautophagy is not sufficient to enhance abnormal accumulation of uptaken α-synuclein in vitro, but may lead to increased production of reactive oxygen species in the presence of fibrillar α-synuclein. Multiple complementary pathways are likely to contribute to GCI formation in MSA.

Keywords: Macroautophagy, Multiple system atrophy, α-Synuclein, Oligodendroglia, Glial cytoplasmic inclusions

Background

Multiple system atrophy (MSA) is a progressive, fatal neurodegenerative disease with unknown etiology. MSA is characterized by α-synuclein (α-syn)-positive glial cytoplasmic inclusions (GCIs) occurring predominantly in oligodendroglial cells [1]. MSA is categorized in the disease group of α-synucleinopathies together with Parkinson's disease (PD) and dementia with Lewy bodies (DLB) which show primarily neuronal α-syn-positive inclusions (Lewy bodies, LBs). Different genetic, neuropathological and experimental studies provide evidence that α-syn plays a major role in the pathogenesis of these disorders [2–9]. Yet, phosphorylated and aggregated α-syn species are not the only constituents of GCIs, but also ubiquitin, heat shock proteins, cytoskeletal proteins and components of the autophagic pathway were identified [10–14]. The formation of GCIs in MSA and the

*Correspondence: lisa.fellner@i-med.ac.at
[1] Department of Neurology, Medical University of Innsbruck, Innrain 66, G2, 6020 Innsbruck, Austria
Full list of author information is available at the end of the article

underlying mechanisms are not elucidated to date [15]. An elevated expression and aggregation of α-syn in oligodendroglial cells is discussed in GCI development, yet contradicting reports exist regarding the expression of α-syn mRNA in oligodendroglial cells [16–19]. Incorporation of α-syn by oligodendroglia either released by dying neurons into the extracellular space or by cell-to-cell propagation represents an alternative mechanism of GCI formation [20–22]. The uptake of α-syn via endocytosis by oligodendroglial cells has been reported in different studies [13, 22–26], but α-syn uptake by oligodendrocytes has not been immediately linked to the formation of GCIs. Furthermore, the degradation of monomeric/soluble α-syn (sol α-syn) by the ubiquitin-proteasome system (UPS) and autophagy has been demonstrated [27–29], whereas autophagy seems to be the favored pathway for the degradation of misfolded α-syn species [30]. Therefore, pathological accumulation of α-syn in the cytoplasm of oligodendroglia might be explained by a primary oligodendroglial injury [31] such as deficits in the cellular protein degradation mechanisms [11, 32, 33].

Three different forms of autophagy are described: macro-, microautophagy and chaperone-mediated autophagy (CMA). Macroautophagy and CMA have been shown to be the most relevant autophagy mechanisms involved in the degradation of α-syn [34]. Macroautophagy (commonly called autophagy) is important for the bulk degradation of cytoplasmic proteins or organelles and thereby involves autophagic vacuoles (autophagosomes) that fuse with lysosomes to form autophagolysosomes where the degradation via hydrolases takes place [35]. The formation of the autophagosome is a complex process which is controlled by various evolutionary conserved ATG (AuTophaGy) genes as well as lipid kinases [36, 37]. A standard assay for macroautophagy is the measurement of autophagosome-associated LC3B protein levels. The processing of microtubule-associated protein 1 light chain 3B (LC3B) creates LC3B-I and after its lipidation LC3B-II develops, which is a robust marker of autophagosomes and correlates with autophagosome numbers [38, 39].

Impaired autophagy associated with deficits in the autophagosome formation has been reported in MSA [40], suggesting that this dysfunction might initiate GCI formation in oligodendroglia [41–43]. In PD brains, macroautophagy was shown to be impaired in nigral neurons [44]. In a recent study, it was found that the autophagosomal protein LC3 and the ubiquitin binding protein p62 are associated with α-syn-positive GCIs in MSA cases and furthermore, LC3 is recruited to α-syn aggregations when the proteasome is impaired in rat oligodendroglial cells [11, 45]. In a transgenic MSA

mouse model, an upregulation of the LC3 protein was demonstrated compared to wild type mice strengthening the assumption of macroautophagy involvement in MSA-like α-synucleinopathy [32]. In addition, dysfunctional macroautophagy caused through mitochondrial impairment or macroautophagy inhibition resulted in the accumulation of α-syn in oligodendroglial cells in vitro respectively [24]. Furthermore, in a different study in neuronal cells a role of CMA and macroautophagy were shown in the degradation process of α-syn [29]. Recently, it was demonstrated that macroautophagy inhibition by using bafilomycin A1 (BAF), a specific inhibitor of vacuolar H + ATPase (V-ATPase) blocking the fusion of the autophagosome and the lysosome [46], reduced intracellular α-syn aggregation, but also led to an enhanced secretion of toxic α-syn oligomers by neuronal cells in vitro and in vivo thereby causing inflammation and neurotoxicity in the microenvironment [42, 47]. These studies underline the involvement of macroautophagy in the aggregation and degradation process of α-syn especially in neuronal, but also in oligodendroglial cells. Yet, the complete mechanisms of α-syn inclusion formation in MSA and the role of autophagy pathways are not elucidated to this date and have to be further investigated to create an overall picture.

In the present study, we investigated the effect of macroautophagy inhibition and exposure to extracellular recombinant α-syn species on the formation of α-syn-positive inclusions in human oligodendroglial cells. Therefore, pharmacological blocking using BAF or genetic knockdown of LC3B was analyzed in oligodendroglial cells exposed to extracellular monomeric/soluble (sol α-syn) or fibrillar α-syn (fib α-syn) species. Macroautophagy block through genetic knockdown of LC3 or BAF treatment was inefficient to increase intracellular accumulation of α-syn in oligodendrocytes exposed to extracellular α-syn. In the current study, no GCI-like formation of α-syn upon macroautophagy blocking was found in the used oligodendroglial cell culture model suggesting that multiple complementary factors are likely to contribute to GCI formation in MSA.

Methods

Preparation, purification and characterization of full length soluble and fibrillar α-syn

The recombinant human full length monomeric sol α-syn was prepared, purified and characterized as described previously [5, 15, 48]. Purification was performed using a histidin-tag attached to the protein. This his-tag leads to a 24 kilodalton (kDa) band when analyzed in western blot analysis. Recombinant human full length fib α-syn was generated and fibrillization was characterized using Thioflavin T (Sigma-Aldrich, St. Louis, MO, USA) as specified before [15]. Furthermore, endotoxin concentration in the α-syn preparations was determined by using the kinetic chromogenic limulus amoebocyte lysate (LAL) endpoint assay by Hyglos GmbH, Bernried, Germany reaching an endotoxin amount under 1 EU/mg in the stock solution as described previously [15].

Cell culture

As part of the current study, a primary murine oligodendroglial cell culture was established using newborn wild type (C57BL/6) mouse cortices (days 1–3). According to national regulations of the Austrian Animal experimentation law (TVG 2012), no ethics approval is necessary for the preparation of primary cell culture. Newborn mice were sacrificed and whole cortices prepared. Meninges were removed and mixed glial cultures were obtained as described before and were kept in culture for 2 weeks [15]. The mixed glial cell culture was shaken consecutively to generate a primary oligodendrocyte precursor cell (OPC) culture by separating OPCs from the underlying astroglial layer. Thereby, murine mixed glial cultures were pre-shaken for 1 h at 180 rpm on a horizontal orbital shaker at 37 °C to remove microglial cells. Medium with microglia was discarded and 10 ml of complete mixed glial medium was added. Then the flasks were shaken at 180 rpm overnight (18–20 h) at 37 °C in a humid atmosphere with 5% CO_2. To separate OPCs from microglia and remaining astroglia, cells were plated onto an untreated petri dish (BD Falcon, BD Biosciences, BD, San Jose, CA, USA) for 40 min to induce adherence of microglia and astroglia to the plastic. OPCs remaining in the medium were centrifuged and replated onto poly-D-lysine (PDL, 20 μg/mL, Gibco, Life Technologies, San Diego, CA, USA) coated 96-well plates (4×10^4 cells per well, TPP, Trasadingen, Switzerland) in OPC-conditioned medium containing basic fibroblast growth factor (bFGF, 10 ng/mL, Life Technologies) and platelet-derived growth factor AA (PDGF-AA, 10 ng/mL, Life Technologies) at 37 °C in a humid atmosphere with 5% CO_2 as described previously [49]. OPCs were differentiated after 5–6 days in culture using a special maturation mix including triiodothyronine (TIT, 15 nM, Sigma-Aldrich), N-acetyl-L-cysteine (NAC, 1×, Sigma-Aldrich) and ciliary neurotrophic factor (CNTF, 10 ng/mL, PeproTech, Hamburg, Germany) as specified by Chen et al. [49].

The human oligodendroglioma cell line MO 3.13 (Cedarlane, Ontario, Canada) was kept in T75 flasks (TPP) in Dulbecco's modified Eagle's medium (DMEM, 4 g/L Glucose, Gibco, Life Technologies) supplemented with 10% fetal calf serum (FCS, Gibco, Life Technologies) and 2 mM Glutamine (Gibco, Life Technologies). Cells were passaged twice a week and kept at 37 °C in a humid atmosphere with 5% CO_2.

α-syn uptake by primary murine oligodendroglial cells and MO 3.13 oligodendroglial cells

Primary murine oligodendroglia were plated into PDL coated 96-well plates (4×10^4 cells per well) and MO 3.13 oligodendroglial cells were plated into 96-well plates (5×10^3 cells per well). After 24 h, the cells were treated with 18 μg/mL recombinant sol and fib α-syn for 1 or 24 h at 37 °C. Cells were washed with PBS, and then fixed with 4% paraformaldehyde (PFA, Sigma-Aldrich) and immunocytochemistry was conducted. The uptake of sol and fib α-syn was analyzed using a DMI 4000B Leica inverse microscope provided with Leica application software and Digital FireWire Color Camera DFC300 FX (Leica Microsystems). All measurements were repeated in at least 4 separate biological replicates and mean values ($\pm$ SEM) were determined.

Induction of macroautophagy dysfunction by pharmacological blocking

Autophagy dysfunction was generated by the addition of BAF (50 nM, Sigma-Aldrich) to the medium, thereby blocking the fusion of the autophagosome with the lysosome. MO 3.13 were plated into 96-well plates (5×10^3 cells per well) for the performance of immunocytochemistry or into 6-well plates (26×10^4 cells per well) for the conduction of western blot. 50 nM BAF was applied for 30 min to induce autophagy dysfunction in MO 3.13 cells. Subsequently, 18 μg/mL sol or fib α-syn was added. Cells were either fixed with 4% PFA and immunocytochemistry was accomplished or lysates were generated.

Sure silencing shRNA plasmids and transfection

To achieve a knockdown of macroautophagy via LC3B silencing using RNA interference in MO 3.13 oligodendroglia, the SureSilencing shRNA plasmids ligated to green fluorescent protein (GFP) were generated according to the manufacturer's instructions (Qiagen, Hilden, Germany). LC3B shRNA plasmid sequence: GCAGCT TCCTGTTCTGGATAA; scrambled shRNA plasmid sequence: ggaatctcattcgatgcatac.

FuGENE Transfection Reagent (Promega, Mannheim, Germany) was applied to perform transfections of MO 3.13 cell cultures as recommended by the manufacturer. Cells were plated 1 day prior to transfection so that they were approximately 80% confluent. 72 h (for Western blot analyses) and 24 h (for confocal microscopy) after transfection with the SureSilencing shRNA plasmids the medium was changed and the cells were treated with 18 μg/mL recombinant human sol α-syn or fib α-syn for 24 h. α-Syn uptake or/and inclusion formation was determined by immunostaining and immunoblotting.

Immunofluorescence

The following primary antibodies were used in this study: rat anti-human α-syn (aa 116-131 human α-syn, 1:500, Enzo Life Sciences, Loerrach, Germany), rabbit anti-human ubiquitin (1:200, Abcam, Cambridge, UK) and rabbit-anti mouse PDGF receptor α (PDGFRα, 1:200, Abcam). Cell culture medium was removed and cells were washed twice with phosphate buffered saline (PBS) prior to fixation with 4% PFA for 20 min at room temperature (RT). Subsequently, cells were blocked in 0.3% Triton-X100, 1% bovine serum albumin (Sigma-Aldrich) and 5% normal goat serum (Gibco, Life Technologies) in PBS for 1 h followed by incubation with primary antibody overnight at 4 °C. Secondary antibodies for immunofluorescence were added for 1 h at RT, including Alexa 488- or Alexa 594-conjugated anti-rat and anti-rabbit IgG (1:500, Jackson Immunoresearch Laboratories, West Grove, PA, USA). Nuclear staining of fixed cells was accomplished using 4′,6-diamidino-2-phenylindole dihydrochloride (DAPI, 1:20,000 Sigma-Aldrich). Membrane staining was achieved by detection of glycoproteins using FITC-conjugated lectin from Triticum vulgaris (wheat germ agglutinin, WGA, 1:1000, Sigma-Aldrich). Cells were visualized using a DMI 4000B Leica inverse microscope and Application Suite V3.1 and Digital Fire Wire Color Camera DFC300 FX by Leica or by confocal microscopy. For confocal microscopy stained oligodendroglial cells were mounted on slides and coverslipped.

Confocal microscopy

Confocal microscopy was conducted at a Leica TCS SP5 laser scanning microscope (Leica Microsystems, Wetzlar, Germany) using a HCX PL APO 63x glycerol immersion objective (N.A. 1.3) and a pinhole of 1 AU. Three-dimensional stacks were acquired according to the Nyquist criterion to allow deconvolution. Image deconvolution was performed using Huygens professional software version 4.1.1 (SVI Scientific Volume Imaging, Hilversum, The Netherlands). Images were processed using the Huygens Object Analyzer Advanced and cells were reconstructed three-dimensionally with the Huygens MIP renderer.

Measurement of ROS

Intracellular superoxide radical generation assessment was accomplished using nitroblue tetrazolium chloride (NBT, Roche Applied Sciences, Basel, Switzerland). Thereby, the formation of a dark blue formazan deposit resulting from superoxide-mediated reduction of NBT can be examined in cell culture visualizing cells positive for ROS production as described previously [15]. Briefly,

MO 3.13 oligodendroglial cells were plated in 96-well plates and treated as described before. Cells were treated with BAF and recombinant α-syn. Untreated cells were used as controls. Subsequently, 1 mg/mL NBT was added at 37 °C for 30 min. Cells were washed with PBS and fixed with 4% PFA at RT. The number of ROS-positive cells per well was analyzed by using a DMI 4000B Leica inverse microscope. All measurements were repeated in at least 4 separate biological replicates and mean values (± SEM) were determined.

SDS-PAGE and western blot

Lysates of treated MO 3.13 oligodendroglia were generated. Cells were washed with PBS once, and lysed in protein lysis buffer containing 1% NP-40, 150 mM NaCl, 50 mM HEPES, 0.8 mM $MgCl_2$, 5 mM EGTA protease inhibitor cocktail (Roche Applied Sciences). Lysates were centrifuged for 15 min at 4 °C and the supernatant was stored at − 80 °C. Protein content of the cell lysates was determined using the BCA protein assay (Sigma-Aldrich). Electrophoresis of cell lysates was accomplished using NuPAGE 10% Bis–Tris gels (Novex Life Technologies) for protein separation. Proteins were electrotransferred to a nitrocellulose membrane (GE Healthcare Bio-Sciences AB, Uppsala, Sweden) and after blocking with 2% milk powder in PBS containing 0.1% Tween-20 (PBS-T), the blots, were incubated with different primary antibodies overnight, including purified monoclonal AS antibody (aa 15-123, 1:1000, BD Transduction Laboratories, San Jose, CA, USA), monoclonal actin antibody (housekeeper, 1:10,000, BD Transduction Laboratories), polyclonal ubiquitin antibody (1:2000, Abcam) and a polyclonal LC3B antibody (1:1000, Cell Signaling, Leiden, The Netherlands). Blots were further incubated with horseradish peroxidase linked anti-mouse or anti-rabbit IgG (1:10,000, GE Healthcare) and incubated for another 2 min with Western Bright enhanced chemiluminescence (ECL, Advansta, Menlo Park, CA, USA). The blots were developed using the imaging system Fusion Fx 7 for Western blot and gel imaging, quantification was performed using the FUSION CAPT V16.09b Software (Vilber Lourmat, Marne La Vallée, France). All measurements were repeated in at least 4 separate biological replicates and mean values (± SEM) were determined.

Statistical analysis

All statistical analyses were carried out using Graph-Pad Prism 5 (Graphpad Software, San Diego, CA, USA) and the results were presented as the mean ± S.E.M. Two-way analysis of variance with post hoc Bonferroni test for the analysis of two independent factors was applied. A p value < 0.05 was considered statistically significant.

Results

Primary murine oligodendrocytes and human oligodendroglial cell line incorporate extracellular α-syn

Previous in vitro studies already suggested the incorporation of α-syn by oligodendroglial cell lines and primary oligodendroglial cells [22, 25, 26]. To determine whether recombinant sol and fib α-syn incorporation from the extracellular space is comparable in primary murine oligodendroglia and human MO 3.13 oligodendroglial cell line, we analyzed different parameters including the percentage of cells with α-syn inclusions (Fig. 1a), the number of inclusions per cell (Fig. 1b) and the total area of inclusion per cell in μm² (Fig. 1c). 24 h after incubation with both α-syn forms, small incorporations of α-syn were found in around 15–20% of the analyzed primary and MO 3.13 oligodendroglia. No differences were detected regarding the cell type and the α-syn species (Fig. 1a). Furthermore, the number of inclusions per cell was similar in primary and MO 3.13 oligodendroglia. Yet,

fib α-syn treatment presented with a significant lower number of inclusions per cell compared to sol α-syn in both cell types (Fig. 1b). Furthermore, we did not observe a statistically significant difference measuring the total area of the inclusions per cell for both α-syn types in primary oligodendroglial cells compared to the oligodendroglial cell line MO 3.13, however a tendency to smaller inclusions in primary oligodendroglial cells was found (Fig. 1c).

BAF-induced dysfunctional macroautophagy in oligodendroglial cells does not trigger GCI-like formation from extracellularly uptaken α-syn

To evaluate the effect of blocking the fusion of the autophagosome and the lysosome on GCI-like formation in oligodendroglia, cells were treated with the pharmacological autophagy inhibitor BAF followed by exposure to sol or fib α-syn. As BAF blocks LC3B-II degradation, successful macroautophagy inhibition

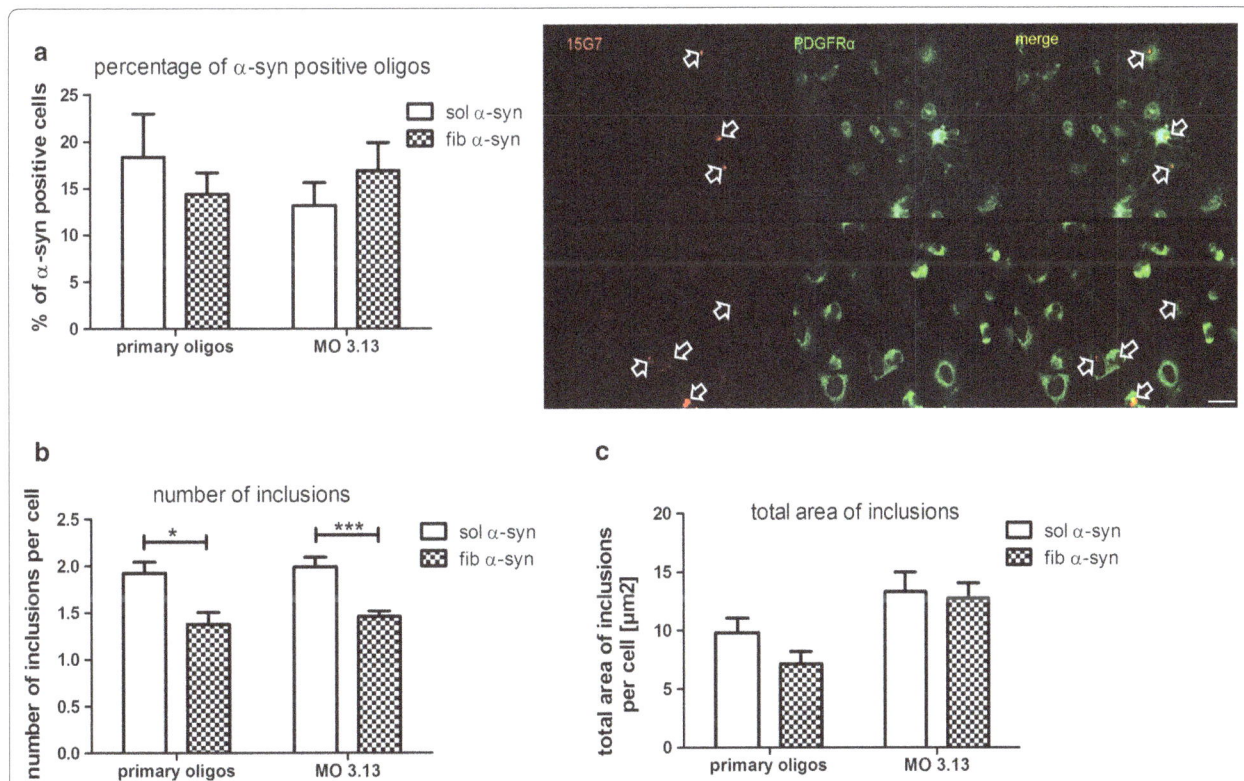

Fig. 1 Incorporation of α-syn by murine primary oligodendroglia as compared to the human oligodendroglioma cell line MO 3.13. Murine primary oligodendroglial cells (primary oligos) and the human oligodendroglial cell line MO 3.13 were treated with 18 μg/mL sol and fib α-syn for 24 h. Immunocytochemistry for α-syn (15G7, red) and PDGFRα (green) were performed and the evaluation was done by an unbiased investigator. The number of α-syn-positive oligodendroglial cells was evaluated and the percentage of α-syn-positive cells was calculated showing no difference between primary and MO 3.13 oligodendroglia. Arrows showing inclusions positively stained for 15G7 in the cytoplasm of primary and MO 3.13 oligodendroglial cells (a). The number of α-syn-positive inclusions per cell was counted revealing fewer inclusions per cell upon fib α-syn compared to sol α-syn exposure in both cell types (b). Moreover, the total area of inclusions per cell (μm²) was measured indicating a slight increase of the area in MO 3.13 compared to primary oligodendroglia; however, the difference did not reach statistical significance (c). Two-way analysis of variance with post hoc Bonferroni test was applied. Data are presented as mean ± SEM *$p < 0.05$; ***$p < 0.001$. Scale bar 20 μm. N number equals 4

can be identified by increased LC3B-II levels [50, 51]. Western blot analysis of BAF-treated oligodendroglia revealed a significant increase of LC3B-II levels in our experiments irrespective of an additional sol or fib α-syn treatment. Comparing untreated cells and sole addition of sol or fib α-syn, no change in the levels of LC3B-II was found indicative of a normal autophagic flux (Fig. 2). Interestingly, we found that blocking of macroautophagy with BAF induces oxidative stress as measured by the formation of ROS (Fig. 3). Treating oligodendroglia with the two types of extracellularly added α-syn only did not induce oxidative stress compared to cells treated with BAF and α-syn as quantified ROS levels reveal. The addition of extracellular recombinant fib α-syn, however not with sol α-syn, showed a significant increase of NBT-positive cells in BAF-treated oligodendroglia compared to untreated cells (Fig. 3).

As shown by other groups, oligodendroglial cells are capable to uptake α-syn from the extracellular space [22, 25, 26]. We confirm here the incorporation of extracellularly added sol and fib α-syn in oligodendroglial cells by confocal microscopy (Fig. 4). BAF treatment induced vesicle formation in the cytoplasm as seen by WGA-stained membranes (Fig. 4a). However, we were not able to generate GCI-like aggregates by blocking the fusion of the autophagosome with the lysosome using 50 nM BAF irrespective of the used extracellular α-syn form after 24 h. Interestingly, sol and fib α-syn were not only distributed in the cytoplasm but also a translocation to the nucleus

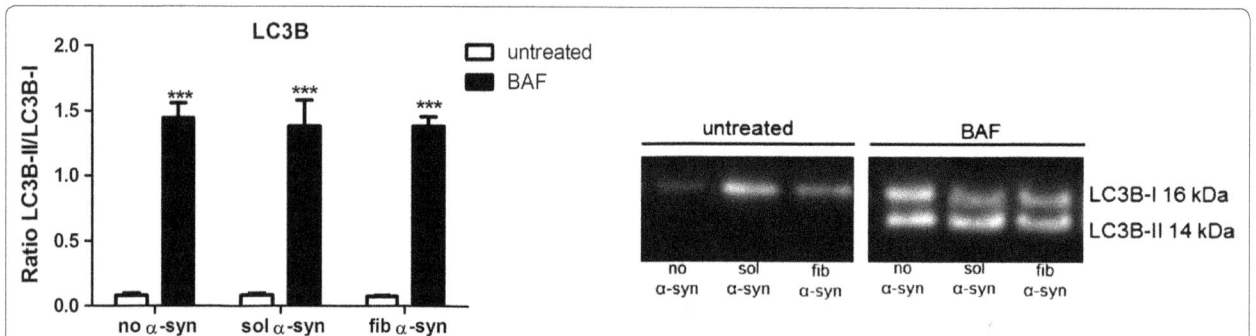

Fig. 2 Confirmation of the block of macroautophagy by treatment with BAF in oligodendroglial cells. Cell lysates were analyzed by Western blotting and the band intensities for LC3B-II were normalized to LC3B-I levels. Increased LC3B-II levels indicate the successful block of the fusion of the autophagosome with the lysosome. Oligodendroglial cells untreated or treated with 18 μg/mL sol or fib α-syn for 24 h showed a low ratio of LC3B-II/LC3B-I, whereas BAF-treated oligodendroglia revealed significantly higher levels of the LC3B-II/LC3B-I ratio independent of the α-syn treatment as compared to oligodendroglia not treated with BAF. Two-way analysis of variance with post hoc Bonferroni test was applied. Data are presented as mean ± SEM. ***$p < 0.001$. N number equals 4

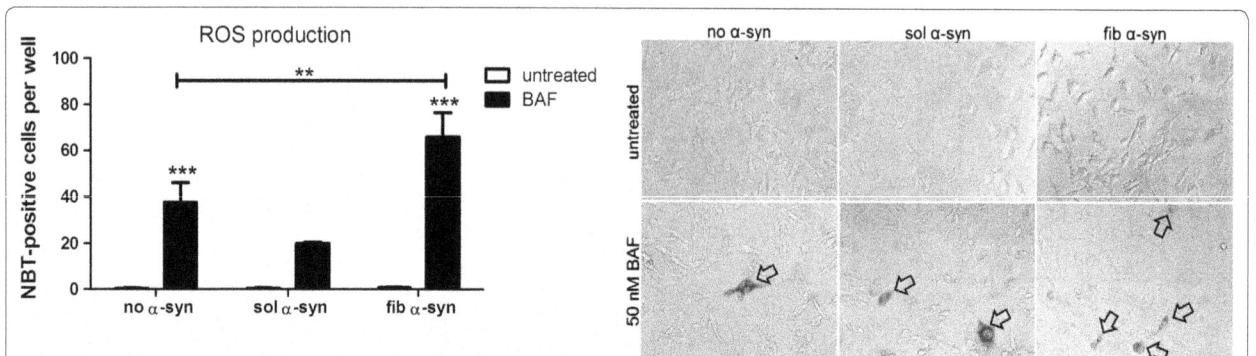

Fig. 3 Blocking macroautophagy with BAF in combination with α-syn treatment results in increased ROS production in oligodendroglial cells. Following treatment, cells were stained for ROS by using nitroblue tetrazolium chloride (NBT) resulting in a blue precipitate in the presence of ROS. We found that treatment with BAF significantly enhances the number of NBT-positive oligodendroglial cells compared to untreated cells. Furthermore, the additional treatment with extracellular fib α-syn for 24 h revealed a significant increase of NBT-positive cells compared to cells treated with BAF only and cells not treated with BAF. However, treatment with sol α-syn did not induce a significant increase of ROS production. Arrows pointing out oligodendroglial cells positively stained for NBT. Two-way analysis of variance with post hoc Bonferroni test was applied. Data are presented as mean ± SEM. **$p < 0.01$; ***$p < 0.001$. Scale bar 20 μm. N number equals 4

of α-syn was found (Fig. 4b). BAF induced the generation of vesicles in the cytoplasm as stained with the lectin compound WGA linked to FITC suggesting inhibited macroautophagy (Fig. 4). Yet, α-syn was not found to co-localize with the WGA-positive vesicles (Fig. 4b).

Western blot analysis of intracellular α-syn supported these morphological observations. Oligodendroglial cells incorporated a significant amount of extracellularly added sol or fib α-syn. Yet, the inhibition of macroautophagy through BAF had no significant effect on the amounts of intracellular α-syn and did not induce a pathological aggregation of α-syn in oligodendroglial cells as no oligomers or fibrils were detected (Fig. 5a). Moreover, the oligodendroglial cells used for these experiments, express a very low amount of endogenous α-syn. However, the blocking of macroautophagy with the pharmacological blocker BAF did not induce an accumulation of the endogenously expressed α-syn. Discrimination between endogenous and extracellular α-syn was possible as the extracellularly added α-syn had due to an attached his-tag an increased size (24 kDa) compared to endogenously expressed α-syn (14 kDa) (Fig. 5).

Furthermore, we analyzed the levels of another protein most common in GCIs, namely ubiquitin [52]. As ubiquitination is abundant in GCIs, higher levels of ubiquitin might indicated GCI-like formation in oligodendroglial cells. In this cell culture model a slight increase of ubiquitin levels upon treatment with BAF and extracellularly added α-syn or with extracellularly added α-syn only was detected. Yet, a significant increase of ubiquitin levels was achieved only by challenging oligodendroglial cells with fib α-syn compared to untreated cells. Macroautophagy blocking using BAF followed by α-syn treatment did not increase ubiquitin levels after 24 h of treatment (Fig. 6a). Furthermore, no co-localization of α-syn and ubiquitin was found upon treatment with BAF and sol or fib α-syn as investigated using fluorescence microscopy (Fig. 6b).

Genetic knockdown of LC3B in oligodendroglial cells does not induce the formation of GCI-like aggregates from extracellularly uptaken α-syn

The genetic knockdown was verified using Western blot analysis revealing a significant reduction of the LC3B protein in oligodendroglial cells transfected with the shRNA against LC3B compared to the scrambled shRNA plasmid (Fig. 7a).

LC3B knockdown in oligodendroglial cells did not reveal a significant effect regarding the levels of incorporated extracellular added α-syn compared to oligodendroglia transfected with a control plasmid. No oligomers

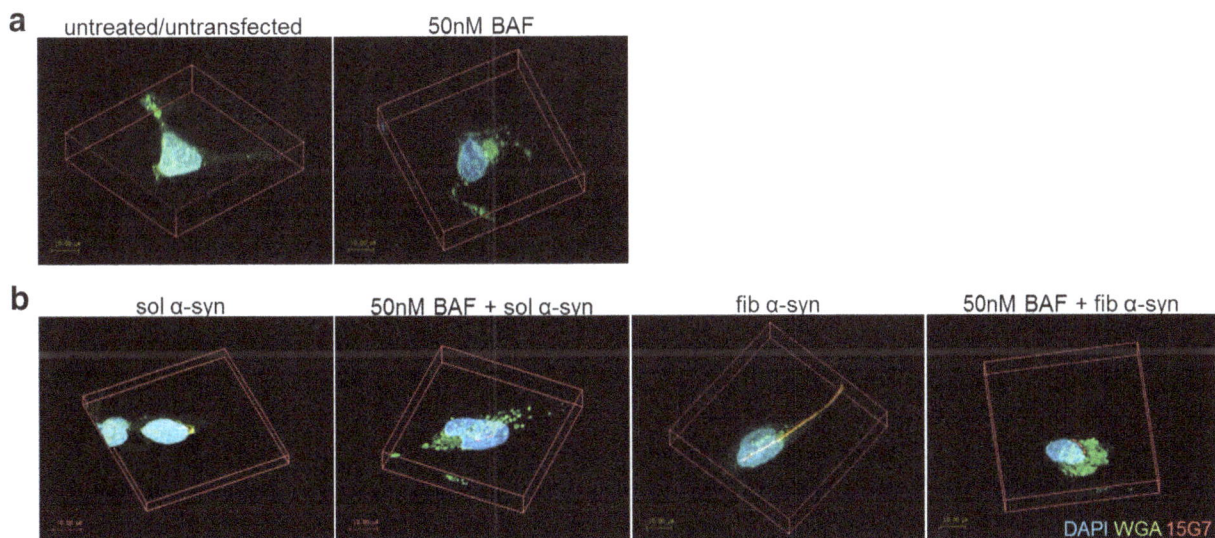

Fig. 4 Morphological analysis of α-syn-positive inclusions upon macroautophagy blocking treatment in oligodendroglial cells. Confocal microscopy was performed to analyze the incorporation and inclusion formation of sol and fib α-syn in oligodendroglial cells challenged with BAF for 24 h. Immunocytochemistry was accomplished following fixation, labelling human α-syn (15G7, red), the membrane using wheat germ agglutinin (WGA, green) and the nucleus using DAPI (blue). Treatment with BAF induced a more pronounced vesicle formation as can be seen by the membrane staining with WGA (**a**). The addition of recombinant sol and fib α-syn for 24 h to the medium induced the incorporation of α-syn by oligodendroglial cells. Yet, simultaneous macroautophagy blocking did not induce an increased amount of α-syn incorporated by these oligodendroglial cells. No GCI-like formation was observed upon macroautophagy block and treatment with extracellularly added sol or fib α-syn. In some cells translocation of α-syn to the nucleus was observed as shown in picture fib α-syn. Moreover, BAF treatment induced an enhanced number of vesicles in the cytoplasm (WGA staining) irrespective of α-syn in the cytoplasm of the cells (**b**). Scale bar 10 μm

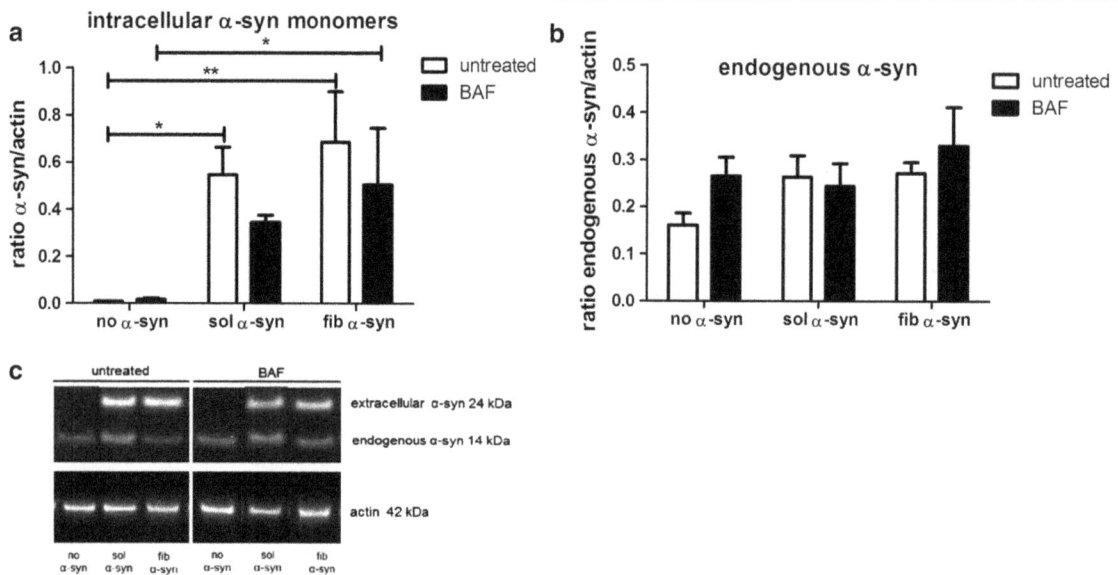

Fig. 5 Incorporation of extracellular monomeric sol and fib α-syn species and inclusion formation in oligodendroglial cells upon macroautophagy blocking with BAF. Intracellular amounts of uptaken α-syn monomers and endogenous α-syn were measured in oligodendroglial cells challenged with extracellular sol or fib α-syn for 24 h combined with macroautophagy blocking for 24 h using Western blot analysis. α-syn levels were normalized to actin. Addition of sol and fib α-syn led to a significantly increased amount of α-syn in oligodendroglial cells (24 kDa band due to his-tag). Moreover, an increased amount of α-syn was found in oligodendroglia treated with BAF compared to cells not treated with α-syn, however a significant change was detected only after fib α-syn exposure. Comparing untreated cells/cells treated with BAF and α-syn a not significant decrease regarding the amounts of α-syn was measured (**a**, **c**). Levels of endogenously expressed α-syn (14 kDa band, no his-tag) remained the same regarding all relevant treatments (**b**, **c**). Two-way analysis of variance with post hoc Bonferroni test was applied. Data are presented as mean ± SEM. *$p < 0.05$; **$p < 0.01$. N number equals 4

and fibrils were detectable. Treatment with sol and fib α-syn of oligodendroglia transfected with the scrambled shRNA plasmid presented with uptake of α-syn, yet the incorporation was not significant. In contrast, LC3B knockdown induced an increased incorporation of α-syn compared to untreated oligodendroglial cells, but only the intracytoplamatic accumulation of fib α-syn was significantly enhanced. Yet, α-syn levels in LC3B knockdown oligodendroglial cells did not reach a significant increase compared to cells transfected with the control plasmid upon α-syn challenge. No oligomers and fibrils were detectable (Fig. 7b, d). Moreover, low amounts of endogenously expressed α-syn were detectable in all shRNA transfected oligodendroglial cells. Knockdown of the LC3B gene did not change levels of endogenous α-syn significantly in oligodendroglia compared to control cells (Fig. 7c, d).

We observed that oligodendroglia transfected with the shRNA plasmid against LC3B were able to incorporate sol and fib α-syn and compared to cells transfected with the scrambled shRNA more punctuate α-syn inclusions were found. Yet, no differences regarding incorporated sol and fib α-syn were found during morphological analyses at the confocal microscope. Furthermore, no GCI

formation was observed in any of the analyzed oligodendroglial cells with LC3B knockdown (Fig. 8).

Discussion

The aggregation of α-syn in oligodendroglial cells, so called GCIs, is the major pathological hallmark of MSA. A connection between the formation of these α-syn-positive inclusions and neuronal degeneration and disease progression respectively has been postulated [31, 53]. However, to date the formation of GCIs in MSA has not been elucidated. Different mechanisms, including autophagy or proteasome dysfunction, are thought to be involved in the development of α-syn-positive inclusions in oligodendroglial cells [11, 32]. In the current study, we investigated the impact of dysfunctional macroautophagy on exposure to extracellular α-syn and formation of α-syn-positive inclusions in oligodendroglia. We observed no GCI-like formation upon pharmacological blocking of the fusion of the autophagosome and the lysosome, as well as genetic knockdown of LC3B combined with the treatment with recombinant extracellular sol and fib α-syn species.

Incorporation of extracellular or neuronal derived α-syn by oligodendroglial cells has already been shown in various studies in vitro and in vivo [22, 24–26]. In our cell

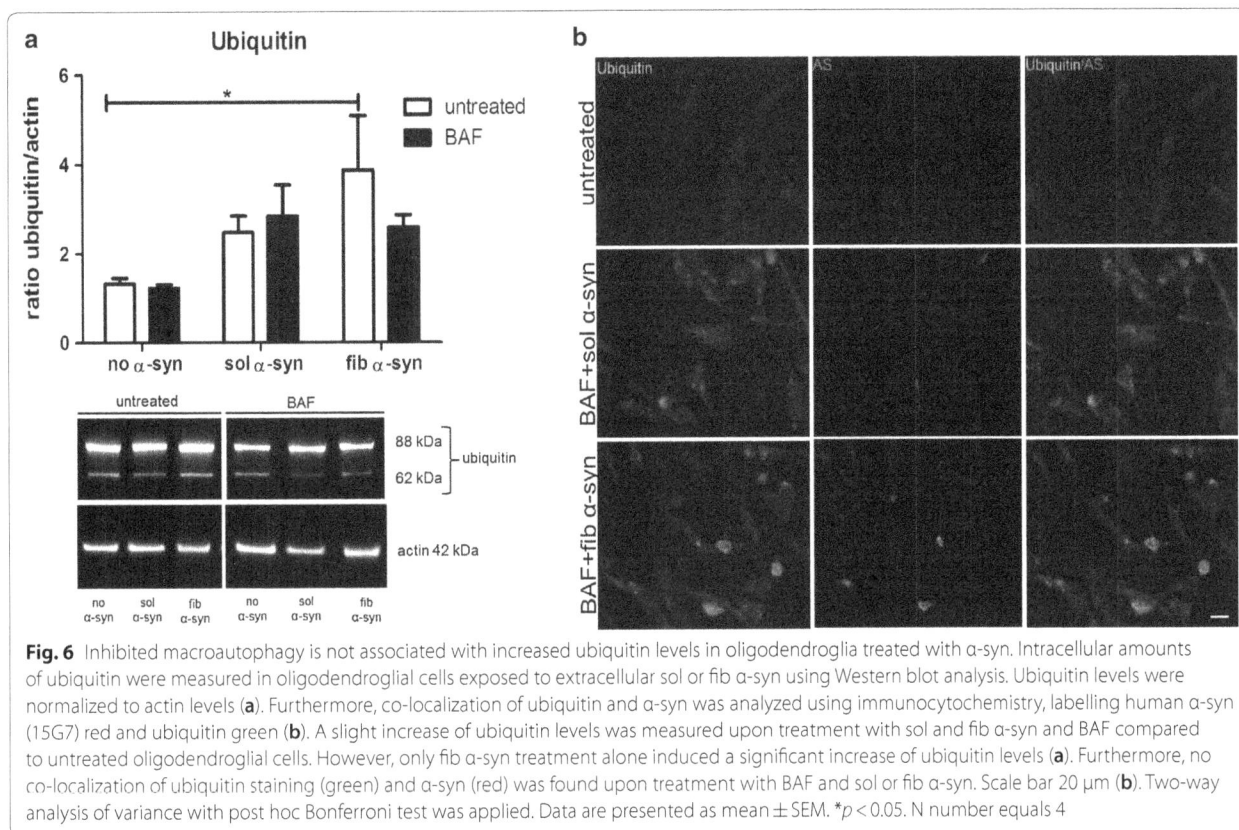

Fig. 6 Inhibited macroautophagy is not associated with increased ubiquitin levels in oligodendroglia treated with α-syn. Intracellular amounts of ubiquitin were measured in oligodendroglial cells exposed to extracellular sol or fib α-syn using Western blot analysis. Ubiquitin levels were normalized to actin levels (**a**). Furthermore, co-localization of ubiquitin and α-syn was analyzed using immunocytochemistry, labelling human α-syn (15G7) red and ubiquitin green (**b**). A slight increase of ubiquitin levels was measured upon treatment with sol and fib α-syn and BAF compared to untreated oligodendroglial cells. However, only fib α-syn treatment alone induced a significant increase of ubiquitin levels (**a**). Furthermore, no co-localization of ubiquitin staining (green) and α-syn (red) was found upon treatment with BAF and sol or fib α-syn. Scale bar 20 μm (**b**). Two-way analysis of variance with post hoc Bonferroni test was applied. Data are presented as mean ± SEM. *$p < 0.05$. N number equals 4

culture model, we were able to demonstrate the uptake of extracellularly added recombinant sol and fib α-syn. Furthermore, we provide evidence that the incorporation of α-syn and the formation of inclusions by MO 3.13 oligodendroglia is comparable to murine primary oligodendroglial cells suggesting that the oligodendroglial cell line is a reliable tool for further experiments. Autophagy mechanisms have been considered as important and efficient α-syn clearance mechanisms [27–29, 41, 43, 44]. An involvement of autophagy pathways regarding α-syn accumulation in oligodendroglial cells in MSA or other α-synucleinopathies seems conclusive [11, 45]. Furthermore, it was shown that extracellularly added α-syn and the overexpression of α-syn alone did not inhibit the autophagic flux in oligodendroglia as suggested by unchanged LC3-II levels among others [24]. Similar results were found in our experiments. The addition of extracellular recombinant sol and fib α-syn did not induce an increase in LC3B-II levels indicating a normal autophagic flux as described previously. Moreover, blocking of macroautophagy with BAF is known to inhibit the degradation of LC3B-II suggesting a successful block of the fusion of the autophagosome with the lysosome in the treated cells [50, 51]. In our experiments, we confirm a successful inhibition of macroautophagy by adding BAF

to oligodendroglial cells irrespective of the treatment with sol or fib α-syn, showing significantly increased LC3B-II levels.

Most cells control their need for energy through autophagy, and oxidative stress or the presence of ROS might interfere with the autophagy pathways as ROS have been associated with an activated autophagy upon nutrient deprivation, yet the connection between oxidative stress and autophagy is far from being elucidated [54]. Furthermore, damage to mitochondria was shown to impair the autophagic flux and lead to α-syn accumulation in oligodendroglial cells [24]. We found that the block of macroautophagy through BAF induces ROS production in oligodendroglia, which can be enhanced by the addition of fib α-syn. Yet, extracellularly added α-syn alone does not induce ROS production in oligodendroglia suggesting an important role of inhibited autophagy in the oxidative stress pathway. In accordance with our data, it was already shown that autophagy deficiency can induce oxidative stress and mitochondrial ROS production [55]. However, although we successfully blocked macroautophagy and thus induced oxidative stress in oligodendroglia, we were not able to detect an accumulation of α-syn and ubiquitin relevant to GCI-like formation in our cell culture model upon treatment

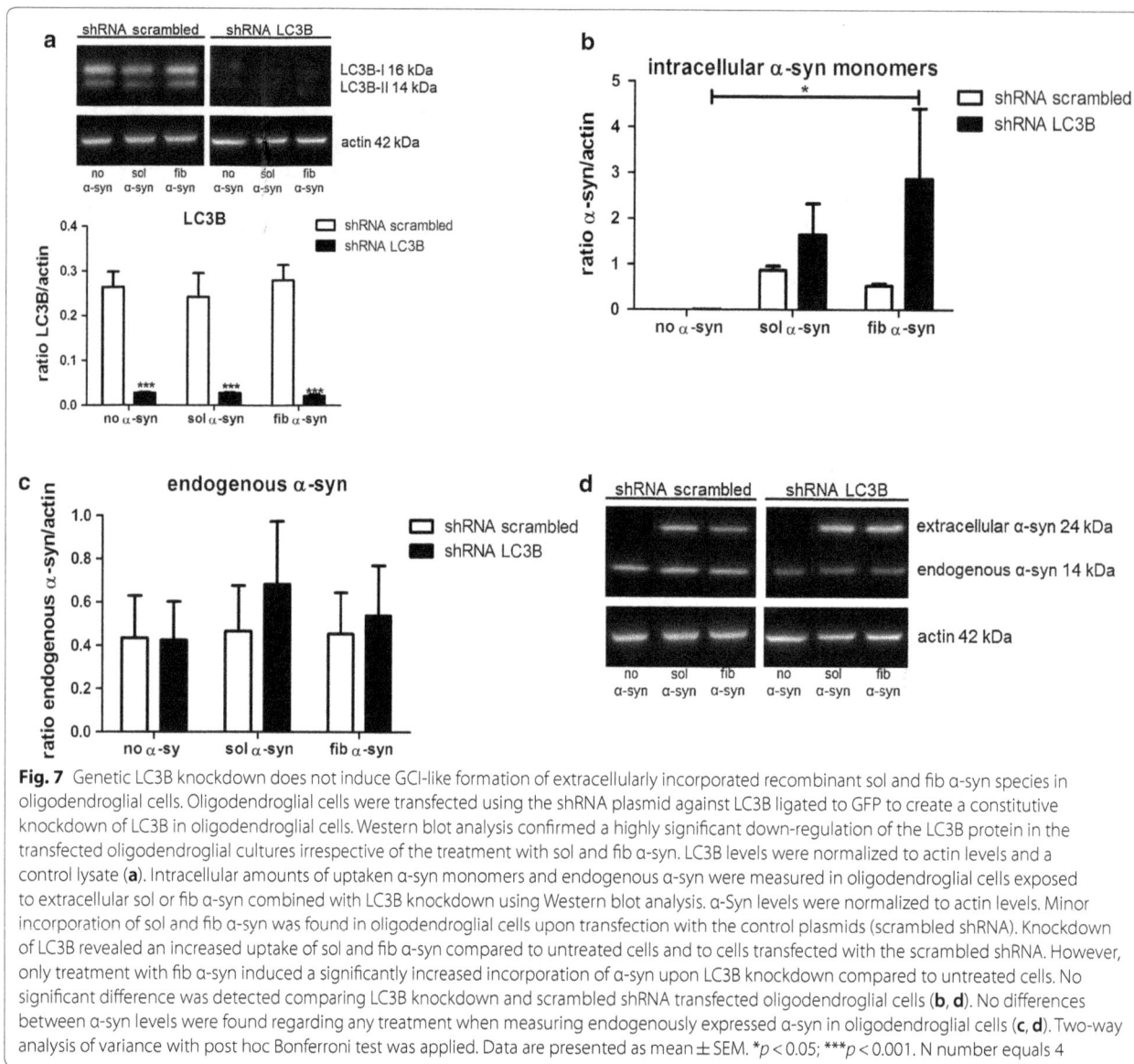

Fig. 7 Genetic LC3B knockdown does not induce GCI-like formation of extracellularly incorporated recombinant sol and fib α-syn species in oligodendroglial cells. Oligodendroglial cells were transfected using the shRNA plasmid against LC3B ligated to GFP to create a constitutive knockdown of LC3B in oligodendroglial cells. Western blot analysis confirmed a highly significant down-regulation of the LC3B protein in the transfected oligodendroglial cultures irrespective of the treatment with sol and fib α-syn. LC3B levels were normalized to actin levels and a control lysate (**a**). Intracellular amounts of uptaken α-syn monomers and endogenous α-syn were measured in oligodendroglial cells exposed to extracellular sol or fib α-syn combined with LC3B knockdown using Western blot analysis. α-Syn levels were normalized to actin levels. Minor incorporation of sol and fib α-syn was found in oligodendroglial cells upon transfection with the control plasmids (scrambled shRNA). Knockdown of LC3B revealed an increased uptake of sol and fib α-syn compared to untreated cells and to cells transfected with the scrambled shRNA. However, only treatment with fib α-syn induced a significantly increased incorporation of α-syn upon LC3B knockdown compared to untreated cells. No significant difference was detected comparing LC3B knockdown and scrambled shRNA transfected oligodendroglial cells (**b, d**). No differences between α-syn levels were found regarding any treatment when measuring endogenously expressed α-syn in oligodendroglial cells (**c, d**). Two-way analysis of variance with post hoc Bonferroni test was applied. Data are presented as mean ± SEM. *$p < 0.05$; ***$p < 0.001$. N number equals 4

with extracellular added α-syn. Analyses at the confocal microscope revealed smaller α-syn inclusions but we did not detect any α-syn aggregates in oligodendroglia treated with recombinant α-syn, as well as they did not resemble GCI-like inclusions as described in MSA brains [56]. In a recent study, the inhibition of macroautophagy with ammonium chloride and chloroquine as well as induced oxidative stress in OLN-t40 oligodendroglia led to the accumulation of α-syn in the cytoplasm [24], yet GCI-like inclusions were also not reported. Only small amounts of incorporated α-syn were found in oligodendroglial cells untreated or treated with BAF. However, we did not induce mitochondrial impairment leading to a halt in the autophagic flux in our model suggesting that

macroautophagy blocking through BAF is not enough to induce GCI-like formation in oligodendroglial cells. Probably more than one pathway dysfunction and in particular a combination of factors is needed to induce GCI formation in oligodendroglial cells and mimic GCIs as seen in MSA. Another limitation of this study could be the difference regarding oligodendroglial features and also GCI formation properties comparing oligodendroglial cells in vivo and in vitro. Macroautophagy dysfunction in oligodendroglia in vivo could reveal a different outcome regarding α-syn accumulation compared to treated oligodendroglial cell lines. Furthermore, it can also be discussed that the results in various studies depend on the oligodendroglial cell type used in the

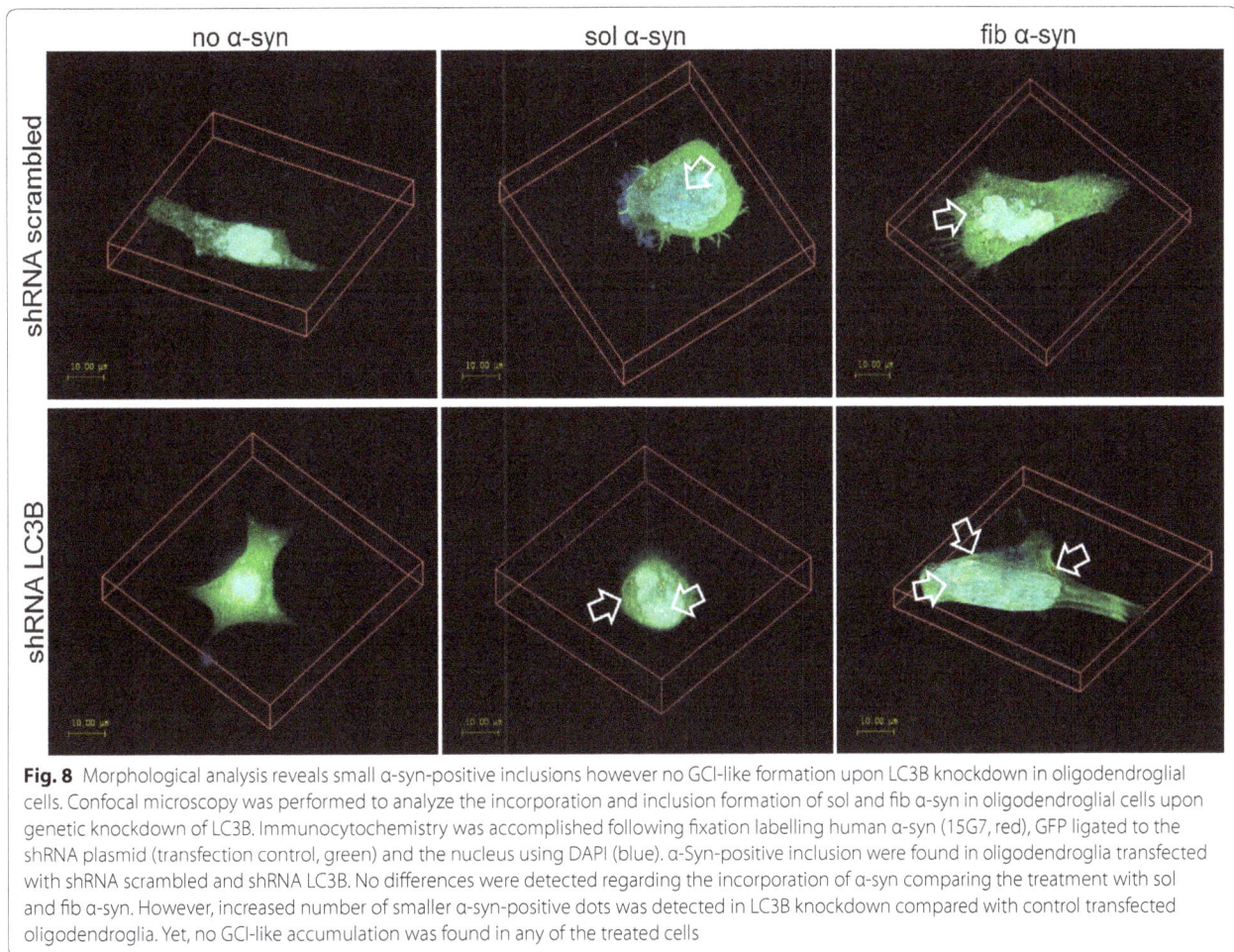

Fig. 8 Morphological analysis reveals small α-syn-positive inclusions however no GCI-like formation upon LC3B knockdown in oligodendroglial cells. Confocal microscopy was performed to analyze the incorporation and inclusion formation of sol and fib α-syn in oligodendroglial cells upon genetic knockdown of LC3B. Immunocytochemistry was accomplished following fixation labelling human α-syn (15G7, red), GFP ligated to the shRNA plasmid (transfection control, green) and the nucleus using DAPI (blue). α-Syn-positive inclusion were found in oligodendroglia transfected with shRNA scrambled and shRNA LC3B. No differences were detected regarding the incorporation of α-syn comparing the treatment with sol and fib α-syn. However, increased number of smaller α-syn-positive dots was detected in LC3B knockdown compared with control transfected oligodendroglia. Yet, no GCI-like accumulation was found in any of the treated cells

experiments and therefore the differing results could indicate different properties of the oligodendroglial cell lines and primary oligodendroglial cells used. Moreover, a 24 h-duration of α-syn treatment and the concentration of 18 μg/mL added, might be not enough for oligodendroglia to build up larger α-syn-positive inclusion, as the incorporation of α-syn has been stated to be time- and concentration-dependent [25, 26]. In a different study, it is suggested that BAF not only potentiates the toxicity of aggregated α-syn species, but also induces a reduction of the α-syn aggregation and furthermore, the secretion of toxic α-syn species by neuronal cells into the extracellular space [42, 47]. This could be an explanation for the low levels of α-syn upon BAF treatment in oligodendroglial cells in our study. However, in future experiments α-syn release would need to be analyzed to support this hypothesis.

In a next step, the genetic knockdown of LC3B was performed in oligodendroglial cells followed by treatment with recombinant sol and fib α-syn. We observed incorporation of α-syn in oligodendroglial cells lacking LC3B compared to cells treated with the control/scrambled shRNA similar to a previously published experiment showing that the down-regulation of Atg5 in oligodendroglial cells leads to an increase of α-syn levels [24]. Furthermore, confocal analysis of the cells revealed more dots of incorporated α-syn in oligodendroglia with reduced LC3B levels suggesting that a genetic knockdown of the macroautophagy gene LC3B might induce accumulation of α-syn. However, no GCI-like formation was observed. As mentioned above, higher α-syn concentration or longer incubation times have to be tested in further experiments. However, the release of α-syn through exosomes by oligodendroglia triggered by macroautophagy dysfunction as described in neurons [42, 47] might be another explanation regarding the lack of GCI-like inclusions.

Conclusion

In conclusion, in this study we demonstrate that blocking of macroautophagy in the presence of sol or fib α-syn does not lead to the formation of α-syn inclusions in oligodendroglia as observed in human MSA. However, we found that macroautophagy blocking leads to higher oxidative stress in combination with fib α-syn treatment. Further studies have to be conducted to clarify the role of macroautophagy in the initiation and progression of MSA. Defects in different pathways might contribute to the formation of MSA-like GCIs. The investigation of the CMA pathway and its role in GCI formation in oligodendroglia could be another interesting next step in future studies, as in neuronal cells CMA is shown to have a leading role in α-syn degradation [43]. Furthermore, it is described that macroautophagy dysfunction induces the release of α-syn through exosomes by neuronal cells [42, 47]. The same mechanism might be also true for oligodendroglial cells, which could be an explanation that macroautophagy blocking does not induce GCI-like formation in our experiments. In summary, our results suggest that macroautophagy dysfunction is not the only pathway involved in the formation process of GCIs in MSA, suggesting a combination of different approaches (e.g. proteasome and autophagy inhibition) in future studies. Furthermore, in-depth studies are required to transfer the relevance of the current findings to the situation in patients.

Abbreviations

α-syn: α-synuclein; BAF: bafilomycin A1; bFGF: basic fibroblast growth factor; CMA: chaperone mediated autophagy; CNTF: ciliary neurotrophic factor; DAPI: 4′,6-diamidino-2-phenylindole dihydrochloride; DLB: dementia with Lewy bodies; DMEM: Dulbecco's modified Eagle's medium; FCS: fetal calf serum; fib α-syn: fibrillar α-synuclein; GCIs: glial cytoplasmic inclusions; GFP: green fluorescent protein; kDa: kilodalton; LAL: limulus amoebocyte lysate; LBs: Lewy bodies; LC3B: microtubule-associated protein 1 light chain 3B; MSA: multiple system atrophy; NAC: N-acetyl-L-cysteine; NBT: nitroblue tetrazolium chloride; OPC: oligodendrocyte precursor cell; PBS: phosphate buffered saline; PBS-T: phosphate buffered saline containing 0.1% Tween-20; PDGF-AA: platelet-derived growth factor AA; PDL: poly-D-lysine; PFA: paraformaldehyde; RT: room temperature; sol α-syn: soluble α-synuclein; TIT: triiodothyronine; UPS: ubiquitin–proteasome system; V-ATPase: vacuolar H + ATPase; WGA: wheat germ agglutinin.

Authors' contributions

Substantial contributions to the conception or design of the work (LF, GKW, NS); or the acquisition, analysis (LF, EB, DB, RI), or interpretation of data for the work (LF, GKW, NS); and Drafting the work (LF) or revising it critically for important intellectual content (EB, DB, RI, GKW, NS); and final approval of the version to be published (LF, EB, DB, RI, GKW, NS); and agreement to be accountable for all aspects of the work in ensuring that questions related to the accuracy or integrity of any part of the work are appropriately investigated and resolved (LF, EB, DB, RI, GKW, NS). All authors read and approved the final manuscript.

Author details

[1] Department of Neurology, Medical University of Innsbruck, Innrain 66, G2, 6020 Innsbruck, Austria. [2] Department of Anatomy, Histology and Embryology, Medical University of Innsbruck, Anichstrasse 35, Innsbruck, Austria.

Acknowledgements
The authors are grateful to Karin Spiss, MSc for her excellent technical assistance and to Priv.-Doz. Dr. Martin Offterdinger for his advice on the confocal microscopy. Confocal microscopy was performed at the Biooptics Core Facility of Medical University of Innsbruck, Austria.

Competing interests
The authors declare that they have no competing interests.

Consent to participate
Not applicable.

Funding
The study is supported by grants P25161 and F4414 of the Austrian Science Fund (FWF) and Grant UNI-0404/1660 of the Tyrolian Science Fund (TWF).

References

1. Kuzdas-Wood D, Stefanova N, Jellinger KA, Seppi K, Schlossmacher MG, Poewe W, et al. Towards translational therapies for multiple system atrophy. Prog Neurobiol. 2014;118:19–35. https://doi.org/10.1016/j.pneurobio.2014.02.007.

2. Al-Chalabi A, Durr A, Wood NW, Parkinson MH, Camuzat A, Hulot JS, et al. Genetic variants of the alpha-synuclein gene SNCA are associated with multiple system atrophy. PLoS ONE. 2009;4(9):e7114. https://doi.org/10.1371/journal.pone.0007114.

3. Scholz SW, Houlden H, Schulte C, Sharma M, Li A, Berg D, et al. SNCA variants are associated with increased risk for multiple system atrophy. Ann Neurol. 2009;65(5):610–4. https://doi.org/10.1002/ana.21685.

4. Fellner L, Stefanova N. The role of glia in alpha-synucleinopathies. Mol Neurobiol. 2013;47(2):575–86. https://doi.org/10.1007/s12035-012-8340-3.

5. Stefanova N, Klimaschewski L, Poewe W, Wenning GK, Reindl M. Glial cell death induced by overexpression of alpha-synuclein. J Neurosci Res. 2001;65(5):432–8. https://doi.org/10.1002/jnr.1171.

6. Stefanova N, Emgard M, Klimaschewski L, Wenning GK, Reindl M. Ultrastructure of alpha-synuclein-positive aggregations in U373 astrocytoma and rat primary glial cells. Neurosci Lett. 2002;323(1):37–40.

7. Stefanova N, Schanda K, Klimaschewski L, Poewe W, Wenning GK, Reindl M. Tumor necrosis factor-alpha-induced cell death in U373 cells overexpressing alpha-synuclein. J Neurosci Res. 2003;73(3):334–40. https://doi.org/10.1002/jnr.10662.

8. Wang T, Pei Z, Zhang W, Liu B, Langenbach R, Lee C, et al. MPP + -induced COX-2 activation and subsequent dopaminergic neurodegeneration. FASEB J. 2005;19(9):1134–6. https://doi.org/10.1096/fj.04-2457fje.

9. Xilouri M, Vogiatzi T, Vekrellis K, Park D, Stefanis L. Abberant alpha-synuclein confers toxicity to neurons in part through inhibition of chaperone-mediated autophagy. PLoS ONE. 2009;4(5):e5515. https://doi.org/10.1371/journal.pone.0005515.

10. Jellinger KA. Neuropathology in Parkinson's disease with mild cognitive impairment. Acta Neuropathol. 2010;120(6):829–30. https://doi.org/10.1007/s00401-010-0755-1.

11. Schwarz L, Goldbaum O, Bergmann M, Probst-Cousin S, Richter-Landsberg C. Involvement of macroautophagy in multiple system atrophy and protein aggregate formation in oligodendrocytes. J Mol Neurosci: MN. 2012;47(2):256–66. https://doi.org/10.1007/s12031-012-9733-5.

12. Tanji K, Odagiri S, Maruyama A, Mori F, Kakita A, Takahashi H, et al. Alteration of autophagosomal proteins in the brain of multiple system atrophy. Neurobiol Dis. 2013;49:190–8. https://doi.org/10.1016/j.nbd.2012.08.017.

13. Fellner L, Jellinger KA, Wenning GK, Stefanova N. Glial dysfunction in the pathogenesis of alpha-synucleinopathies: emerging concepts. Acta Neuropathol. 2011;121(6):675–93. https://doi.org/10.1007/s00401-011-0833-z.

14. Wenning GK, Jellinger KA. The role of alpha-synuclein and tau in neurodegenerative movement disorders. Curr Opin Neurol. 2005;18(4):357–62.

15. Fellner L, Irschick R, Schanda K, Reindl M, Klimaschewski L, Poewe W, et al. Toll-like receptor 4 is required for alpha-synuclein dependent

activation of microglia and astroglia. Glia. 2013;61(3):349–60. https://doi.org/10.1002/glia.22437

16. Asi YT, Simpson JE, Heath PR, Wharton SB, Lees AJ, Revesz T, et al. Alpha-synuclein mRNA expression in oligodendrocytes in MSA. Glia. 2014;62(6):964–70. https://doi.org/10.1002/glia.22653.

17. Djelloul M, Holmqvist S, Boza-Serrano A, Azevedo C, Yeung MS, Goldwurm S, etal. Alpha-synuclein expression in the oligodendrocyte lineage: an in vitro and in vivo study using rodent and human models. Stem Cell Rep. 2015;5(2):174–84. https://doi.org/10.1016/j.stemcr.2015.07.002.

18. Miller DW, Johnson JM, Solano SM, Hollingsworth ZR, Standaert DG, Young AB. Absence of alpha-synuclein mRNA expression in normal and multiple system atrophy oligodendroglia. J Neural Transm (Vienna). 2005;112(12):1613–24. https://doi.org/10.1007/s00702-005-0378-1.

19. Ozawa T, Okuizumi K, Ikeuchi T, Wakabayashi K, Takahashi H, Tsuji S. Analysis of the expression level of alpha-synuclein mRNA using postmortem brain samples from pathologically confirmed cases of multiple system atrophy. Acta Neuropathol. 2001;102(2):188–90.

20. Emmanouilidou E, Melachroinou K, Roumeliotis T, Garbis SD, Ntzouni M, Margaritis LH, et al. Cell-produced alpha-synuclein is secreted in a calcium-dependent manner by exosomes and impacts neuronal survival. J Neurosci. 2010;30(20):6838–51. https://doi.org/10.1523/JNEUROSCI.5699-09.2010.

21. Hansen C, Angot E, Bergstrom AL, Steiner JA, Pieri L, Paul G, et al. α-Synuclein propagates from mouse brain to grafted dopaminergic neurons and seeds aggregation in cultured human cells. J Clin Investig. 2011;121(2):715–25. https://doi.org/10.1172/JCI43366.

22. Reyes JF, Rey NL, Bousset L, Melki R, Brundin P, Angot E. Alpha-synuclein transfers from neurons to oligodendrocytes. Glia. 2014;62(3):387–98. https://doi.org/10.1002/glia.22611.

23. Bruck D, Wenning GK, Stefanova N, Fellner L. Glia and alpha-synuclein in neurodegeneration: a complex interaction. Neurobiol Dis. 2016;85:262–74. https://doi.org/10.1016/j.nbd.2015.03.003.

24. Pukass K, Goldbaum O, Richter-Landsberg C. Mitochondrial impairment and oxidative stress compromise autophagosomal degradation of alpha-synuclein in oligodendroglial cells. J Neurochem. 2015;135(1):194–205. https://doi.org/10.1111/jnc.13256.

25. Konno M, Hasegawa T, Baba T, Miura E, Sugeno N, Kikuchi A, et al. Suppression of dynamin GTPase decreases alpha-synuclein uptake by neuronal and oligodendroglial cells: a potent therapeutic target for synucleinopathy. Mol neurodegener. 2012;7:38. https://doi.org/10.1186/1750-1326-7-38.

26. Kisos H, Pukass K, Ben-Hur T, Richter-Landsberg C, Sharon R. Increased neuronal alpha-synuclein pathology associates with its accumulation in oligodendrocytes in mice modeling alpha-synucleinopathies. PLoS ONE. 2012;7(10):e46817. https://doi.org/10.1371/journal.pone.0046817.

27. Webb JL, Ravikumar B, Atkins J, Skepper JN, Rubinsztein DC. Alpha-Synuclein is degraded by both autophagy and the proteasome. J Biol Chem. 2003;278(27):25009–13. https://doi.org/10.1074/jbc.M300227200.

28. Cuervo AM, Stefanis L, Fredenburg R, Lansbury PT, Sulzer D. Impaired degradation of mutant alpha-synuclein by chaperone-mediated autophagy. Science. 2004;305(5688):1292–5. https://doi.org/10.1126/science.1101738.

29. Vogiatzi T, Xilouri M, Vekrellis K, Stefanis L. Wild type alpha-synuclein is degraded by chaperone-mediated autophagy and macroautophagy in neuronal cells. J Biol Chem. 2008;283(35):23542–56. https://doi.org/10.1074/jbc.M801992200.

30. Martinez-Vicente M, Vila M. Alpha-synuclein and protein degradation pathways in Parkinson's disease: a pathological feed-back loop. Exp Neurol. 2013;247:308–13. https://doi.org/10.1016/j.expneurol.2013.03.005.

31. Wenning GK, Stefanova N, Jellinger KA, Poewe W, Schlossmacher MG. Multiple system atrophy: a primary oligodendrogliopathy. Ann Neurol. 2008;64(3):239–46. https://doi.org/10.1002/ana.21465.

32. Stefanova N, Kaufmann WA, Humpel C, Poewe W, Wenning GK. Systemic proteasome inhibition triggers neurodegeneration in a transgenic mouse model expressing human alpha-synuclein under oligodendrocyte promoter: implications for multiple system atrophy. Acta Neuropathol. 2012;124(1):51–65. https://doi.org/10.1007/s00401-012-0977-5.

33. Ebrahimi-Fakhari D, Cantuti-Castelvetri I, Fan Z, Rockenstein E, Masliah E, Hyman BT, et al. Distinct roles in vivo for the ubiquitin-proteasome system and the autophagy-lysosomal pathway in the degradation of alpha-synuclein. J Neurosci. 2011;31(41):14508–20.

34. Xilouri M, Vogiatzi T, Vekrellis K, Stefanis L. alpha-synuclein degradation by autophagic pathways: a potential key to Parkinson's disease pathogenesis. Autophagy. 2008;4(7):917–9.

35. Rubinsztein DC, DiFiglia M, Heintz N, Nixon RA, Qin ZH, Ravikumar B, et al. Autophagy and its possible roles in nervous system diseases, damage and repair. Autophagy. 2005;1(1):11–22.

36. Mizushima N, Yoshimori T, Ohsumi Y. The role of Atg proteins in autophagosome formation. Annu Rev Cell Dev Biol. 2011;27:107–32. https://doi.org/10.1146/annurev-cellbio-092910-154005.

37. Gukovskaya AS, Gukovsky I. Autophagy and pancreatitis. Am J Physiol Gastrointest Liver Physiol. 2012;303(9):G993–1003. https://doi.org/10.1152/ajpgi.00122.2012.

38. Winslow AR, Chen CW, Corrochano S, Acevedo-Arozena A, Gordon DE, Peden AA, et al. alpha-Synuclein impairs macroautophagy: implications for Parkinson's disease. J Cell Biol. 2010;190(6):1023–37. https://doi.org/10.1083/jcb.201003122.

39. Kabeya Y, Mizushima N, Ueno T, Yamamoto A, Kirisako T, Noda T, et al. LC3, a mammalian homologue of yeast Apg8p, is localized in autophagosome membranes after processing. EMBO J. 2000;19(21):5720–8. https://doi.org/10.1093/emboj/19.21.5720.

40. Wakabayashi K, Tanji K. Multiple system atrophy and autophagy. Rinsho shinkeigaku = Clin Neurol. 2014;54(12):966–8.

41. Xilouri M, Stefanis L. Autophagic pathways in Parkinson disease and related disorders. Expert Rev Mol Med. 2011;13:e8. https://doi.org/10.1017/S1462399411001803.

42. Klucken J, Poehler AM, Ebrahimi-Fakhari D, Schneider J, Nuber S, Rockenstein E, et al. Alpha-synuclein aggregation involves a bafilomycin A_1-sensitive autophagy pathway. Autophagy. 2012;8(5):754–66. https://doi.org/10.4161/auto.19371.

43. Xilouri M, Brekk OR, Landeck N, Pitychoutis PM, Papasilekas T, Papadopoulou-Daifoti Z, et al. Boosting chaperone-mediated autophagy in vivo mitigates α-synuclein-induced neurodegeneration. Brain. 2013;136(Pt 7):2130–46. https://doi.org/10.1093/brain/awt131.

44. Anglade P, Vyas S, Javoy-Agid F, Herrero MT, Michel PP, Marquez J, et al. Apoptosis and autophagy in nigral neurons of patients with Parkinson's disease. Histol Histopathol. 1997;12(1):25–31.

45. Masui K, Nakata Y, Fujii N, Iwaki T. Extensive distribution of glial cytoplasmic inclusions in an autopsied case of multiple system atrophy with a prolonged 18-year clinical course. Neuropathology. 2012;32(1):69–76. https://doi.org/10.1111/j.1440-1789.2011.01222.x.

46. Yamamoto A, Tagawa Y, Yoshimori T, Moriyama Y, Masaki R, Tashiro Y. Bafilomycin A1 prevents maturation of autophagic vacuoles by inhibiting fusion between autophagosomes and lysosomes in rat hepatoma cell line, H-4-II-E cells. Cell Struct Funct. 1998;23(1):33–42.

47. Poehler AM, Xiang W, Spitzer P, May VE, Meixner H, Rockenstein E, et al. Autophagy modulates SNCA/alpha-synuclein release, thereby generating a hostile microenvironment. Autophagy. 2014;10(12):2171–92. https://doi.org/10.4161/auto.36436.

48. Stefanova N, Fellner L, Reindl M, Masliah E, Poewe W, Wenning GK. Toll-like receptor 4 promotes alpha-synuclein clearance and survival of nigral dopaminergic neurons. Am J Pathol. 2011;179(2):954–63. https://doi.org/10.1016/j.ajpath.2011.04.013.

49. Chen Y, Balasubramaniyan V, Peng J, Hurlock EC, Tallquist M, Li J, et al. Isolation and culture of rat and mouse oligodendrocyte precursor cells. Nat Protoc. 2007;2(5):1044–51. https://doi.org/10.1038/nprot.2007.149.

50. Rubinsztein DC, Cuervo AM, Ravikumar B, Sarkar S, Korolchuk V, Kaushik S, et al. In search of an "autophagomometer". Autophagy. 2009;5(5):585–9.

51. Sarkar S, Perlstein EO, Imarisio S, Pineau S, Cordenier A, Maglathlin RL, et al. Small molecules enhance autophagy and reduce toxicity in Huntington's disease models. Nat Chem Biol. 2007;3(6):331–8. https://doi.org/10.1038/nchembio883.

52. Wakabayashi K, Yoshimoto M, Tsuji S, Takahashi H. Alpha-synuclein immunoreactivity in glial cytoplasmic inclusions in multiple system atrophy. Neurosci Lett. 1998;249(2–3):180–2.

53. Ozawa T, Paviour D, Quinn NP, Josephs KA, Sangha H, Kilford L, et al. The spectrum of pathological involvement of the striatonigral and olivopontocerebellar systems in multiple system atrophy: clinicopathological correlations. Brain. 2004;127(Pt 12):2657–71. https://doi.org/10.1093/brain/awh303.

54. Filomeni G, De Zio D, Cecconi F. Oxidative stress and autophagy: the clash between damage and metabolic needs. Cell Death Differ. 2015;22(3):377–88. https://doi.org/10.1038/cdd.2014.150.

55. Tal MC, Sasai M, Lee HK, Yordy B, Shadel GS, Iwasaki A. Absence of autophagy results in reactive oxygen species-dependent amplification of RLR signaling. Proc Natl Acad Sci USA. 2009;106(8):2770–5. https://doi.org/10.1073/pnas.0807694106.

56. Wenning GK, Jellinger KA. The role of alpha-synuclein in the pathogenesis of multiple system atrophy. Acta Neuropathol. 2005;109(2):129–40. https://doi.org/10.1007/s00401-004-0935-y.

17

An effort toward molecular biology of food deprivation induced food hoarding in gonadectomized NMRI mouse model: focus on neural oxidative status

Noushin Nikray[1], Isaac Karimi[1,2]* (ID), Zahraminoosh Siavashhaghighi[3], Lora A. Becker[4] and Mohammad Mehdi Mofatteh[5]

Abstract

Background: Environmental uncertainty, such as food deprivation, may alter internal milieu of nervous system through various mechanisms. In combination with circumstances of stress or aging, high consumption of unsaturated fatty acids and oxygen can make neural tissues sensitive to oxidative stress (OS). For adult rats, diminished level of gonadal steroid hormones accelerates OS and may result in special behavioral manifestations. This study was aimed to partially answer the question whether OS mediates trade-off between food hoarding and food intake (fat hoarding) in environmental uncertainty (e.g., fluctuations in food resource) within gonadectomized mouse model in the presence of food deprivation-induced food hoarding behavior.

Results: Hoarding behavior was not uniformly expressed in all male mice that exposed to food deprivation. Extended phenotypes including hoarder and non-hoarder mice stored higher and lower amounts of food respectively as compared to that of low-hoarder mice (normal phenotype) after food deprivation. Results showed that neural oxidative status was not changed in the presence of hoarding behavior in gonadectomized mice regardless of tissue type, however, glutathione levels of brain tissues were increased in the presence of hoarding behavior. Decreased superoxide dismutase activity in brain and spinal cord tissues and increased malondialdehyde in brain tissues of gonadectomized mice were also seen.

Conclusions: Although, food deprivation-induced hoarding behavior is a strategic response to food shortage in mice, it did not induce the same amount of hoarding across all colony mates. Hoarding behavior, in this case, is a response to the environmental uncertainty of food shortage, therefore is not an abnormal behavior. Hoarding behavior induced neural OS with regard to an increase in brain glutathione levels but failed to show other markers of neural OS. Decreased superoxide dismutase activity in brain and spinal cord tissues and increased malondialdehyde levels in brain tissues of gonadectomized mice could be a hallmark of debilitated antioxidative defense and more lipid peroxidation due to reduced amount of gonadal steroid hormones during aging.

Keywords: Gonadectomy, Hoarding behavior, Neural tissue, Oxidative stress

*Correspondence: isaac_karimi2000@yahoo.com; karimiisaac@razi.ac.ir
[2] Department of Biology, Faculty of Science, Razi University, Kermanshah 67149-67346, Iran
Full list of author information is available at the end of the article

Background

Based on natural selection theory, animals in their natural habitats should adapt to varying environmental conditions for survival [1] and their adaptation may have morphological, physiological or behavioral features [2]. The major adaptive strategies of animals to environmental uncertainty include decrease of energy costs and its maintenance, migration, weight gain, hibernation or aestivation, increasing fat storage and at least hoarding behavior [2–4]. Hoarder animals prefer to either save food for the future or consume food rapidly [5]. Generally, hoarding is influenced by environment, internal milieu of animals, and their interactions. Environmental uncertainties such as food shortage, low food availability, coldness, and short day-length trigger hoarding [3, 6]. Furthermore, internal factors such as endogenous fat depots, internal energy, gonadal steroids, metabolic hormones, glucocorticoids, neuropeptide regulators of food intake, and catecholamines especially dopamine are all known to alter hoarding behavior [6–9]. However, it remains an open question whether oxidative stress (OS) mediates the trade-off between food hoarding and food intake (fat hoarding) in times of food shortage as an example of environmental uncertainty.

To the best of our knowledge, oxidative status of the central nervous system (CNS) was not broadly investigated in human hoarders or animal models. More recently, our laboratory reported an increase (~ 50-fold) in encephalic xanthine oxidoreductase (XOR) gene, as a key player in cellular oxidative status, in female high-hoarder vs. female low-hoarder while a decrease (0.026-fold) in encephalic XOR in male high-hoarder vs. male low-hoarder mice [10]. Accordingly, we concluded that food deprivation is associated with sex-dependent alteration in XOR expression. The OS is caused by an imbalance between production of oxidants (e.g., reactive oxygen species: ROS) and antioxidants (e.g., glutathione: GSH) and leads to progressive loss of control over biological homeostasis or rheostasis that results in functional impairments and cell death [11]. Antioxidative capacity decreases in almost all aged mammals [12, 13]. Free radicals are formed in the CNS as part of normal metabolic processes [14], while high oxygen uptake and low antioxidative defenses increase vulnerability of CNS to OS [13]. It is known that neuronal susceptibility to OS can be affected by steroid hormones. In this context, Ahlbom and coworkers demonstrated that testosterone triggers antioxidative defenses of cerebellar granule cells [15].

Food hoarding behavior has marked associations with endocrine system output, especially sex steroid hormones. For instance, Nyby and coworkers demonstrated that castration increased food hoarding in male Mongolian gerbil (Meriones unguiculatus Milne-Edwards,

1867) [16]. Likewise, infantile food and water deprivation resulted in impaired testicular development and lower androgen levels which may increase hoarding behavior [16]. Hence, the aim of this study was to investigate the relationship between food hoarding behavior and oxidative status of neural tissue in gonadectomized mouse model.

Methods

Animal housing

Male Naval Medical Research Institute (NMRI) mice (Mus musculus L.; $n = 80$; 2-month-old; 30–40 g) were prepared from our historical colony (Laboratory Animal House, School of Veterinary Medicine, Razi University, Kermanshah, Iran) and housed in metallic cages carpeted with wood shavings in groups consisting of 5–8 individuals. The room temperature was 22 ± 1 °C and 12 h light and dark cycles were maintained. All animals had ad libitum access to tap water and commercial standard rodent pelleted diet (Dan-e-pars Co., Iran). Animal maintenance and all research protocols were approved and reviewed by ethical committee of Razi University and followed the NIH Guide for the Care and Use of Laboratory Animals.

Hoarding test

Evaluation of hoarding behavior was performed using hoarding apparatus that was shown in Fig. 1. It composed of medium-density fibreboard (MDF) to make a home furnished with 4 chambers ($13.0 \times 32.0 \times 6.5$ cm^3) and a hole (4 cm) in the front of each box. In addition, four wire-mesh end-sealed tubes used as food storing tubes (45 cm long, 4 cm external diameter). The wire-meshes were rolled in order to prevent food pellet dropping. Plastic tubes (10 cm long) were embedded in holes of boxes and storing tubes connected to them. The proximal end of hole was blocked with a removable plastic plug. A wire mesh used as the roof of MDF made home. Each box was equipped with a water bottle. For at least one night, we considered a limestone-made lodge in home box which furnished by wood shaving bedding to simulate natural nest for mice (Fig. 1).

Each mouse weighed and introduced to home box in the morning. Food pellets (100 g) were placed in the wire-mesh tube (storing tube) while access to food was restricted via an interface plastic plug. The plugs were removed just before the start of the dark and food-restricted mice were allowed to access obtainable food in storing tube. The next morning, body weights and weight of food pellets which each mouse had been hoarded into the home base box were recorded. Of course animals had ad libitum access to water during the experiment [17]. Mice that hoarded less than 5 g of food were considered "non-hoarders" while mice that hoarded more than

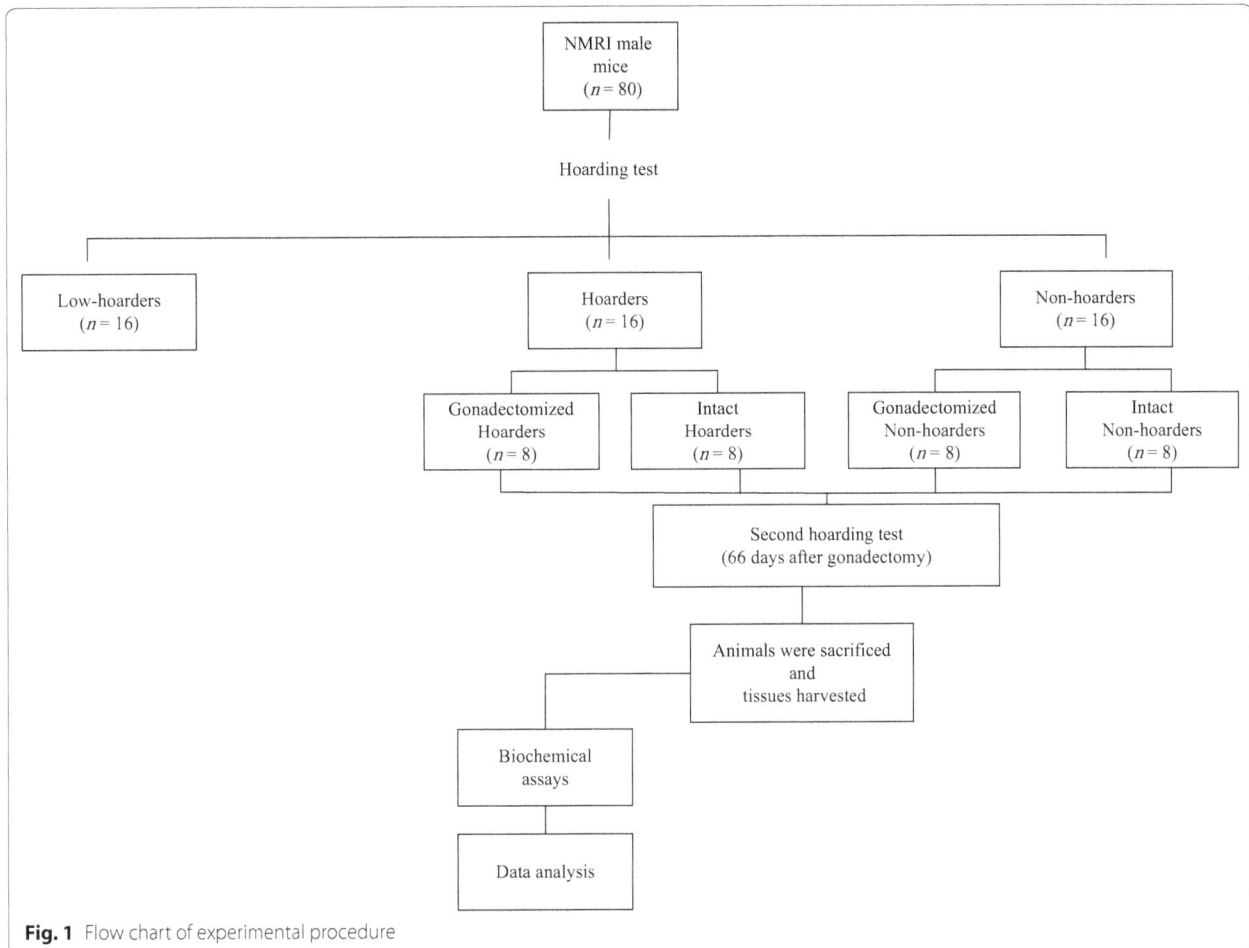

Fig. 1 Flow chart of experimental procedure

20 g of food were considered "hoarders" [10]. Mice that hoarded between 5 and 20 g of food were considered as "low-hoarder" subjects and excluded from study.

Gonadectomy

After screening of hoarder ($n = 16$) and non-hoarder ($n = 16$) mice using hoarding apparatus (vide supra), half of the mice were randomly underwent gonadectomy. The model used in present study was accelerated aging and animals were gonadectomized through bilateral orchiectomy. For this purpose, animals were anesthetized by intraperitoneal (i.p.) injection of ketamine (80 mg/kg)/diazepam (0.5 mg/kg) cocktail. During surgical procedure, animals receiving abdominal incision and both testes and their associated epididymides were removed.

Treatment groups

Mice were divided into four groups of eight including intact hoarder, gonadectomized hoarder, intact non-hoarder and gonadectomized non-hoarder male mice. For comparison, hoarding behavior between

gonadectomized and intact mice, hoarding test was repeated 66 days post-gonadectomy (Fig. 2). Biochemical assays were performed only on hoarder and non-hoarder mice (vide infra).

Preparation of tissue homogenates

All mice in our screened population were weighed and sacrificed by decapitation using a guillotine without anesthesia after 12–14 h fasting. Brain and spinal cord tissues have been harvested over ice blocks, weighed, wrapped in aluminum foil, snap-frozen in liquid nitrogen and stored at -70 °C until use for biochemical assays.

Frozen brains and spinal cords were thawed and homogenized over ice by a tissue homogenizer (WiseTis model HG-15D; Korea) in potassium phosphate buffer solution (50 mM; pH 7.4) for 3 times, at 3,000 rpm. Then, tissue homogenates were centrifuged at 12,000 g at 4 °C for 15 min using super-speed refrigerated centrifuge bridges (Sigma, model 3–30 K; Germany) and resulting tissue extracts (supernatants) were stored at -20 °C for biochemical assays [18].

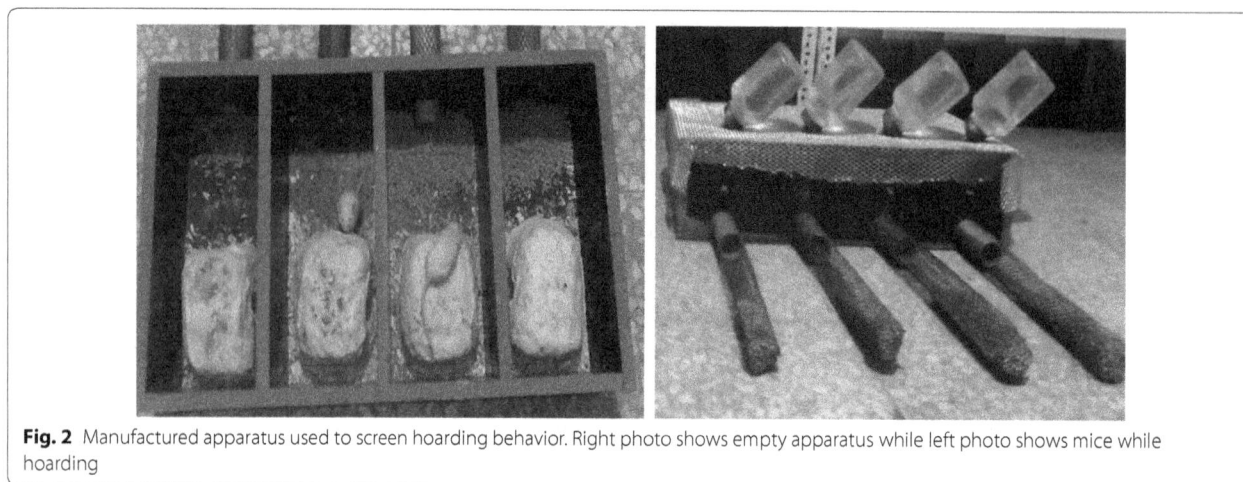

Fig. 2 Manufactured apparatus used to screen hoarding behavior. Right photo shows empty apparatus while left photo shows mice while hoarding

Estimation of glutathione (GSH) levels

Trichloroacetic acid (TCA; 5%; 0.5 ml) solution was added to tissue extract (0.5 ml) to precipitate proteins and centrifuged at 3000 rpm for 20 min. Sodium phosphate buffer solution (1 ml; pH 8.0) and 5,5'-dithiobis(2-nitrobenzoic acid) (DTNB; 1 mM; 0.5 ml) were added to the supernatant (0.1 ml). The absorbance of the yellow color developed was measured at 412 nm [19]. The GSH concentration (μM) was determined using GSH dissolved in diluted metaphosphoric acid as standard.

Estimation of catalase (CAT) activity

The CAT (hydrogen peroxide oxidoreductase) activity was assayed based on its ability to oxidize hydrogen peroxide [20]. Briefly, potassium phosphate buffer (2.25 ml; 65 mM; pH 7.8) was mixed to tissue extract (0.1 ml) and incubated at 25 °C for 30 min. Then, 3 ml of hydrogen peroxide (30% w/v) was added to the mixture and the decline in absorbance was measured at 240 nm for 3 min by UV–Vis spectrophotometer [21]. The CAT activity was measured based on its ability to decompose 1 mM of hydrogen peroxide per min per protein (mg) at 25 °C.

Estimation of superoxide dismutase (SOD) activity

The activity of superoxide dismutase was determined based on methodology of Misra and Fridowich (1977) with some modifications [22]. Nitroblue tetrazolium (NBT; 0.4 ml; 25 mM), and hydroxylamine HCl (0.02 ml; 0.1 mM) were added to sodium bicarbonate solution (1 ml; 50 mM). Tissue extract (0.1 ml) was added to the mixture and its absorbance was measured at 560 nm after 2 min using UV–Vis spectrophotometer. The SOD activity was measured based on its ability

to prevent photo-reduction of 1 mM of NBT per min per protein (mg) at 25 °C.

Estimation of total antioxidant status (TAS)

Concisely, 0.1 ml of tissue extract was deproteinated using 1 ml of methanol, vortexed for 30 s, then centrifuged at 3000 rpm for 30 min. Stable free radical α,α-diphenyl-β-picryl hydrazyl (DPPH; 0.5 ml; 0.2 mM) was prepared in methanol (1.5 ml), then added to the supernatant, mixed thoroughly and absorbance was measured at 517 nm against blank. The standard graph was plotted using different concentrations of ascorbic acid and the antioxidative status values were expressed in terms of nM of ascorbic acid [23].

Estimation of lipid peroxidation (malondialdehyde (MDA) assay)

The magnitude of lipid peroxidation was determined by measuring MDA which is thiobarbituric acid reactive substance (TBARS). To precipitate the proteins, TCA (30%; 0.5 ml) was added to tissue extract (0.5 ml), vortexed for 30 s, and finally centrifuged at 3000 rpm for 5 min. Thiobarbitoric acid (TBA; 1%; 500 μl) solution and 500 μl of distilled water were added to the supernatant and the resulting mixture heated for 1 h at 98 °C, then cooled to room temperature and kept in ice for 5 min. At last, the absorbance of pink mixture recorded at 532 nm. Standard graph was plotted using 1,1,3,3-tetraethoxy propane (TEP) to estimate MDA values [24].

Protein content of tissue extract

Each assay was performed at least in triplicate and protein concentration was determined by the method of Bradford (1976) using bovine serum albumin as the standard [25].

Statistical analyses

Statistical analyses performed using SPSS version 20.0 software for Windows (SPSS, Chicago, IL, USA). Normal distribution of data was assessed using the Shapiro–Wilk normality test. The data with normal distribution were analyzed using one- or two-way analysis of variance (ANOVA) and data were not normally distributed, submitted to nonparametric statistics, Kruskal–Wallis H test. Post hoc LSD test was used for additional comparison. Body weights were compared before and after hoarding evaluation, using paired samples T test. Pearson correlation test was used for evaluation of the correlation (r) between the body weight before and after the hoarding with the amount of hoarded food. A p value ≤ 0.05 was considered as statistically significant and results were expressed as mean $\pm$ standard error of the mean (SEM).

Results

Hoarding test

Classifying of animals into hoarder, low-hoarder and non-hoarder groups showed that there was no significant correlation between the body weight before hoarding and the amount of hoarded food in screened population (r = 0.274, p = 0.097). There was also no significant relationship between body weight after hoarding and the amount of hoarded food (r = 0.056, p = 0.737). However, hoarder, low-hoarder and non-hoarder groups had significant difference based on amounts of hoarded food (F(2,37) = 47.520, p = 1.057e^{-10}). Post hoc LSD test showed that there was a significant difference in amount of hoarded food between hoarder group in comparison with low hoarder group (p = 3.475e^{-6}) and non-hoarder group (p = 2.144e^{-11}; Table 1). Also the low-hoarder group compared to non-hoarder group (p = 0.016) had significant increase in amount of hoarded food (Table 1).

This significant difference in the amounts of hoarded food among these groups confirmed precise classification based on hoarded food in colony. There was no significant difference between the animal's body weight before and after hoarding using paired-samples T-test (t = − 0.234, p = 0.817, df = 37) which indicated food intake during the hoarding test was not different among groups. There was no significant difference in the amount of hoarded food between gonadectomized and intact mice in second hoarding test at the end of study (F(1,10) = 0.534, p = 0.483). However, the amount of hoarded food by gonadectomized mice was tended to be higher than intact mice (data not shown).

The interaction between gonadectomy and the presence of hoarding behavior on neural antioxidative profile

Using two-way ANOVA, it has been revealed that tissue, gonadectomy, presence or absence of hoarding behavior and the interaction between them have not a significant impacts on the CAT, SOD, TAS, MDA, and total protein content in the neural tissue while GSH levels were significantly varied in tissues (F(1,29) = 51.683, p = 0.039; Table 2).

Evaluation of neural antioxidant status

The GSH levels had significant difference in brain tissues of studied groups (F(3,17) = 3.926, p = 0.032; Table 3). Post hoc LSD test showed that GSH levels were significantly higher in brain tissues of intact hoarder group in comparison with intact non-hoarder group (p = 0.007) and in gonadectomized hoarder group in comparison with intact non-hoarder group (p = 0.022).

Table 2 Interaction between gonadectomy and hoarding behavior on glutathione levels (μM) in neural tissues

Parameter	F(1,29)	P$_{ANOVA}$
Glutathione	2.998	0.333
Hoarding	1.697	0.417
Gonadectomy	0.895	0.518
Tissue	51.683	0.039*
Hoarding × gonadectomy	0.582	0.585
Hoarding × tissue	3.891	0.299
Gonadectomy × tissue	7.409	0.224
Hoarding × gonadectomy × tissue	0.137	0.714

Parameters with significant difference at P$_{ANOVA}$ ≤ 0.05 in each row have marked with * sign

Table 1 Hoarded food (g) in food deprived colony mate mice used to classify mice based on hoarding test

Parameter	P$_{ANOVA}$	F(2,37)	Groups		
			Hoarder	Low-hoarder	Non-hoarder
BW (g) before hoarding	0.378	1.000	23.92 ± 0.95	21.62 ± 1.28	22.81 ± 0.97
BW (g) after hoarding	0.572	0.567	22.64 ± 1.29	22.12 ± 1.74	23.93 ± 0.89
Hoarded food (g) in day 0	1.057e−10	47.520	37.35 ± 4.41a	12.37 ± 1.32b	1.20 ± 0.32c

Results shown as mean ± SEM and parameters that are significantly different at P$_{ANOVA}$ ≤ 0.05 are displayed with different letters among groups

BW body weight

Table 3 Glutathione levels in the brain tissues of studied groups

Group	Glutathione (µM)
Intact hoarder	1428.78 ± 22.17ac
Intact non-hoarder	1292.99 ± 22.96b
Gonadectomized hoarder	1414.01 ± 44.51c
Gonadectomized non-hoarder	1355.41 ± 23.69ab

Results shown as mean ± SEM; in columns, values with different letters are significantly different

Table 4 Effect of hoarding on antioxidative profile of brain tissues in male mice

Parameter	Group	Quantity	F value	P_{ANOVA}
GSH	Hoarder	1422.87 ± 20.83	$F(1,17) = 9.66$	0.007*
	Non-hoarder	1332.00 ± 19.68		
CAT	Hoarder	0.148 ± 0.067	$F(1,13) = 0.639$	0.440
	Non-hoarder	0.219 ± 0.057		
SOD	Hoarder	4.04 ± 0.411	$F(1,19) = 0.979$	0.336
	Non-hoarder	3.39 ± 0.512		
TAS	Hoarder	1229.36 ± 40.86	$F(1,18) = 0.002$	0.965
	Non-hoarder	1226.75 ± 38.49		
MDA	Hoarder	47.76 ± 4.16	$F(1,19) = 0.276$	0.606
	Non-hoarder	51.07 ± 4.49		
Protein	Hoarder	2.38 ± 0.046	$F(1,21) = 4.327$	0.056
	Non-hoarder	2.21 ± 0.071		

Data are expressed as mean ± SEM and parameters with $P_{ANOVA} \leq 0.05$ are significantly different and displayed with * sign

GSH glutathione (µM), *CAT* catalase (1 mM of H2O2/min/mg protein), *SOD* superoxide dismutase (1 mM of NBT/min/mg protein), *TAS* total antioxidant status (nM of ascorbic acid), *MDA* malondialdehyde (nM/mg protein), protein (mg/ml)

GSH levels of spinal cord tissues showed no significant differences among groups $(F(3,18) = 0.509, p = 0.682)$. The CAT levels in the brain tissues $(F(3,13) = 1.062, p = 0.408)$ and spinal cord $(F(3,13) = 1.582, p = 0.255)$ were not different in studied groups. The SOD levels did not show any significant difference in the brain tissues of the studied groups $(F(3,19) = 1.960, p = 0.161)$. Post hoc LSD test showed a significant reduction in the SOD levels of brain in gonadectomized non-hoarder group compared to intact non-hoarder group $(p = 0.048)$. No significant difference was found in the SOD levels of spinal cord among studied groups $(F(3,20) = 2.053, p = 0.145)$. However, a significant reduction in the SOD levels of spinal cord in gonadectomized non-hoarder group compared with intact non-hoarder group was observed using Post hoc LSD test $(p = 0.049)$. There was no significant differences in TAS of brain $(F(3,18) = 1.158, p = 0.358)$ and spinal cord $(F(3,20) = 1.004, p = 0.415)$ tissues of studied groups. The amount of MDA in the brain tissues showed no significant difference between groups $(F(3,19) = 2.818, p = 0.072)$. Post hoc LSD test showed that MDA levels in the brain of gonadectomized non-hoarder group has been significantly increased in comparison with intact hoarder group $(p = 0.034)$. The MDA levels in the spinal cord had no significant difference between groups $(F(3,23) = 0.872, p = 0.472)$. The protein content of brain tissues did not show any significant change in studied groups $(F(3,21) = 2.022, p = 0.147)$. Shapiro–Wilk normality test showed that protein content in spinal cord tissues were not normally distributed, so the non-parametric Kruskal–Wallis H test was used. Total protein content in the spinal cord of studied groups showed no significant difference (Chi square = 1.749, asymptotic significance = 0.626, df = 1).

Effect of hoarding on neural antioxidative profile

Presence of hoarding behavior had significant effect on the GSH levels in the brain tissues of studied mice $(F(1,17) = 9.66, p = 0.007)$. This means that the GSH levels in the brain tissues of hoarder mice were higher than those of non-hoarder mice (Table 4).

Hoarding behavior had no significant effect on the antioxidative profile of spinal cord tissue (Table 5). Shapiro–Wilk normality test showed that protein content in spinal cord tissues was not normally distributed, therefore the protein content in the spinal cord of male mice were analyzed using Kruskal–Wallis H test. Hoarding behavior had no significant effect on the protein content of spinal cord tissue; hoarder mice (1.901 ± 0.097) vs non-hoarder mice $(1.857 \pm 0.091;$ Chi Square = 0.431; Asymp. Sig = 0.511; df = 1).

Effect of gonadectomy on neural antioxidative profile of male mice

Amongst all studied parameters of antioxidative profile, MDA levels in brain tissues were significantly affected by gonadectomy $(F(1,19) = 9.067, p = 0.008)$. MDA levels were higher in brain tissues of gonadectomized mice than intact mice (Table 6).

Gonadectomy had significant effect on the SOD levels in spinal cord tissue $(F(1,20) = 5.45, p = 0.031)$ but not on any other measure. In this regard, SOD levels in gonadectomized mice have been significantly decreased in comparison with intact mice (Table 7).

Gonadectomy had no significant effect on the overall protein content in spinal cord tissue. Shapiro–Wilk normality test showed that protein content in spinal cord tissues was non-parametrically distributed, so analysis was carried out with Kruskal–Wallis H test; gonadectomized mice (1.813 ± 0.080) and intact mice (1.995 ± 0.104) did not differ (Chi Square = 1.269; Asymp. Sig = 0.260; df = 1).

Table 5 Effect of hoarding on antioxidative profile of spinal cord tissues male mice

Parameter	Group	Quantity	F value	P_{ANOVA}
GSH	Hoarder	5447.98 ± 558.67	$F_{(1,18)} = 0.547$	0.470
	Non-hoarder	4838.94 ± 482.72		
CAT	Hoarder	1.62 ± 0.380	$F_{(1,13)} = 1.957$	0.187
	Non-hoarder	1.057 ± 0.203		
SOD	Hoarder	22.12 ± 3.42	$F_{(1,20)} = 0.209$	0.653
	Non-hoarder	19.76 ± 3.85		
TAS	Hoarder	9078.00 ± 1095.09	$F_{(1,20)} = 0.139$	0.713
	Non-hoarder	9859.66 ± 1937.34		
MDA	Hoarder	441.26 ± 69.09	$F_{(1,23)} = 0.266$	0.611
	Non-hoarder	389.59 ± 72.00		

Data are expressed as mean ± SEM and parameters with $P_{ANOVA} \leq 0.05$ are significantly different and displayed with * sign

GSH glutathione (μM), *CAT* catalase (1 mM of H2O2/min/mg protein), *SOD* superoxide dismutase (1 mM of NBT/min/mg protein), *TAS* total antioxidant status (nM of ascorbic acid), *MDA* malondialdehyde (nM/mg protein)

Table 6 Effect of gonadectomy on antioxidative profile of brain tissues in male mice

Parameter	Group	Mean ± SEM	F value	P_{ANOVA}
GSH	Gonadectomized	1383.51 ± 27.58	$F_{(1,17)} = 0.003$	0.956
	Intact	1381.45 ± 24.33		
CAT	Gonadectomized	0.240 ± 0.068	$F_{(1,13)} = 2.501$	0.140
	Intact	0.108 ± 0.027		
SOD	Gonadectomized	3.48 ± 0.398	$F_{(1,19)} = 1.118$	0.304
	Intact	4.16 ± 0.517		
TAS	Gonadectomized	1275.00 ± 32.51	$F_{(1,18)} = 3.55$	0.077
	Intact	1176.33 ± 41.73		
MDA	Gonadectomized	55.99 ± 3.38	$F_{(1,19)} = 9.067$	0.008*
	Intact	40.65 ± 3.82		
Protein	Gonadectomized	2.36 ± 0.063	$F_{(1,21)} = 1.512$	0.233
	Intact	2.26 ± 0.055		

Data are expressed as mean ± SEM and parameters with $P_{ANOVA} \leq 0.05$ are significantly different and displayed with * sign

GSH glutathione (μM), *CAT* catalase (1 mM of H2O2/min/mg protein), *SOD* superoxide dismutase (1 mM of NBT/min/mg protein), *TAS* total antioxidant status (nM of ascorbic acid), *MDA* malondialdehyde (nM/mg protein), protein (mg/ml)

Discussion

Hoarding behavior is more prevalent in older adults [26]. The CNS is exclusively vulnerable to oxidative damage because of its high energy needs, oxygen consumption, and iron content and relatively low efficient antioxidative systems [27]. In addition, the ability of brain to repair its damaged cells is curtailed with age because it composed of postmitotic neurons and differentiated glial cells [28]. If the amount of free radicals in brain was in their physiological levels, the innate antioxidative defense neutralizes this assault. Otherwise, CNS antioxidative defense against oxidants fails and subsequently, the activity of

neurons as well as cognitive functions will be severely affected [29]. Many attempts have been made to translate hoarding behavior in animal models, however a thorough and reliable mechanism and model has not been identified. In this study, examined a potential relationship between hoarding behavior and oxidative status in a gonadectomized mouse model.

We did not find any significant difference between body weights of mice before and after hoarding screening. Since weight control is a long-term physiological phenomenon so within 12 h of fasting and access to food did not change. Studied groups had a significant difference in amount of hoarded food in day 0. This difference in hoarding behavior among colony members remains unanswered by us and other previous studies [5, 6, 10, 17, 30–32]. Previous studies have focused more on presenting and describing hoarding behavior while this study initially has a molecular insight to antioxidative status in the presence of hoarding behavior. This study suggests that changes in antioxidative status between individuals may be the cause of these differences. Since behavioral changes are consequence of overt biological changes, we excluded the low-hoarder group from the study so that we decide to find biological connection in both lower and upper boundaries of hoarding expression.

Animals have an innate defense system including endogenous antioxidants to neutralize harmful effects of oxidative insults [33]. It is noteworthy that the glutathione is one of the most important antioxidants found in cells [34]. This tripeptide (Glu-Cys-Gly) contains cysteine residue which its "thiol" group acts as a reducing agent [35] and converts free radicals into non-toxic substances such as water and oxygen [36]. Glutathione exists in 2 forms: reduced (GSH) and oxidized (GSSG), which an increase of GSSG to GSH is an index of OS [37]. Disturbance in glutathione metabolism complicates the pathogenicity of various psychiatric disorders [38–40]. It seems that GSH levels in neural tissues has tissue-specific activity which may be due to difference in protein contents of neural tissues. In present study, GSH levels have been significantly increased in brain tissues of intact and gonadectomized hoarders in comparison to intact non-hoarders. One of striking feature of present study was higher GSH levels in brain tissues of hoarders in comparison with non-hoarders. This finding may be due to the functional changes of gamma-glutamylcysteine synthetase and GSH synthetase or through the interference in de novo GSH synthesis by glutathione reductase function [41]. If hoarding is considered a "coping behavior" which occurs in response to stresses, such as food shortage [42], then increased antioxidant levels could be a mechanism used to confront this stress.

Table 7 Effect of gonadectomy on antioxidative profile of spinal cord tissues in male mice

Parameter	Group	Mean ± SEM	F value	P_{ANOVA}
GSH	Gonadectomized	4900.63 ± 644.09	F(1,18) = 0.742	0.401
	Intact	5582.44 ± 426.33		
CAT	Gonadectomized	1.37 ± 0.349	F(1,13) = 0.179	0.679
	Intact	1.19 ± 0.161		
SOD	Gonadectomized	16.52 ± 2.98	F(1,20) = 5.45	0.031*
	Intact	27.23 ± 3.49		
TAS	Gonadectomized	8386.33 ± 1583.51	F(1,20) = 1.39	0.252
	Intact	10781.88 ± 994.22		
MDA	Gonadectomized	357.16 ± 64.59	F(1,23) = 2.23	0.149
	Intact	502.16 ± 70.63		

Data are expressed as mean ± SEM and parameters with P_ANOVA ≤ 0.05 are significantly different and displayed with * sign

GSH glutathione (µM), CAT catalase (1 mM of H2O2/min/mg protein), SOD superoxide dismutase (1 mM of NBT/min/mg protein), TAS total antioxidant status (nM of ascorbic acid), MDA malondialdehyde (nM/mg protein)

The brain consumes about 20% of total body oxygen [43] which increases the possibility of superoxide production. The SOD has a key role in antioxidative defense and mice lacking SOD enzyme die a few days after birth [44]. Three main families of SOD are known in human and most vertebrates which are categorized based on their relevant metal cofactor and cellular location [45, 46]. In this line, SOD1 (Cu/Zn SOD) is found in cytoplasm, SOD2 (Mn SOD) is located in mitochondria, and SOD3 (Cu/Zn SOD) is active in extracellular space [47]. In present study, SOD levels were significantly lower in brain and spinal cord tissues of gonadectomized non-hoarders than intact non-hoarders. The SOD activity was significantly lower in spinal cord tissues of gonadectomized mice in comparison with intact mice. Accordingly, we can conclude that induction of gonadectomy in mice is one of the main factors that reduces SOD activity in neural tissues of gonadectomized mice. Androgens have both neuroprotective [47–49] and neurotoxic effects [50] depending on biological systems and their concentrations [46, 48]. For instance, testosterone has antioxidative properties in human prostate [51] and rat nervous system [15, 52] nevertheless high testosterone levels produce oxidation in testicular tissues of rats and rabbits [53, 54], muscles of rats [55], and placenta of women [56]. These findings indicate that pro-oxidative effect of testosterone depends on type of tissue and testosterone levels [57]. Neuroprotective properties of testosterone may be related to its conversion to estradiol that has protective role on dopamine neurons in experimental studies [58–60]. It seems that either directly or through aromatization to estrogen, testosterone exerts its protective effect

on nerve cells [61]. Gonadectomy is associated with reduction of testosterone, dihydrotestosterone and estradiol levels. These hormones have a key role in activation of cytoplasmic SOD (SOD1) [62] and reduced levels of aforementioned hormones can be considered as main reason of reduced activity of SOD enzyme in brain and spinal cord tissues of gonadectomized mice in comparison to intact mice. In a similar study that examined the impact of orchiectomy on SOD levels in hippocampus of rat, decrease in SOD activity was detected in gonadectomized group compared to sham group that caused oxidative damage and morphological changes in hippocampal tissue [63]. In a comparative study on 21–92 years old men, an age-related decrease in SOD activity in thoracic segment and cervical intumescence of spinal cord was seen [64]. In other study, a decline in the activities of antioxidant enzymes and a non-significant decrease of SOD activity were observed in brain tissues of 4–24 months old rats [65]. However, an increase in SOD activity in various parts of neural tissue by aging has been reported in other studies [12, 66]. Taken in sum, we can conclude that SOD activity is different in various parts of CNS and decreased steroid sex hormones following gonadectomy can reduce SOD activity and subsequently lead to weakness in antioxidative defense of neural tissue.

As mentioned earlier, CAT is an enzyme that converts hydrogen peroxide to water and oxygen and this enzyme has been characterized in rat brain as a peroxisomal marker enzyme which is involved in antioxidative defense [67]. However, its main role is still unknown because mice lacking CAT seem normal [68]. In present study, CAT activity in neural tissue was varied independent to tissue, gonadectomy, hoarding behavior and their interactions. The CAT activities tended to be higher in brain and spinal cord tissues of gonadectomized mice in comparison with intact mice. In this line, an age-related increase in CAT activity in cervical and lumbosacral intumescence of spinal cord has been reported in 21–92 years old men [64]. Nonetheless, reduction in CAT activity due to aging has been reported in several studies [12, 65, 69]. The CAT activity and its mRNA in brain tissues of male Fisher rats were correlated and significantly decreased with aging [70]. Hence, CAT activity could be attributed to the expression and distribution of this enzyme in different tissues. Although the amounts of produced hydrogen peroxide in various tissues can influence CAT activity.

The MDA is an organic compound produced through decomposition of multiple unsaturated lipids and usually considered as a biomarker of lipid peroxidation [71]. The MDA reacts with free amino groups of proteins, phospholipids and nucleic acids and leads to structural changes [72]. Neuronal membranes are rich in polyunsaturated fatty acids, substrates of ROS, which increase the susceptibility of neurons to OS [73]. In present investigation, MDA levels were significantly higher in brain tissues of gonadectomized non-hoarder group than the intact hoarder group. Gonadectomy also caused a significant increase in MDA levels in brain tissues of gonadectomized mice in comparison with intact mice. In this context, chronic stresses built up lipid peroxidation and MDA production in brain tissues of rats and weakened antioxidative defense [74]. As well as estrogen and testosterone which possess antioxidative properties may be declined post-gonadectomy which culminates to membrane lipid peroxidation and MDA production [75]. In other comparable study, an increase of lipid peroxidation and MDA in hippocampus of gonadectomized rats has been reported compared to sham group [63]. Accordingly, we can conclude that probable decline in steroid sex hormones that occurred following the gonadectomy may lead to weakened antioxidative defense and increased lipid peroxidation and MDA production.

Conclusion

Overall, our results showed that food deprivation-induced hoarding behavior in mice cannot be simply a strategic response to food shortage because all colony mates exposed to food deprivation in this study did not show hoarding behavior. On the other hand, hoarding behavior is considered a naturally occurring action in response to an environmental cue, food shortage, and not a disorder. In addition, decreased gonadal steroid hormones, which physiologically occurs during andropause, may increase the incidence of this behavior because of the gonadectomized mice hoarded non-significantly more food in comparison to intact mice. Decreased SOD activity in brain and spinal cord tissues and increased MDA levels in brain tissues of gonadectomized mice could be a sign of weakened antioxidative defense and more lipid peroxidation due to reduced amount of gonadal steroid hormones during aging. Current results showed that hoarding behavior does not have a significant impact on the neural antioxidative profile except the increase in brain GSH levels. Increased brain GSH levels in the presence of hoarding behavior may indicate the effect of this behavior on improving brain antioxidative defense or may imply on the increase of OS in the presence of this behavior. Therefore, GSH could be a good candidate in studying molecular biology of hoarding behavior.

Abbreviations

OS: oxidative stress; CNS: central nervous system; ROS: reactive oxygen species; GSH: glutathione; NMRI: Naval Medical Research Institute; i.p.: intraperitoneal; MDF: medium-density fibreboard; TCA: trichloroacetic acid; DTNB:

5,5'-dithiobis(2-nitrobenzoic acid); CAT: catalase; SOD: superoxide dismutase; NBT: nitroblue tetrazolium; TAS: total antioxidant status; DPPH: α,α-diphenyl-β-picryl hydrazyl; MDA: malondialdehyde; TBARS: thiobarbituric acid reactive substance; TBA: thiobarbitoric acid; TEP: 1,1,3,3-tetraethoxy propane.

Authors' contributions

This study was designed by IK and MMM. NN and ZMSH raised mice and performed biochemical assay. NN, IK and LAB analyzed data and prepared manuscript. All authors read and approved the final manuscript.

Author details

[1] Laboratory of Molecular and Cellular Biology 1214, Department of Basic Veterinary Sciences, School of Veterinary Medicine, Razi University, Kermanshah, Iran. [2] Department of Biology, Faculty of Science, Razi University, Kermanshah 67149-67346, Iran. [3] Department of Pathobiology, Faculty of Veterinary Medicine, Razi University, Kermanshah, Iran. [4] Department of Psychology, University of Evansville, Evansville, IN 47722, USA. [5] Department of Accounting, School of Economics and Accounting, Islamic Azad University South Tehran Branch, Tehran, Iran.

Acknowledgements

This paper emanates from Doctor of Veterinary Medicine thesis of first author, School of Veterinary Medicine, Razi University, Kermanshah, Iran. Authors acknowledge David Alimoradian and Tahereh Sajadipour for technical assistance.

Competing interests

The authors declare that they have no competing interests.

Ethics approval

Animals used in this study were bred in the animal facility of the Department of Basic Veterinary Sciences, School of Veterinary Medicine, Razi University, Kermanshah, Iran. All protocols were approved by the regional animal care and use committee of Razi University and followed the NIH Guide for the Care and Use of Laboratory Animals.

Funding

This work was supported financially by Razi University.

References

1. Darwin C. On the origin of species by means of natural selection, or the preservation of favoured races in the struggle for life. London. 1859;1:859.
2. Smith E. Illumination and food deprivation as determinants for hoarding in golden hamsters. Honors projects 35 (http://digitalcommons.iwu.edu/psych_honproj/35). 2002. p. 35.
3. Zhang H, Wang Y. Differences in hoarding behavior between captive and wild sympatric rodent species. Curr Zool. 2011;57(6):725–30.
4. Daly M, Jacobs LF, Wilson MI, Behrends PR. Scatter hoarding by kangaroo rats (*Dipodomys merriami*) and pilferage from their caches. Behav Ecol. 1992;3(2):102–11.
5. Pravosudov VV, Smulders TV. Integrating ecology, psychology and neurobiology within a food-hoarding paradigm. Philos Trans R Soc Lond B Biol Sci. 2010;365:859–67.

6. Keen-Rhinehart E, Dailey MJ, Bartness T. Physiological mechanisms for food-hoarding motivation in animals. Philos Trans R Soc Lond B Biol Sci. 2010;365(1542):961–75.

7. Bartness TJ, Keen-Rhinehart E, Dailey MJ, Teubner BJ. Neural and hormonal control of food hoarding. Am J Physiol Regul Integr Comp Physiol. 2011;301(3):R641–55.

8. Teubner BJ, Bartness TJ. Cholecystokinin-33 acutely attenuates food foraging, hoarding and intake in Siberian hamsters. Peptides. 2010;31(4):618–24.

9. Salamone JD, Farrar AM, Font L, Patel V, Schlar DE, Nunes EJ, Collins LE, Sager TN. Differential actions of adenosine A 1 and A 2A antagonists on the effort-related effects of dopamine D 2 antagonism. Behav Brain Res. 2009;201(1):216–22.

10. Karimi I, Motamedi S, Becker LA. An effort toward molecular neuroeconomics of food deprivation induced food hoarding in mice: focus on xanthine oxidoreductase gene expression and xanthine oxidase activity. Metab Brain Dis. 2018;33(1):325–31.

11. Gandhi S, Abramov AY. Mechanism of oxidative stress in neurodegeneration. Oxid Med Cell Longev. 2012;2012.

12. Siqueira IR, Fochesatto C, de Andrade A, Santos M, Hagen M, Bello-Klein A, Netto CA. Total antioxidant capacity is impaired in different structures from aged rat brain. Int J Dev Neurosci. 2005;23(8):663–71.

13. Harman D. Free radical involvement in aging. Drugs Aging. 1993;3(1):60–80.

14. Halliwell B. Reactive oxygen species and the central nervous system. J Neurochem. 1992;59(5):1609–23.

15. Ahlbom E, Prins GS, Ceccatelli S. Testosterone protects cerebellar granule cells from oxidative stress-induced cell death through a receptor mediated mechanism. Brain Res. 2001;892(2):255–62.

16. Nyby J, Wallace P, Owen K, Thiessen DD. An influence of hormones on hoarding behavior in the Mongolian gerbil (Meriones unguiculatus). Horm Behav. 1973;4(4):283–8.

17. Deacon RM. Assessing hoarding in mice. Nat Protoc. 2006;1(6):2828.

18. Wang X, Wang CP, Hu QH, Lv YZ, Zhang X, OuYang Z, Kong LD. The dual actions of Sanmiao wan as a hypouricemic agent: down-regulation of hepatic XOD and renal mURAT1 in hyperuricemic mice. J Ethnopharmacol. 2010;128(1):107–15.

19. Beutler E, Duron O. Kelly BM. Improved method for the determination of blood glutathione. J Lab Clin Med. 1963;61(5):882–8.

20. Beers RF, Sizer IW. A spectrophotometric method for measuring the breakdown of hydrogen peroxide by catalase. J Biol Chem. 1952;195(1):133–40.

21. Hugo A. Catalase. In: methods of enzymatic analysis (Bergmeyer). Academic press. 1963. pp. 672–683.

22. Misra HP, Fridovich I. Superoxide dismutase: a photochemical augmentation assay. Arch Biochem Biophys. 1977;181(1):308–12.

23. Blois MS. Antioxidant determinations by the use of a stable free radical. Nature. 1958;181(4617):1199.

24. Ohkawa H, Ohishi N, Yagi K. Assay for lipid peroxides in animal tissues by thiobarbituric acid reaction. Anal Biochem. 1979;95(2):351–8.

25. Bradford MM. A rapid and sensitive method for the quantitation of microgram quantities of protein utilizing the principle of protein-dye binding. Anal Biochem. 1976;72(1–2):248–54.

26. Diefenbach GJ, DiMauro J, Frost R, Steketee G, Tolin DF. Characteristics of hoarding in older adults. Am J Geriatr Psychiatry. 2013;21(10):1043–7.

27. Rodriguez-Capote K, Cespedes E, Arencibia R, Gonzalez-Hoyuela M. Indicators of oxidative stress in aging rat brain. The effect of nerve growth factor. Rev Neurol. 1998;27(157):494–500.

28. Simpson T, Pase M, Stough C. Bacopa monnieri as an antioxidant therapy to reduce oxidative stress in the aging brain. Evid Based Complementary Altern Med. 2015;2015, Article ID 615384, 9 pages http://dx.doi.org/10.1155/2015/615384.

29. Garbarino VR, Orr ME, Rodriguez KA, Buffenstein R. Mechanisms of oxidative stress resistance in the brain: lessons learned from hypoxia tolerant extremophilic vertebrates. Arch Biochem Biophys. 2015;576:8–16.

30. Fantino M, Cabanac M. Body weight regulation with a proportional hoarding response in the rat. Physiol Behav. 1980;24(5):939–42.

31. Charron I, Cabanac M. Influence of pellet size on rat's hoarding behavior. Physiol Behav. 2004;82(2–3):447–51.

32. Healy SD, de Kort SR, Clayton NS. The hippocampus, spatial memory and food hoarding: a puzzle revisited. Trends Ecol Evol. 2005;20(1):17–22.

33. Evelson P, Travacio M, Repetto M, Escobar J, Llesuy S, Lissi EA. Evaluation of total reactive antioxidant potential (TRAP) of tissue homogenates and their cytosols. Arch Biochem Biophys. 2001;388(2):261–6.

34. Pompella A, Visvikis A, Paolicchi A, De Tata V, Casini AF. The changing faces of glutathione, a cellular protagonist. Biochem Pharmacol. 2003;66(8):1499–503.

35. White CC, Viernes H, Krejsa CM, Botta D, Kavanagh TJ. Fluorescence-based microtiter plate assay for glutamate–cysteine ligase activity. Anal Biochem. 2003;318(2):175–80.

36. Meister AM, Anderson ME. Glutathione. Annu Rev Biochem. 1983;52:711–60.

37. Couto N, Malys N, Gaskell SJ, Barber J. Partition and turnover of glutathione reductase from Saccharomyces cerevisiae: a proteomic approach. J Proteome Res. 2013;12(6):2885–94.

38. Raffa M, Barhoumi S, Atig F, Fendri C, Kerkeni A, Mechri A. Reduced antioxidant defense systems in schizophrenia and bipolar I disorder. Progress Neuro-Psychopharmacol Biol Psychiatry. 2012;39(2):371–5.

39. Kantarci KJ, Jack CR, Xu YC, Campeau NG, O'Brien PC, Smith GE, Ivnik RJ, Boeve BF, Kokmen E, Tangalos EG, Petersen RC. Regional metabolic patterns in mild cognitive impairment and Alzheimer's disease a 1 h mrs study. Neurology. 2000;55(2):210–7.

40. Sian J, Dexter DT, Lees AJ, Daniel S, Agid Y, Javoy-Agid F, Jenner P, Marsden CD. Alterations in glutathione levels in Parkinson's disease and other neurodegenerative disorders affecting basal ganglia. Ann Neurol. 1994;36(3):348–55.

41. Kenchappa RS, Ravindranath V. γ-Glutamyl cysteine synthetase is up-regulated during recovery of brain mitochondrial complex I following neurotoxic insult in mice. Neurosci Lett. 2003;350(1):51–5.

42. Gutman R, Yosha D, Choshniak I, Kronfeld-Schor N. Two strategies for coping with food shortage in desert golden spiny mice. Physiol Behav. 2007;90(1):95–102.

43. Demopoulos HB, Flamm E, Seligman M, Pietronigro DD. Oxygen free radicals in central nervous system ischemia and trauma. Pathology of Oxygen. (Autor AP, Ed.). New York: Academic Press. 1982;127–55.

44. Li Y, Huang TT, Carlson EJ, Melov S, Ursell PC, Olson JL, Noble LJ, Yoshimura MP, Berger C, Chan PH, Wallace DC. Dilated cardiomyopathy and neonatal lethality in mutant mice lacking manganese superoxide dismutase. Nat Genet. 1995;11(4):376.

45. Richter C. Oxidative damage to mitochondrial DNA and its relationship to ageing. Int J Biochem Cell Biol. 1995;27(7):647–53.

46. Bajaj NP, Irving NG, Leigh PN, Miller CC. Alzheimer's disease, amyotrophic lateral sclerosis, and transgenic mice. J Neurol Neurosurg Psychiatry. 1998;64:711–5.

47. Hammond J, Le Q, Goodyer C, Gelfand M, Trifiro M, LeBlanc A. Testosterone-mediated neuroprotection through the androgen receptor in human primary neurons. J Neurochem. 2001;77(5):1319–26.

48. Ramsden M, Shin TM, Pike CJ. Androgens modulate neuronal vulnerability to kainate lesion. Neurosci. 2003;122(3):573–8.

49. Nguyen TV, Yao M, Pike CJ. Androgens activate mitogen-activated protein kinase signaling: role in neuroprotection. J Neurochem. 2005;94(6):1639–51.

50. Gavrielides MV, Gonzalez-Guerrico AM, Riobo NA, Kazanietz MG. Androgens regulate protein kinase Cδ transcription and modulate its apoptotic function in prostate cancer cells. Cancer Res. 2006;66(24):11792–801.

51. Tam NN, Gao Y, Leung YK, Ho SM. Androgenic regulation of oxidative stress in the rat prostate: involvement of NAD (P) H oxidases and antioxidant defense machinery during prostatic involution and regrowth. Am J Pathol. 2003;163(6):2513–22.

52. Guzmán DC, Mejía GB, Vázquez IE, García EH, del Angel DS, Olguín HJ. Effect of testosterone and steroids homologues on indolamines and lipid peroxidation in rat brain. J Steroid Biochem Mol Biol. 2005;94(4):369–73.

53. Chainy GB, Samantaray S, Samanta L. Testosterone-induced changes in testicular antioxidant system. Andrologia. 1997;29(6):343–9.

54. Aydilek N, Aksakal M, Karakılçık AZ. Effects of testosterone and vitamin E on the antioxidant system in rabbit testis. Andrologia. 2004;36(5):277–81.

55. Pansarasa O, D'antona G, Gualea M, Marzani B, Pellegrino M, Marzatico F. Oxidative stress: effects of mild endurance training and

testosterone treatment on rat gastrocnemius muscle. Eur J Appl Physiol. 2002;87(6):550–5.

56. Zhu XD, Bonet B, Knopp RH. 17β-Estradiol, progesterone, and testosterone inversely modulate low-density lipoprotein oxidation and cytotoxicity in cultured placental trophoblast and macrophages. Am J Obstet Gynecol. 1997;177(1):196–209.

57. Alonso-Alvarez C, Bertrand S, Faivre B, Chastel O, Sorci G. Testosterone and oxidative stress: the oxidation handicap hypothesis. Proc R Soc Lond B Biol Sci. 2007;274(1611):819–25.

58. D'Astous M, Morissette M, Di Paolo T. Effect of estrogen receptor agonists treatment in MPTP mice: evidence of neuroprotection by an ERα agonist. Neuropharmacology. 2004;47(8):1180–8.

59. Bains M, Cousins JC, Roberts JL. Neuroprotection by estrogen against MPP +-induced dopamine neuron death is mediated by ERalpha in primary cultures of mouse mesencephalon. Exp Neurol. 2007;204(2):767–76.

60. Morissette M, Jourdain S, Al Sweidi S, Menniti FS, Ramirez AD, Di Paolo T. Role of estrogen receptors in neuroprotection by estradiol against MPTP toxicity. Neuropharmacology. 2007;52(7):1509–20.

61. Saldanha CJ, Duncan KA, Walters BJ. Neuroprotective actions of brain aromatase. Front Neuroendocrinol. 2009;30(2):106–18.

62. Wenzel P, Schuhmacher S, Kienhöfer J, Müller J, Hortmann M, Oelze M, Schulz E, Treiber N, Kawamoto T, Scharffetter-Kochanek K, Münzel T. Manganese superoxide dismutase and aldehyde dehydrogenase deficiency increase mitochondrial oxidative stress and aggravate age-dependent vascular dysfunction. Cardiovasc Res. 2008;80(2):280–9.

63. Meydan S, Kus I, Tas U, Ogeturk M, Sancakdar E, Dabak DO, Zararsız I, Sarsılmaz M. Effects of testosterone on orchiectomy-induced oxidative damage in the rat hippocampus. J Chem Neuroanat. 2010;40(4):281–5.

64. Volchegorskii IA, Teleshova IB, Turygin VV. Comparative study of age-related activity of monoamine oxidase-B, antioxidant defense enzymes, and tolerance to oxidative stress in various segments of human spinal cord. Bull Exp Biol Med. 2003;135(1):40–2.

65. Haider S, Saleem S, Perveen T, Tabassum S, Batool Z, Sadir S, Liaquat L, Madiha S. Age-related learning and memory deficits in rats: role of altered brain neurotransmitters, acetylcholinesterase activity and changes in antioxidant defense system. Age. 2014;36(3):9653.

66. Hussain S, Slikker W, Ali SF. Age-related changes in antioxidant enzymes, superoxide dismutase, catalase, glutathione peroxidase and glutathione in different regions of mouse brain. Int J Dev Neurosci. 1995;13(8):811–7.

67. Schad A, Fahimi HD, Völkl A, Baumgart E. Expression of catalase mRNA and protein in adult rat brain: detection by nonradioactive in situ hybridization with signal amplification by catalyzed reporter deposition (ISH–CARD) and immunohistochemistry (IHC)/immunofluorescence (IF). J Histochem Cytochem. 2003;51(6):751–60.

68. Ho YS, Xiong Y, Ma W, Spector A, Ho DS. Mice lacking catalase develop normally but show differential sensitivity to oxidant tissue injury. J Biol Chem. 2004;279(31):32804–12.

69. Tiana L, Caib Q, Wei H. Alterations of antioxidant enzymes and oxidative damage to macromolecules in different organs of rats during aging. Free Radic Biol Med. 1998;24(9):1477–84.

70. Rao G, Xia E, Richardson A. Effect of age on the expression of antioxidant enzymes in male Fischer F344 rats. Mech Ageing Dev. 1990;53(1):49–60.

71. Pryor WA, Stanley JP. Letter: a suggested mechanism for the production of malondialdehyde during the autoxidation of polyunsaturated fatty acids. Nonenzymatic production of prostaglandin endoperoxides during autoxidation. J Org Chem. 1975;40:3615–7.

72. Nair V, O'Neil CL, Wang PG. Malondialdehyde. e-EROS Encyclopedia of Reagents for Organic Synthesis. 2008.

73. Shichiri M. The role of lipid peroxidation in neurological disorders. J Clin Biochem Nutr. 2014;54(3):151–60.

74. Che Y, Zhou Z, Shu Y, Zhai C, Zhu Y, Gong S, Cui Y, Wang JF. Chronic unpredictable stress impairs endogenous antioxidant defense in rat brain. Neurosci Lett. 2015;584:208–13.

75. Sugioka K, Shimosegawa Y, Nakano M. Estrogens as natural antioxidants of membrane phospholipid peroxidation. FEBS Lett. 1987;210(1):37–9.

18

Riboflavin and pyridoxine restore dopamine levels and reduce oxidative stress in brain of rats

Armando Valenzuela Peraza[1], David Calderón Guzmán[1], Norma Osnaya Brizuela[1], Maribel Ortiz Herrera[2], Hugo Juárez Olguín[3*] (iD), Miroslava Lindoro Silva[3], Belén Juárez Tapia[3] and Gerardo Barragán Mejía[1]

Abstract

Background: Neurological disorders suggest that the excitotoxicity involves a drastic increase in intracellular Ca^{2+} concentrations and the formation of reactive oxygen species. The presence of these free radicals may also affect the dopaminergic system. The aim of this work was to determine if riboflavin (B_2) and pyridoxine (B_6) provide protection to the brain against free radicals generated by 3-nitropropionic acid (3-NPA) by measuring the levels of dopamine (DA) and selected oxidative stress markers.

Methods: Male Fisher rats were grouped (n = 6) and treated as follows: group 1, control (NaCl 0.9%); group 2, 3-NPA (20 mg/kg); group 3, B_2 (10 mg/kg); group 4, B_2 (10 mg/kg) + 3-NPA (20 mg/kg); group 5, B_6 (10 mg/kg) and group 6, B_6 + 3-NPA. All treatments were administered every 24 h for 5 days by intraperitoneal route. After sacrifice, the brain was obtained to measure DA, GSH, and lipid peroxidation, Ca^{2+}, Mg^{2+}, ATPase and H_2O_2.

Main findings: Levels of dopamine increased in cortex, striatum and cerebellum/medulla oblongata of animals that received 3-NPA alone. The lipid peroxidation increased in cortex, striatum, and cerebellum/medulla oblongata, of animals treated with B_2 vitamin alone. ATPase dependent on Ca^{+2}, Mg^{+2} and H_2O_2 increased in all regions of animals that received 3-NPA alone.

Conclusion: The results confirm the capacity of 3-NPA to generate oxidative stress. Besides, the study suggests that B_2 or B_6 vitamins restored the levels of DA and reduced oxidative stress in brain of rats. We believe that these results would help in the study of neurodegenerative diseases.

Keywords: Brain, Huntington animal model, Oxidative stress, Riboflavin, Pyridoxine

Background

The main incident in neurological disorders is excitotoxicity which entails an extensive upsurge in the concentrations of intracellular Ca^{2+} and the production of reactive species such as ROS and RNS by lethal pathways [1]. In addition, there are alterations of the mitochondrial ultrastructure and DNA damage caused by nitric oxide- (NO-)

dependent oxidative stress [2]. This damage is the primary event in 3-nitropropionic acid (3-NPA) toxicity.

In Wistar rats, it has been reported that 3-nitropropionic acid leads to neurodegeneration and that the intravenous administration in rats provides valuable insight of Huntington's disease model [3]. There is evidence that metabolism of transmitter dopamine by monoamine oxidase enzyme may promote striatal damage in mitochondrial toxin induced models of Huntington's disease (HD) [4], and that HD is a devastating neurodegenerative disorder that reflect neuronal dysfunction and ultimately death in selected brain regions with striatum and cerebral cortex being the principal targets [5]. Some nutrients are known to act as antioxidants; and although neglected as

*Correspondence: juarezol@yahoo.com; adrianos27@hotmail.com
[3] Laboratorio de Farmacología, Instituto Nacional de Pediatría (INP), y Facultad de Medicina, Universidad Nacional Autónoma de México, Av Imán #1, 3er piso, Col Cuicuilco, CP 04530 Mexico City, Mexico
Full list of author information is available at the end of the article

an antioxidant, riboflavin is one of such nutrients that independently or as a component of the glutathione redox cycle has an important antioxidant action [6]. On the other hand, pyridoxine alters serotonin metabolism [7]. Both compounds are water-soluble vitamins that possess antioxidant activity [8].

Neuromodulation activity of the NO- is a documented fact, however, an excess amount of it can produce oxidative damage or nitroso-glutathione (NOGSH) inside the cell, thus; causing the damage of the cell [9]. It is known that free radicals (FR) induce damage to the components of the cell [10]. Such FR-induced damage particularly affects the plasma membrane lipids [11]. In addition, the cells of the central nervous system are extremely susceptible to these unpaired electron molecular species. Nitric oxide (NO) acts on hypothalamic neurocircuits and on higher brain circuits, e.g. dopaminergic system to regulate energy and glucose homeostasis [12]. Therefore, the presence of FR may upset this regulatory function of NO. The structural proteins in the lipid bilayer are contiguous with brain plasma membrane phospholipids [13] and the ionic inflow and outflow through the lipid bilayer is maintained by Na^+, K^+ ATPase enzyme which stimulates Na^+ and K^+ flows [14]. It is know that when the activity of the enzyme Na^+, K^+ ATPase is inhibited, it triggers the release of excitatory amino acid in the CNS [15].

In view of all the aforementioned, the objective of the present work was to make a comparative analysis of the protective effects derivable from riboflavin (B_2) and pyridoxine (B_6) on 5-HIAA and dopamine levels, as well as on selected markers of oxidative stress in rats' brain regions after an induction of Huntington's disease (HD). Literature reports suggest that these substances may participate in the neutralization of excess free radicals in oxidation mechanisms. The production of free radicals, a usual biological phenomenon, is regulated by different metabolic routes, which constitute the first line of defence in the human body.

The aim of this work was to determine if riboflavin (B_2) and pyridoxine (B_6) provide protection to the brain against free radicals generated by 3-nitropropionic acid (3-NPA) by measuring the levels of dopamine (DA) and selected oxidative stress markers.

Materials and methods

Thirty-six male Wistar rats (250 g) were procured from Bioterium of Metropolitan University of Mexico City and housed in clean plastic cages, separated into 6 groups and treated as follows: group 1, control (NaCl 0.9%); group 2, 3-NPA (20 mg/kg); group 3, B_2 (10 mg/kg); group 4, B_2 (10 mg/kg) + 3-NPA (20 mg/kg); group 5, B_6 (10 mg/kg); group 6, B_6 (10 mg/kg) + 3-NPA (20 mg/kg), each group N = 6. The administration of treatments was by i.p. The

animals received the drugs every 24 h during 3 days. At the end of the treatment period and 30 min after the last drug administration, the animals were sacrificed with guillotine without anaesthetic procedure. The animal brains were immediately extirpated and put in saline solution (NaCl 0.9%) at 4 °C. Tissues were immediately dissected in regions and used to evaluate reduced glutathione (GSH), H_2O_2, lipid peroxidation, ATPase, and the levels of DA and 5-hydroxyindolacetic acid (5-HIAA).

The rats or breeds employed in the study were subjected to a selection process based on phenotypic variety; genetic, environmental and compartmental factors. Longitudinal weight curves, weight and physical exploration were the means employed to select a breed for inclusion or exclusion in the study. Also, to select a breed, it is fundamental that inbreeding is non-existence, thus having a hereditary control of traits with continuous variation.

The selected animals were kept in cool and dry place at a temperature of 15–16 °C and with air filter and humidity of between 50 and 60. The place was maintained clean and was continuously sterilized to avoid bacterial and fungal growth.

The breeds were fed with standardized diet based on 3800 kcal/kg, proteins 12%, fat 5%, vitamins and minerals. The selected animals were 3 months old male Wistar of approximately 250 g weight.

Brain extraction

On sacrificing the animals, the brains were excised from the base. Then, the brain tissue was dissected in cortex, striatum and cerebellum/medulla oblongata, weighed and homogenised in 5 volumes of 0.05 M tris–HCl, pH 7.4. An aliquot of the homogenized brain tissue was obtained and again homogenised in 0.1 M perchloric acid ($HClO_4$) (50:50 v/v) using Yamato homogenizer (Yamato lh-21 LSC Lab, Dallas, USA) and stored at − 20 °C until analysed.

Animal management and care was conducted in accordance to the international guidelines for animal care and to the Mexican Guidelines ZOO-062. Besides, the study was approved by the Laboratory Animals Use and Care Committee of National Institute of Pediatrics.

Measurement of Dopamine (DA)

The DA levels were measured in the supernatant of tissue homogenized in HClO4 after centrifugation at 5000g for 10 min in a microcentrifuge (Hettich Zentrifugen, model Mikro 12-42, Tuttlingen, Germany), with a version of the technique reported by Calderon et al. [16]. An aliquot of the HClO4 supernatant, and 1.9 mL of buffer (0.003 M octyl-sulphate, 0.035 M KH_2PO_4, 0.03 M citric acid, 0.001 M ascorbic acid), were placed in a test tube. The mixture was incubated for 5 min at room temperature in total darkness, and subsequently, the samples were read in a spectrofluorometer (Perkin Elmer LS 55, Buckinghamshire, England) with 282 nm excitation and 315 nm emission lengths. The FL Win Lab version 4.00.02 software was used. Values were inferred in a previously standardized curve and reported as nMoles/g of wet tissue.

Measurement of 5-HIAA

5-HIAA levels were measured in the supernatant of tissue homogenized in $HClO_4$ after centrifugation at 5000g for 10 min in a microcentrifuge (Hettich Zentrifugen), with a modified version of the technique reported by Beck et al. [17]. An aliquot of the $HClO_4$ supernatant, and 1.9 mL of acetate buffer 0.01 M pH 5.5 were placed in a test tube. The mixture was incubated for 5 min at room temperature in total darkness, and subsequently, the samples were read in a spectrofluorometer (Perkin Elmer LS 55) with 296 nm excitation and 333 nm emission lengths. The FL Win Lab version 4.00.02 software was used. Values were inferred in a previously standardized curve and reported as nMoles/g of wet tissue.

Measurement of reduced glutathione (GSH)

GSH levels were measured from the supernatant of the perchloric acid homogenised tissue, obtained after centrifuging at 5000g for 5 min (Hettich Zentrifugen) according to a modified method of Hissin and Hilf [18]. A 1.8 mL phosphate buffer pH 8.0 with EDTA 0.2% plus a 20 µL aliquot of the supernatant and 100 mL of orthophthaldehyde (OPT) 1 mg/mL in methanol were put in a test tube and mixed. The mixture was then incubated for 15 min at room temperature in absolute darkness. At the end of the incubation time, the samples were read in a spectrophotometer (Perkin Elmer LS 55), with excitation and emission wavelengths of 350 and 420, respectively. FL Win Lab version 4.00.02 software was used. Values were inferred from a previously standardised curve and expressed as nM/g.

Measurement of lipid peroxidation

The lipid peroxidation across the reactive substances to the thiobarbituric acid (Tbars) determination was carried out using the modified technique of Gutteridge and Halliwell [11], as described below: From the homogenized brain in tris–HCl 0.05 M pH 7.4, 1 mL was taken and to it was added 2 mL of thiobarbituric acid (Tba) containing 1.25 g of Tba, 40 g of trichloroacetic acid (Tca), and 6.25 mL of concentrated chlorhydric acid (HCl) diluted in 250 mL of deionized H_2O. The mixture was heated to boiling point for 30 min. (Thermomix 1420) and then cooled in an ice bath for 5 min. after which it was centrifuged at 700g for 15 min. (Sorvall RC-5B Dupont). The absorbance of the floating tissues was read in triplicate at 532 nm in a spectrophotometer (Helios de UNICAM). The concentration of TBARS was expressed in µM of Malondialdehyde/g of wet tissue.

Measurement of total ATPase

The activity of ATPase was assayed according to the method proposed by Calderón et al. [19]. 1 mg (10%) w/v of homogenised brain and heart tissues in tris–HCl 0.05 M pH 7.4 was incubated for 15 min in a solution containing 3 mM $MgCl_2$, 7 mM KCl, and 100 mM NaCl. To this was added 4 mM tris-ATP and incubated for another 30 min at 37 °C in a shaking water bath (Dubnoff Labconco, TX, USA). 100 µL trichloroacetic acid at 10% w/v was used to stop the reaction and the samples were centrifuged at 100g for 5 min at 4 °C. Inorganic phosphate (Pi) was measured in triplicates using one supernatant aliquot as proposed by Fiske and Subarrow [20]. Supernatant absorbance was read at 660 nm in a Helios-α, UNICAM spectrophotometer and expressed as mM Pi/g wet tissue per minute.

Measurement of H_2O_2

The determination of H_2O_2 was made using the modified technique of Asru [21]. Each brain region (cortex, striatum, cerebellum/medulla oblongata) was homogenized in 3 mL of tris–HCl 0.05 M pH 7.4 buffers. From the diluted homogenates, 100 µL was taken and mixed with 1 mL of potassium dichromate solution ($K_2Cr_2O_7$). The mixtures were heat to boiling point for 15 min (Thermomix 1420, CA, USA). The samples were later placed in an ice bath for 5 min and centrifuged at 3000g for 5 min (Hettich Zentrifugen). The absorbance of the floating was read in triplicate at 570 nm in a spectrophotometer (Heλios-α of UNICAM, Bristol, UK). The concentration of H_2O_2 was expressed in µMoles.

Statistical analysis

One way analysis of variance (ANOVA) or Non parametric Kruskal–Wallis test was used after the data have been subjected to variances homogeneity test. Post hoc Tukey–Kramer or Steel–Dwass contrast was employed. The values of $p < 0.05$ were considered statistically significant [22]. JMP Statistical Discovery Software version 10.0 from SAS was used.

Results

In cortex, the administration of 3-NPA produced a significant increase in the levels of dopamine as well as a significant decrease in the levels of 5-HIAA (Fig. 1). GSH decreased in all animals groups that received the treatments however, the decrease of GSH had statistical significant difference only in those treated with

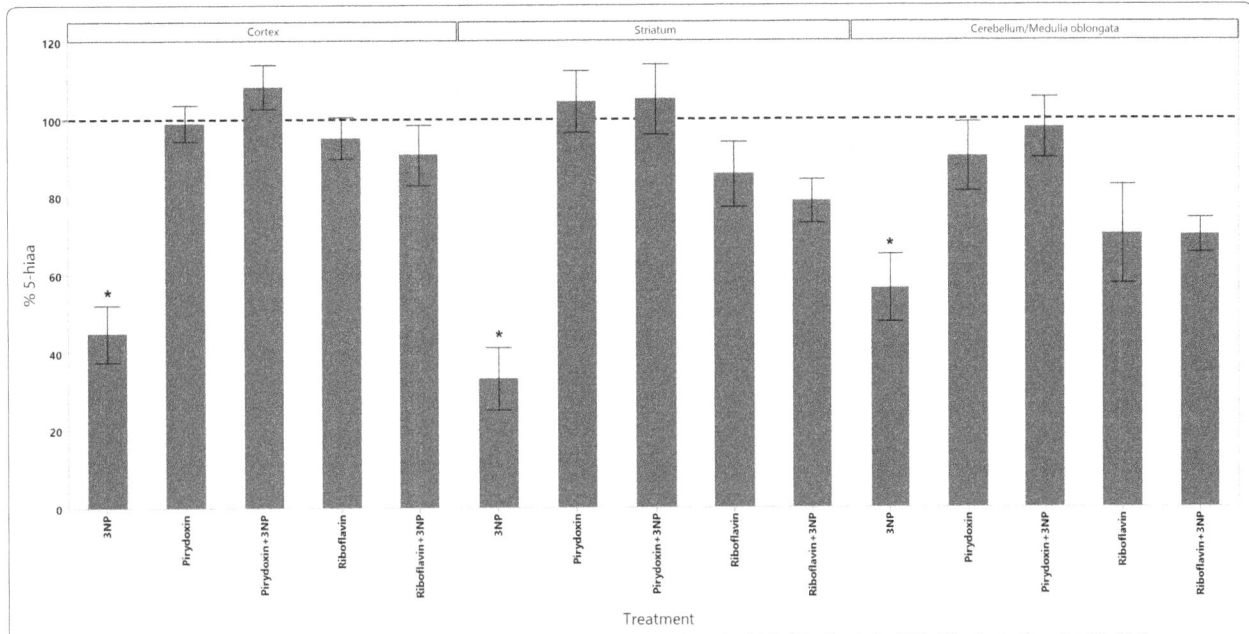

Fig. 1 5-HIAA levels in brain of rats treated with NaCl (G1), 3-Nitropropionic acid 3-NPA (G2), Riboflavin B_2 (G3), Riboflavin B_2 + 3-NPA (G4), Pyridoxine B_6 (G5) and Pyridoxine B_6 + 3-NPA (G6). Data presented as Mean ± SD values of percentage with respect to NaCl control group. Assays were made by triplicate. Cortex: Anova F = 11.06; $p < 0.0001$; *$p < 0.0004$ 3-NPA versus control, B_2, B_2 + 3-NPA, B_6, B_6 + 3-NPA. Striatum: Anova F = 10.3; $p < 0.0001$; *$p < 0.006$ 3-NPA versus control, B_2, B_2 + 3-NPA, B_6, B_6 + 3-NPA. Cerebellum/medulla oblongata: Anova F = 4.9; $p = 0.002$; *$p < 0.02$ 3-NPA versus control and B_6 + 3-NPA

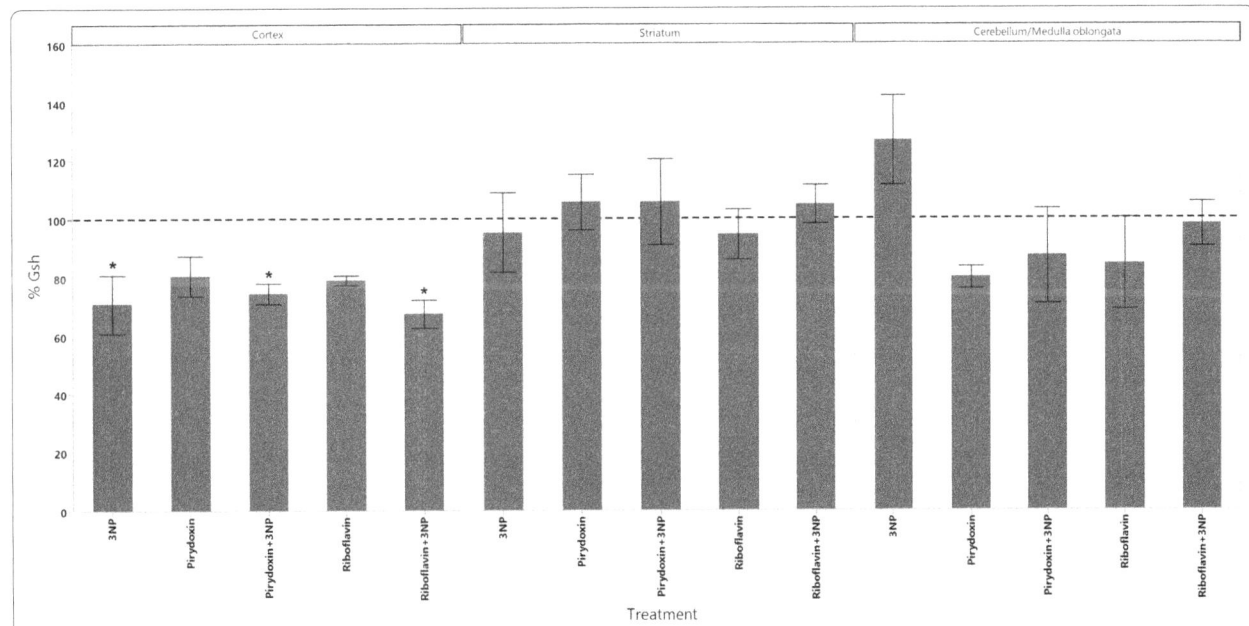

Fig. 2 GSH levels in brain of rats treated with NaCl (G1), 3-Nitropropionic acid 3-NPA (G2), Riboflavin B_2 (G3), Riboflavin B_2 + 3-NPA (G4), Pyridoxine B_6 (G5) and Pyridoxine B_6 + 3-NPA (G6). Data presented as Mean ± SD values of percentage with respect to NaCl control group. Assays were made by triplicate. Cortex: Anova F = 3.97; $p = 0.008$; *$p < 0.05$ control versus 3-NPA, B_2 + 3-NPA, B_6 + 3-NPA. Striatum: Anova F = 0.02; $p = 0.95$. Cerebellum/medulla oblongata: Anova F = 1.8; $p < 0.13$

Rivoflavin (B_2), Rivoflavin (B_2) + 3-NPA and Pyridoxine (B_6) + 3-NPA when compared with the control group (Fig. 2). Significant lipid peroxidation was appreciated in animals treated with Rivoflavin in comparison with control, B_2 + 3-NPA and B_6 + 3-NPA groups (Fig. 3). Calcium Magnesium dependent ATPase activity increased significantly in the group of animals that received 3-NPA when compared with other treatments (Fig. 4). In this region, the changes in H_2O_2 levels did not have statistical differences among treated and control groups (Fig. 5).

In striatum similar results as those observed in cortex were found. 3-NPA decreased 5-HIAA concentration (Fig. 1). Rivoflavin administration produced an increase in lipid peroxidation and 3-NPA treated animals showed significant increase in ATPase activity (Fig. 4).

In the cerebellum/Medulla oblongata of the animals that received 3-NPA alone, Dopamine, H_2O_2 and ATPase activity increased while 5-HIAA levels were found to. In this region significant lipid peroxidation increment was observed in Rivoflavin treated group when compared with the rest of the treated animals decrease (Figs. 1, 4, 5, 6).

Discussion

Evidence has shown that Huntington's disease (HD) can be caused by mitochondrial toxin produced as a result of striatal damaged that is provoked when the transmitter

dopamine is metabolized by monoamine oxidase enzymes [4]. Also, HD is a destructive neurodegenerative disorder and indicates dysfunction in the neurons that may eventually lead to death of selected brain regions; especially, the striatum and cerebral cortex [5]. In recent studies, the dendritic spine density of striatal projection neurons was reported to be seriously decreased after 3-nitropropionic acid treatment [23]. This finding is in conformity with the results of the present study where dopamine levels increased in cortex, striatum and cerebellum/medulla oblongata regions of animals that received 3-nitropropionic acid treatment. Moreover, it is possible that the increase in dopamine turnover produces an increase in oxygen radical by monoamine oxidase activity.

H_2O_2 concentration increased in cerebellum/medulla oblongata regions in animals treated with 3-NPA. This demonstrates that reactive oxygen species is the primary event in 3-NPA toxicity. In the same brain regions, lipid peroxidation increased in animals treated with riboflavin. Such increase may be due to the association of this substance with increased mitochondrial energy metabolism that is probably responsible for the high rate of oxidative metabolic activity in the brain which gives rise to intense production of reactive oxygen metabolite and subsequently to the generation of free radicals implicated in the pathogenesis of neurological disorders. These results

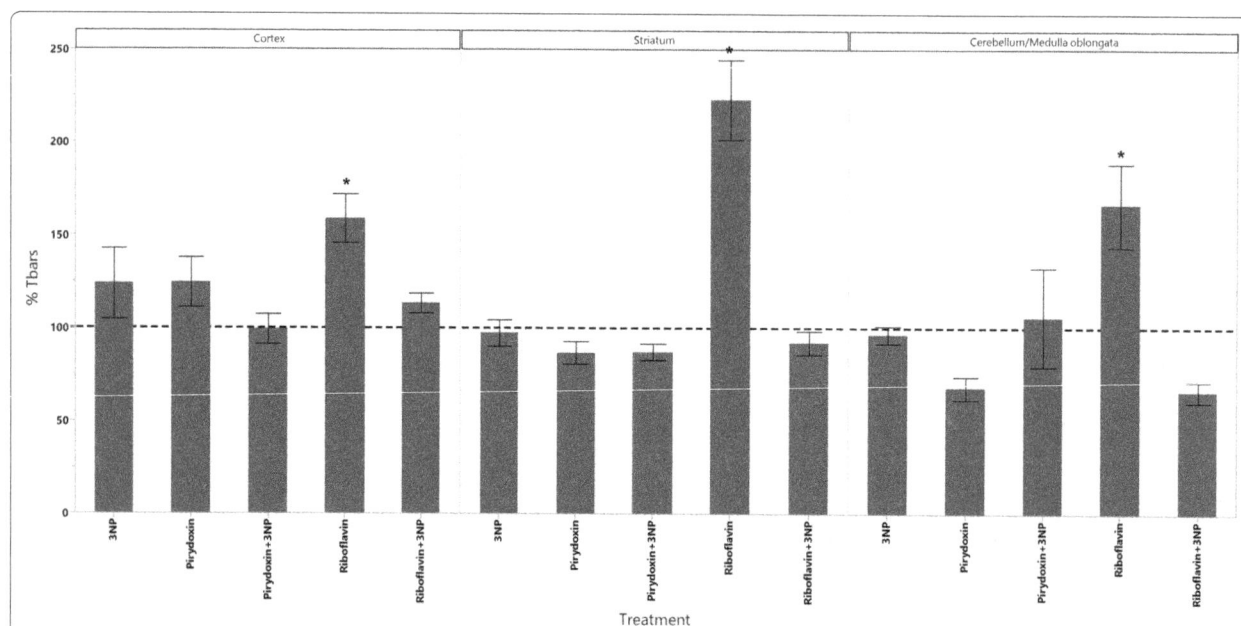

Fig. 3 TBARS levels in brain of rats treated with NaCl (G1), 3-Nitropropionic acid 3-NPA (G2), Riboflavin B_2 (G3), Riboflavin B_2 + 3-NPA (G4), Pyridoxine B_6 (G5) and Pyridoxine B_6 + 3-NPA (G6). Data presented as Mean ± SD values of percentage with respect to NaCl control group. Assays were made by triplicate. Cortex: Anova F = 4.60; $p = 0.003$; *$p < 0.05$ B_2 versus control, B_2 + 3-NPA, B_6 + 3-NPA. Striatum: Anova F = 21.5; $p < 0.0001$; *$p < 0.0001$ B_2 versus control, 3-NPA, B_2 + 3-NPA, B_6, B_6 + 3-NPA. Cerebellum/medulla oblongata: Anova F = 5.21; $p = 0.002$; *$p < 0.05$ B2 versus control, 3-NPA, B_2 + 3-NPA, B_6

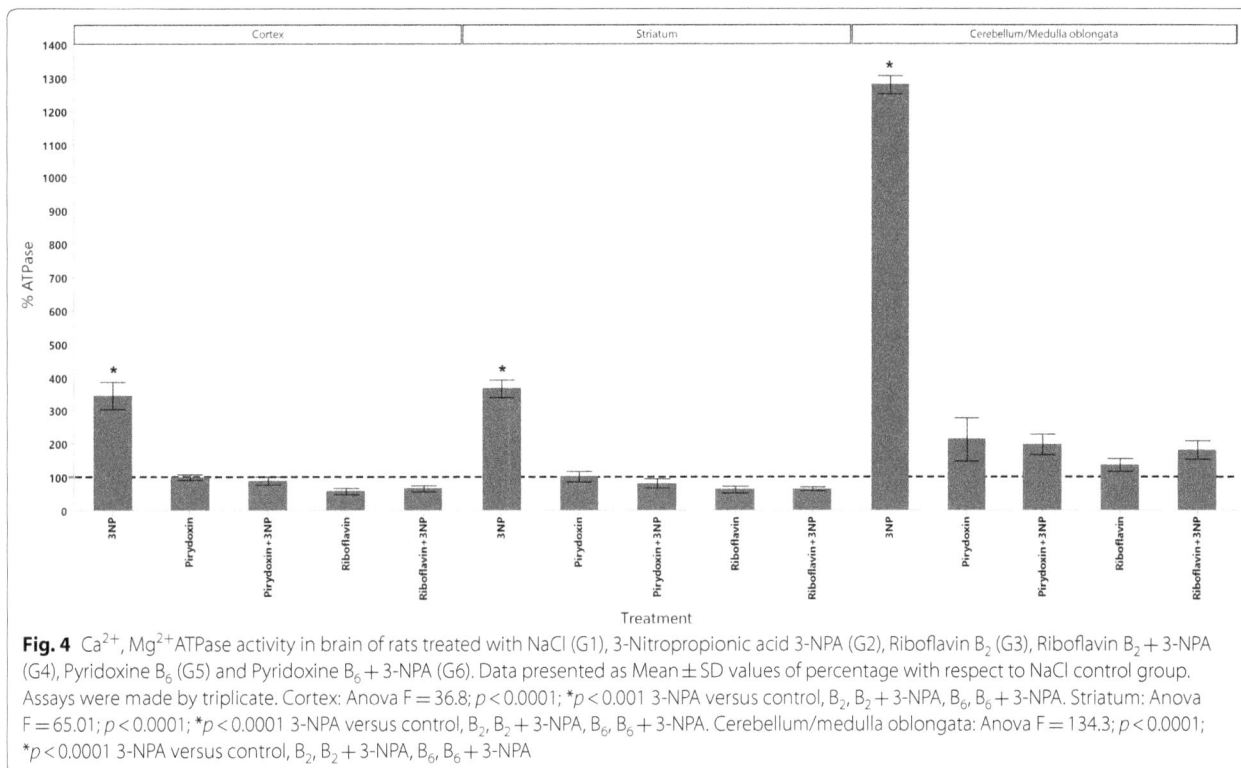

Fig. 4 Ca^{2+}, Mg^{2+}ATPase activity in brain of rats treated with NaCl (G1), 3-Nitropropionic acid 3-NPA (G2), Riboflavin B_2 (G3), Riboflavin B_2 + 3-NPA (G4), Pyridoxine B_6 (G5) and Pyridoxine B_6 + 3-NPA (G6). Data presented as Mean ± SD values of percentage with respect to NaCl control group. Assays were made by triplicate. Cortex: Anova F = 36.8; $p < 0.0001$; *$p < 0.001$ 3-NPA versus control, B_2, B_2 + 3-NPA, B_6, B_6 + 3-NPA. Striatum: Anova F = 65.01; $p < 0.0001$; *$p < 0.0001$ 3-NPA versus control, B_2, B_2 + 3-NPA, B_6, B_6 + 3-NPA. Cerebellum/medulla oblongata: Anova F = 134.3; $p < 0.0001$; *$p < 0.0001$ 3-NPA versus control, B_2, B_2 + 3-NPA, B_6, B_6 + 3-NPA

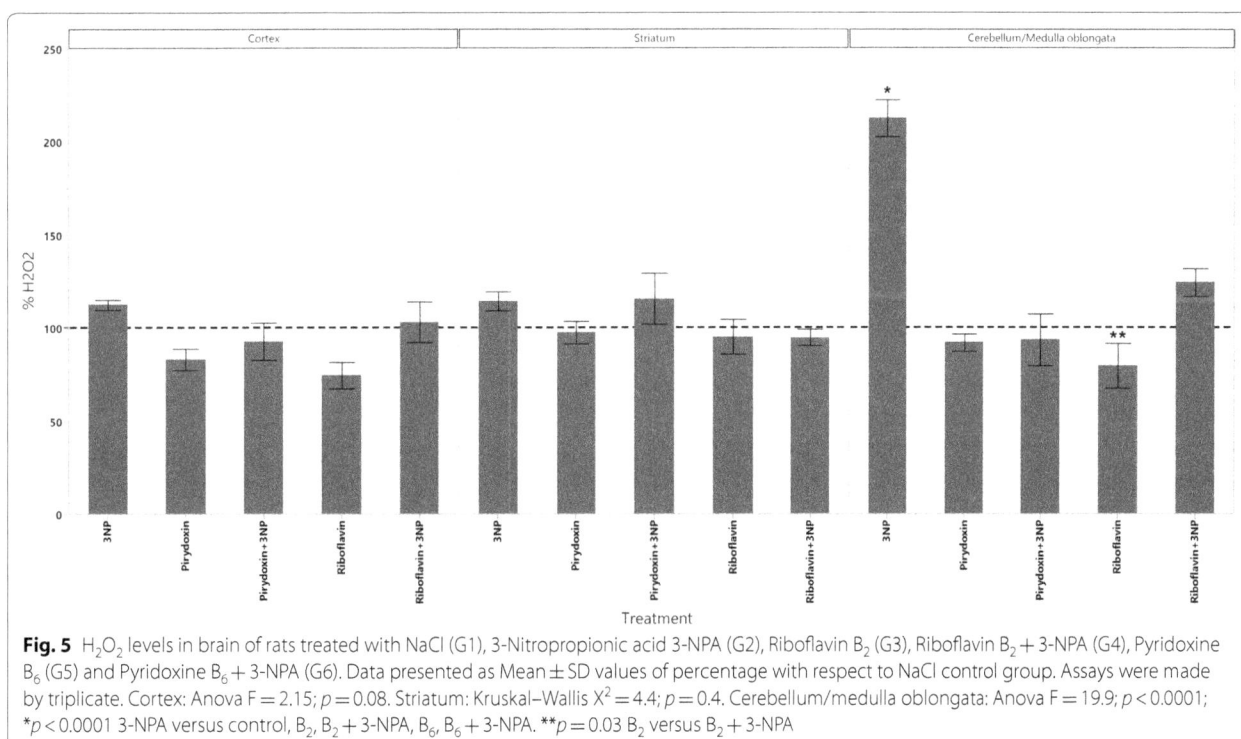

Fig. 5 H_2O_2 levels in brain of rats treated with NaCl (G1), 3-Nitropropionic acid 3-NPA (G2), Riboflavin B_2 (G3), Riboflavin B_2 + 3-NPA (G4), Pyridoxine B_6 (G5) and Pyridoxine B_6 + 3-NPA (G6). Data presented as Mean ± SD values of percentage with respect to NaCl control group. Assays were made by triplicate. Cortex: Anova F = 2.15; $p = 0.08$. Striatum: Kruskal–Wallis $X^2 = 4.4$; $p = 0.4$. Cerebellum/medulla oblongata: Anova F = 19.9; $p < 0.0001$; *$p < 0.0001$ 3-NPA versus control, B_2, B_2 + 3-NPA, B_6, B_6 + 3-NPA. **$p = 0.03$ B_2 versus B_2 + 3-NPA

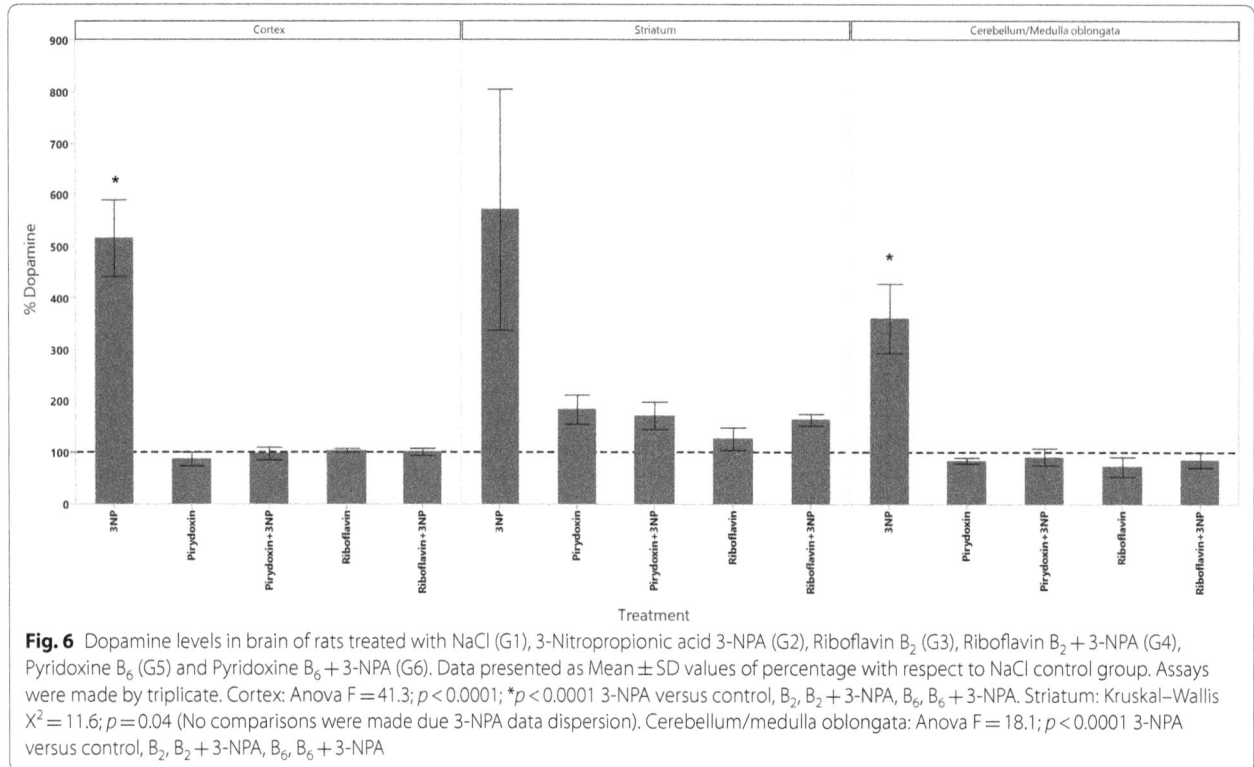

Fig. 6 Dopamine levels in brain of rats treated with NaCl (G1), 3-Nitropropionic acid 3-NPA (G2), Riboflavin B_2 (G3), Riboflavin B_2 + 3-NPA (G4), Pyridoxine B_6 (G5) and Pyridoxine B_6 + 3-NPA (G6). Data presented as Mean ± SD values of percentage with respect to NaCl control group. Assays were made by triplicate. Cortex: Anova F = 41.3; $p < 0.0001$; *$p < 0.0001$ 3-NPA versus control, B_2, B_2 + 3-NPA, B_6, B_6 + 3-NPA. Striatum: Kruskal–Wallis $X^2 = 11.6$; $p = 0.04$ (No comparisons were made due 3-NPA data dispersion). Cerebellum/medulla oblongata: Anova F = 18.1; $p < 0.0001$ 3-NPA versus control, B_2, B_2 + 3-NPA, B_6, B_6 + 3-NPA

may have relation with the reports of Kumar et al. [24] and Kaur et al. [25], which suggest that 3-NPA depleted GSH in cortex, although the present study was made with young animal models.

Calcium and magnesium-dependent ATPase activity increased in cortex, striatum and cerebellum/medulla oblongata regions of the animals that received 3-NPA alone. This could be attributed to changes in the affinity of the enzyme [26]. These results may have relation with the reports of Naziroğlu et al. [27], which suggest that increase in Ca^{2+}-ATPase activities may have protective effects against substances that induce brain injury by inhibiting free radical production, regulating calcium-dependent processes and supporting the antioxidant redox system.

Conclusion

The results of the present study suggest that the partial increase in antioxidant capacity in brain due to B_2 and B_6 vitamins promotes an effect in dopamine or serotonin metabolisms when we consider 3-NPA capacity to generate oxidative stress.

We recommend that further studies be carried out to investigate the possible relationship between B_2 and B_6 vitamins on dopamine and serotonin levels in different animal models. Undoubtedly, we believe that this would help in the study of neurodegenerative diseases.

Abbreviations

AO: antioxidant; CNS: central nervous system; DA: dopamine; DNA: deoxyribonucleic acid; EAA: excitatory amino acids; FR: free radicals; GSH: glutathione; HD: Huntington's disease; 5-HIAA: 5-hydroxyindole-acetic acid; NOGSH: nitroso-glutathione; 3-NPA: 3-nitropropionic acid; L-DOPA: L-3,4-dihydroxyphenylalanine; OPT: ortho-phthaldehyde; RNS: reactive nitrogen species; ROS: reactive oxygen species; Tbars.: thiobarbituric acid reactive substances.

Authors' contributions

AVP: contributed in the conception and design, critically revised the manuscript for important intellectual content, drafted manuscript. DCG: Contributed in the acquisition, analysis and interpretation of data, critically revised the manuscript for important intellectual content, drafted manuscript. NOB, MOH, BJT, GBM: Contributed in the acquisition, analysis and interpretation of data, drafted manuscript. HJO, MLS: Critically revised the manuscript for important intellectual content, drafted manuscript. All authors read and approved the final manuscript.

Author details

[1] Laboratorio de Neurociencias, Instituto Nacional de Pediatría (INP), Mexico City, Mexico. [2] Laboratorio de Bacteriología Experimental, INP, Mexico City, Mexico. [3] Laboratorio de Farmacología, Instituto Nacional de Pediatría (INP), y Facultad de Medicina, Universidad Nacional Autónoma de México, Av Imán #1, 3er piso, Col Cuicuilco, CP 04530 Mexico City, Mexico.

Acknowledgements

We thank Dr. Cyril Ndidi Nwoye, a native English speaker and language professor, for the critical review and translation of this manuscript.

Competing interests

The authors declare that they have no competing interests.

Funding
This manuscript was not funded by any organization.

References

1. Rami A, Ferger D, Krieglstein J. Blockade of calpain proteolytic activity rescues neurons from glutamate excitotoxicity. Neurosci Res. 1997;27:93–7.
2. Aliev G, Obrenovich ME, Tabrez S, Jabir NR, Reddy VP, Li Y, et al. Link between cancer and Alzheimer disease via oxidative stress induced by nitric oxide-dependent mitochondrial DNA overproliferation and deletion. Oxid Med Cell Longev. 2013;2013:962984. https://doi.org/10.1155/2013/962984 **(Epub 2013 Apr 3)**.
3. Szabó A, Papp A, Nagymajtényi L. Effects of 3-nitropropionic acid in rats: general toxicity and functional neurotoxicity. Arh Hig Rada Toksikol. 2005;56:297–302.
4. Smith RR, Dimayuga ER, Keller JN, Maragos WF. Enhanced toxicity to the catecholamine tyramine in polyglutamine transfected SH-SY5Y cells. Neurochem Res. 2005;30:527–31.
5. Browne SE, Beal MF. Oxidative damage in Huntington's disease pathogenesis. Antioxid Redox Signal. 2006;8:2061–73.
6. Ashoori M, Saedisomeolia A. Riboflavin (vitamin B2) and oxidative stress: a review. Br J Nutr. 2014;20:1–7.
7. Calderón-Guzmán D, Hernández-Islas JL, Espitia-Vázquez I, Barragán-Mejía G, Hernández-García E, Santamaría-del Angel D, et al. Pyridoxine, regardless of serotonin levels, increases production of 5-hydroxytryptophan in rat brain. Arch Med Res. 2004;35:271–4.
8. Tupe RS, Agte VV. Effect of water soluble vitamins on Zn transport of Caco-2 cells and their implications under oxidative stress conditions. Eur J Nutr. 2010;49:53–61.
9. Hogg N, Singh RJ, Kalyanaraman B. The role of glutathione in the transport and catabolism of nitric oxide. FEBS Lett. 1996;382:223–8.
10. Beckman JS, Beckman TW, Chen J, Marshall PA, Freeman BA. Apparent hydroxyl radical production by peroxynitrite: implications for endothelial injury from nitric oxide and superoxides. Proc Natl Acad Sci USA. 1990;87:1624–9.
11. Gutteridge JM, Halliwell B. The measurement and mechanism of lipid peroxidation in biological systems. Trends Biochem Sci. 1990;15:129–35.
12. Vogt MC, Brüning JC. CNS insulin signaling in the control of energy homeostasis and glucose metabolism: from embryo to old age. Trends Endocrinol Metab. 2013;24:76–84.
13. Swapna I, Sathya KV, Murthy CR, Senthilkumaran B. Membrane alterations and fluidity changes in cerebral cortex during ammonia intoxication. NeuroToxicol. 2005;335:700–4.
14. Stefanello FM, Chiarani F, Kurek AG. Methionine alters Na^+, K^+ ATPase activity, lipid peroxidation and nonenzymatic antioxidant defenses in rat hippocampus. Int J Dev Neurosci. 2005;23:651–6.
15. Calderon GD, Juarez OH, Hernandez GE, Labra RN, Barragan MG, Trujillo JF, et al. Effect of an antiviral and vitamins A, C, D on dopamine and some oxidative stress markers in rat brain exposed to ozone. Arch Biol Sci Belgrade. 2013;65:1371–9.
16. Calderón GD, Osnaya BN, García AR, Hernández GE, Guillé PA. Levels of glutathione and some biogenic amines in the human brain putamen after traumatic death. Proc West Pharmacol Soc. 2008;51:25–7.
17. Beck O, Palmskog G, Hultman E. Quantitative determination of 5-hydroxyindole-3-acetic acid in body fluids by HPLC. Clin Chim Acta. 1977;79:149–54.
18. Hissin PJ, Hilf R. A flurometric method for determination of oxidized and reduced glutathione in tissue. Anal Biochem. 1974;4:214–26.
19. Calderón-Guzmán D, Espitia-Vázquez I, López-Domínguez A, Hernández-García E, Huerta-Gertrudis B, Juárez-Olguín H. Effect of toluene and nutritional status on serotonin, lipid peroxidation levels and Na^+/K^+ATPase in adult rat brain. Neurochem Res. 2005;30:619–24.
20. Fiske CH, Subbarow Y. The colorimetric determination of phosphorus. J Biol Chem. 1925;66:375–400.
21. Asru KS. Colorimetric assay of catalase. Anal Biochem. 1972;47:389–94.
22. Castilla-Serna L. Practical statistic guide for human health. 1st ed. México: Editorial Trillas; 2011.
23. Mu S, Lin E, Liu B, Ma Y, OuYang L, Li Y, Chen S, Zhang J, Lei W. Melatonin reduces projection neuronal injury induced by 3-nitropropionic acid in the rat striatum. Neurodegener Dis. 2014;14(3):139–50.
24. Kumar P, Kalonia H, Kumar A. Protective effect of sesamol against 3-nitropropionic acid-induced cognitive dysfunction and altered glutathione redox balance in rats. Basic Clin Pharmacol Toxicol. 2010;107:577–82.
25. Kaur N, Jamwal S, Deshmukh R, Gauttam V, Kumar P. Beneficial effect of rice bran extract against 3-nitropropionic acid induced experimental Huntington's disease in rats. Toxicol Rep. 2015;2:1222–32.
26. Hoskins B, Ho IK, Meydrech EF. Effects of aging and morphine administration on calmodulin and calmodulin-regulated enzymes in striata of mice. J Neurochem. 1985;44:1069–73.
27. Naziroğlu M, Kutluhan S, Yilmaz M. Selenium and topiramate modulates brain microsomal oxidative stress values, Ca^{2+}-ATPase activity, and EEG records in pentylentetrazol-induced seizures in rats. J Membr Biol. 2008;225:39–49.

19

Social defeat stress before pregnancy induces depressive-like behaviours and cognitive deficits in adult male offspring: correlation with neurobiological changes

Sheng Wei[1,2,3,4], Zifa Li[3,4], Meng Ren[4], Jieqiong Wang[1], Jie Gao[1], Yinghui Guo[1], Kaiyong Xu[4], Fang Li[1,5], Dehao Zhu[3], Hao Zhang[3], Rongju Lv[3] and Mingqi Qiao[1]*

Abstract

Background: Epidemiological surveys and studies with animal models have established a relationship between maternal stress and affective disorders in their offspring. However, whether maternal depression before pregnancy influences behaviour and related neurobiological mechanisms in the offspring has not been studied.

Results: A social defeat stress (SDS) maternal rat model was established using the resident-intruder paradigm with female specific pathogen-free Wistar rats and evaluated with behavioural tests. SDS maternal rats showed a significant reduction in sucrose preference and locomotor and exploratory activities after 4 weeks of stress. In the third week of the experiment, a reduction in body weight gain was observed in SDS animals. Sucrose preference, open field, the elevated-plus maze, light–dark box, object recognition, the Morris water maze, and forced swimming tests were performed using the 2-month-old male offspring of the female SDS rats. Offspring subjected to pre-gestational SDS displayed enhanced anxiety-like behaviours, reduced exploratory behaviours, reduced sucrose preference, and atypical despair behaviours. With regard to cognition, the offspring showed significant impairments in the retention phase of the object recognition test, but no effect was observed in the acquisition phase. These animals also showed impairments in recognition memory, as the discrimination index in the Morris water maze test in this group was significantly lower for both 1 h and 24 h memory retention compared to controls. Corticosterone, adrenocorticotropic hormone, and monoamine neurotransmitters levels were determined using enzyme immunoassays or radioimmunoassays in plasma, hypothalamus, left hippocampus, and left prefrontal cortex samples from the offspring of the SDS rats. These markers of hypothalamic–pituitary–adrenal axis responsiveness and the monoaminergic system were significantly altered in pre-gestationally stressed offspring. Brain-derived neurotrophic factor (BDNF), cyclic adenosine monophosphate response element binding protein (CREB), phosphorylated CREB (pCREB), and serotonin transporter (SERT) protein levels were evaluated using western blotting with right hippocampus and right prefrontal cortex samples. Expression levels of BDNF, pCREB, and SERT in the offspring were also altered in the hippocampus and in the prefrontal cortex; however, there was no effect on CREB.

Conclusion: We conclude that SDS before pregnancy might induce depressive-like behaviours, cognitive deficits, and neurobiological alterations in the offspring.

*Correspondence: qmingqi@163.com
[1] Laboratory of Traditional Chinese Medicine Classical Theory, Ministry of Education, Shandong University of Traditional Chinese Medicine, #4655 University Road, University Science Park, Changqing District, Jinan 250355, China
Full list of author information is available at the end of the article

Keywords: Social defeat stress, Stress before pregnancy, Offspring, Behavioural phenotype, Neurobiochemistry

Background

Epidemiological surveys and animal experiments have established connections between maternal stress and changes in the mood and behaviour of their offspring [1–5]. For example, it has been reported that the risks for anxiety, depression, and addiction disorders, are increased in the children of depressed parents compared to those of non-depressed parents [3], and a considerable number of animal experiments have shown that maternal stress during the prenatal period leads to increased depressive and anxiety-like behaviours in the offspring [6–9]. However, the neurobiological mechanisms through which maternal depression prior to pregnancy has these effects on the offspring have not been well studied.

It has been reported that when female rats are exposed to chronic unpredictable stress (CUS) prior to being pregnant, their male offspring are at increased risk of developing depressive-like behaviours, and it has been suggested that such behaviours are due to altered expression of phosphorylated cyclic adenosine monophosphate response element binding protein (pCREB), brain-derived neurotrophic factor (BDNF), and N-methyl-D-aspartate receptor (NMDA-R) subunits in the hippocampus [4, 5]. In most experiments, CUS is implemented through the administration of electric shocks or by physically restraining the animal [4, 5], but such physical stressors are more or less artificial and might be regarded as irrelevant to the situations and stressors that humans and animals encounter in everyday life [10]. In contrast to the paradigm mentioned above, the use of social defeat stress (SDS) as a naturalistic psychosocial stressor might be more suitable for inducing maternal depressive-like behaviours [11]. The resident-intruder paradigm is often used to induce SDS in rodents [12, 13], and in such experiments an adult rodent (the intruder) is placed in the cage of an unfamiliar and aggressive individual (the resident). The animals will instinctively fight, and the intruder will usually lose. These experiments are terminated as soon as the intruder shows signs of submissive behaviour so as to minimize injury while ensuring that the psychosocial components of stress are maximized. In rats, social defeat by an aggressive male is a more natural stressor than the physical stressors mentioned above, and such stress results in a variety of molecular, physiological, and behavioural changes in the intruder animal, and many of these changes exist for a long time.

However, the evidence to support the effects of maternal chronic SDS before pregnancy on offspring is still weak. Therefore, there is much interest in understanding the abnormal behaviours of the offspring and the underlying mechanisms induced by the social stress experienced by the mother before pregnancy. The hypothalamic-pituitary-adrenal (HPA)-axis, is responsible for an individual's ability to cope with stress, and it does so by regulating the production and release of various hormones [14, 15]. Hyperactivity of the HPA axis has been observed in the majority of patients with depression [16, 17]. Furthermore, it is also well documented that corticosteroids modulate emotional behaviours and cognition in animals and humans in a complex manner [18]. On the other hand, the serotonergic and adrenergic systems play critical roles in modulating the functional neural circuits in brain [19, 20] and have been implicated in hippocampal-dependent memory. It has also been shown that the hippocampus, hypothalamus, and prefrontal cortex are involved in the stress response and are the areas most relevant to depression [21, 22] and that these regions play a primary role in the neuroendocrine control of feeding, emotion, and metabolism in adult life [23]. In addition, monoaminergic signalling pathways mainly act via G-proteins that in turn activate adenylyl cyclase, protein kinase A (PKA), and the transcription factor CREB. pCREB can regulate multiple target genes involved in the pathophysiology of depression [4, 6, 24]. Taken together, the HPA axis, serotonergic and adrenergic systems, and monoaminergic signalling pathways have been investigated in the hippocampus, hypothalamus, and prefrontal cortex to evaluate the mechanisms involved in depression.

In this study, we hypothesized that (1) the SDS experienced by dams before pregnancy causes behavioural abnormalities in their male offspring and (2) the behavioural abnormalities observed in the male offspring are related to abnormalities in the HPA axis, monoaminergic system, and signal transduction pathways. To test these hypotheses, dams were subjected to social defeat on a daily basis for 4 weeks (1 week of social isolation and 3 weeks of defeat stress) and then subjected to a series of behavioural tests. Subsequently, the offspring delivered by the stressed dams were selected for behavioural testing (open-field, sucrose preference, elevated plus maze, light–dark box, forced swim, object recognition, and Morris water maze (MWM) tests). The levels of neurotransmitters in different brain regions; the expression of pCREB, serotonin transporter (SERT), and BDNF; and the correlation between behavioural and molecular changes were examined.

Methods
Study design

A maternal SDS rat model was established using the resident-intruder paradigm with female specific pathogen-free Wistar rats and was evaluated by behavioural tests. The maternal SDS procedure and the behavioural analysis process are shown in Fig. 1a. Seven days after the end of the SDS exposure, two female rats were housed with one sexually experienced males of the same strain. These male rats for mating had similar scores on the open-field and sucrose preference tests. The day when sperm were observed in vaginal smears was designated as embryonic day 0. The female rats were then housed separately and allowed to nest and give birth without being disturbed. The day of delivery was designated as postnatal day 0. The pups were removed from their dams at 22 days of age and housed in groups of three or four with males and females kept separate. All experiments described below were performed in the male offspring at 2 months of age. Eight pups from the control and SDS dams were used, with one or two pups used from each dam. The behavioural tests used with the offspring are shown in Fig. 1b. Some methods detailed below (including sucrose preference test, open field test, elevated plus maze, object recognition task, morris water maze test and monoamine neurotransmitter concentration analyses) mainly refer to our previously published work [25].

Animals and grouping

Twelve female specific pathogen-free (SPF) Wistar rats (resident) weighing 120–150 g and aged 6 weeks, twelve female SPF Wistar rats (intruder) weighing 150–180 g and aged 6 weeks, and six male SPF Wistar rats (used for mating) weighing 180–220 g were provided by Beijing Vital River Experimental Animal Technology Co. Ltd. (SCXK [JING] 2007-0001; Beijing, China).

All animals were housed under a reversed 12/12 h light/dark cycle (lights off at 8:00 a.m. and on at 8:00 p.m.), and food and water were available ad libitum except during the behavioural experiments. The animals were handled daily for 1 week to habituate them to the experimental conditions. The room temperature was maintained at 22 ± 1 °C with 50% humidity. Rats were minimally handled, and soiled bedding was periodically only partially replaced, without removing the rats, so that home-cage odours, nests, etc., were minimally disrupted [26]. All experiments were conducted during the dark phase of the light/dark cycle under dim red light conditions (10:00 a.m. to 5:00 p.m.). Animals were tested using a matched block design with roughly equal numbers of animals in each treatment group in a series of several blocks. The operators were blinded to the experimental design.

Prior to the experiments, all female rats were checked to ensure they had a regular oestrous cycle of 4–5 days and that they showed an equal distribution of the different stages of the oestrous cycle. The oestrous cycle was again examined during the last week of SDS using vaginal smears, as has been previously described [5, 27]. In general, aggressive females with strong bodies and rich

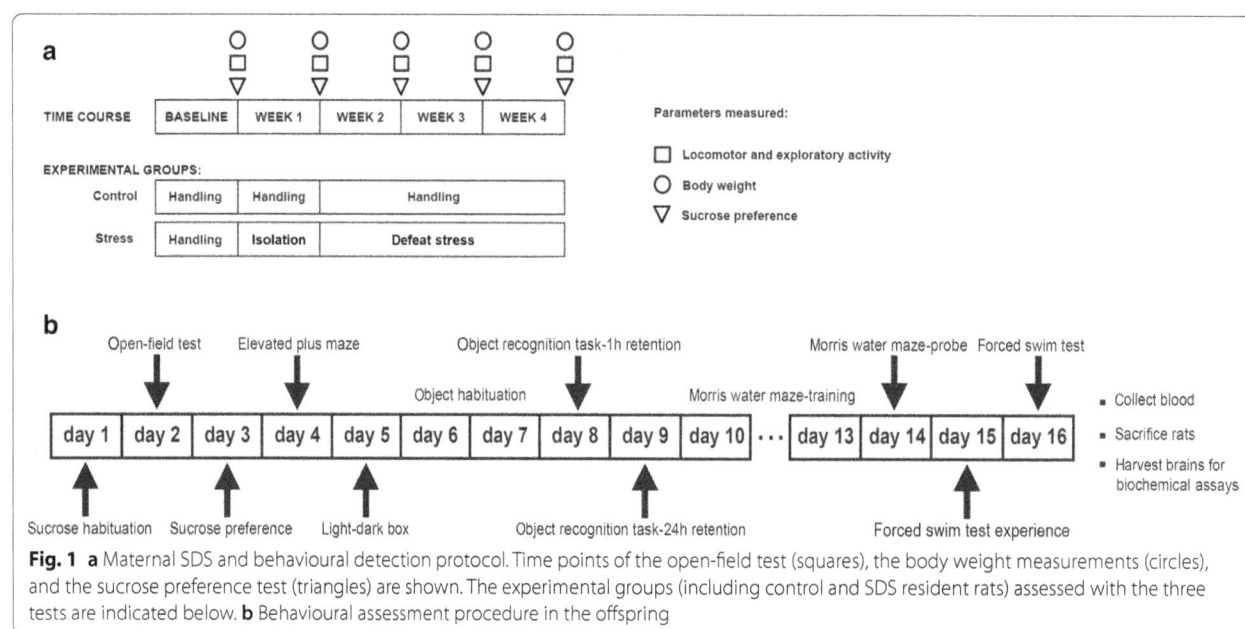

Fig. 1 **a** Maternal SDS and behavioural detection protocol. Time points of the open-field test (squares), the body weight measurements (circles), and the sucrose preference test (triangles) are shown. The experimental groups (including control and SDS resident rats) assessed with the three tests are indicated below. **b** Behavioural assessment procedure in the offspring

fighting experience in non-receptive phases were selected as intruders. Because females in non-receptive phases exhibited aggressive behaviour more than females in other phases [28], these intruders always defeated the resident rats. The intruder rats were housed individually in a separate room under identical conditions as the resident rats. Prior to all stress-inducing procedures, the resident rats were divided into the control group (n = 6) and SDS group (n = 6).

Weight of female rats

The body weight of each female rat was measured before the start of the SDS (W0) paradigm, and once per week (W1, W2, W3) during the protocol (Fig. 1a). Weight was taken at 9:00 a.m. to 12:00 p.m. every day.

Sucrose preference test (SPT)

SPTs were performed weekly during the SDS experiment, with the first test being performed at baseline. Two bottles of liquid were provided for the rats to choose from over a 24 h period. One bottle contained a 0.8% sucrose solution and the other contained tap water, and the bottle positions were switched after 12 h. The sucrose preference was determined as the percentage of the total amount of liquid consumed [29]. SPTs were performed in the same manner with the male offspring.

Open field test (OFT)

The OFT was performed in an open-topped Plexiglas arena (100 cm × 100 cm × 50 cm), Each animal was placed in the centre of the arena and was allowed to explore it for 6 min, and all movements of the animals within the arena were automatically recording using the XR-SuperMaze video tracking and analysis system (Shanghai SOFTMAZE Information Technology Co., Ltd, Shanghai, China). The behaviours within the arena were analysed according to the total distance moved, the distance travelled in the centre and peripheral areas, the time spent in the centre [30, 31], and the number of rearings. The arena was carefully cleaned with 70% ethanol after every test.

Social defeat stress

The resident-intruder social stress paradigm was used with modifications in which the intruder was the aggressor and the resident was the defeated subject. The social defeat test was conducted for 4 weeks, including 1 week of social isolation (in which dams were fed separately) and 3 weeks of defeat stress (Fig. 1a). The control rats were housed at three rats per cage over the course of the 4 weeks. Experiments were performed using a dark red light (< 2 lx) during the dark period. Female rats in non-receptive phases (metestrus and diestrus) with obvious

aggressive behaviour and that were larger in size and heavier in body weight than the residents were selected as intruders [28]. The cage was moved to an observation table, and after approximately 15 min of adaptation a female intruder was transferred from her home cage and introduced into the resident's cage for a period of 15 min. All fights between intruders and resident rats were observed, and the outcomes of the fights were recorded. The defeat test was conducted once per day for 3 weeks. To avoid individual differences in defeat intensity, residents were confronted each day with a different intruder in a Latin square design.

The defeat sessions were monitored. The quality of the defeat sessions was precisely controlled in order to overcome individual variability within the stress group. 'Defeat' was defined as one rat being 'on top', or as 'pinning behaviour', lasting for approximately 2 s. While the residents and intruders met during the 15 min, they fought many times with different outcomes. Although the intruders were more aggressive and stronger and had more experience in fighting, it was hard to ensure that the residents were defeated every time. Hence, a 'defeat ratio' was introduced to make sure that social defeat stress would outweigh individual variability. The defeat ratio was the number of defeats of a resident divided by the total number of fights. Only the residents whose defeat ratio was greater than 80% every day were assigned to the stress group as the pairing dams.

Control animals (n = 6) were handled daily throughout the entire experiment. Handling consisted of picking up each rat, transferring it to the experimental room, and returning it to its home cage.

Elevated plus maze (EPM) test

The EPM was made of black Perspex with a 10 cm × 10 cm central area and arms 50 cm long and 10 cm wide, and the maze was 50 cm above the floor. The closed arms were enclosed by a 40 cm wall, and the open arms had 0.5 cm edges in order to maximize entries into the open arm [32]. The animals were placed in the centre of the maze facing an open arm [33, 34] and were allowed to explore the maze for 5 min. The time spent in an arm of the maze was recorded starting when two paws had crossed the line into the arm. The number of entries into the arms and the time spent in the arms were used as a measure of the locomotor activity of the rat in the maze.

Light–dark box (LDB) test

The LDB was made of Plexiglas and consisted of two compartments. The larger section was the bright section (25 cm long × 25 cm wide × 30 cm high) and was illuminated by a 75 W white-light bulb (about 200 lx). The smaller section was the dark section (18 cm long × 25 cm wide × 30 cm high) and was illuminated by a 40 W red-light bulb (about 30 lx). Both bulbs were 45 cm above the floor of the box. The compartments were separated by a wall with a 6.5 cm × 6.5 cm doorway. For each test, the animal was placed in the centre of the bright compartment facing the separating wall. An entry was recorded when the rat moved through the doorway and placed all four paws in the other compartment. The total number of transitions between compartments and the time spent in the illuminated compartment were recorded and used as an indicator of overall activity and anxiety level. The frequencies of grooming, wall climbing, and rearing were also recorded [35].

Object recognition task (ORT)

Male offspring were tested for four consecutive days in the open-field arena following a previously described ORT protocol [36, 37]. At 10.00 a.m. on days 1 and 2, the animals were habituated to the apparatus by allowing them to freely explore the arena. The open field apparatus was a square box 40 cm wide × 40 cm long × 40 cm high. On day 3, the animals were subjected to a 5 min training session in which they were presented with two identical metal cans that were placed against one wall of the arena. Each rat was released in the middle of the opposite wall with its back to the two cans and allowed to explore the arena and the cans on its own. The time spent exploring each object was recorded using the SuperMaze video tracking system. The time spent exploring the cans was recorded as the time the animal's nose was within a 2 cm^2 area surrounding the cans. After the training session, the animals were returned to their home cage for 1 h. The animals were then returned to the arena, only now it contained two different objects. One object was identical to the metal cans used in the training session but that had not been previously used, while the other was a novel metal, glass, or hard plastic object. The time spent exploring each object was recorded over a period of 5 min. On day 4, the rats were tested again for 5 min with the familiar object and a different novel object from that used on day 3. The novel objects were randomized and counterbalanced among all of the tested animals. All objects employed in this experiment were used only once in order to eliminate olfactory cues. Familiar objects were always of the same material, colour, size, and shape, and the unfamiliar objects were always different between day 3 and day 4. The objects and the arena were thoroughly cleaned with 70% ethanol at the end of each experimental session.

The recognition index (RI) is calculated as the time spent investigating the novel object divided by the total time spent exploring the novel and familiar objects [RI = TN/(TN + TF)] and is a measure of novel object recognition and is the main index used for analysing memory (or the response to novelty). An RI greater than 50% indicates more time spent exploring the novel object, while an RI less than 50% indicates more time spent exploring the familiar object. An RI of 50% indicates a null preference.

Morris water maze (MWM) test

The MWM consisted of a light-blue swimming pool 160 cm in diameter with 70 cm walls filled with tap water to a depth of 50 cm. The water temperature was maintained at 23 ± 2 °C. The SuperMaze system was used to divide the pool into four quadrants (North-West [NW], North-East [NE], South-West [SW], and South-East [SE]) of equal size. A removable square escape platform (10 cm × 10 cm) could be positioned in the quadrants, and the centre of the platform was 30 cm away from the wall and 1.5 cm below the surface of the water such that it was not visible to the swimming rat. The pool was placed in an experiment room that had several external visual cues such as bookshelves and posters, and the pool was kept in the same position throughout the entire experimental period. The SuperMaze video system was used to record the animal's movements in the pool, including measures of the time until finding the escape platform, the total path length of swimming, and the time spent in each quadrant.

The animals were subjected to a training protocol as described by Plescia et al. [36]. Place learning was conducted over 4 days by training the rats to escape from the water by reaching the hidden platform placed in the SE zone where it was maintained throughout the experimental session. Rats were placed in the pool facing the walls of each quadrant in the following order: SW, NW, NE, and SE. Each animal underwent four trials per day over four consecutive days, and they were allowed to swim until the escape platform was found (escape latency) for a maximum of 120 s. When the platform was reached, they were allowed to rest on it for 15 s. If the animal did not find the escape platform within 120 s, the experimenter guided it gently to the platform where it was allowed to rest for 15 s in order to reinforce the information from the visuo-spatial cues in the environment of the experiment room. The animals were returned to their cages and briefly warmed under a heating lamp during the 5 min interval between trials. The video tracking software recorded the escape latency (s) as a measure of the acquisition and retrieval of the spatial information necessary to reach the platform location, and the path length (m) was recorded as an additional element in the search strategies.

The day after the animal had completed the 4-day place-learning task, it was placed in the pool but without the escape platform. The time spent in each quadrant was recorded (transfer test) to determine the degree of learning in the animals with respect to where the escape platform had been located during the place-learning task.

Forced swimming test (FST)

The FST was performed as described previously [38]. The animals were individually placed into glass cylinders 18 cm in diameter and 40 cm tall containing 18 cm of water at 23 °C. After a pre-test of 15 min swimming, the rats were transferred to a 30 °C drying environment for 30 min before being returned to their cages. The animals were then returned to the cylinder 24 h later for a 5 min test that was recorded with a video camera. Fresh water was used for each rat, and the cylinder was cleaned after each use. All experiments were performed between 12:00 p.m. and 4:00 p.m, and the videotapes were reviewed by an experimenter who was blinded to the group allocation of the animals. Immobility time was measured, which was defined as when the animal was floating and only moving enough to keep its nostrils above the surface of the water [29].

Tissue and blood collection

Rats were taken from their home cages on the next day after FST in order to collect tissue and blood samples, and they were sacrificed via decapitation between 8:00 a.m. and 10:00 a.m. Trunk blood was collected into ethylenediaminetetraacetic acid (EDTA) tubes, centrifuged at $1250 \times g$ (15 min, 4 °C), and plasma was collected and frozen until ACTH and corticosterone levels were determined. The brains were removed from the skull and placed on ice. Using the bregma as a reference landmark, the hippocampus, hypothalamus, and prefrontal cortex were dissected out. The hypothalamus, left hippocampus, and left prefrontal cortex were used for the detection of monoamine neurotransmitters via radioimmunoassays, and the right hippocampus and right prefrontal cortex were used to examine BDNF, CREB, pCREB, and serotonin transporter (SERT) protein levels using western blotting.

Plasma corticosterone and ACTH analyses

Corticosterone levels were determined using 30 μl of plasma with a commercially available enzyme immunoassay kit (CUSABIO®, China), and ACTH levels were assessed using 200 μl of plasma with the HS-ACTH radioimmunoassay kit (CUSABIO®, China) as previously described [33]. The inter- and intra-assay coefficients of variation (CVs) for ACTH level determination were both 15%, and the inter- and intra-assay CVs for corticosterone determination were 8% and 10%, respectively.

Monoamine neurotransmitter concentration analyses

Norepinephrine (NE), serotonin (5-HT), and dopamine (DA) levels in the hypothalamus, hippocampus, and prefrontal cortex were measured in brain tissue samples of recommended volume using commercially available enzyme immunoassay kits (CUSABIO®, China) specific for each compound as previously described [33]. The inter- and intra-assay CVs for neurotransmitter concentration measurements were 8% and 10% for NE, 15% and 15% for 5-HT, and 8% and 10% for DA, respectively.

Western blotting

Tissue samples from the hippocampus and prefrontal cortex of offspring were homogenized in extraction buffer (C500006, Sangon Biotech, Shanghai, China) according to the manufacturer's instructions. Each sample was adjusted to a final protein concentration of 1 μg/μl, mixed with Laemmeli's sample buffer, and boiled for 5 min. Samples (40 mg) were loaded onto 8% bisacrylamide gels and separated by sodium dodecyl sulphate polyacrylamide gel electrophoresis (SDS-PAGE). Proteins were electrophoretically transferred from gels to polyvinylidene fluoride (PVDF) membranes that were then incubated with the following primary antibodies: anti-BDNF (1:200 dilution, AV41970, Sigma-Aldrich, St. Louis, MO, USA), anti-SERT (1:200, AG1204, Abgent, San Diego, CA, USA), anti-CREB (1:500 dilution, ab31387, Abcam, Cambridge, MA, USA), anti-pCREB (1:500 dilution, ab32096, Abcam), and anti-GAPDH (1:2500 dilution, ab9485, Abcam). Dilutions of peroxidase-conjugated goat anti-rabbit IgG secondary antibody (1:2000 dilution, sc-2004, Santa Cruz Biotechnology, Dallas, TX, USA) were prepared following the manufacturer's instructions. Immuno-positive bands were visualized using a chemiluminescent method (G:BOX chemiXR5, SYNGEN, Sacramento, CA, USA), and the band densities were determined with the Gel-Pro32 software [39]. All western blotting experiments were repeated at least three times.

Statistical analysis

Data were analysed using GraphPad Prism version 7.0.4 (GraphPad Software, Inc., San Diego, California, USA). Outliers were defined as two or more standard deviations from the mean, and these were removed from the analysis [26]. The data were tested for normality (Kolmogorov–Smirnov test) and homoscedasticity (Levene's test) before being analysed using either unpaired t-tests or parametric repeated measures analysis of variance (ANOVA). The results from the behavioural tests were analysed using unpaired t-tests or two-way ANOVA, and neurochemical and biochemical data were analysed using unpaired *t*-tests. For all analyses, Bonferroni post hoc tests were performed following ANOVA where appropriate. Data are presented as mean ± standard error of the mean (SEM), and the level of significance for differences determined via ANOVA and post hoc testing was set at $p < 0.05$.

Results

Effects of SDS on body weight gain and behaviour of dams

The body weight gain of dams exposed to SDS was found to be significantly reduced compared to controls after 4 weeks of stress (Fig. 2). Statistical analyses revealed a significant effect of stress [$F(1, 9) = 5.516$, $p = 0.0434$] and a significant stress × time interaction [$F(4, 36) = 5.689$, $p = 0.0012$]. Subsequent Bonferroni post hoc tests confirmed a significant reduction in body weight gain in SDS animals after 3 weeks [$t(45) = 2.703$, $p = 0.0483$] or 4 weeks [$t(45) = 4.533$, $p = 0.0002$] of experimentation compared to controls.

At baseline and after 3 weeks of stress, both the SDS and control animals showed similar preferences for sucrose (Fig. 3). However, 4 weeks of stress reduced this preference in SDS animals (Fig. 3), and subsequent Bonferroni post hoc tests showed that the consumption of the 0.8% sucrose solution was significantly lower in the SDS group [$t(50) = 4.133$, $p = 0.0007$] than in control rats (Fig. 3). Two-way ANOVA revealed a significant effect of stress [$F(1, 10) = 7.04$, $p = 0.0242$].

In the OFT, there was a significant difference in the total distance and in the distance travelled in peripheral areas between the control and SDS groups after 4 weeks of stress. Subsequent Bonferroni post hoc tests

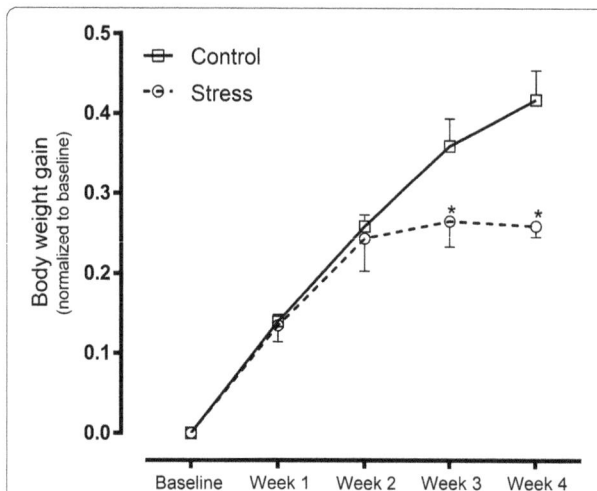

Fig. 3 Sucrose preference in maternal rats exposed to SDS as well as control rats at 4 weeks after induced stress. Control: control group (hollow square, n = 6); stress: SDS dams (hollow circle, n = 6); *p < 0.05

revealed that the SDS group showed a reduction in the total distance moved and in the distance travelled in the peripheral areas compared to controls (Fig. 4a–c). Two-way ANOVA revealed a significant effect of stress [total distance: $F(1, 10) = 19.3$, $p = 0.0014$; Peripheral area distance: $F(1, 10) = 19.87$, $p = 0.0012$]. There were also significant differences in the distance travelled in the centre area, in the time spent in the centre area, and in the number of rearings between the groups after 4 weeks of stress, and Bonferroni post hoc tests showed a significant decrease in those measures in the SDS group compared to controls [distance travelled: $t(50) = 3.086$, $p = 0.0165$; Time in centre area: $t(50) = 3.608$, $p = 0.0036$; Rearings: $t(50) = 3.002$, $p = 0.0209$] (Fig. 4a, d–f). Two-way ANOVA revealed a significant effect of stress [$F(1, 10) = 10.29$, $p = 0.0094$] on the distance travelled in the centre area, a significant effect of stress × time interaction [$F(4, 40) = 3.852$, $p = 0.0097$] and time [$F(4, 40) = 5.299$, $p = 0.0016$] on the time spent in the centre area, and a significant effect of time [$F(4, 40) = 3.577$, $p = 0.0138$] on the number of rearings.

Behavioural characterization of offspring subjected to pre-gestational SDS

In the OFT, locomotor activity was modified by pre-gestational SDS (Student's *t*-test). The total path length travelled was $40,277 \pm 1062$ mm for the control offspring and $20,607 \pm 3590$ mm for the stressed offspring (Fig. 5a, b). There was no significant difference in the maximum speed between the groups ($t(14) = 2.054$, $p = 0.0591$ [Student's *t*-test], SDS offspring: 533.6 ± 53.95 mm/s vs. control offspring: 676.2 ± 43.68 mm/s; Fig. 5c). The offspring subjected to pre-gestational SDS travelled a reduced

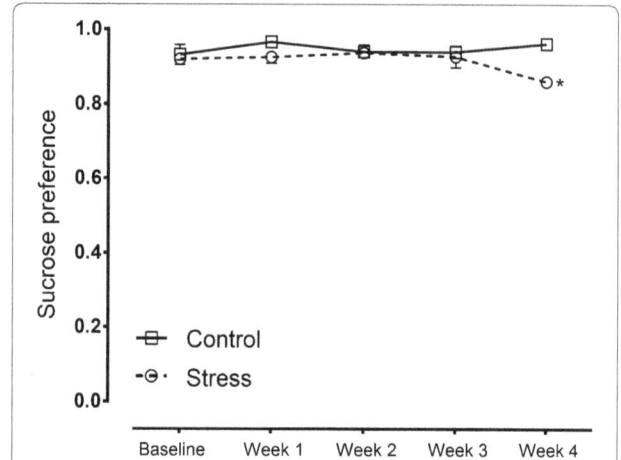

Fig. 2 Body weight gain of maternal rats exposed to SDS as well as control rats at 4 weeks after induced stress. Control: control group (hollow square, n = 6); stress: SDS dams (hollow circle, n = 5, outlier number = 1); *p < 0.05

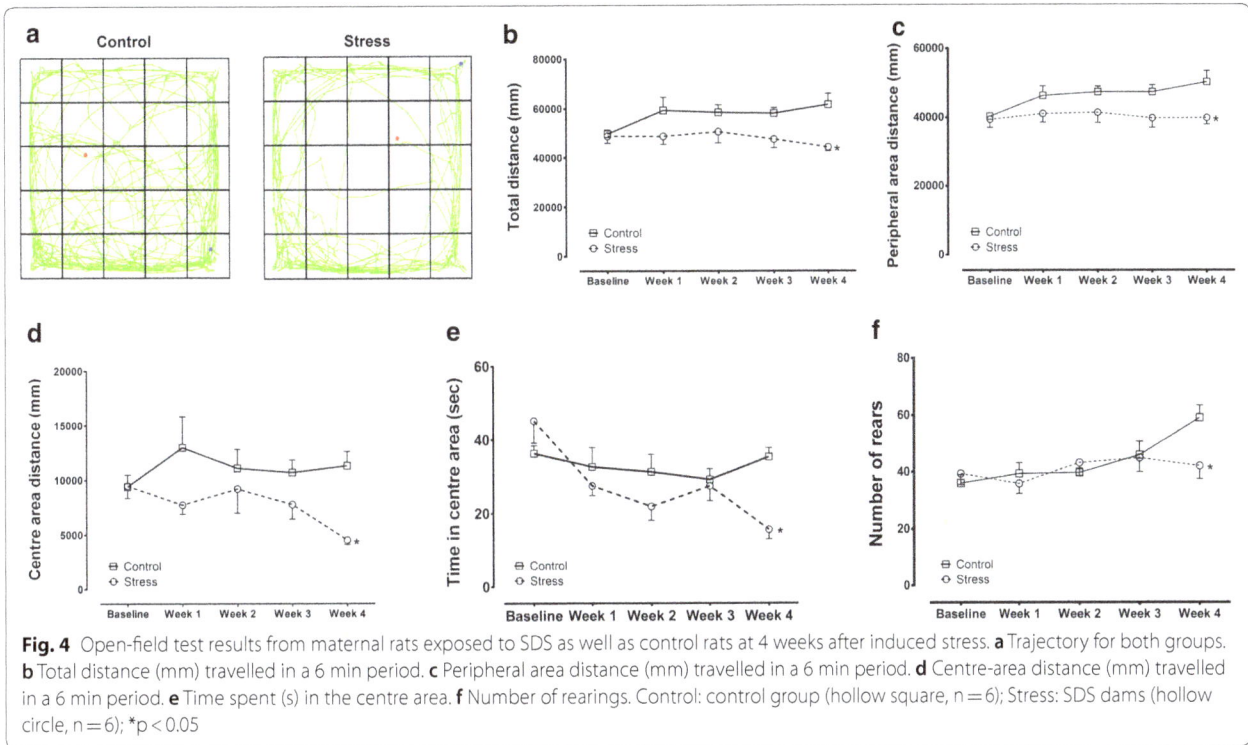

Fig. 4 Open-field test results from maternal rats exposed to SDS as well as control rats at 4 weeks after induced stress. **a** Trajectory for both groups. **b** Total distance (mm) travelled in a 6 min period. **c** Peripheral area distance (mm) travelled in a 6 min period. **d** Centre-area distance (mm) travelled in a 6 min period. **e** Time spent (s) in the centre area. **f** Number of rearings. Control: control group (hollow square, n=6); Stress: SDS dams (hollow circle, n=6); *p<0.05

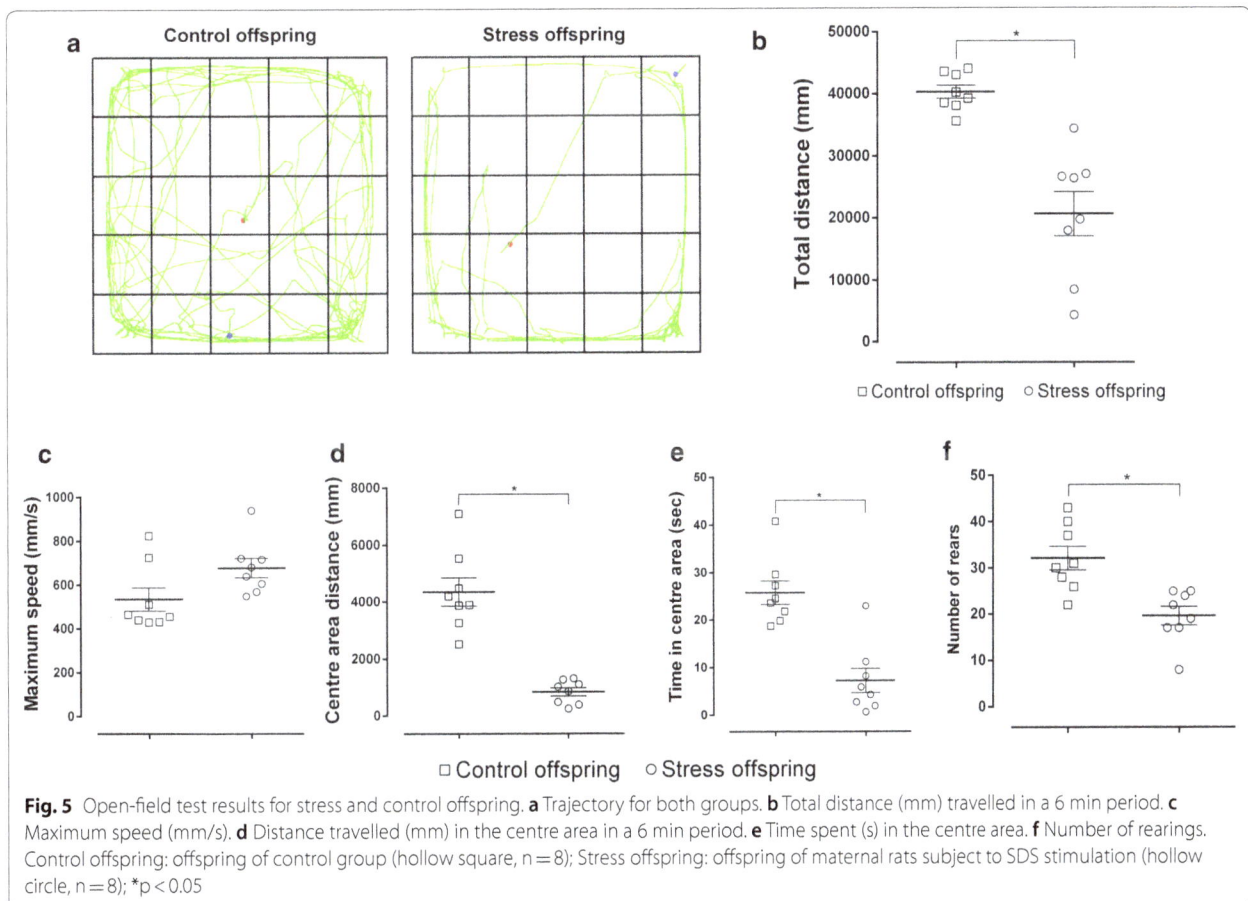

Fig. 5 Open-field test results for stress and control offspring. **a** Trajectory for both groups. **b** Total distance (mm) travelled in a 6 min period. **c** Maximum speed (mm/s). **d** Distance travelled (mm) in the centre area in a 6 min period. **e** Time spent (s) in the centre area. **f** Number of rearings. Control offspring: offspring of control group (hollow square, n=8); Stress offspring: offspring of maternal rats subject to SDS stimulation (hollow circle, n=8); *p<0.05

distance in the centre area and spent less time in the centre area than the control offspring (distance travelled: t(14)=6.754, p<0.05, SDS offspring=4349±500.3 mm vs. control offspring=829.4±145.4 mm; Time in centre area: t(14)=5.185, p<0.05 [Student's *t*-test], SDS offspring=25.74±2.499 s vs. control offspring=7.221±2.553 s; Fig. 5a, d, e). The pre-gestationally stressed offspring also reared less than the controls (t(14)=3.823, p=0.0019 [Student's *t*-test], SDS offspring=32.13±2.560 rearings vs. control offspring=19.63±2.035 rearings; Fig. 5a, f).

In the SPT, although all animals tested showed preference for the sucrose solution compared to water, sucrose intake (sucrose preference index and relative sucrose intake) was reduced in the offspring of SDS dams compared with controls (sucrose preference index: t(14)=5.782, p<0.05, SDS offspring=0.9656±0.008635 g/g bwt [body weight] vs. control offspring=0.8581±0.01647 g/g bwt; relative sucrose intake: t(14)=4.717, p=0.0003 [Student's *t*-test], SDS offspring=0.3245±0.02641 g/g bwt vs. control offspring=0.1679±0.02012 g/g bwt; Fig. 6a, b).

In the EPM, there was no significant difference in the distance travelled in the closed arm between the offspring subjected to pre-gestational SDS and control offspring (t(14)=0.799, p=0.4376, SDS offspring=13,281±1488 mm vs. control offspring=11,975±677.2 mm) (Fig. 7a, b). The total distance travelled in both the closed and open arms was 22,127±1228 mm for the control offspring and

17,130±1461 mm for the stressed offspring [t(14)=2.617, p=0.0203] (Fig. 7a, c). The total number of arm crosses was 29±2.507 for the control offspring and 20±2.471 for the stressed offspring [t(14)=2.557, p=0.0228] (Fig. 7d). Additionally, the offspring subjected to pre-gestational SDS showed a decrease in the percentage of open-arm staying time (OT%) and in the percentage of open-arm entries (OE %) compared to the control offspring (OT%: t(14)=6.290, p<0.05, SDS offspring=10.56±2.052% vs. control offspring=38.74±3.982%; OE%: t(14)=3.906, p=0.0016 [Student's *t*-test], SDS offspring=15.55±3.113% vs. control offspring=40.87±5.685%; Fig. 7a, e, f).

In the LDB, no difference was observed in the distance travelled in the dark compartment (t(14)=0.01819, p=0.9857, SDS offspring=9461±1088 mm vs. control offspring=9485±669.7 mm) (Fig. 8a, b). However, there was a remarkable reduction in the total distance travelled between the SDS offspring and controls (t(14)=3.718, p=0.0023 [Student's *t*-test], SDS offspring=11,316±1282 mm vs. control offspring=18,108±1302 mm; Fig. 8a, c). The offspring subjected to pre-gestational SDS spent less time in the light, made less light-side entries, and moved less in the light side compared with the controls (time in light: t(14)=5.895, p<0.05, SDS offspring=20.69±4.662 s vs. control offspring=103±13.15 s; Light-side entries: t(14)=4.425, p=0.0006, SDS offspring=2.125±0.6105 vs. control offspring=6.125±0.6665; Distance travelled in light area: t(14)=5.4, p<0.05 [Student's *t*-test],

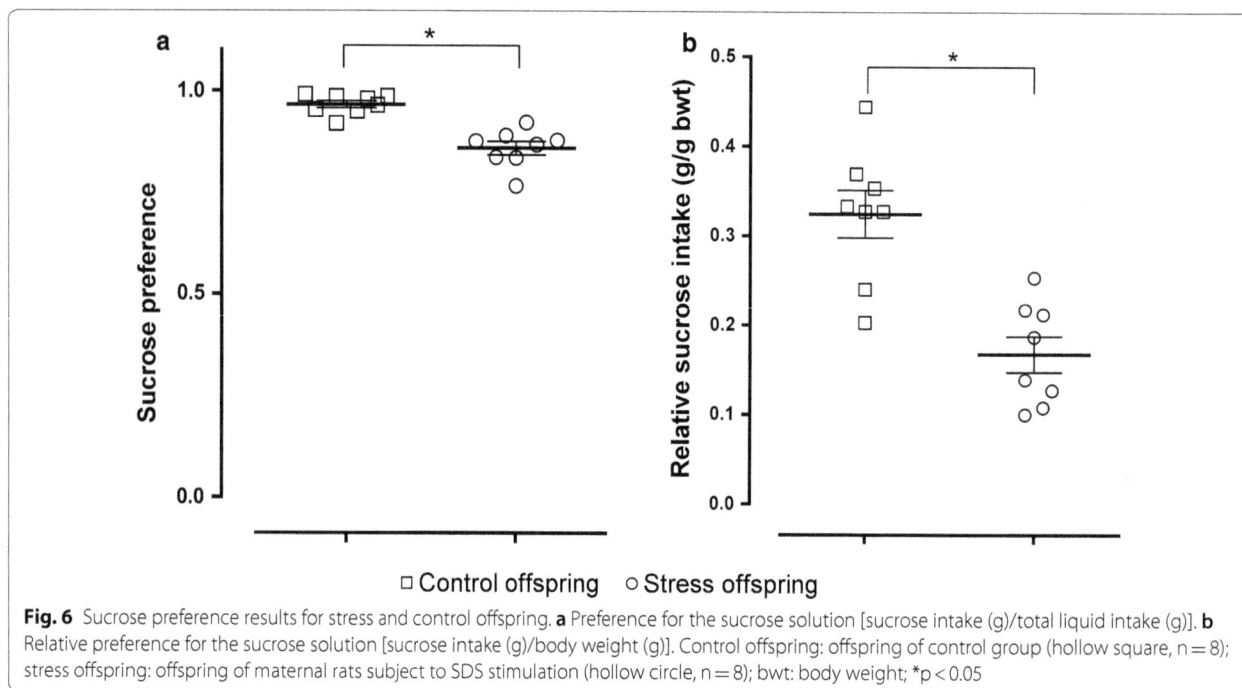

Fig. 6 Sucrose preference results for stress and control offspring. **a** Preference for the sucrose solution [sucrose intake (g)/total liquid intake (g)]. **b** Relative preference for the sucrose solution [sucrose intake (g)/body weight (g)]. Control offspring: offspring of control group (hollow square, n=8); stress offspring: offspring of maternal rats subject to SDS stimulation (hollow circle, n=8); bwt: body weight; *p<0.05

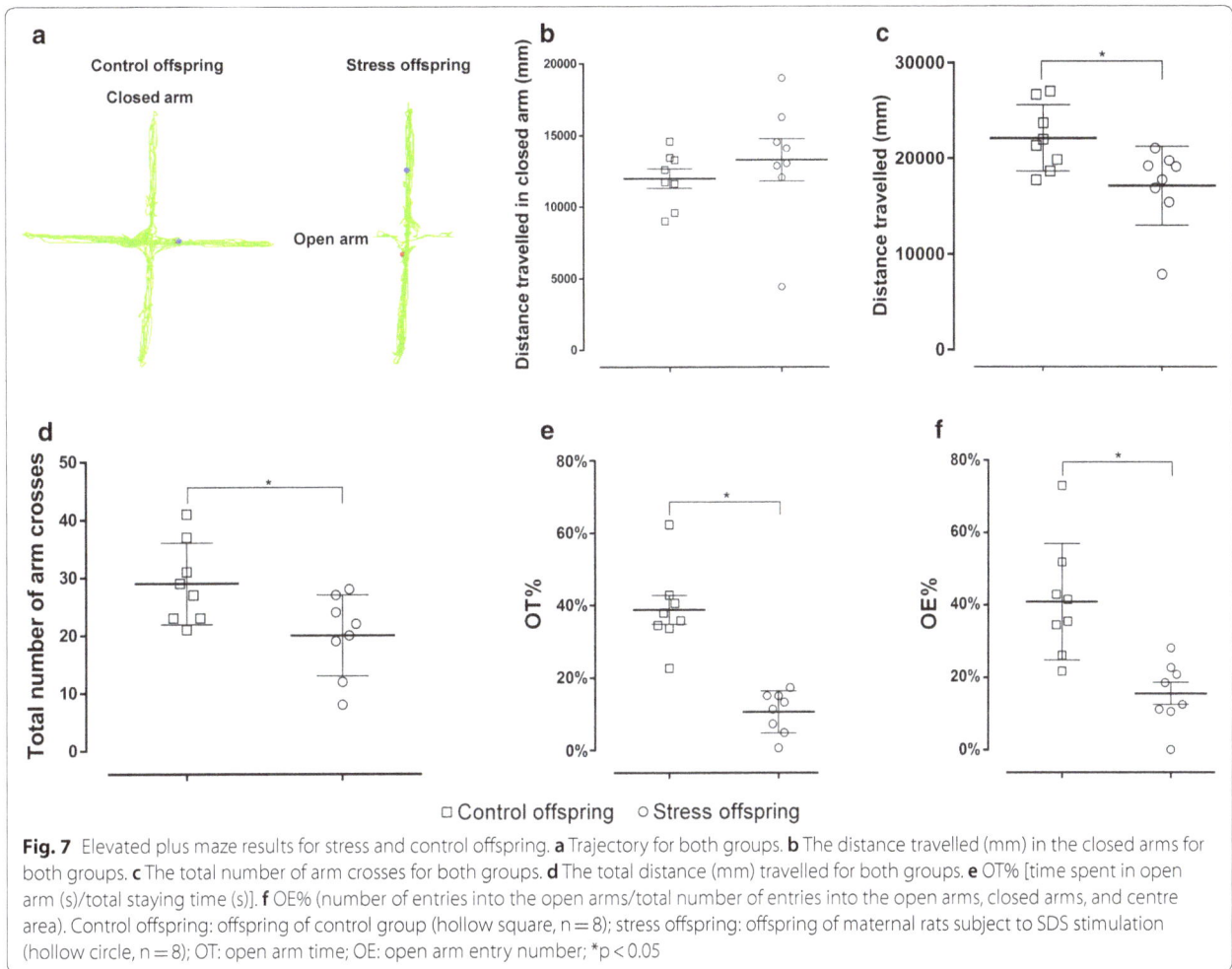

Fig. 7 Elevated plus maze results for stress and control offspring. **a** Trajectory for both groups. **b** The distance travelled (mm) in the closed arms for both groups. **c** The total number of arm crosses for both groups. **d** The total distance (mm) travelled for both groups. **e** OT% [time spent in open arm (s)/total staying time (s)]. **f** OE% (number of entries into the open arms/total number of entries into the open arms, closed arms, and centre area). Control offspring: offspring of control group (hollow square, n = 8); stress offspring: offspring of maternal rats subject to SDS stimulation (hollow circle, n = 8); OT: open arm time; OE: open arm entry number; *p < 0.05

SDS offspring = 1855 ± 463.2 mm vs. control offspring = 6123 ± 640.6 mm; Fig. 8a, d–f).

In the FST, the offspring of SDS dams showed increased immobility and a decreased latency to immobility compared to the controls (immobility: t(14) = 5.475, p < 0.05, SDS offspring = 78 ± 2.368 s vs. control offspring = 51 ± 4.326 s; latency to immobility: t(14) = 3.752, p = 0.0021 [Student's t-test], SDS offspring = 3.362 ± 0.5545 s vs. control offspring = 17.89 ± 3.834 s; Fig. 9a, b).

Effect of offspring subjected to pre-gestational SDS on cognition

In the acquisition phase of the MWM task, the overall analysis (repeated measures ANOVA) revealed no significant effect of pre-gestational stress on escape latency, distance swum to find the platform, or time spent in the SE zone (Fig. 10a–c). However, pre-gestational stress induced a significant impairment in the retention phase, that is, the stressed offspring had a prolonged escape latency compared to controls (t(14) = 4.984, p = 0.0002 [Student's t-test], SDS offspring = 10.03 ± 0.8083 s vs. control

offspring = 4.394 ± 0.7917 s; Fig. 10d, e). The distance swum by animals searching for the platform, time spent in the SE zone, and platform crossings were significantly lower in the offspring of SDS dams compared to controls (distance swum: t(14) = 5.516, p < 0.05, SDS offspring = 10,668 ± 382.3 mm vs. control offspring = 13,819 ± 424.5 mm; time spent in the SE zone: t(14) = 4.32, p = 0.0007, SDS offspring = 37.28 ± 2.047 s vs. control offspring = 50.58 ± 2.301 s; Platform crossings: t(14) = 2.763, p = 0.0152 [Student's t-test], SDS offspring = 8.125 ± 0.8543 vs. control offspring = 11.75 ± 0.9955; Fig. 10f–h).

In the novel object recognition test, offspring of stressed rats showed recognition memory deficits because the discrimination index was significantly lower for both the object recognition task with 1 h and 24 h memory retention (1 h retention: t(14) = 4.472, p = 0.0005, SDS offspring = 0.4844 ± 0.03877 vs. control offspring = 0.6935 ± 0.02613; 24 h retention: p = 0.0002 [Student's t-test], SDS offspring = 0.4987 ± 0.01535 vs. control offspring = 0.6314 ± 0.02255, t(14) = 4.868; Fig. 11).

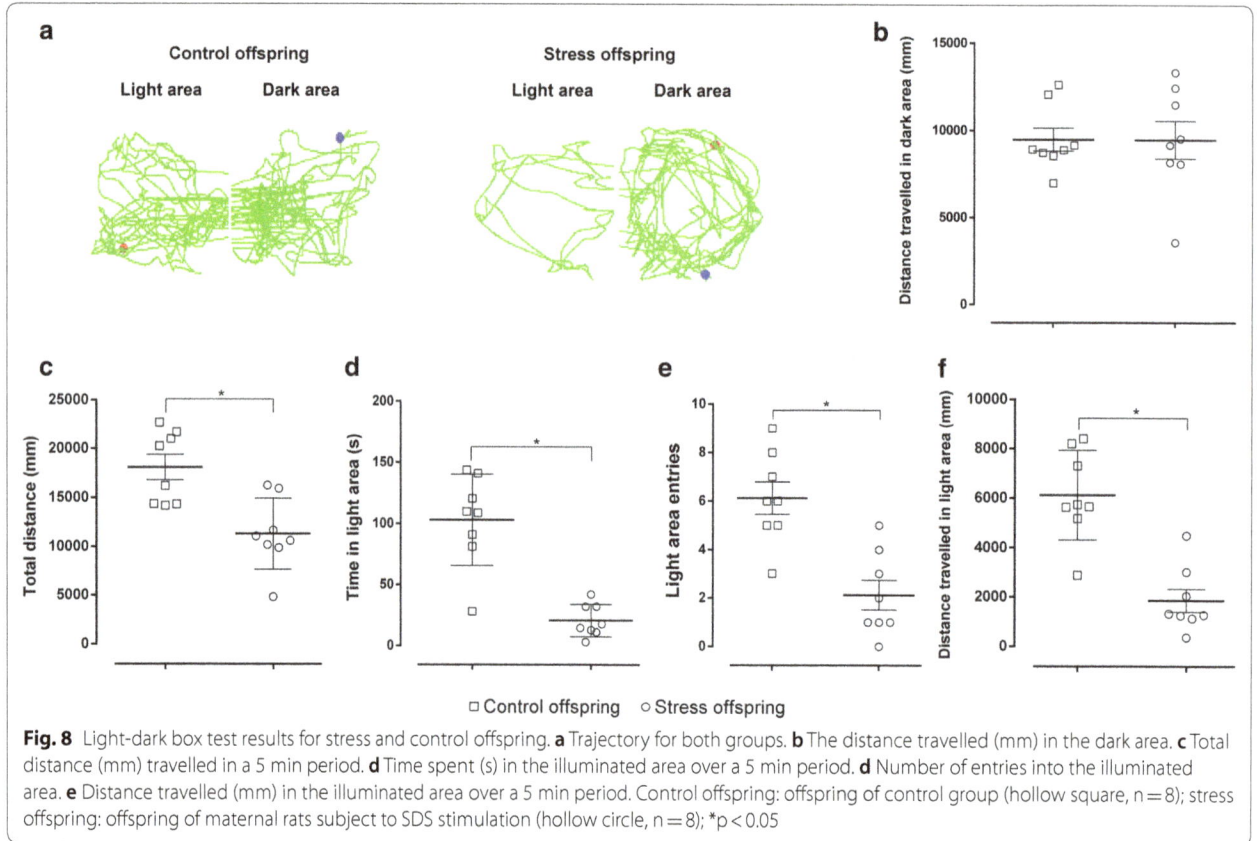

Fig. 8 Light-dark box test results for stress and control offspring. **a** Trajectory for both groups. **b** The distance travelled (mm) in the dark area. **c** Total distance (mm) travelled in a 5 min period. **d** Time spent (s) in the illuminated area over a 5 min period. **d** Number of entries into the illuminated area. **e** Distance travelled (mm) in the illuminated area over a 5 min period. Control offspring: offspring of control group (hollow square, n = 8); stress offspring: offspring of maternal rats subject to SDS stimulation (hollow circle, n = 8); *p < 0.05

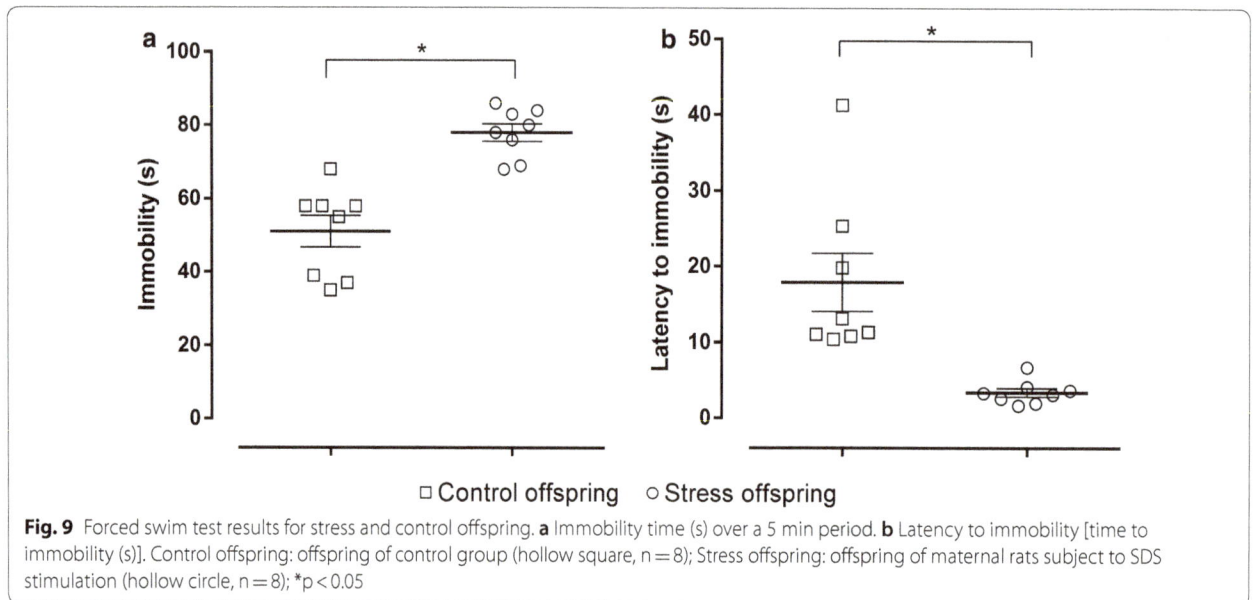

Fig. 9 Forced swim test results for stress and control offspring. **a** Immobility time (s) over a 5 min period. **b** Latency to immobility [time to immobility (s)]. Control offspring: offspring of control group (hollow square, n = 8); Stress offspring: offspring of maternal rats subject to SDS stimulation (hollow circle, n = 8); *p < 0.05

HPA responsiveness in offspring

As shown in Fig. 12, corticosterone and ACTH levels in the pre-gestationally stressed offspring were significantly higher than those of the control offspring (corticosterone: t(11) = 3.875, p = 0.0026, ACTH: t(14) = 3.045, p = 0.0087 [Student's t-test]).

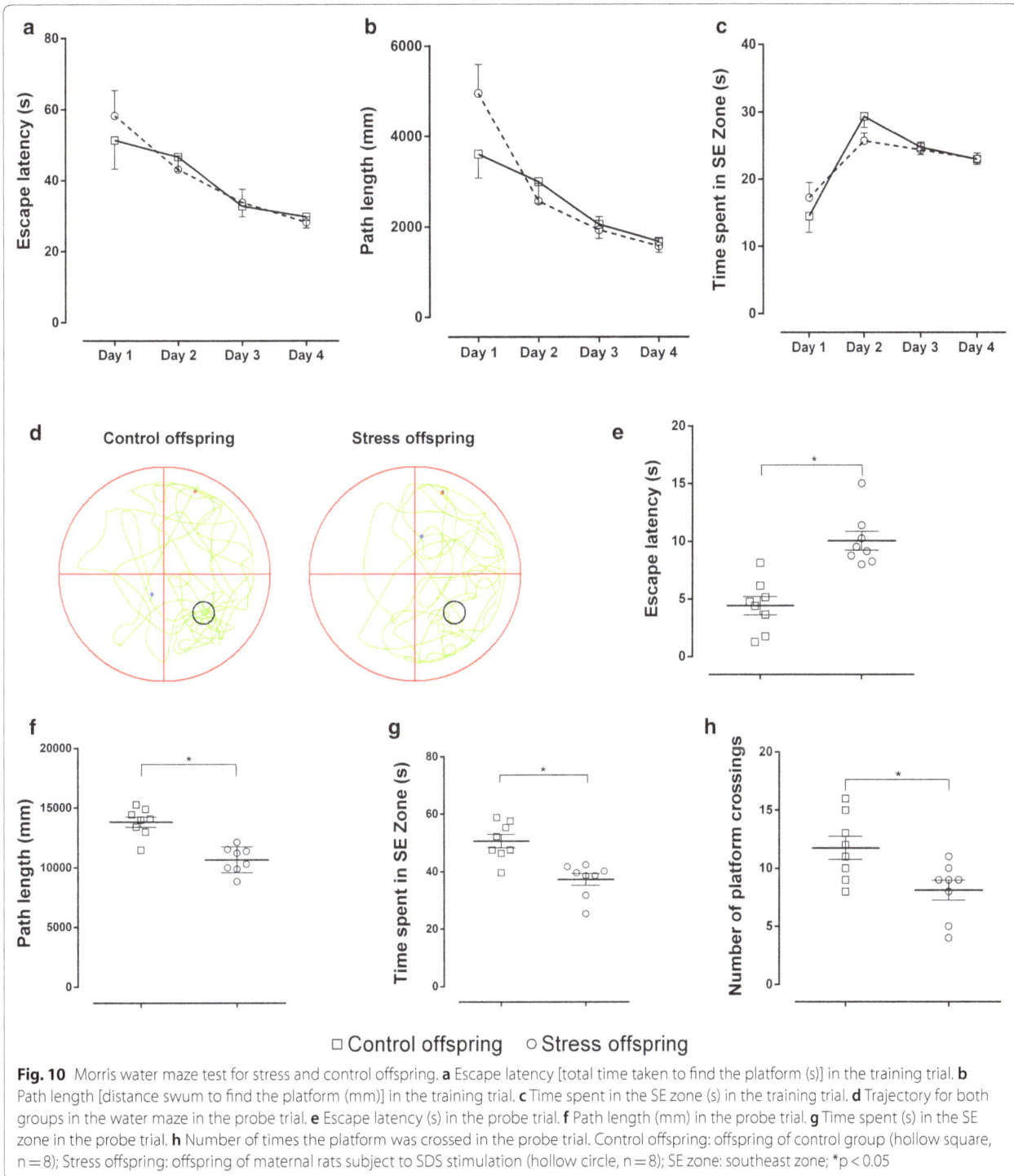

Fig. 10 Morris water maze test for stress and control offspring. **a** Escape latency [total time taken to find the platform (s)] in the training trial. **b** Path length [distance swum to find the platform (mm)] in the training trial. **c** Time spent in the SE zone (s) in the training trial. **d** Trajectory for both groups in the water maze in the probe trial. **e** Escape latency (s) in the probe trial. **f** Path length (mm) in the probe trial. **g** Time spent (s) in the SE zone in the probe trial. **h** Number of times the platform was crossed in the probe trial. Control offspring: offspring of control group (hollow square, n = 8); Stress offspring: offspring of maternal rats subject to SDS stimulation (hollow circle, n = 8); SE zone: southeast zone; *p < 0.05

The corticosterone levels were 170.7 ± 16.14 ng/ml and 99.52 ± 5.892 ng/ml for pre-gestationally stressed and control offspring, respectively, while ACTH values were 3.619 ± 0.1173 pg/ml and 2.918 ± 0.198 pg/ml, respectively.

Involvement of the monoaminergic system in the effects of pre-gestational stress in offspring

5-hydroxytryptamine levels were significantly lower in offspring of SDS dams compared to control offspring in the hippocampus (t(13) = 4.382, p = 0.0007, SDS offspring = 682 ± 38.57 ng/g vs.

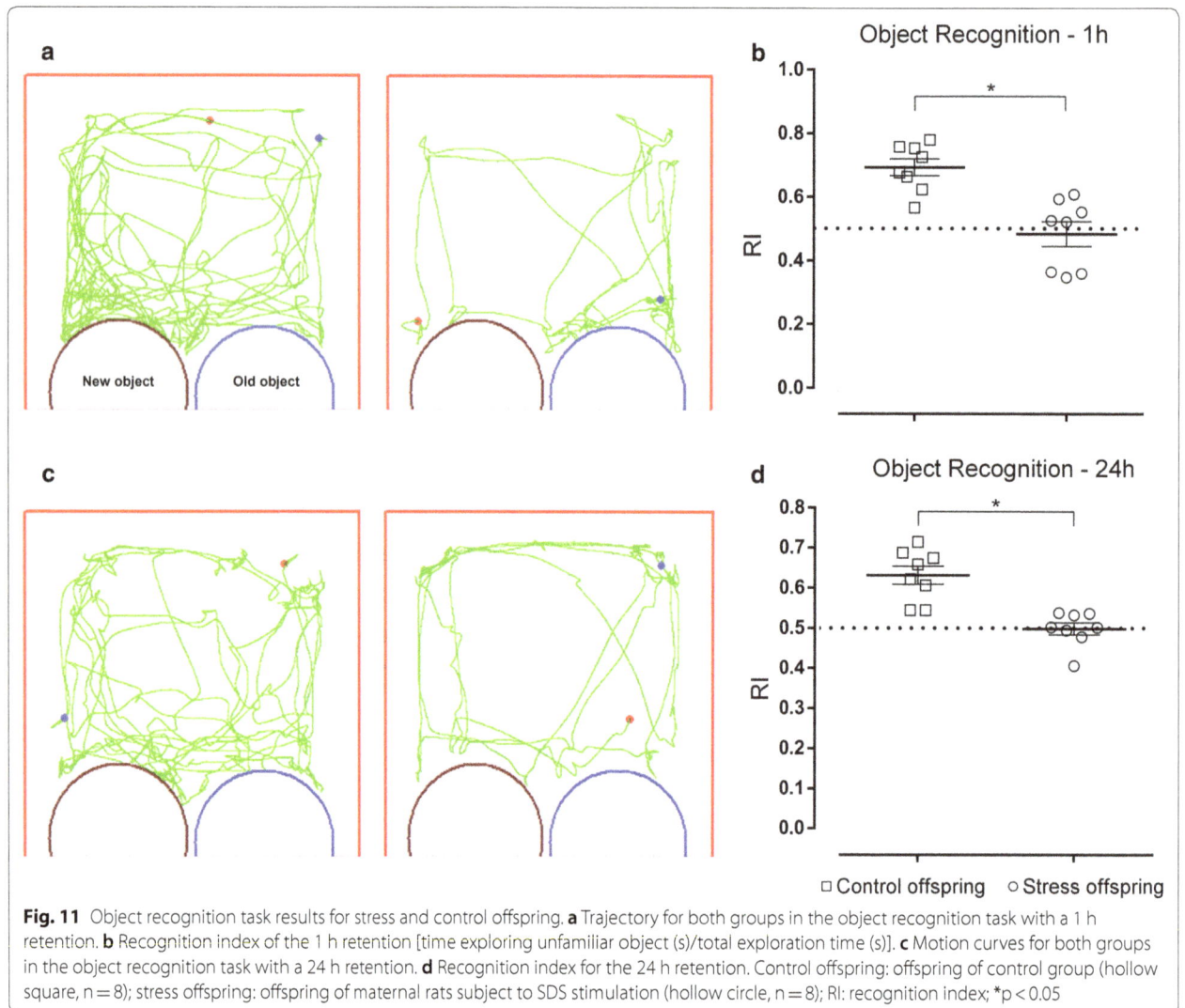

Fig. 11 Object recognition task results for stress and control offspring. **a** Trajectory for both groups in the object recognition task with a 1 h retention. **b** Recognition index of the 1 h retention [time exploring unfamiliar object (s)/total exploration time (s)]. **c** Motion curves for both groups in the object recognition task with a 24 h retention. **d** Recognition index for the 24 h retention. Control offspring: offspring of control group (hollow square, n = 8); stress offspring: offspring of maternal rats subject to SDS stimulation (hollow circle, n = 8); RI: recognition index; *p < 0.05

control offspring = 950.8 ± 48.64 ng/g), the hypothalamus (t(13) = 3.826, p = 0.0021, SDS offspring = 704.6 ± 28.38 ng/g vs. control offspring = 998 ± 75.64 ng/g), and the prefrontal cortex (t(11) = 3.273, p = 0.0074 [Student's t-test], SDS offspring = 782.2 ± 46.36 ng/g vs. control offspring = 1035 ± 63.81 ng/g; Fig. 13a–c).

However, noradrenaline and dopamine levels were significantly higher in the offspring of pre-gestationally stressed rats compared to the offspring of control rats both in the hippocampus (noradrenaline: t(13) = 4.533, p = 0.0006, SDS offspring = 1012 ± 78.51 pg/g vs. control offspring = 611.4 ± 46.49 pg/g; dopamine: t(10) = 4.565, p = 0.001, SDS offspring = 146.6 ± 7.996 ng/g vs. control offspring = 91.45 ± 9.052 ng/g) and in the prefrontal cortex (noradrenaline: t(9) = 2.979, p = 0.0155, SDS offspring = 1036 ± 62.13 pg/g vs. control offspring = 703.8 ± 87.13 pg/g; dopamine: t(8) = 3.352, p = 0.01

[Student's t-test], SDS offspring = 31.84 ± 2.055 ng/g vs. control offspring = 24.04 ± 1.091 ng/g; Fig. 13d, g, f, i).

Effects of pre-gestational SDS on the expression of BDNF, pCREB, and SERT in the hippocampus and the prefrontal cortex of offspring

As shown in Fig. 14a, c, the relative optical density of BDNF and pCREB in the hippocampus and the prefrontal cortex of pre-gestationally stressed offspring was significantly lower in controls (BDNF hippocampus: t(6) = 8.228, p = 0.0002, SDS offspring = 0.1099 ± 0.05645 vs. control offspring = 1.037 ± 0.09748; BDNF prefrontal cortex: t(6) = 7.413, p = 0.0003, SDS offspring = 0.3782 ± 0.0363 vs. control offspring = 0.8606 ± 0.05401; pCREB hippocampus: t(6) = 6.239, p = 0.0008, SDS

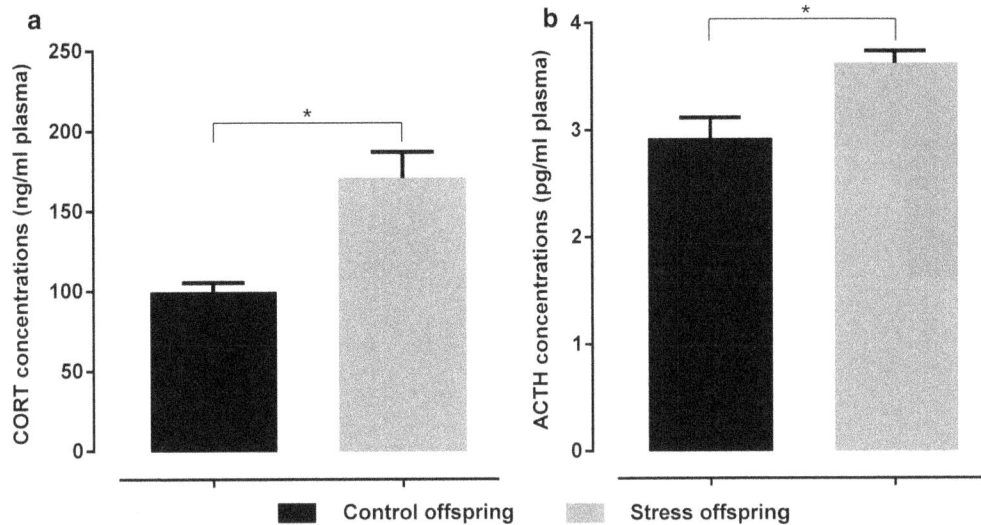

Fig. 12 a CORT plasma concentrations (ng/ml plasma) in stress and control offspring (n = 6, outlier number = 2 for Control offspring; n = 7, outlier number = 1 for Stress offspring). **b** ACTH plasma concentrations (pg/ml plasma) in stress and control offspring (n = 8 for Control offspring; n = 8 for Stress offspring). Control offspring: offspring of control group (black); Stress offspring: offspring of maternal rats subject to SDS stimulation (grey); CORT: corticosterone; ACTH: adrenocorticotropic hormone; *p < 0.05

offspring = 0.2464 ± 0.09318 vs. control offspring = 1.026 ± 0.08334; pCREB prefrontal cortex: t(6) = 4.038, p = 0.0068 [Student's t-test], SDS offspring = 0.217 ± 0.05386 vs. control offspring = 0.8223 ± 0.1399).

As shown in Fig. 14b, there was no significant difference between the relative optical density of CREB in the hippocampus and prefrontal cortex of pre-gestationally stressed offspring and controls (hippocampus: t(6) = 0.2529, p = 0.8088, SDS offspring = 1.342 ± 0.0916 vs. control offspring = 1.307 ± 0.103; prefrontal cortex: t(6) = 0.3728, p = 0.7221 [Student's t-test], SDS offspring = 1.101 ± 0.05346 vs. control offspring = 1.13 ± 0.05984).

There was a significant increase in the relative optical density of SERT in the hippocampus and prefrontal cortex of SDS offspring compared to controls (hippocampus: t(6) = 17.95, p < 0.0001, SDS offspring = 1.07 ± 0.04871 vs. control offspring = 0.1014 ± 0.02325; prefrontal cortex: t(6) = 13.18, p < 0.0001 [Student's t-test], SDS offspring = 0.8166 ± 0.03799 vs. control offspring = 0.1496 ± 0.03341; Fig. 14d).

Discussion

Chronic SDS in dams induces depressive-like behaviours

The first step in our investigation was to analyse whether the stress paradigm was effective or not in triggering the stress response in adult female rats. The dams exposed to social isolation and defeat stress showed lower body weight gain than the control group (Fig. 2), and this was

comparable to results that have previously been reported in studies using a similar stress paradigm [40–42]. The limbic brain regions of the rats exposed to chronic stress were reported to show increased glutamate release [43], which in turn increased the demand for energy provided through lipid catabolism [44].

OFT was also designed to confirm the effect of our social defeat stress. Both the affective and motivational status of an animal can be determined by the initial activity of the animal when placed in an unfamiliar environment [29, 45], and it is generally believed that the responses of animals to an open but inescapable area are reflections of both the stress and reward induced by unfamiliar things [29]. In rats, reduced exploratory behaviour in an unfamiliar environment reflects a 'refractory loss of interest' [46] that is related to anhedonia [46, 47] because strange things are normally seen as rewarding in rats [47]. Exploratory behaviour, defined as the time taken by animals to explore unfamiliar environments, is very sensitive to past stress experiences [48]; however, the effects of physical stress tend to become attenuated following increased exposure to the stressors [49]. In the current paradigm, we explored the effects of chronic and sub-chronic social stress on open-field activities. Four weeks of social isolation and defeat stress significantly reduced the activity of stressed rats (Fig. 4b), and similar results have also been shown in a different SDS paradigm with adult rats and mice [29, 40, 42, 43]. Reduced exploratory behaviour in unfamiliar environments is also associated

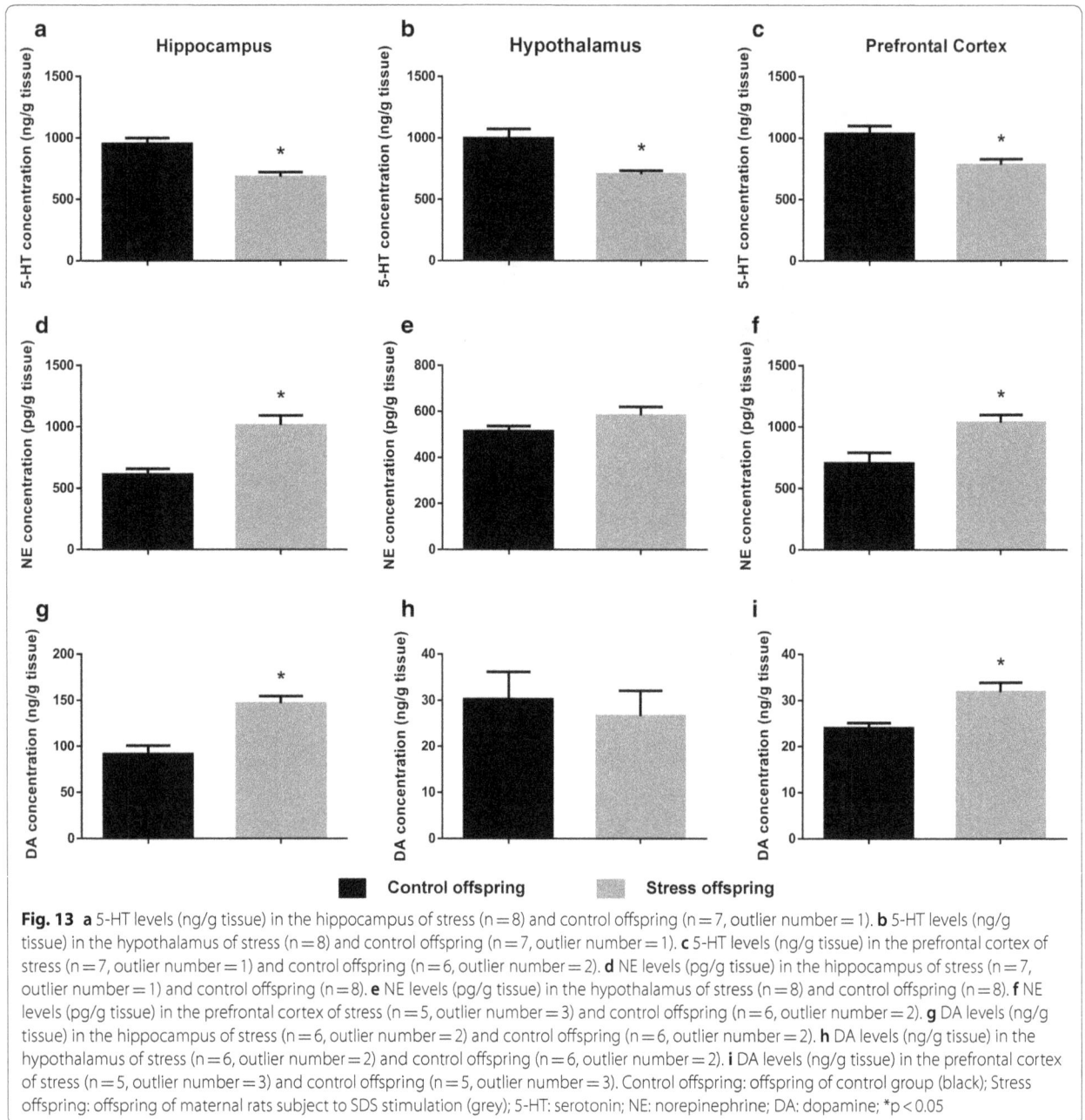

Fig. 13 **a** 5-HT levels (ng/g tissue) in the hippocampus of stress (n = 8) and control offspring (n = 7, outlier number = 1). **b** 5-HT levels (ng/g tissue) in the hypothalamus of stress (n = 8) and control offspring (n = 7, outlier number = 1). **c** 5-HT levels (ng/g tissue) in the prefrontal cortex of stress (n = 7, outlier number = 1) and control offspring (n = 6, outlier number = 2). **d** NE levels (pg/g tissue) in the hippocampus of stress (n = 7, outlier number = 1) and control offspring (n = 8). **e** NE levels (pg/g tissue) in the hypothalamus of stress (n = 8) and control offspring (n = 8). **f** NE levels (pg/g tissue) in the prefrontal cortex of stress (n = 5, outlier number = 3) and control offspring (n = 6, outlier number = 2). **g** DA levels (ng/g tissue) in the hippocampus of stress (n = 6, outlier number = 2) and control offspring (n = 6, outlier number = 2). **h** DA levels (ng/g tissue) in the hypothalamus of stress (n = 6, outlier number = 2) and control offspring (n = 6, outlier number = 2). **i** DA levels (ng/g tissue) in the prefrontal cortex of stress (n = 5, outlier number = 3) and control offspring (n = 5, outlier number = 3). Control offspring: offspring of control group (black); Stress offspring: offspring of maternal rats subject to SDS stimulation (grey); 5-HT: serotonin; NE: norepinephrine; DA: dopamine; *p < 0.05

with enhanced anxiety levels in stressed animals [29], which is shown by reductions in the distance travelled in the central area and the time spent in the central area in stressed animals compared to controls (Fig. 4d, e). Similar results were also found [50] using Lewis rats exposed to SDS, in line with our findings. The unidirectional effects of social stress on locomotion (Fig. 4b, d, e) and rearing (Fig. 4f) suggest that the parameters chosen for exploratory activity should be dependent on the overall activity of the animals [29]. This is consistent

with a report by Thiel et al. [51], who suggested that rearing and locomotor activity are related. It is noteworthy that there are also reports on the absence of any relationships between those two behaviours [52], and that is why we analysed all parameters of the OFT separately.

Over time, the rats exposed to chronic social stress showed decreased sucrose preference (Fig. 3), indicating a reduction in the sensitivity of stressed rats to reward, which is possibly homologous to anhedonia [53]. Similar

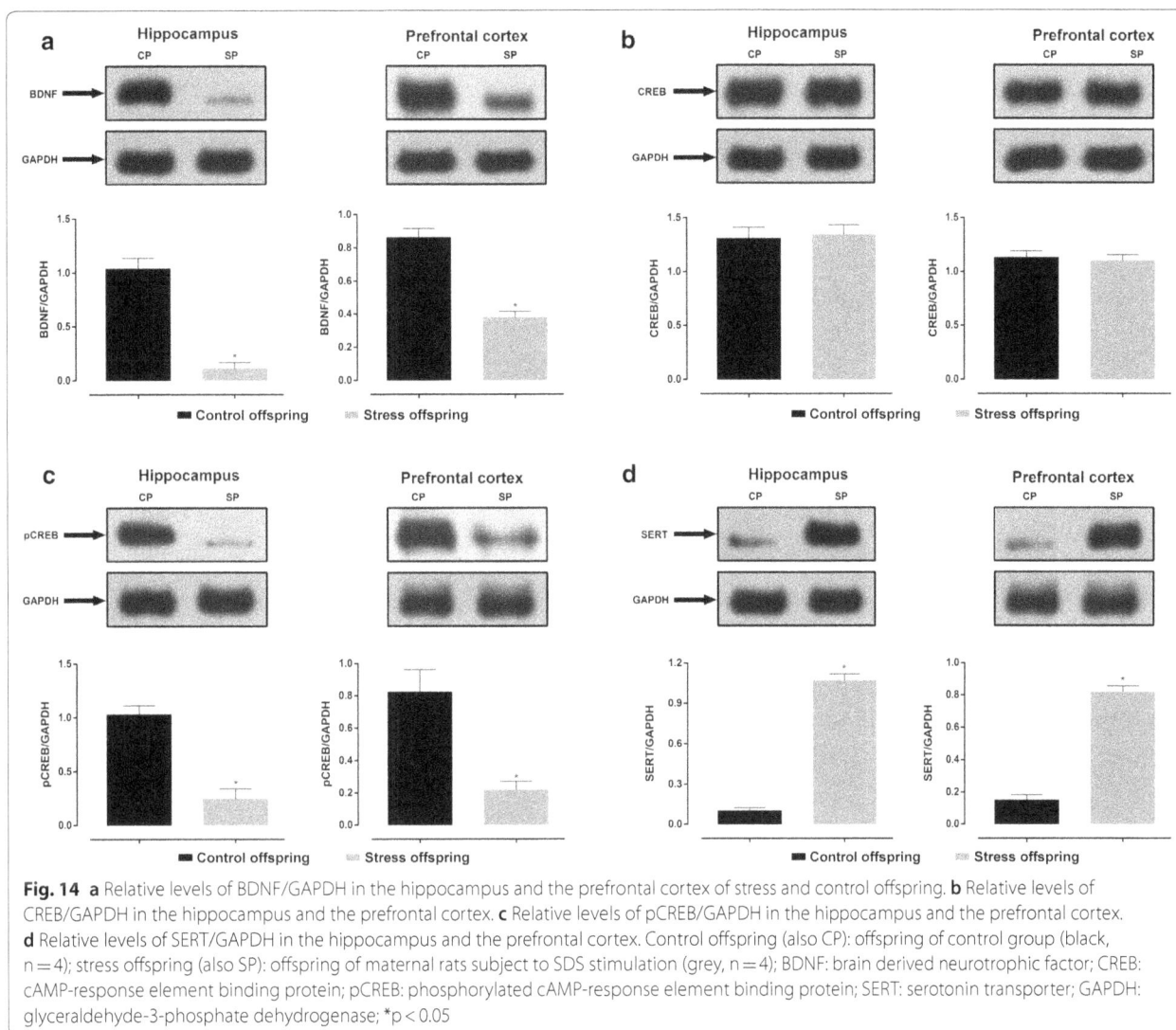

Fig. 14 a Relative levels of BDNF/GAPDH in the hippocampus and the prefrontal cortex of stress and control offspring. **b** Relative levels of CREB/GAPDH in the hippocampus and the prefrontal cortex. **c** Relative levels of pCREB/GAPDH in the hippocampus and the prefrontal cortex. **d** Relative levels of SERT/GAPDH in the hippocampus and the prefrontal cortex. Control offspring (also CP): offspring of control group (black, n = 4); stress offspring (also SP): offspring of maternal rats subject to SDS stimulation (grey, n = 4); BDNF: brain derived neurotrophic factor; CREB: cAMP-response element binding protein; pCREB: phosphorylated cAMP-response element binding protein; SERT: serotonin transporter; GAPDH: glyceraldehyde-3-phosphate dehydrogenase; *p < 0.05

effects have also been observed in other SDS paradigms [29, 40, 54].

Our data show that the chronic SDS experienced by rats induces depressive-like behavioural changes similar to those observed in humans [53, 55]. According to the DSM-IV criteria of the American Psychiatric Association, anhedonia occurs in patients with depression and opioid withdrawal and is characterised by a loss of interest and an incapacity to feel pleasure and joy, even in the case of normal positive stimuli. In our model, the reduced sucrose preference suggests desensitisation of the brain's reward mechanism, while reduced locomotor activity and exploratory behaviours represent a lack of interest in unfamiliar stimuli, which may be indicative of motivational deficits. Anhedonia is one of the core symptoms of depression, and our results suggest that the current SDS

paradigm might reliably simulate human depressive-like symptoms in rats.

Chronic SDS in dams induces anxiety- and depressive-like behavioural changes accompanied by cognitive impairments in offspring

The male offspring of the dams exposed to SDS showed a profound decrease in the total path length travelled, path length travelled in the central area, time spent in the central area, and number of rearings in the open field compared with the offspring of the control group. This indicates that the offspring of stressed rats have significantly decreased locomotor and exploratory activities. These behavioural changes are consistent with those of stressed dams.

The offspring of the stressed dams showed a reduction in sucrose preference and relative sucrose preference, which was analysed to eliminate the effects of body weight on sucrose intake [5] (Fig. 6a, b). The decrease in sucrose intake represents a lack of preference for the sucrose solution [56], which is considered to be indicative of anhedonia [24]. Therefore, the results of our sucrose preference experiment show that the offspring of dams displaying depressive-like behaviours are at risk for developing depressive-like behaviours themselves.

The LDB and EPM are the most commonly used unconditioned tests to measure spontaneous approach-avoidance behaviours [57–59]. The time spent in the illuminated area, the number of entries into the illuminated area, and the distance travelled in the illuminated area in the LDB, as well as the OT% and OE% in the EPM, are mainly related to anxiety-like behaviours of animals [35, 60]. It has been shown that stressed male rats display significantly enhanced anxiety-like behaviours compared with controls and that SDS significantly decreased OT% in the EPM in rats [61]. On the other hand, the total path length travelled in the LDB and the EPM mainly reflects the overall activity of the animals [60], and we found that the offspring of stressed dams seemed to be significantly less active than the offspring of the control group, which is consistent with the results shown with regard to the total distance travelled in the OFT (Figs. 5, 7, 8). In order to overcome the problem of locomotor activity observed in the EPM and the LDB, we also measured the distance travelled in the closed arms of the EPM as well as in the dark compartment of the LDT, and found no difference in these measures between the groups (Figs. 7b, 8b). This suggests that stressed offspring indeed display an anxiety-like phenotype that is not due to a locomotor activity deficit. Thus, our results from the EPM and LDB indicate that the offspring of stressed dams show depressive and anxiety-like behaviours that were induced and occurred in their mothers.

The FST is the most widely used tool for the preclinical evaluation of antidepressant activity, and immobility in the FST is thought to reflect the failure of persistent escape-oriented behaviours and the development of passive behaviours from an active coping style towards stressful stimuli in animals. The reduction in immobility time after antidepressant treatment reflects the antidepressant activity of a drug [10]. In our experiment, the offspring of the stressed group showed increased immobility and a decreased latency to immobility compared to controls (Fig. 9). This can be explained by the hypothesis that the increase in immobility time induced by psychosocial stress is indicative of depressive-like behaviour [62, 63], which is representative of the loss of motivation and behavioural despair observed in patients with depression [10].

The spatial memory test showed that the memory acquisition ability of the offspring of the stressed group in the MWM was normal but that their ability to retrieve memories was impaired. As such, although there were no differences in escape latency, platform quadrant swimming distance, and the time spent swimming between the offspring of the stressed and control groups in the training phase (Fig. 10a–c), the benefits obtained from the previous long-term retention test were decreased. This manifested as a prolonged escape latency in the probe phase of the MWM and a significant decrease in swimming distance, time in the target quadrant, and number of platform crossings (Fig. 10f–h).

The ORT is used to assess recognition memory in animals, namely, non-spatial memories of facts and events [36]. In the ORT training phase, the offspring from the different treatment groups spent the same amount of time exploring the same two objects (RI > 50%), which indicates that exploration of unfamiliar objects takes longer than the exploration of familiar objects. However, after 1 h and 24 h memory retention, the offspring from the stressed group showed a significant decrease in the RI value, indicating a lower preference for unfamiliar objects compared to the offspring from the control group (Fig. 11).

In general, our data show that chronic SDS in dams can induce anxiety- and depressive-like behavioural changes accompanied by cognitive impairments in their offspring.

Behavioural abnormalities in offspring of stressed dams are related to changes in the hypothalamic–pituitary–adrenal (HPA)-axis, the monoaminergic system, and transcriptional factors

In rats, reduced body weight gain and increased adrenal gland weight are reliable indicators of stress [10, 64]. It has been reported that rats following SDS and chronic unpredictable mild stress (CUMS) paradigms have increased adrenal gland weight [10, 65]. The increased adrenal gland weight in stressed animals may reflect hyperactivation of the HPA axis [10]. This is also shown by the significant increase in plasma concentrations of ACTH and CORT in the offspring of stressed rats compared to controls (Fig. 12). These results suggest that the offspring of dams exposed to SDS have an over-activated HPA axis and increased ACTH and CORT secretion.

The serotonergic system and the noradrenergic system play key roles in regulating the functional neural circuits of the brain and are involved in hippocampal-dependent memory [19, 20]. All brain regions involved in the stress response, such as the hippocampus, the hypothalamus, and the prefrontal cortex, represent the most relevant areas for depression [21, 22]. A decrease in levels of 5-HT was observed in the hypothalamus, the hippocampus, and the prefrontal cortex (Fig. 13a–c), but an increase in NE levels was observed only in the hippocampus and the prefrontal cortex (Fig. 13e, f) of the offspring of the stressed group compared with controls. Substantial evidence has shown that there are abnormalities in the NE and 5-HT neurotransmitter systems in depression and anxiety, and most of the evidence supports an underactivation of the 5-HT system and complex dysfunction of the NE system (most of the results indicate overactivation of this system) [4, 66].

An earlier study has shown that the DA system in the brain plays a key role in modulating the social behaviours of experimental animals [67]. Defeat promotes dopamine metabolism in the mesencephalic cortex and mesencephalic marginal zones in rats and mice [68, 69]. In addition, social defeat-related clues shown to rodents that have previously experienced defeat increase the release of DA in the mesencephalic cortex zone and meso-nucleus accumbens [69, 70]. Our experimental results also confirmed this change (Fig. 13g–i). In fact, activation of the DA system in the mesencephalic cortex region is a well-known stress response, and a number of studies have shown that the conditional increase in the metabolism and release of DA in the mesencephalic cortical zone and meso-nucleus accumbens is related to aversive experiences [71, 72]. The DA projection in the midbrain prefrontal cortex is selectively affected by a variety of mild stressors [73–75]. Some reports have suggested that the activation of dopaminergic neurons in the prefrontal cortex reflects emotionality and anticipatory fear. It has been argued that the release of dopamine in stress-related brain regions may be involved in the execution of cognitive activities aimed at eliminating or responding to stressors [74, 76], while another hypothesis attributes changes in dopamine to emotional arousal and the attempt to deal with the social stressor [69].

Notably, these abnormalities of the HPA-related monoaminergic system were observed in offspring of SDS dams, not the SDS dams themselves, in the present study. Our experiments show that the exposure of dams to chronic SDS alters the emotional behaviour, learning, and memory functions of their offspring. This is also accompanied by in vivo abnormalities in HPA-related hormones, the monoaminergic system, and transcriptional regulation factors (Fig. 14) such as CREB and BDNF. The above findings are consistent with the report by Zhang et al. [18], who also showed that the oral administration of CORT to rats unexposed to SDS increased SERT protein levels in the dorsal raphe nuclei, the hippocampus, the frontal cortex, and the amygdala. Furthermore, they also found that using antagonists of the glucocorticoid receptor, mifepristone and spironolactone (both alone and in combination), inhibited the increase in SERT protein levels in cerebral regions induced by SDS or orally administered CORT. Therefore, the increase in SERT protein levels in the dorsal raphe nuclei and forebrain limbic structures induced by SDS is primarily induced by CORT via the corticosteroid receptors [18]. This links changes in HPA axis-modulating hormones to changes in monoamine neurotransmitter levels in the offspring in this study. We speculate that chronic SDS causes an imbalance in the parental neuro-endocrine-immune network that affects the secretion of HPA axis regulatory hormones through the mother-placenta-foetus interface.

It has been suggested that in addition to serving as a neurotrophic factor during development BDNF regulates synaptic plasticity [77] and is involved in stress-induced hippocampal adaptation and the pathogenesis of depression [78]. This viewpoint is supported by the following facts: (a) exogenous BDNF exerts antidepressant activity [79, 80], and (b) antidepressant therapy inhibits the stress-induced reduction in BDNF mRNA and protein in the hippocampus [81]. Stress-induced increases in glucocorticoids are accompanied by structural changes in certain brain regions, neuronal damage, as well as decreased BDNF expression in the hippocampus, which can be blocked by chronic electroconvulsive shock and antidepressant treatments [82]. The monoaminergic signalling pathway mainly acts through G proteins leading to changes in adenylate cyclase activity [83] and increases in circulating cAMP causing the activation of protein kinase A (PKA), which is reportedly increased after chronic antidepressant treatment [84]. A key molecule related to the long-term protein expression changes observed following the activation of PKA and other signal transduction pathways is the constitutively expressed transcription factor CREB [85]. pCREB can regulate a variety of target genes involved in the pathophysiology of depressive disorders [24, 85]. In our experiment, the relative levels of pCREB/GAPDH in the hippocampus and prefrontal cortex of the male offspring of stressed dams were significantly lower than that of controls (Fig. 14c). This result is in keeping with the findings of Honghai et al. [4, 22]. The possible mechanism therein is that CREB acts as a third messenger and through its activated form, pCREB, acts on the promoters (the so-called fourth messengers) of target genes (e.g., BDNF, dynorphin, fos, and corticotropin releasing factor [CRF]) via its cognate gene regulatory element CRE (cAMP response element), thus causing/mediating subsequent physiological responses [85]. Taking previously reported works and our findings together, we also speculate that abnormal fluctuations in these neurosteroids induce a change in the levels of proteins such as SERT via the glucocorticoid receptor, thus affecting levels of neurotransmitters such as 5-HT,

NE, and DA. These neurotransmitters are involved in the activation of CREB as a first messenger and influence the expression and regulation of multiple genes relevant to depressive- and anxiety-like behaviours, ultimately leading to abnormal behavioural phenotypes in the male offspring of SDS dams. In fact, our results from the association analysis between offspring behavioural phenotype and neurochemical indices also showed that the total distance travelled in the OFT, sucrose preference in the SPT, and the recognition index in the ORT were significantly positively correlated with BDNF and pCREB levels and were significantly negatively correlated with SERT.

Summary and limitations of current study

In summary, our results show that (a) the maternal social defeat paradigm may reliably imitate human depressive-like symptoms; (b) the maternal rats experiencing SDS pass their anxiety- and depressive-like behaviours on to their offspring; and (c) the abnormal behaviours observed in the offspring may involve HPA axis regulatory hormones, the monoaminergic system, and changes in transcriptional regulation factors such CREB and BDNF. Moreover, there is evidence to suggest that dams exposed to SDS also experience the same physiological and biochemical changes, showing a homology of behavioural phenotypes and neurobiochemical profiles between the dams and their offspring. Recently, many studies have presented evidence that parental influences on offspring occur through changes in the epigenetic modification in germline stem cells [86–89]. We were not sure if the influence of maternal SDS before pregnancy on offspring behaviours and neurological damages occurs in a similar manner, and this needs to be further studied.

This work has some potential limitations. First, we did not examine maternal care behaviours (e.g. nursing, grooming, etc.), which could have also been affected by SDS. The SDS dams also did not cross-foster the pups. As a result, the "passing on" behavioural deficits could be a mixture of nature and nurture.

Interestingly, other groups found that offspring of the socially defeated paternal side also display anxiety- and depression-related behaviours [90]. Although we used separately fed paternal rats with sexual experience and statistically equal open-field and sucrose preference scores as the mating partners of SDS maternal rats, we failed to thoroughly eliminate the adverse effect of individual variability in paternal stress history.

Another concern might be that blood and brain tissues were collected after a series of behavioural experiments. We did not assess whether the neurobiological outcomes would have been influenced by the behavioural tests. In other words, the previous experiments,

especially the FST experiment [91], could have affected the results of the subsequent experiments.

In addition, only male offspring were experimentally evaluated in the current study to avoid interference of hormones with the behaviour of the offspring. However, exclusion of females could be a significant point against this study's clinical relevance because depression and anxiety are more prevalent in women than in men. Actually, we noticed that some subtypes of depression or anxiety were related to fluctuating hormones [92, 93]. Evaluating only male offspring could focus more on the "passing on" behavioural deficits caused by maternal chronic SDS.

Conclusion

Our findings show that maternal SDS before pregnancy can affect behaviour and related neurobiological mechanisms in the offspring. This results in a tendency for emotional disorders/diseases in the offspring, and such a tendency extends to adult stage even though the maternal rats subject to SDS stimulation might recover as time passes. This extends our understanding of the influence of parental stress on offspring, both before and during pregnancy.

Abbreviations

SPF: specific pathogen-free; SDS: social defeat stress; CUS: chronic unpredictable stress; MWM: Morris water maze; SPT: sucrose preference test; OFT: open field test; EPM: elevated plus maze; LDB: light–dark box; ORT: object recognition task; RI: recognition index; FST: forced swimming test; CV: coefficient of variation; ANOVA: analysis of variance; HPA: hypothalamic–pituitary–adrenal; ACTH: adrenocorticotropic hormone; CORT: corticosterone; BDNF: brain-derived neurotrophic factor; CREB: cyclic adenosine monophosphate response element binding protein; pCREB: phosphorylated CREB; SERT: serotonin transporter; PKA: protein kinase A; NE: norepinephrine; 5-HT: serotonin; DA: dopamine.

Authors' contributions

MQ and SW designed the work, interpreted the data, performed the statistical analysis and drafted the manuscript. SW, ZL, MR and JW fed and nursed animals in facility. ZL, MR and KX contributed to establishment of SDS maternal rat model and its behavioural evaluation. SW, ZL, MR JW and KX were responsible for offspring caring, grouping and following behavioural experiments. KX, FL JG and YG sacrificed animals, sampled tissues, disposed animal bodies, extracted proteins and performed western blotting. DZ, HZ and RL sacrificed animals, sampled tissues, collected blood and carried out ELISA and RIA experiments. They also provided essential assistance such as discussing on HPA researches and supporting for technical matters of molecular biology. MQ directed the team, managed facility, gave key advice and provided the funds. He was also responsible for data administration and providing samples, materials and datasets used and/or analysed during current study on reasonable request. All authors read and approved the final manuscript.

Author details

[1] Laboratory of Traditional Chinese Medicine Classical Theory, Ministry of Education, Shandong University of Traditional Chinese Medicine, #4655 University Road, University Science Park, Changqing District, Jinan 250355, China.
[2] Department of Neurosurgery, Qilu Hospital of Shandong University and Brain Science Research Institute, Shandong University, Jinan 250012, China.
[3] Laboratory of Behavioural Brain Analysis, Shandong University of Traditional

Chinese Medicine, Jinan 250355, China. [4] Experimental Center, Shandong University of Traditional Chinese Medicine, Jinan 250355, China. [5] Fengtai Maternal and Children's Health Hospital of Beijing, Beijing 100069, China.

Acknowledgements

We are grateful to Dr Mathias Schmidt for valuable discussions and his expert comments during the preparation of this manuscript. We also thank Adam & Stone Bio-Medicals Ltd Co. (Soochow, China) and Dr. Matthew Hogg from Green Mountain Editing Services (www.gmediting.com/index) for language rephrasing and polishing.

Competing interests

All authors have discussed the results and approved the manuscript. There is no competing interest to declare.

Ethics approval

Animal experiments were performed in accordance with the Guide for the Care and Use of Laboratory Animals, formulated by the National Institutes of Health, USA, and were approved by the Institutional Committee for Animal Care and Use of Shandong University of Traditional Chinese Medicine (Approval ID: DWSY201404013).

Funding

The study was supported by the National Natural Science Foundation of China (No. 81573854 and 81202617).

References

1. Foster CJ, Garber J, Durlak JA. Current and past maternal depression, maternal interaction behaviors, and children's externalizing and internalizing symptoms. J Abnorm Child Psychol. 2008;36(4):527–37.
2. Gao W, Paterson J, Abbott M, Carter S, Iusitini L. Maternal mental health and child behaviour problems at 2 years: findings from the Pacific Islands Families Study. Aust N Z J Psychiatry. 2007;41(11):885–95.
3. Weissman MM, Wickramaratne P, Nomura Y, Warner V, Pilowsky D, Verdeli H. Offspring of depressed parents: 20 years later. Am J Psychiatry. 2006;163(6):1001–8.
4. Li H, Zhang L, Fang Z, Lin L, Wu C, Huang Q. Behavioral and neurobiological studies on the male progeny of maternal rats exposed to chronic unpredictable stress before pregnancy. Neurosci Lett. 2010;469(2):278–82.
5. Huang Y, Shi X, Xu H, Yang H, Chen T, Chen S, Chen X. Chronic unpredictable stress before pregnancy reduce the expression of brain-derived neurotrophic factor and N-methyl-D-aspartate receptor in hippocampus of offspring rats associated with impairment of memory. Neurochem Res. 2010;35(7):1038–49.
6. Guan L, Jia N, Zhao X, Zhang X, Tang G, Yang L, Sun H, Wang D, Su Q, Song Q. The involvement of ERK/CREB/Bcl-2 in depression-like behavior in prenatally stressed offspring rats. Brain Res Bull. 2013;99:1–8.
7. Wilson CA, Vazdarjanova A, Terry AV. Exposure to variable prenatal stress in rats: effects on anxiety-related behaviors, innate and contextual fear, and fear extinction. Behav Brain Res. 2013;238:279–88.
8. Kapoor A, Kostaki A, Janus C, Matthews SG. The effects of prenatal stress on learning in adult offspring is dependent on the timing of the stressor. Behav Brain Res. 2009;197(1):144–9.
9. O'Donnell K, O'Connor T, Glover V. Prenatal stress and neurodevelopment of the child: focus on the HPA axis and role of the placenta. Dev Neurosci. 2009;31(4):285–92.
10. Rygula R, Abumaria N, Domenici E, Hiemke C, Fuchs E. Effects of fluoxetine on behavioral deficits evoked by chronic social stress in rats. Behav Brain Res. 2006;174(1):188–92.
11. Björkqvist K. Social defeat as a stressor in humans. Physiol Behav. 2001;73(3):435–42.
12. Koolhaas J, De Boer S, De Rutter A, Meerlo P, Sgoifo A. Social stress in rats and mice. Acta Physiol Scand Suppl. 1996;640:69–72.
13. Miczek KA, Covington HE, Nikulina EM, Hammer RP. Aggression and defeat: persistent effects on cocaine self-administration and gene expression in peptidergic and aminergic mesocorticolimbic circuits. Neurosci Biobehav Rev. 2004;27(8):787–802.
14. Garcia-Bueno B, Caso JR, Leza JC. Stress as a neuroinflammatory condition in brain: damaging and protective mechanisms. Neurosci Biobehav Rev. 2008;32(6):1136–51.
15. Joels M, Baram TZ. The neuro-symphony of stress. Nat Rev Neurosci. 2009;10(6):459–66.
16. Sandstrom A, Peterson J, Sandstrom E, Lundberg M, Nystrom IL, Nyberg L, Olsson T. Cognitive deficits in relation to personality type and hypothalamic–pituitary–adrenal (HPA) axis dysfunction in women with stress-related exhaustion. Scand J Psychol. 2011;52(1):71–82.
17. de Kloet ER, Joels M, Holsboer F. Stress and the brain: from adaptation to disease. Nat Rev Neurosci. 2005;6(6):463–75.
18. Zhang J, Fan Y, Li Y, Zhu H, Wang L, Zhu M-Y. Chronic social defeat up-regulates expression of the serotonin transporter in rat dorsal raphe nucleus and projection regions in a glucocorticoid-dependent manner. J Neurochem. 2012;123(6):1054–68.
19. Ressler KJ, Nemeroff CB. Role of serotonergic and noradrenergic systems in the pathophysiology of depression and anxiety disorders. Depress Anxiety. 2000;12(S1):2–19.
20. Brocardo PS, Budni J, Kaster MP, Santos AR, Rodrigues ALS. Folic acid administration produces an antidepressant-like effect in mice: evidence for the involvement of the serotonergic and noradrenergic systems. Neuropharmacology. 2008;54(2):464–73.
21. Mizoguchi K, Ishige A, Aburada M, Tabira T. Chronic stress attenuates glucocorticoid negative feedback: involvement of the prefrontal cortex and hippocampus. Neuroscience. 2003;119(3):887–97.
22. Li H, Zhang L, Huang Q. Differential expression of mitogen-activated protein kinase signaling pathway in the hippocampus of rats exposed to chronic unpredictable stress. Behav Brain Res. 2009;205(1):32–7.
23. Baquedano E, Garcia-Caceres C, Diz-Chaves Y, Lagunas N, Calmarza-Font I, Azcoitia I, Garcia-Segura LM, Argente J, Chowen JA, Frago LM. Prenatal stress induces long-term effects in cell turnover in the hippocampus–hypothalamus–pituitary axis in adult male rats. PLoS ONE. 2011;6(11):e27549.
24. Qi X, Lin W, Li J, Pan Y, Wang W. The depressive-like behaviors are correlated with decreased phosphorylation of mitogen-activated protein kinases in rat brain following chronic forced swim stress. Behav Brain Res. 2006;175(2):233–40.
25. Wei S, Xiao XY, Wang JQ, Sun SG, Li ZF, Xu KY, Li F, Gao J, Zhu DH, Qiao MQ. Impact of anger emotional stress before pregnancy on adult male offspring. Oncotarget. 2017;8(58):98837–52.
26. Zaidan H, Gaisler-Salomon I. Prereproductive stress in adolescent female rats affects behavior and corticosterone levels in second-generation offspring. Psychoneuroendocrinology. 2015;58:120–9.
27. Sfikakis A, Galanopoulou P, Konstandi M, Tsakayannis D. Stress through handling for vaginal screening, serotonin, and ACTH response to ether. Pharmacol Biochem Behav. 1996;53(4):965–70.
28. Ho HP, Olsson M, Westberg L, Melke J, Eriksson E. The serotonin reuptake inhibitor fluoxetine reduces sex steroid-related aggression in female rats: an animal model of premenstrual irritability? Neuropsychopharmacology. 2001;24(5):502–10.
29. Rygula R, Abumaria N, Flügge G, Fuchs E, Rüther E, Havemann-Reinecke U. Anhedonia and motivational deficits in rats: impact of chronic social stress. Behav Brain Res. 2005;162(1):127–34.
30. Prut L, Belzung C. The open field as a paradigm to measure the effects of drugs on anxiety-like behaviors: a review. Eur J Pharmacol. 2003;463(1–3):3–33.

31. Grivas V, Markou A, Pitsikas N. The metabotropic glutamate 2/3 receptor agonist LY379268 induces anxiety-like behavior at the highest dose tested in two rat models of anxiety. Eur J Pharmacol. 2013;715(1–3):105–10.

32. Casarrubea M, Faulisi F, Sorbera F, Crescimanno G. The effects of different basal levels of anxiety on the behavioral shift analyzed in the central platform of the elevated plus maze. Behav Brain Res. 2015;281:55–61.

33. Aisa B, Tordera R, Lasheras B, Del Rio J, Ramirez MJ. Cognitive impairment associated to HPA axis hyperactivity after maternal separation in rats. Psychoneuroendocrinology. 2007;32(3):256–66.

34. van Zyl PJ, Dimatelis JJ, Russell VA. Behavioural and biochemical changes in maternally separated Sprague-Dawley rats exposed to restraint stress. Metab Brain Dis. 2016;31(1):121–33.

35. Acevedo MB, Nizhnikov ME, Molina JC, Pautassi RM. Relationship between ethanol-induced activity and anxiolysis in the open field, elevated plus maze, light-dark box, and ethanol intake in adolescent rats. Behav Brain Res. 2014;265:203–15.

36. Plescia F, Marino RA, Navarra M, Gambino G, Brancato A, Sardo P, Cannizzaro C. Early handling effect on female rat spatial and non-spatial learning and memory. Behav Proc. 2014;103:9–16.

37. Bevins RA, Besheer J. Object recognition in rats and mice: a one-trial non-matching-to-sample learning task to study 'recognition memory'. Nat Protoc. 2006;1(3):1306–11.

38. Porsolt RD, Anton G, Blavet N, Jalfre M. Behavioural despair in rats: a new model sensitive to antidepressant treatments. Eur J Pharmacol. 1978;47(4):379–91.

39. Murphy EK, Spencer RL, Sipe KJ, Herman JP. Decrements in nuclear glucocorticoid receptor (GR) protein levels and DNA binding in aged rat hippocampus. Endocrinology. 2002;143(4):1362–70.

40. Becker C, Zeau B, Rivat C, Blugeot A, Hamon M, Benoliel J. Repeated social defeat-induced depression-like behavioral and biological alterations in rats: involvement of cholecystokinin. Mol Psychiatry. 2007;13(12):1079–92.

41. Meerlo P, Overkamp G, Daan S, Van Den Hoofdakker R, Koolhaas J. Changes in behaviour and body weight following a single or double social defeat in rats. Stress. 1996;1(1):21–32.

42. de Jong JG, Wasilewski M, van der Vegt BJ, Buwalda B, Koolhaas JM. A single social defeat induces short-lasting behavioral sensitization to amphetamine. Physiol Behav. 2005;83(5):805–11.

43. Reznikov LR, Grillo CA, Piroli GG, Pasumarthi RK, Reagan LP, Fadel J. Acute stress-mediated increases in extracellular glutamate levels in the rat amygdala: differential effects of antidepressant treatment. Eur J Neurosci. 2007;25(10):3109–14.

44. Negrón-Oyarzo I, Pérez MÁ, Terreros G, Muñoz P, Dagnino-Subiabre A. Effects of chronic stress in adolescence on learned fear, anxiety, and synaptic transmission in the rat prelimbic cortex. Behav Brain Res. 2014;259:342–53.

45. Katz RJ, Roth KA, Carroll BJ. Acute and chronic stress effects on open field activity in the rat: implications for a model of depression. Neurosci Biobehav Rev. 1981;5(2):247–51.

46. Roth KA, Katz RJ. Stress, behavioral arousal, and open field activity- a reexamination of emotionality in the rat. Neurosci Biobehav Rev. 1980;3(4):247–63.

47. Bevins RA, Bardo MT. Conditioned increase in place preference by access to novel objects: antagonism by MK-801. Behav Brain Res. 1999;99(1):53–60.

48. D'Aquila PS, Peana AT, Carboni V, Serra G. Exploratory behaviour and grooming after repeated restraint and chronic mild stress: effect of desipramine. Eur J Pharmacol. 2000;399(1):43–7.

49. Puglisi-Allegra S, Kempf E, Schleef C, Cabib S. Repeated stressful experiences differently affect brain dopamine receptor subtypes. Life Sci. 1991;48(13):1263–8.

50. Berton O, Durand M, Aguerre S, Mormede P, Chaouloff F. Behavioral, neuroendocrine and serotonergic consequences of single social defeat and repeated fluoxetine pretreatment in the Lewis rat strain. Neuroscience. 1999;92(1):327–41.

51. Thiel C, Müller C, Huston J, Schwarting R. High versus low reactivity to a novel environment: behavioural, pharmacological and neurochemical assessments. Neuroscience. 1999;93(1):243–51.

52. Pawlak CR, Schwarting RK. Object preference and nicotine consumption in rats with high vs. low rearing activity in a novel open field. Pharmacol Biochem Behav. 2002;73(3):679–87.

53. Willner P, Muscat R, Papp M. Chronic mild stress-induced anhedonia: a realistic animal model of depression. Neurosci Biobehav Rev. 1992;16(4):525–34.

54. Iñiguez SD, Riggs LM, Nieto SJ, Dayrit G, Zamora NN, Shawhan KL, Cruz B, Warren BL. Social defeat stress induces a depression-like phenotype in adolescent male c57BL/6 mice. Stress. 2014;17(3):247–55.

55. Moreau J. Validation of an animal model of anhedonia, a major symptom of depression. Encephale. 1996;23(4):280–9.

56. Jayatissa MN, Bisgaard C, Tingström A, Papp M, Wiborg O. Hippocampal cytogenesis correlates to escitalopram-mediated recovery in a chronic mild stress rat model of depression. Neuropsychopharmacology. 2006;31(11):2395–404.

57. Cryan JF, Holmes A. The ascent of mouse: advances in modelling human depression and anxiety. Nat Rev Drug Discov. 2005;4(9):775–90.

58. Lister RG. The use of a plus-maze to measure anxiety in the mouse. Psychopharmacology. 1987;92(2):180–5.

59. Costall B, Jones B, Kelly M, Naylor RJ, Tomkins D. Exploration of mice in a black and white test box: validation as a model of anxiety. Pharmacol Biochem Behav. 1989;32(3):777–85.

60. Arrant AE, Schramm-Sapyta NL, Kuhn CM. Use of the light/dark test for anxiety in adult and adolescent male rats. Behav Brain Res. 2013;256:119–27.

61. Nakayasu T, Ishii K. Effects of pair-housing after social defeat experience on elevated plus-maze behavior in rats. Behav Proc. 2008;78(3):477–80.

62. D'Aquila PS, Panin F, Serra G. Long-term imipramine withdrawal induces a depressive-like behaviour in the forced swimming test. Eur J Pharmacol. 2004;492(1):61–3.

63. Gregus A, Wintink AJ, Davis AC, Kalynchuk LE. Effect of repeated corticosterone injections and restraint stress on anxiety and depression-like behavior in male rats. Behav Brain Res. 2005;156(1):105–14.

64. Sapolsky RM, Romero LM, Munck AU. How do glucocorticoids influence stress responses? Integrating permissive, suppressive, stimulatory, and preparative actions. Endocr Rev. 2000;21(1):55–89.

65. Muscat R, Willner P. Suppression of sucrose drinking by chronic mild unpredictable stress: a methodological analysis. Neurosci Biobehav Rev. 1992;16(4):507–17.

66. Lee J-H, Kim HJ, Kim JG, Ryu V, Kim B-T, Kang D-W, Jahng JW. Depressive behaviors and decreased expression of serotonin reuptake transporter in rats that experienced neonatal maternal separation. Neurosci Res. 2007;58(1):32–9.

67. Cabib S, D'Amato FR, Puglisi-Allegra S, Maestripieri D. Behavioral and mesocorticolimbic dopamine responses to non aggressive social interactions depend on previous social experiences and on the opponent's sex. Behav Brain Res. 2000;112(1):13–22.

68. Mos J, Van Valkenburg C. Specific effect on social stress and aggression on regional dopamine metabolism in rat brain. Neurosci Lett. 1979;15(2–3):325.

69. Puglisi-Allegra S, Cabib S. Effects of defeat experiences on dopamine metabolism in different brain areas of the mouse. Aggress Behav. 1990;16(3–4):271–84.

70. Tidey JW, Miczek KA. Social defeat stress selectively alters mesocorticolimbic dopamine release: an in vivo microdialysis study. Brain Res. 1996;721(1):140–9.

71. Wedzony K, Mackowiak M, Fijal K, Golembiowska K. Evidence that conditioned stress enhances outflow of dopamine in rat prefrontal cortex: a search for the influence of diazepam and 5-HT1A agonists. Synapse. 1996;24(3):240–7.

72. Young A, Joseph M, Gray J. Latent inhibition of conditioned dopamine release in rat nucleus accumbens. Neuroscience. 1993;54(1):5–9.

73. Bradberry CW, Gruen RJ, Berridge CW, Roth RH. Individual differences in behavioral measures: correlations with nucleus accumbens dopamine measured by microdialysis. Pharmacol Biochem Behav. 1991;39(4):877–82.

74. Claustre Y, Rivy JP, Dennis T, Scatton B. Pharmacological studies on stress-induced increase in frontal cortical dopamine metabolism in the rat. J Pharmacol Exp Ther. 1986;238(2):693–700.

75. Kaneyuki H, Yokoo H, Tsuda A, Yoshida M, Mizuki Y, Yamada M, Tanaka M. Psychological stress increases dopamine turnover selectively in meso-prefrontal dopamine neurons of rats: reversal by diazepam. Brain Res. 1991;557(1):154–61.

76. D'Angio M, Serrano A, Driscoll P, Scatton B. Stressful environmental stimuli increase extracellular DOPAC levels in the prefrontal cortex of hypoe-motional (Roman high-avoidance) but not hyperemotional (Roman low-avoidance) rats. An in vivo voltammetric study. Brain research. 1988;451(1):237–47.

77. Thoenen H. Neurotrophins and neuronal plasticity. Science. 1995;270(5236):593–8.

78. Duman RS, Heninger GR, Nestler EJ. A molecular and cellular theory of depression. Arch Gen Psychiatry. 1997;54(7):597–606.

79. Siuciak JA, Lewis DR, Wiegand SJ, Lindsay RM. Antidepressant-like effect of brain-derived neurotrophic factor (BDNF). Pharmacol Biochem Behav. 1997;56(1):131–7.

80. Duman RS. Depression: a case of neuronal life and death? Biol Psychiatry. 2004;56(3):140–5.

81. Nibuya M, Morinobu S, Duman RS. Regulation of BDNF and trkB mRNA in rat brain by chronic electroconvulsive seizure and antidepressant drug treatments. J Neurosci. 1995;15(11):7539–47.

82. Vollmayr B, Faust H, Lewicka S, Henn F. Brain-derived-neurotrophic-factor (BDNF) stress response in rats bred for learned helplessness. Mol Psychia-try. 2001;6(4):471–474, 358.

83. Nutt DJ. The neuropharmacology of serotonin and noradrenaline in depression. Int Clin Psychopharmacol. 2002;17:S1–12.

84. Tardito D, Perez J, Tiraboschi E, Musazzi L, Racagni G, Popoli M. Signaling pathways regulating gene expression, neuroplasticity, and neurotrophic mechanisms in the action of antidepressants: a critical overview. Pharma-col Rev. 2006;58(1):115–34.

85. Gass P, Riva MA. CREB, neurogenesis and depression. BioEssays. 2007;29(10):957–61.

86. Martinez D, Pentinat T, Ribo S, Daviaud C, Bloks VW, Cebria J, Villalmanzo N, Kalko SG, Ramon-Krauel M, Diaz R, et al. In utero undernutrition in male mice programs liver lipid metabolism in the second-generation offspring involving altered Lxra DNA methylation. Cell Metab. 2014;19(6):941–51.

87. Gapp K, Jawaid A, Sarkies P, Bohacek J, Pelczar P, Prados J, Farinelli L, Miska E, Mansuy IM. Implication of sperm RNAs in transgenerational inheritance of the effects of early trauma in mice. Nat Neurosci. 2014;17(5):667–9.

88. Morgan CP, Bale TL. Early prenatal stress epigenetically programs dysmas-culinization in second-generation offspring via the paternal lineage. J Neurosci. 2011;31(33):11748–55.

89. Zaidan H, Leshem M, Gaisler-Salomon I. Prereproductive stress to female rats alters corticotropin releasing factor type 1 expression in ova and behavior and brain corticotropin releasing factor type 1 expression in offspring. Biol Psychiatry. 2013;74(9):680–7.

90. Dietz DM, Laplant Q, Watts EL, Hodes GE, Russo SJ, Feng J, Oosting RS, Vialou V, Nestler EJ. Paternal transmission of stress-induced pathologies. Biol Psychiatry. 2011;70(5):408–14.

91. Lesse A, Rether K, Groger N, Braun K, Bock J. Chronic postnatal stress induces depressive-like behavior in male mice and programs second-hit stress-induced gene expression patterns of OxtR and AvpR1a in adult-hood. Mol Neurobiol. 2017;54(6):4813–9.

92. Qiao M, Sun P, Wang H, Wang Y, Zhan X, Liu H, Wang X, Li X, Wang X, Wu J, et al. Epidemiological distribution and subtype analysis of premenstrual dysphoric disorder syndromes and symptoms based on TCM theories. Biomed Res Int. 2017;2017:4595016.

93. Li F, Feng J, Gao D, Wang J, Song C, Wei S, Qiao M. Shuyu capsules relieve premenstrual syndrome depression by reducing 5-HT3AR and 5-HT3BR expression in the rat brain. Neural Plast. 2016;2016:7950781.

Permissions

The contributors of this book come from diverse backgrounds, making this book a truly international effort. This book will bring forth new frontiers with its revolutionizing research information and detailed analysis of the nascent developments around the world.

We would like to thank all the contributing authors for lending their expertise to make the book truly unique. They have played a crucial role in the development of this book. Without their invaluable contributions this book wouldn't have been possible. They have made vital efforts to compile up to date information on the varied aspects of this subject to make this book a valuable addition to the collection of many professionals and students.

This book was conceptualized with the vision of imparting up-to-date information and advanced data in this field. To ensure the same, a matchless editorial board was set up. Every individual on the board went through rigorous rounds of assessment to prove their worth. After which they invested a large part of their time researching and compiling the most relevant data for our readers.

The editorial board has been involved in producing this book since its inception. They have spent rigorous hours researching and exploring the diverse topics which have resulted in the successful publishing of this book. They have passed on their knowledge of decades through this book. To expedite this challenging task, the publisher supported the team at every step. A small team of assistant editors was also appointed to further simplify the editing procedure and attain best results for the readers.

Apart from the editorial board, the designing team has also invested a significant amount of their time in understanding the subject and creating the most relevant covers. They scrutinized every image to scout for the most suitable representation of the subject and create an appropriate cover for the book.

The publishing team has been an ardent support to the editorial, designing and production team. Their endless efforts to recruit the best for this project, has resulted in the accomplishment of this book. They are a veteran in the field of academics and their pool of knowledge is as vast as their experience in printing. Their expertise and guidance has proved useful at every step. Their uncompromising quality standards have made this book an exceptional effort. Their encouragement from time to time has been an inspiration for everyone.

The publisher and the editorial board hope that this book will prove to be a valuable piece of knowledge for researchers, students, practitioners and scholars across the globe.

List of Contributors

Vladimir N. Babenko, Dmitry A. Afonnikov, Elena V. Ignatieva and Anton V. Klimov
The Federal Research Center Institute of Cytology and Genetics of Siberian Branch of the Russian Academy of Sciences, Center of Neurobiology and Neurogenetics, Lavrentieva str. 10, Novosibirsk, Russia 630090
Novosibirsk State University, Pirogova Str, 2, Novosibirsk, Russia 630090. 3 Vavilov Institute of General Genetics RAS, Gubkina str

Fedor E. Gusev
Moscow, Russia 119991

Evgeny I. Rogaev
The Federal Research Center Institute of Cytology and Genetics of Siberian Branch of the Russian Academy of Sciences, Center of Neurobiology and Neurogenetics, Lavrentieva str. 10, Novosibirsk, Russia 630090
Moscow, Russia 119991
Department of Psychiatry, University of Massachusetts Medical School, BNRI, Worcester, MA 15604, USA
Faculty of Biology, Faculty of Bioengineering and Bioinformatics, Lomonosov Moscow State University, Moscow, Russia 119234

Laura Aldavert-Vera, Ignacio Morgado-Bernal and Pilar Segura-Torres
Departament de Psicobiologia i de Metodologia de les Ciències de la Salut, Institut de Neurociències, Universitat Autónoma de Barcelona, 08193 Bellaterra, Barcelona, Spain

Elisabet Kádár
Departament de Biologia, Universitat de Girona, 17071 Girona, Spain
Department of Biology, Sciences Faculty, University of Girona, C/Mª Aurèlia Capmany 40, Camous Montilivi, 17003 Girona, Spain

Eva Vico Varela
Departament de Psicobiologia i de Metodologia de les Ciències de la Salut, Institut de Neurociències, Universitat Autónoma de Barcelona, 08193 Bellaterra, Barcelona, Spain
Douglas Mental Health University Institute, McGill University, Montreal, QC H4H 1R3, Canada

Gemma Huguet
Departament de Biologia, Universitat de Girona, 17071 Girona, Spain

Jesús Martínez-Sámano, Alan Flores-Poblano, Marco Antonio Juárez-Oropeza and Patricia V. Torres-Durán
Departamento de Bioquímica, Facultad de Medicina, Universidad Nacional Autónoma de México, Circuito Escolar s/n, Ciudad Universitaria, C.P. 04510 Mexico City, Mexico

Leticia Verdugo-Díaz
Departamento de Fisiología, Facultad de Medicina, Universidad Nacional Autónoma de México, Circuito Escolar s/n, Ciudad Universitaria, C.P. 04510 Mexico City, Mexico

Thorsten Fehr and Manfred Herrmann
Center for Cognitive Sciences, University of Bremen, Bremen, Germany
University of Bremen, Hochschulring 18, 28359 Bremen, Germany
Center for Advanced Imaging, Universities of Bremen and Magdeburg, Bremen, Germany

Angelica Staniloiu and Hans J. Markowitsch
Physiological Psychology, University of Bielefeld, Bielefeld, Germany
Hanse Institute for Advanced Study (HWK), Delmenhorst, Germany

Peter Erhard
Center for Cognitive Sciences, University of Bremen, Bremen, Germany
Center for Advanced Imaging, Universities of Bremen and Magdeburg, Bremen, Germany
AG in vivo MR, University of Bremen, Bremen, Germany

Hiroshi Ueno
Department of Medical Technology, Kawasaki University of Medical Welfare, 288, Matsushima, Kurashiki, Okayama 701-0193, Japan
Department of Medical Technology, Graduate School of Health Sciences, Okayama University, Okayama 700-8558, Japan

Motoi Okamoto
Department of Medical Technology, Graduate School of Health Sciences, Okayama University, Okayama 700-8558, Japan

Shunsuke Suemitsu, Shinji Murakami, Naoya Kitamura, Kenta Wani, Shozo Aoki and Takeshi Ishihara
Department of Psychiatry, Kawasaki Medical School, Kurashiki 701-0192, Japan

Yosuke Matsumoto
Department of Neuropsychiatry, Graduate School of Medicine, Dentistry and Pharmaceutical Sciences, Okayama University, Okayama 700-8558, Japan

Christoph Justen
University of Tuebingen, Tuebingen, Germany
Institute of Psychology and Education, Applied Emotion and Motivation Research, University of Ulm, Ulm, Germany

Cornelia Herbert
Institute of Psychology and Education, Applied Emotion and Motivation Research, University of Ulm, Ulm, Germany

Mushfiquddin Khan and Tajinder S. Dhammu
Department of Pediatrics, 508 Children's Research Institute, Medical University of South Carolina, 173 Ashley Ave, Charleston, SC 29425, USA

Inderjit Singh
Department of Pediatrics, 508 Children's Research Institute, Medical University of South Carolina, 173 Ashley Ave, Charleston, SC 29425, USA
Ralph H Johnson VA Medical Center, Charleston, SC, USA

Avtar K. Singh
Ralph H Johnson VA Medical Center, Charleston, SC, USA
Department of Pathology and Laboratory Medicine, Medical University of South Carolina, Charleston, SC, USA

Hyejung Lee
Acupuncture and Meridian Science Research Center, College of Korean Medicine, Kyung Hee University, 26, Kyungheedae-ro, Dongdaemun-gu, Seoul 02447, Republic of Korea

Bombi Lee and Dae-Hyun Hahm
Acupuncture and Meridian Science Research Center, College of Korean Medicine, Kyung Hee University, 26, Kyungheedae-ro, Dongdaemun-gu, Seoul 02447, Republic of Korea
Center for Converging Humanities, Kyung Hee University, Seoul 02447, Republic of Korea

Insop Shim
Acupuncture and Meridian Science Research Center, College of Korean Medicine, Kyung Hee University, 26, Kyungheedae-ro, Dongdaemun-gu, Seoul 02447, Republic of Korea
Department of Physiology, College of Medicine, Kyung Hee University, Seoul 02447, Republic of Korea

YiLong Dong, KangJing Pu and HuiCheng Chen
School of Medicine, Yunnan University, 2 Cuihu Bei Road, Kunming 650091, Yunnan, People's Republic of China

WenJing Duan, LiXing Chen and YanMei Wang
The First Affiliated Hospital of Kunming Medical University, 295 Xichang Road, Kunming 650031, Yunnan, People's Republic of China

Kenji Ishibashi and Kenji Ishii
Research Team for Neuroimaging, Tokyo Metropolitan Institute of Gerontology, 35-2 Sakae-cho, Itabashi-ku, Tokyo 173-0015, Japan

Keita Sakurai, Keigo Shimoji and Aya M. Tokumaru
Department of Diagnostic Radiology, Tokyo Metropolitan Geriatric Hospital, 35-2 Sakae-cho, Itabashi-ku, Tokyo 173-0015, Japan

Jue Huang and Tilman Hensch
Department of Psychiatry and Psychotherapy, University of Leipzig, Semmelweisstrasse 10, 04103 Leipzig, Germany

Christine Ulke, Christian Sander, Philippe Jawinski, Janek Spada and Ulrich Hegerl
Department of Psychiatry and Psychotherapy, University of Leipzig, Semmelweisstrasse 10, 04103 Leipzig, Germany
Depression Research Centre, German Depression Foundation, Leipzig, Germany

Magdalena Zygmunt, Dżesika Hoinkis, Jacek Hajto, Marcin Piechota, Jan Rodriguez Parkitna and Michał Korostyński
Department of Molecular Neuropharmacology, Institute of Pharmacology of the Polish Academy of Sciences, Smetna 12, 31-343 Krakow, Poland

Bożena Skupień-Rabian and Urszula Jankowska
Laboratory of Proteomics and Mass Spectrometry, Malopolska Centre of Biotechnology, Jagiellonian University, Krakow, Poland

Sylwia Kędracka-Krok
Department of Physical Biochemistry, Faculty of Biochemistry, Biophysics and Biotechnology, Jagiellonian University, Krakow, Poland

Angelo Costa, Nicola Gilberti and Mauro Magoni
Stroke Unit, Azienda Socio Sanitaria Territoriale "Spedali Civili", "Spedali Civili" Hospital, Piazza Spedali Civili 1, 25123 Brescia, Italy

Alberto Benussi, Valentina Cantoni, Alessandro Padovani and Barbara Borroni
Neurology Unit, Department of Clinical and Experimental Sciences, University of Brescia, Brescia, Italy

Enrico Premi
Stroke Unit, Azienda Socio Sanitaria Territoriale "Spedali Civili", "Spedali Civili" Hospital, Piazza Spedali Civili 1, 25123 Brescia, Italy
Neurology Unit, Department of Clinical and Experimental Sciences, University of Brescia, Brescia, Italy

Antonio La Gatta
cNVR Consorzio Veneto di Ricerca, Padua, Italy

Stefano Visconti
Rehabilitation Unit, Casa di Cura "Villa Barbarano", Salò, Brescia, Italy

Wei Chen, Qing-Qing Hao, Li–Li Ren, Wei Ren, Wei-Wei Guo and Shi-Ming Yang
Department of Otolaryngology, Head and Neck Surgery, Institute of Otolaryngology, Chinese PLA General Hospital, Beijing Key Laboratory of Hearing Impairment Prevention and Treatment, Key Laboratory of Hearing Impairment Science, Chinese PLA Medical School, Ministry of Education, Beijng, China

Hui-sang Lin
Department of Biotechnology, Dalian Medical University, Dalian 116044, Liaoning, China

Hye Joo Son, Young Jin Jeong, Hyun Jin Yoon and Sang Yoon Lee
Department of Nuclear Medicine, Dong-A University Medical Center, Dong-A University College of Medicine, 26 Daesingongwon-ro, Seo-gu, Busan 602-812, Korea

Go-Eun Choi and Kook Cho
Institute of Convergence Bio-Health, Dong-A University, Busan, Korea

Do-Young Kang
Department of Nuclear Medicine, Dong-A University Medical Center, Dong-A University College of Medicine, 26 Daesingongwon-ro, Seo-gu, Busan 602-812, Korea
Institute of Convergence Bio-Health, Dong-A University, Busan, Korea

Ji-Ae Park, Min Hwan Kim, Kyo Chul Lee and Yong Jin Lee
Division of RI-Convergence Research, Korea Institute of Radiological and Medical Sciences, Seoul, Korea

Mun Ki Kim
Pohang Center of Evolution of Biomaterials, Pohang Technopark, Pohang, Korea

Lisa Fellner, Edith Buchinger, Dominik Brueck, Gregor K. Wenning and Nadia Stefanova
Department of Neurology, Medical University of Innsbruck, Innrain 66, G2, 6020 Innsbruck, Austria

Regina Irschick
Department of Anatomy, Histology and Embryology, Medical University of Innsbruck, Anichstrasse 35, Innsbruck, Austria

Noushin Nikray
Laboratory of Molecular and Cellular Biology 1214, Department of Basic Veterinary Sciences, School of Veterinary Medicine, Razi University, Kermanshah, Iran

Isaac Karimi
Laboratory of Molecular and Cellular Biology 1214, Department of Basic Veterinary Sciences, School of Veterinary Medicine, Razi University, Kermanshah, Iran
Department of Biology, Faculty of Science, Razi University, Kermanshah 67149-67346, Iran

Zahraminoosh Siavashhaghighi
Department of Pathobiology, Faculty of Veterinary Medicine, Razi University, Kermanshah, Iran

Lora A. Becker
Department of Psychology, University of Evansville, Evansville, IN 47722, USA

Mohammad Mehdi Mofatteh
Department of Accounting, School of Economics and Accounting, Islamic Azad University South Tehran Branch, Tehran, Iran

Armando Valenzuela Peraza, David Calderón Guzmán, Norma Osnaya Brizuela and Gerardo Barragán Mejía
Laboratorio de Neurociencias, Instituto Nacional de Pediatría (INP), Mexico City, Mexico

Maribel Ortiz Herrera
Laboratorio de Bacteriología Experimental, INP, Mexico City, Mexico

Hugo Juárez Olguín, Miroslava Lindoro Silva and Belén Juárez Tapia
Laboratorio de Farmacología, Instituto Nacional de Pediatría (INP), y Facultad de Medicina, Universidad Nacional Autónoma de México, Av Imán #1, 3er piso, Col Cuicuilco, CP 04530 Mexico City, Mexico

Jieqiong Wang, Jie Gao, Yinghui Guo and Mingqi Qiao
Laboratory of Traditional Chinese Medicine Classical Theory, Ministry of Education, Shandong University of Traditional Chinese Medicine, #4655 University Road, University Science Park, Changqing District, Jinan 250355, China

Dehao Zhu, Hao Zhang and Rongju Lv
Laboratory of Behavioural Brain Analysis, Shandong University of Traditional Chinese Medicine, Jinan 250355, China

Sheng Wei
Laboratory of Traditional Chinese Medicine Classical Theory, Ministry of Education, Shandong University of Traditional Chinese Medicine, #4655 University Road, University Science Park, Changqing District, Jinan 250355, China
Department of Neurosurgery, Qilu Hospital of Shandong University and Brain Science Research Institute, Shandong University, Jinan 250012, China
Laboratory of Behavioural Brain Analysis, Shandong University of Traditional Chinese Medicine, Jinan 250355, China
Experimental Center, Shandong University of Traditional Chinese Medicine, Jinan 250355, China

Zifa Li
Laboratory of Behavioural Brain Analysis, Shandong University of Traditional Chinese Medicine, Jinan 250355, China
Experimental Center, Shandong University of Traditional Chinese Medicine, Jinan 250355, China

Meng Ren and Kaiyong Xu
Experimental Center, Shandong University of Traditional Chinese Medicine, Jinan 250355, China

Fang Li
Laboratory of Traditional Chinese Medicine Classical Theory, Ministry of Education, Shandong University of Traditional Chinese Medicine, #4655 University Road, University Science Park, Changqing District, Jinan 250355, China
Fengtai Maternal and Children's Health Hospital of Beijing, Beijing 100069, China

Index

www.ingramcontent.com/pod-product-compliance
Lightning Source LLC
Chambersburg PA
CBHW080510200326

41458CB00012B/4158